Drugs, Society, and Human Behavior

Ninth Edition

Oakley Ray, Ph.D.

Professor, Departments of Psychology and Psychiatry
Associate Professor, Department of Pharmacology
Vanderbilt University and
Vanderbilt University School of Medicine
Nashville, Tennessee

Charles Ksir, Ph.D.

Professor, Department of Psychology
University of Wyoming
Laramie, Wyoming

McGraw Hill

Boston   Burr Ridge, IL   Dubuque, IA   Madison, WI   New York   San Francisco   St. Louis
Bangkok   Bogotá   Caracas   Kuala Lumpur   Lisbon   London   Madrid   Mexico City
Milan   Montreal   New Delhi   Santiago   Seoul   Singapore   Sydney   Taipei   Toronto

McGraw-Hill Higher Education

A Division of The McGraw-Hill Companies

DRUGS, SOCIETY, AND HUMAN BEHAVIOR, NINTH EDITION

Published by McGraw-Hill, a business unit of The McGraw-Hill Companies, Inc., 1221 Avenue of the Americas, New York, New York, NY 10020. Copyright © 2002, 1999, 1996, 1993, 1987, 1983, 1978, 1972 by The McGraw-Hill Companies, Inc. All rights reserved. No part of this publication may be reproduced or distributed in any form or by any means, or stored in a data base or retrieval system, without the prior written consent of The McGraw-Hill Companies, Inc., including, but not limited to, in any network or other electronic storage or transmission, or broadcast for distance learning.

Some ancillaries, including electronic and print components, may not be available to customers outside the United States.

This book is printed on acid-free paper.

1 2 3 4 5 6 7 8 9 0 VNH/VNH 0 9 8 7 6 5 4 3 2 1

ISBN 0-07-231963-1

Vice president and editor-in-chief: *Thalia Dorwick*
Executive editor: *Vicki Malinee*
Senior developmental editor: *Melissa Martin*
Senior marketing manager: *Pamela S. Cooper*
Project manager: *Mary Lee Harms*
Production supervisor: *Sherry L. Kane*
Coordinator of freelance design: *Michelle D. Whitaker*
Freelance cover/interior designer: *Kim Rokusek/Rokusek Design*
Cover image: © *Jody Winger/Stock Illustration Source*
Photo research coordinator: *John C. Leland*
Photo research: *Connie Gardner Picture Research*
Senior supplement producer: *David A. Welsh*
Media technology producer: *Judi David*
Compositor: *GAC/Indianapolis*
Typeface: *10/12 Garth Graphic*
Printer: *Von Hoffmann Press, Inc.*

The credits section for this book begins on page 516 and is considered an extension of the copyright page.

Library of Congress Cataloging-in-Publication Data

Ray, Oakley Stern.
Drugs, society, and human behavior / Oakley Ray, Charles Ksir.—9th ed.
   p.   cm.
Includes index.
ISBN 0–07–231936–1
1. Drugs of abuse. 2. Drug abuse—Social aspects. 3. Neuropsychopharmacology.
I. Ksir, Charles. II. Title.
RM316.R39 2002
362.29—dc21

2001030409
CIP

The web addresses listed in this text were accurate at the time of publication. The inclusion of a web address does not constitute an endorsement of the site's content by the authors or by The McGraw-Hill Companies. Furthermore, The McGraw-Hill Companies does not guarantee the accuracy of the information presented at these websites.

www.mhhe.com

Contents in Brief

Contents

Section VI
Restricted Drugs,   375

Preface

Today's media-oriented college students are aware of critical issues relating to substance abuse. Nearly every day we hear about new pharmaceuticals, club drugs, HIV and AIDS, and the effects of tobacco and alcohol, and most of us have had some personal experience with these issues through family, friends, or coworkers. This course is one of the most exciting you will take because it will help you relate the latest information on drugs to their effect on society and human behavior. You will then be able to examine your attitudes toward drugs and have the ability to modify your behavior to improve your health.

Much has changed in the nearly 30 years since *Drugs, Society, and Human Behavior* was first published. The 1970s were a period of widespread experimentation with marijuana and hallucinogens, while the 1980s brought increased concern about illegal drugs and conservatism, along with decreased use of alcohol and all illicit drugs. Not only did drug-using behavior change, but so did attitudes and knowledge. And, of course, each decade the particular drugs of immediate social concern have changed: LSD gave way to angel dust, then to heroin, then to cocaine and crack. In the 1990s we saw increased use of LSD and marijuana, but not to the levels of the 1970s. Methamphetamine use—associated with the so-called speed freaks of the late 1960s—also increased, but the drug was more often smoked than injected.

Update trends through 2000

The new millenium has brought with it a focus on the "club drugs," especially ecstacy and GHB. While we cannot predict the next drug on which we will focus our attention, we can confidently predict that there will be a next one. As these changes have occurred, our old standbys, alcohol and tobacco, have remained with us and have continued to be serious social problems. Although regulations have changed, new scientific information has become available, new approaches to prevention and treatment are being tried, and these substances continue to be the most widely used drugs in our society.

This text approaches drugs and drug use from a variety of perspectives—behavioral, pharmacological, historical, social, legal, and clinical—which will help you apply the content to your own needs.

SPECIAL FEATURES

Updated Content

Throughout each chapter we have included the very latest information and statistics, and the Drugs in the Media feature has allowed us to comment on breaking news right up to press time. In addition, we have introduced many timely topics and issues that are sure to pique your interest and stimulate class discussion.

HealthQuest Activities

Each chapter contains a new activities box to complement the *HealthQuest* 3.0 CD-ROM that accompanies the text. These activities and *HealthQuest*'s exciting graphics and interactive approach will help you assess your knowledge of drugs and lifestyle in many different areas.

Web Watch Activities

Today we can find reliable health and drug information at our fingertips when we search the web. New Web Watch activities at the end of each chapter direct you to important websites related to the material. The activities, including many assessments and quizzes, will help you think critically about valuable health information.

Taking Sides

These boxes discuss a particular drug-related issue or problem and ask you to take a side in the debate. This thought-provoking material will help you apply what you learned in the chapter. Each box also refers you to a special McGraw-Hill website, www.dushkin.com/takingsides, for current news and valuable links, in case you wish to pursue the topic in more depth.

Online Learning Center Resources

Online Learning Center Resources boxes, found on the opening page of each chapter, direct you toward the useful resources available on the Online Learning Center that accompanies this text. These resources include chapter key terms and definitions, learning objectives, question-and-answer sites, and chapter quizzes. The Online Learning Center Resources boxes also list some of the web links that you will find on the OLC.

Drugs in the Media

Your world revolves around media of all types—TV, films, radio, print media, and the web. To meet you on familiar ground, we've included Drugs in the Media boxes (see inside front cover for a list of boxes), which take an informative and critical look at these media sources of drug information. This feature appears on the first page of each chapter.

Exploring Your Spirituality

Spirituality has become an important focus in health courses. The new Exploring Your Spirituality boxes highlight the spiritual dimension of dealing with substance use, abuse, and addiction. This new feature includes topics such as spiritual resources as alternatives to drugs, a rewarding social life without alcohol and other drugs, and the search for humane drug policies.

Targeting Prevention

The new Targeting Prevention boxes offer perspective and provoke thought regarding what drug-related behaviors we, as a society, want to reduce or prevent. These boxes will help you better evaluate prevention strategies and messages.

Drugs in Depth

The Drugs in Depth boxes examine specific, often controversial drug-related issues and are a perfect starting point for class or group discussions.

Try It!

These self-assessments help you put health concepts into practice. Each Try It! asks you to answer questions and analyze your own habits and behavior.

Attractive Design and Updated Illustration Package

The inviting new look, bold colors, and exciting graphics in *Drugs, Society, and Human Behavior* will draw you in at every turn of the page. Sharp and appealing photographs, attractive drawings, and informative tables support and clarify the chapter material.

New or Expanded Topics

Following is a sampling of topics in each chapter that are new or have been significantly expanded:

Chapter 1
Drug and alcohol use patterns and statistics
Risk factors and protective factors for substance abuse

Chapter 2
Drug toxicity
Drug use among those arrested for nondrug crimes

Chapter 3
Substance-abuse treatment admissions for various drugs
Success of treatment for adolescents

Chapter 4
The Institute of Medicine's new prevention model
Successful family-oriented prevention programs

Chapter 5
Regulation of legal pharmaceuticals
Regulation of tobacco and alcohol
Drug-related imprisonment
New regulations on club drugs

Chapter 6
Effects of behavior on brain chemistry
Sexual dysfunction among drug addicts

Chapter 7
Drug interactions

Chapter 8
How ADHD affects drug treatment

Chapter 9
Trends in use of club drugs

Chapter 10
New drugs to treat mental disorders

Chapter 11
Trends in beer, wine, and liquor sales
New findings about alcohol and health

Chapter 12
Alcohol use reported state-by-state
Alcohol-related crashes in the United States

Pedagogical Aids

Definition Boxes
Key terms are set in boldface type and are defined in corresponding boxes. Other important terms in the text are set in italics for emphasis. Both approaches facilitate your vocabulary comprehension.

Chapter Summaries
Each chapter concludes with a bulleted summary of key concepts and their significance or application. You can then return to any topic in the chapter for clarification or study.

Review Questions
A set of questions appears at the end of each chapter to aid you in review and analysis of chapter content.

Appendices
The appendices include handy references on brand and generic names of prescription drugs; drug organizations and resources; and drug categories, uses, and effects.

Owner's Manual

Are you looking for drug information in the media? working to change your attitude and health for the better? trying to improve your grade? The great features in *Drugs, Society, and Human Behavior* will help you do all this and more! Let's take a look.

Online Learning Center
Want to get a better grade? This box reminds you about the study aids and other resources avail-able at our free Online Learning Center and describes some of the useful web links you'll find there.

Drugs in the Media
How can you tell whether to trust drug information in the media? These boxes take a critical look at coverage of drug issues on the web, on television, in film, and in print.

HealthQuest Activities

You received a free *HealthQuest* 3.0 CD-ROM with your new copy of *Drugs, Society, and Human Behavior.* This feature provides activities to help you explore *HealthQuest* and assess your behavior in relation to drugs and alcohol.

Exploring Your Spirituality

A healthy body and a healthy mind go hand-in-hand. This feature helps you consider the spiritual dimension of health in your own attitudes toward alcohol and other drug use.

Web Watch Activities

Get healthier and smarter by surfing the web! These fun activities guide you to interactive self-assessments on the web. Do you know drug slang? Do you need advice on a drug-related problem? Has your "social drinking" gone too far? Log on and find out.

Try It!

Taking these self-assessments will help you analyze your behavior and habits and apply health concepts to your personal life.

Taking Sides

Is there a medical need for marijuana? Are alternatives to drugs *really* alternatives? Is methadone maintenance an effective treatment or an admission of failure? Read these articles and decide where you stand on controversial issues.

Targeting Prevention

These boxes will provoke thinking about what drug-related behaviors it's important to reduce or prevent. They'll help you evaluate prevention strategies and messages.

Drugs in Depth

Want to take a closer look? These articles examine specific drug-related issues and are a great starting point for discussion.

ANCILLARIES

Course Integrator Guide

This comprehensive manual is a traditional instructor's manual combined with a useful guide to incorporating McGraw-Hill supplements into the course. It incorporates all these useful features and more:

- Chapter outlines and special supplements outlines with teaching suggestions, key terms, and relevant Presentation Manager illustrations noted at relevant points
- Current resources lists, including annotated readings, websites, journals, and films

Test Bank

This printed manual includes a test bank of multiple choice, true/false, matching, and critical thinking questions. It has been rewritten to enhance clarity, and it now includes more applications questions.

Computerized Test Bank

Test questions from the printed test bank are available on our computerized testing and grading program, MicroTest III, for Windows or Macintosh.

HealthQuest 3.0. CD
By Bob Gold and Nancy Meyer

Packaged free with new copies of *Drugs, Society, and Human Behavior,* this interactive CD may be used with any personal health text and includes coverage of alcohol and other drugs. This edition of *Drugs, Society, and Human Behavior* includes *HealthQuest* Activities boxes to integrate multimedia into the course.

Health and Human Performance Discipline Page www.mhhe.com/hhp

McGraw-Hill's Health and Human Performance Discipline Page provides a wide variety of information for instructors and students, including monthly articles about current issues, monthly articles that celebrate our diversity, downloadable text supplements, a "how to" guide to McGraw-Hill technology, study tips, and more. The page lists professional organizations, convention schedules, career possibilities, and information for instructors on how to become a McGraw-Hill author. Additional features of the discipline page include the following:

- This Just In—This feature presents the latest hot topics, the best web resources, and more—all updated monthly!
- Faculty Support—Instructors can access downloadable course supplements such as

lecture outlines and PowerPoint presentations, and create their own course website with PageOut!

- Student Success Center—Find online study guides and other resources to improve your academic performance. Explore scholarship opportunities and learn how to launch your career!
- Author Arena—Interested in writing a textbook or a supplement for the college market? Read the McGraw-Hill proposal guidelines, find links to the Editorial and Marketing teams, and meet and talk with our current authors!

McGraw-Hill Online Learning Center

The Online Learning Center provides instructors with downloads of helpful ancillaries. For students, the OLC offers self-scoring quizzes, review material for exam preparation, and access to web links and updated material.

PowerWeb

PowerWeb is a password-protected website developed by McGraw-Hill/Dushkin. It offers current articles from *Annual Editions*—peer-reviewed articles from some of the most important magazines, journals, and newspapers published today. Self-scoring quizzes allow students to gauge their understanding of the material in each article. Dozens of additional web links are organized by topic. Each online text includes a glossary of standard terms with a self-testing feature. PowerWeb also offers surveys, interactive illustrations, current news updates, study tips, interview tips, and a résumé builder. Students and faculty receive $25 worth of free research time on NorthernLight.com, which provides access to more than 6,300 journals.

Visual Resource Library to Accompany *Drugs, Society, and Human Behavior*

The Visual Resource Library is a bank of images for use in the classroom and in the accompanying PowerPoint presentation. It's easy to import useful illustrations right into the pre-packaged PowerPoint lecture, which you can customize to fit your needs.

WebCT

WebCT, a product of Universal Learning Technology, makes it even easier for instructors to take their course online. McGraw-Hill content is delivered through one of the most popular and easy-to-use platforms available. With the adoption of *Focus on Health,* McGraw-Hill will pre-pay the WebCT student site license, and the school may use our Online Learning Center free of charge. In addition, McGraw-Hill offers our *Instructor Advantage* program to all McGraw-Hill/WebCT customers. This program provides unlimited technical support by phone and e-mail directly from WebCT. (Other WebCT customers have access to e-mail support from WebCT and are charged for phone support.) Each technical support representative has been specially trained to work with McGraw-Hill customers.

Overhead Transparency Acetates

Seventy-two full-color key illustrations and graphics from the text are available as transparency acetates. These useful tools facilitate learning and classroom discussion. They were chosen specifically to help explain complex concepts. This ancillary is provided free to all instructors who wish to use acetates.

McGraw-Hill PageOut: The Course Website Development Center

PageOut is a program that enables instructors to easily develop websites for their courses. The site includes the following:

- A course home page
- An instructor home page
- A syllabus (the syllabus is interactive and customizable, allows quizzing and the addition of instructor notes, and can be linked to the Online Learning Center)
- Web links
- Online discussion areas (multiple discussion areas per class)
- Online grade book
- An area to list links to students' web pages
- Sixteen design templates to choose from

ACKNOWLEDGMENTS

We would like to express our appreciation to the following instructors who reviewed the seventh and eighth editions and helped lay the groundwork for the improvements and changes that were needed in the ninth edition:

Brian A. Adrian, Ph.D.
Grand Valley State University

Scott Alpert
University of Maryland

Martin Ayim, Ph.D.
Grambling State University

Karen Ball, Ph.D.
Alma College

Robert W. Bell
Texas Tech University

Angela K. Bray
Illinois State University

Joseph Brown, Ph.D.
Austin Peay State University

Gary L. Chandler, Ed.D.
Gardner-Webb University

Diane L. Clemen
Illinois Wesleyan University

Akbar Davami
California State University–Sacramento

Lou Ebrite, Ph.D.
University of Central Oklahoma

Dale W. Evans, Ph.D.
California State University

Getene Gebrewold, Ph.D.
Western Illinois University

William T. Hey, Ph.D.
Delta State University

Ping Hu, Ph.D.
Florida Atlantic University

Howard Ishisaka, Ed.D.
Indiana State University

John Janowiak, Ph.D.
Appalachian State College

Linda Kryel, RPH
Drake College

Jerry W. Lee, Ph.D.
Loma Linda University

Linda Ludovico, MS
Tyler Junior College

Jennifer McLean
Corning Community College

Edward Meister, Ph.D.
Worcester State College

Patricia A. Miller
Anderson University

Ed Mink
University of Arkansas

Ranjita Misra
Ohio University

Patsy Queen
Gaston College

Kerry Redican, Ph.D.
Virginia Tech

Laurna Robinson, Ph.D.
University of Illinois

Thomas Rowe
University of Wisconsin

Glenn B. Schmidt
Mississippi University for Women

Israel M. Schwartz, Ph.D.
Hofstra University

Sharon Simson
University of Maryland

Barry A. Staples
Lacawanna Junior College

George T. Taylor
University of Missouri–St. Louis

Peggy Trueman, MSN
Gaston College

Martin Turnauer
Radford University

Ralph Wood
Southeastern Louisiana University

Special thanks to Carl Hart, College of Physicians and Surgeons, Columbia University, who gave us detailed suggestions for chapters 8 and 16, and Roland D. Shytle, University of South Florida, who gave us valuable advice for chapters 17 and 18.

Keeping up with all the changes in this field is a formidable task, one in which we are aided immensely by our continuing to teach courses based on the text and receiving feedback and new information from our students, from students at other institutions, and from other faculty members who use the text. We appreciate (and need!) all that input. Although we also welcome regular mail, in keeping with the information age we invite comments, questions, and criticisms to be sent by electronic mail to cksir@uwyo.edu.

Oakley Ray
Charles Ksir

Section I

Drug Use in Modern Society

The interaction between drugs and behavior can be approached from two general perspectives. Certain drugs, the ones we call psychoactive, have profound effects on behavior. So part of what a book on this topic should do is describe the effects of these drugs on behavior, *and later chapters do that in some detail. Another perspective, however, views drug taking* as behavior. *The psychologist sees drug-taking behaviors as interesting examples of human behavior that are influenced by many psychological, social, and cultural variables. In the first section of this text, we focus on drug taking as behavior that can be studied in the same way that other behaviors, such as aggression, learning, and human sexuality, can be studied.*

*D*rug Use: An Overview

KEY TERMS

- drug
- club drug
- illicit drug
- deviant drug use
- drug misuse
- drug abuse
- addiction
- psychoactive
- marijuana
- psychopharmacology
- correlate
- antecedent
- longitudinal study
- gateway
- reinforcement

Online Learning Center Resources

www.mhhe.com/ray

Log on to our Online Learning Center (OLC) for access to these additional resources.

- Chapter key terms and definitions
- Learning objectives
- Additional behavior change objectives
- Student interactive questions and answer sites
- Self-scoring chapter quiz

The OLC also offers web links for study and exploration of health topics. Here are some examples of what you'll find:

www.healthcentral.com/cooltools/
CT_drugsandalcohol/
CT_drugsandalcohol.cfm

Take the assessment entitled "Alcohol and Substance Abuse Mini-Profile" at this website. Whether you have questions about caffeine use, illicit drugs, OTC drugs, or your personal approach to substances, this assessment covers a broad range of subjects and includes detailed information on each one.

www.health.org/govestudy/bkd376/

Check out the U.S. government's 1999 National Survey Results at this website. You may wish to compare these scientific results with your assumptions about the percentages of Americans using drugs.

health.cybear.com/atoz/teen/
tsindex.asp

Learn about the current issues related to teen substance abuse. This site includes a variety of articles, quizzes, warning signs, and tips for a healthy lifestyle. Plus, send a health-themed e-card or post a message on the Teen Substance Abuse message board.

Drugs in the Media

Reporting on the "Drug du Jour"

At the beginning of this millennium, newspaper and television stories about drugs are dominated by the

Drugs in the Media Continued. . .

so-called **club drugs,** such as Ecstasy and GHB. Before that there was a wave of media reports about crystal meth and other forms of methamphetamine. In the mid-1980s, it was crack cocaine. Of course these waves of media focus are associated with waves of drug use, but the news media all seem to jump on the latest "drug du jour" (drug of the day) at the same time. For example, the U.S. Drug Enforcement Administration (DEA) announced in the year 2000 that the club drugs were its highest priority, and this means more news stories about arrests of distributors for these types of drugs.

One question that doesn't get asked much is this: What role does such media attention play in popularizing the current drug fad, perhaps making it spread farther and faster than would happen without all the publicity? About 30 years ago, in a chapter entitled "How to Create a Nationwide Drug Epidemic," journalist E. M. Brecher described a sequence of news stories that he believed were the key

factor in spreading the practice of sniffing the glues sold to kids for assembling plastic models of cars and airplanes (see *volatile solvents* in Chapter 9). He argued that, without the well-meant attempts to warn people of the dangers of this practice, it would probably have remained isolated to a small group of youngsters in Pueblo, Colorado. Instead, sales of model glue skyrocketed across America, leading to widespread restrictions on sales to minors.

Thinking about the kinds of things such articles often say about the latest drug problem, are there components of those articles that you would include if you were writing an advertisement to promote use of the drug? Do you think such articles actually do more harm than good, as Brecher suggested? If so, does the important principle of a free press mean there is no way to reduce the impact of such journalism?

"THE DRUG PROBLEM"

Talking About Drug Use

"Drug use on the rise" is a headline that has been seen quite regularly over the years. It gets our attention, but "drug use" can't always be rising, can it? No, but at any given time the unwanted use of some kind of drug can be found to be increasing, at least in some group of people. How big a problem does the current headline represent?

Before you can meaningfully evaluate the extent of such a problem or propose possible solutions, it helps to define what you're talking about. In other words, it helps to be more specific about just what the problem is. Most of us don't really view drug use as the problem, if

that includes your Aunt Margie's taking two aspirins when she has a headache. What we really mean is that some drugs being used by some people or in some situations constitute problems with which our society must deal.

---

club drugs: drugs associated with use at all-night dance parties, known as "raves," held in dance clubs, abandoned warehouses, and increasingly in more traditional night clubs as the rave-party generation moves into its twenties. The drugs most commonly included in this group include the hallucinogen MDMA ("Ecstasy"; Chapter 17) and the depressants GHB and rohypnol ("roofies"; Chapter 9).

Journalism students are told that an informative news story must answer the questions *who, what, when, where, why,* and *how.* Let's see how answering the same questions plus one more question—*how much*—can help us analyze problem drug use.

• *Who* is taking the drug? We are more concerned about a 15-year-old girl drinking a beer than we are about a 21-year-old woman doing the same thing. We worry more about a 10-year-old boy chewing tobacco than we do about a 40-year-old man chewing it (unless we happen to be riding right behind him when he spits out the window). And, although we don't like anyone taking heroin, we undoubtedly get more upset when we hear about the girl next door becoming an addict.

• *What* drug are they taking? This question should be obvious, but often it is overlooked.

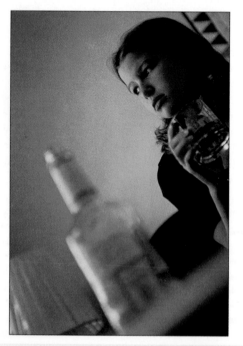

Our concern about the use of a substance often depends on who is using it.

A simple claim that a high percentage of students are "drug users" doesn't tell us if there has been an epidemic of crack smoking or if the drug referred to is alcohol (more likely). If someone begins to talk about a serious "drug problem" at the local high school, the first question should be "what drug or drugs?"

• *When and where* is the drug being used? The situation in which the drug use occurs often makes all the difference. The clearest example is the drinking of alcohol; if it is confined to appropriate times and places, most people accept drinking as normal behavior. When an individual begins to drink on the job, at school, or in the morning, that behavior is evidence of a drinking problem. Even subcultures that accept the use of illegal drugs might distinguish between acceptable and unacceptable situations; some college-age groups might accept marijuana smoking at a party but not just before going to a calculus class!

• *Why* a person takes a drug or does anything else is a tough question to answer. Nevertheless, we can see that it is important in some cases. If a person takes a narcotic drug because her doctor prescribed it for the knee injury she got while skiing, most of us would not be concerned. If, on the other hand, she takes that drug on her own, just because she likes the way it makes her feel, then we should begin to worry about her developing a dependency. The motives for drug use, as with motives for other behaviors, can be complex. Even the person taking the drug might not be aware of all the motives involved. One of the ways a psychologist can try to answer *why* questions is to look for consistency in the situations in which the behavior occurs (when and where). If a person drinks only with other people who are drinking, we may suspect social motives; if a person often drinks alone, we may suspect that the person is trying to deal with personal problems by drinking.

Drugs in Depth

Some Important Definitions—and a Caution!

Some terms that are commonly used in discussing drugs and drug use are difficult to define with precision, partly because they are so widely used for many different purposes. Therefore, any definition we offer should be viewed with caution because each represents a compromise between leaving out something important versus including so much that the defined term is "watered down."

The word **drug** will be defined as "any substance, natural or artificial, other than food, that by its chemical nature alters structure or function in the living organism." One obvious difficulty is that we haven't defined *food*, and how we draw that line can sometimes be arbitrary. Alcoholic beverages, such as wine and beer, may be seen as either drug, food, or both. Are we discussing how much sherry wine to include in beef Stroganoff, or are we discussing how many ounces of wine can be consumed before becoming intoxicated? Since this is not a cookbook but, rather, a book on the use of psychoactive chemicals, we will view all alcoholic beverages as drugs.

Illicit drug is a term used to refer to a drug that is unlawful to possess or use. This is complicated by the fact that many of these drugs are available by prescription, but when they are manufactured or sold illegally they are illicit. Traditionally, alcohol and tobacco have not been considered illicit substances even when used by minors, probably because of their widespread legal availability to adults. On the other hand, common household chemicals, such as glues and paints, take on some characteristics of illicit substances when people inhale them to get "high."

Deviant drug use is drug use that is not common within a social group *and* that is disapproved of by the majority, causing members of the group to take corrective action when it occurs. The corrective action may be informal (making fun of the behavior, criticizing the behavior) or formal (incarceration, treatment). Some examples of drug use might be deviant in the society at large but accepted or even expected in particular subcultures. We still consider this behavior to be deviant, since it makes more sense to apply the perspective of the larger society.

Drug misuse generally refers to the use of prescribed drugs in greater amounts than, or for purposes other than, those prescribed by a physician or dentist. For nonprescription drugs or chemicals such as paints, glues, or solvents, misuse might mean any use other than the use intended by the manufacturer.

Drug abuse consists of the use of a substance in a manner, amounts, or situations such that the drug use causes problems or greatly increases the chances of problems occurring. The problems may be social (including legal), occupational, psychological, or physical. Once again, this definition gives us a good idea of what we're talking about, but it isn't precise. For example, some would consider any use of an illicit drug to be abuse because of the possibility of legal problems, but many people who have tried marijuana on occasion would argue that they had no problems and therefore didn't abuse it. Another problem is that the use of almost any drug, even under the orders of a physician, has at least some potential for causing problems. The question might come down to how great the risk is and whether the user is recklessly disregarding the risk. How does cigarette smoking fit this definition? In your opinion, should all cigarette smoking be considered drug abuse?

Drug **addiction** is a very controversial term, and in Chapter 3 we review evidence that the scientific view of addiction has changed over the past several years. We find it most convenient to use the term in its original dictionary sense, to "give oneself up to a habit." Drug addiction is thus characterized by frequent use of the drug (usually at least daily) and by the fact that a great deal of the individual's behavior is focused on using the drug, obtaining the drug, or talking about the drug or, is focused on the paraphernalia associated with the drug's use. We mean this only in a descriptive, behavioral way, not necessarily implying anything about physiology or disease. It should be obvious that one could apply this definition to other kinds of behavior, such as playing golf or surfing the Internet, and in common parlance we often use the term *addiction* in reference to such activities. The controversy discussed in Chapter 3 is mainly over whether the addiction to drugs is somehow fundamentally different from these other "addictions."

It might seem that we don't need all of these definitions, since our stereotypical view of addiction usually

---

Drugs in Depth Continued. . .

involves both deviant drug use and drug abuse. However, these definitions allow for the possibility that one might abuse a drug without being an addict (driving while intoxicated is a good example) or that one might be addicted to coffee drinking without engaging in deviant drug use. One of the most active current controversies about cigarettes is that, when they are being used in the manner intended by the manufacturer (therefore not misused), they are still potentially dangerous and addictive.

- *How* the drug is taken can often be critical. South American Indians who chew coca leaves absorb cocaine slowly over a long period of time. The same total amount of cocaine "snorted" into the nose produces a more rapid, more intense effect of shorter duration and probably leads to much stronger dependence. Smoking cocaine in the form of "crack" produces an even more rapid, intense, and brief effect, and dependence occurs very quickly.
- *How much* of the drug is being used? This isn't one of the standard journalism questions, but it is important when describing drug use. Often the difference between what one considers normal use and what one considers abuse of, for example, alcohol or a prescription drug comes down to how much a person takes.

Four Principles of Psychoactive Drugs

Now that we've seen how helpful it can be to be specific when talking about drug use, let's look for some organizing principles.

Are there any general statements that can be made about **psychoactive** drugs—those compounds that alter consciousness and affect mood? In fact, there are four basic principles that seem to apply to all of these drugs.

1. *Drugs, per se, are not good or bad.* There are no "bad drugs." When drug abuse, drug addiction, and deviant drug use are talked about, it is the behavior, the way the drug is being used, that is being referred to. This statement sounds controversial and has angered some prominent political figures and drug educators. It therefore requires some defense. From the point of view of a pharmacologist, it is difficult to view the drug, the chemical substance itself, as somehow possessing evil intent. It sits there in its bottle and does nothing until we put it into a living system. From the perspective of a psychologist who treats drug addicts, it is difficult to imagine what good there might be in heroin or cocaine. However, heroin is a perfectly good painkiller, at least as effective as morphine, and it is used medically in many countries. Cocaine is a good local anesthetic and is still used for medical procedures, even in the United States. Each of these drugs can also produce bad effects when people abuse them. In the cases of heroin and cocaine, our society has weighed its perception of the risks of bad consequences against the potential benefits and decided that we should severely restrict the availability of these substances. It is wrong, though, to place all of the blame for these bad consequences on the drugs themselves and to conclude that they are simply "bad" drugs. This is very important because many people have a tendency to view some of these substances as possessing an almost magical power to produce evil. When we blame the substance itself, our efforts to correct drug-related problems tend to focus exclusively on eliminating the substance, perhaps ignoring all of the factors that led to the abuse of the drug.

2. *Every drug has multiple effects.* Although a user might focus on a single aspect of a drug's effect, we do not yet have compounds that alter only one aspect of consciousness. All psychoactive drugs act on more than one place in the brain, so we might expect them to produce complex psychological effects. Also, virtually every drug that acts in the brain also has effects on the rest of the body, influencing blood pressure, intestinal activity, or other functions.

3. *Both the size and the quality of a drug's effect depend on the amount the individual has taken.* The relationship between dose and effect works in two ways. By increasing the dose, there is usually an increase in the same effects noticed at lower drug levels. Also, and frequently this is a more important relationship, at different dose levels there is often a change in the kind of effect, an alteration in the character of the experience.

4. *The effect of any psychoactive drug depends on the individual's history and expectations.* Because these drugs alter consciousness and thought processes, the effect they have on an individual depends on what was there initially. An individual's attitude can have a major effect on his or her perception of the drug experience. The fact that some people can experience a high when smoking oregano and dry oak tree leaves—thinking it's good **marijuana**—should come as no surprise to anyone who has arrived late at a party and felt a "buzz" after one drink rather than the usual two or three. It is not possible, then, to talk about many of the effects of these drugs independent of the user's attitude and the setting.

HOW DID WE GET HERE?

Have Things Really Changed?

Drug use is not new. Humans have been using alcohol and plant-derived drugs for thousands of years—as far as we know, since *Homo sapiens* first appeared on the planet. What recorded history we have indicates that some of these drugs were used not just for their presumed therapeutic effects but also for recreational purposes. In some of the highly developed ancient cultures, psychoactive plants played important economic and religious roles. There is also evidence that some people have always overused, misused, or abused these substances.

Drugs play a much different role in modern society than they did even 100 years ago. Major events have occurred in pharmacology and medicine that have produced revolutionary changes in the way in which we view drugs. In addition, recent cultural revolutions have influenced our attitudes and behavior regarding drugs and drug use.

Four Pharmacological Revolutions

One hundred years ago, most Americans had a very different view of medicines than we have today. There were only a few drugs that had powerful effects, and these were used to treat a wide variety of ailments. The idea that a drug could be a specific treatment for a specific disease was only a dream. As a consequence, most people had limited faith in the power of drugs and were cautious about using them. Our modern attitudes about drugs are based to a great extent on several important advances in pharmacology.

The first revolution brought some major communicable diseases well under control. The use of *vaccines,* which began with Pasteur, Jenner, and Koch in the nineteenth century, certainly has had a major impact on our society. The deadly disease smallpox was almost entirely eliminated, and other serious diseases are virtually a thing of the past; diphtheria, polio, and whooping cough are unheard of, except when we refer to the vaccines for them. Measles, mumps, and tetanus also are preventable now through the development of specific vaccines. *Vaccines helped convince the public that medicine is capable of producing drugs with very powerful and very selective beneficial effects.*

The second pharmacological revolution resulted from the introduction of *antibiotics:*

Taking Sides

Can We Predict or Control Trends in Drug Use?

Looking at the overall trends in drug use, it is clear that significant changes have occurred in the number of people using marijuana, cocaine, alcohol, and tobacco. However, while it's easy to describe the changes once they have happened, it's much tougher to predict what will come next. Maybe even harder than predicting trends in drug use is knowing what social policies are effective in controlling these trends. The two main kinds of activities that we usually look to as methods to prevent or reduce drug use are legal controls and education (including advertising campaigns). How effective do you think laws have been in helping prevent or reduce drug use? Be sure to consider laws regulating sales of alcohol and tobacco to minors in your analysis. What

about the public advertising campaigns you are familiar with? How about school-based prevention programs? As you go through the remainder of this book, these questions will come up again, along with more information about specific laws, drugs, and prevention programs. For now, choose which side you would rather take in a debate on the following proposition: broad changes in drug use reflect shifts in society and are not greatly influenced by drug-control laws, antidrug advertising, or drug-prevention programs in schools.

For more on this topic, log on to www.dushkin.com/online for current news and links to other popular and informative sites, as well as time-saving web search strategies and study tools.

"sulfa" drugs, penicillin, and then others. First proven effective during World War II, they continue to save lives daily. These drugs not only cure such previously dreaded diseases as syphilis and pneumonia but can also prevent or treat infections resulting from injury or surgery, thus saving both lives and limbs. *Antibiotics helped give us faith in drugs as effective cures for serious illnesses.* We now expect that when we get sick we will go to a physician who will prescribe a drug that will make us better.

The first two revolutions might be too pervasive and too close to home for most of us to appreciate their importance. This is not the case with the third pharmacological revolution—the development of **psychopharmacology** that began in the 1950s (see Chapter 10). The most important single event was the introduction of the antipsychotic drugs for the treatment of schizophrenia and other major psychotic disorders. These drugs have freed thousands of patients from long-term hospitalization and have helped restructure our society's approach to mental illness on several levels. One important, but little-studied, effect on our culture came about

because these drugs have their primary effect on mental processes. *Because of advances in psychopharmacology, we came to accept the notion that drugs can have powerful and selective effects on our mind, our emotions, and our perceptions.* Perhaps the psychopharmacological revolution of the 1950s helped set the stage for the "psychedelic" experimentation of the 1960s.

The fourth pharmacological revolution, the development of the *oral contraceptive,* contributed to the sexual revolution, which was beginning to occur in the 1950s and has not yet stabilized. It is probably true that the opportunity for unmarried couples to engage in sex without fear of pregnancy contributed to a greater sexual freedom in the 1960s and 1970s. That a married woman could be relatively certain for the first time of having several years of her life uninterrupted by pregnancy made it possible for her to commit to attaining more education and to developing her career. Perhaps those social changes were ready to happen without "the pill," but we all began to think in terms of *planning* for pregnancy and childbirth. In fact, this control factor might be one of the most pervasive and subtle influences of the oral contraceptive on our society's view of drugs. *With oral contraceptives, powerful chemicals clearly labeled as drugs were not being used to prevent or treat disease but were being used by healthy people to gain chemical control over their own bodies.* This may have helped pave the way for attempts to control emotions and thoughts by using chemistry in the 1960s.

Recent Cultural Change

America bounded out of World War II with a belief in the future that was untarnished by minor setbacks, such as the Iron Curtain, the Korean War, and an economic recession here and there. Everything seemed to be moving up after the depression of the 1930s and the war of the 1940s. This was the time to make it big, to make up for not having. The bright-eyed boys and girls who applauded the American flag when it appeared in the movies during the world war grew up, got married, and moved to the suburbs. They knew where they were headed. The formula was simple: work hard, and you'll get ahead. Advancement meant a nicer home, a new car, and a college education for the kids. Blue-collar workers also got their share. In the 1950s, miners and assembly-line workers could make their take-home pay cover a house payment and a car payment, with a bit left over to save up for that TV set. This was the good life—and their kids would have it even better!

When those kids of the postwar baby-boom generation began to turn 17 or 18 in the early 1960s, American society underwent a rapid change. The kids who grew up in that affluent society without fear of poverty and hunger did not understand the driving ambition of their parents. Partly, television and the information age made it clear that the society their parents had built was far from perfect. In particular, institutionalized racial discrimination in the form of segregated schools and colleges; segregated public transportation, hotels, restrooms, and restaurants; and discriminatory voter registration procedures all

existed in 1960. The picture being painted of hard work leading to the better life apparently didn't apply to everyone. The Vietnam War contributed in a major way. Why were we being asked to risk our lives over there? Who were the good guys and who were the bad guys, and why? Automatic acceptance of authority wasn't going to work anymore. It was time to fix American society, to open it up. We needed more understanding and acceptance of those who were different, not more conformity and materialism. Thus was born the hang-loose ethic of the 1960s and 1970s. The so-called Protestant ethic, in which a person's worthiness is indicated partly by material success, was replaced by a more existential approach, which focused on how people responded to the experiences of life and how well they got along with others. *Peace, love,* and *happiness* were the watchwords. Could experiences be more profound, feelings more intense, with the help of psychoactive drugs? Hopeful and unafraid, young people experimented with a wide variety of hallucinogens, stimulants, and depressants.

Perhaps it's true that, when the social pendulum swings that far that fast, it will always swing back again. Maybe it's just that each new generation has to reject their parents' values to forge their own. That's what we started to do in the late 1970s. The shift to conservatism began about when the large baby-boom generation entered their 30s and began to constitute the establishment they had earlier criticized. The expansion of individual liberties and civil rights faltered and bogged down.

---

psychoactive: having effects on thoughts, emotions, or behavior.

psychopharmacology: the study of the behavioral effects of drugs.

marijuana: (**mare i** *wan* **ah**) also spelled "marihuana." Dried leaves of the *cannabis* plant.

The mood of the country changed fairly quickly. American society in the 1980s became less tolerant of differences, foreigners, pornography, experimental drug use, and young people questioning America's traditional ideals. Congress debated a constitutional amendment to ban the burning of the American flag. Penalties for violating drug laws, which had been loosened in the 1970s, were increased and broadened. The drinking age, which most states had lowered during the 1970s, was increased to 21 again. Authority was back, along with conformity and materialism. College students were being criticized for their focus on the dollar value of their degree rather than on the experience of learning.

If the 1970s were the decade of the "hippie," then the 1980s were the decade of the "yuppie": the young, upwardly mobile professional. The ideal yuppie appeared to be someone with a very nice job, very nice clothes, a very nice car, and a very nice apartment. Married or unmarried, the ideal yuppie had a meaningful relationship with a very nice member of the opposite sex, who also had a very nice job, very nice clothes, and so on.

The stereotypical 1980s person was more interested in personal health than were previous generations; running shoes, Jazzercise, fitness centers, and home exercise equipment became significant indicators of that change. You would expect that these health-conscious individuals would use fewer drugs, and they might have: light beers, low-alcohol beverages, decaffeinated coffee, and soft drinks grew rapidly in popularity. Average consumption of alcohol and cigarettes declined along with drops in per capita intake of sugar and red meat.[1] But the stereotypical yuppies were also status conscious. Imported bottled water quenched their thirst, but sales of designer chocolates and imported cheese also increased. It is ironic that expensive imported beers also sold well, even though they contained more alcohol and calories than their domestic counterparts.[1]

So the yuppie seemed capable of balancing concerns about health with a little self-indulgence, especially if the indulgence was in

HealthQuest Activities

On the *HealthQuest 2.0*, go to the Wellboard and answer the Lifestyle Questions concerning tobacco, alcohol, and other drugs. After answering each question, click on the question mark icon to discover why these questions are relevant to you. You will receive a pop-up box with information about tobacco, alcohol, or drugs and related topics such as drinking and driving. How do your answers reflect on your health and lifestyle? Return to the start of the Wellboard assessment and complete it. As you read the assessment, pay special attention to the summaries you receive regarding your use of tobacco, alcohol, and drugs. Keep this assessment in mind as you continue through this textbook.

something chic and expensive. In that context, what was the major new drug of abuse for this generation? until the 1980s, considered by many to be relatively safe and nonaddicting? expensive, supposedly glamorous, used by film and TV stars and sport figures? a drug not intended to expand consciousness but to give that extra energy, effort, the competitive edge? "Coke" was it (and not the kind in the red and white cans).

It's always easier to look back and characterize a decade than it is to describe one when it is happening. Would the 1990s be a continuation of the conservative 1980s, or would the pendulum swing again? By the year 2000, the jury was in: marijuana use was rising, and five states had passed initiatives in favor of medical use of marijuana. The only question now is how far the pendulum will swing, and for how long?

DRUGS AND DRUG USE TODAY

Extent of Drug Use

In trying to get an overall picture of drug use in today's society, we quickly discover that it's not easy to get accurate information. It's not possible to measure with great accuracy the use of, let's say, cocaine in the United States. We don't really know how much is imported and sold, because most of it is illegal. We don't really know how many cocaine users there are in the country, because we have no good way of counting them. For some things, such as prescription drugs, tobacco, and alcohol, we have a wealth of sales information and can make much better estimates of rates of use. Even there, however, our information might not be complete (home-brewed beer would not be counted, for example, and prescription drugs might be bought and then left unused in the medicine cabinet).

Let us look at some of the kinds of information we do have. A large number of survey questionnaire studies have been conducted in junior highs, high schools, and colleges, partly because this is one of the easiest ways to get a lot of information with a minimum of fuss. Researchers have always been most interested in drug use by adolescents and young adults, because this age is when drug use usually begins and reaches its highest levels.

There are a couple of drawbacks to this type of research. The first is that we can use this technique only on the students who are in class-rooms. We can't get this information from high school dropouts. That causes a bias, because those who skip school or have dropped out are more likely to use drugs.

A second limitation is that we must assume that most of the self-reports are done honestly. In most cases, we have no way of checking to see if Johnny really did smoke marijuana last week, as he claimed on the questionnaire. Nevertheless, if every effort is made to encourage honesty (including assurances of anonymity), we expect that this factor is minimized. To the extent that tendencies to overreport or under-report drug use are relatively constant from one year to the next, we can use such results to reflect trends in drug use over time and to compare relative reported use of various drugs.

Let's look first at the drugs most commonly reported by young college students in a recent nationwide sample. Table 1.1 presents data from

TABLE 1.1

Percentage of College Students One to Four Years Beyond High School Reporting Use of Seven Types of Drugs (1999)

Drug	Ever used	Used in past 30 days	Used daily for past 30 days
Alcohol	87	66.0	4.5
Cigarettes	NA	28.0	15.2
Marijuana/hashish	46	18.0	3.7
Inhalants	12	1.0	0.0
Stimulants	11	2.0	0.2
Hallucinogens	14	2.0	0.0
Cocaine (all)	6	2.0	0.0
Crack	1	0.2	0.0

Source: Monitoring the Future Project, University of Michigan.[3]

one of the best and most complete research programs of this type, the Monitoring the Future Project at the University of Michigan. Data are collected each year from more than 15,000 high school seniors in schools across the United States, so that nationwide trends can be assessed. Data are also gathered from 8th- and 10th-graders and from college students. We are presenting three numbers for each drug: the percentage of college students (1 to 4 years beyond high school) who have *ever* used the drug, the smaller percentage who report having used it within the past *30 days,* and the still smaller percentage who report *daily* use for the past 30 days.[2] Note that almost all of these college students have tried alcohol at some time in their lives. Fewer than half have tried marijuana, and most students report never having tried the rest of the drugs listed. Also note that daily use of any of these drugs other than cigarettes can be considered somewhat rare. One especially valuable aspect of this project is that the high school senior survey has been conducted annually since 1975. Figure 1.1 shows trends from 1975 to 1999 in the reported use within the past

Drugs in Depth

Methamphetamine Use in Your Community

Assume that you have just been appointed to a community-based committee that is looking into drug problems. A high school student on the committee has just returned from a residential treatment program and reports that methamphetamine use has become "very common" in local high schools. Some members of the committee want to call in some experts immediately to give schoolwide assemblies describing the dangers of methamphetamine. You have asked for a little time to check out the student's story to find out what you can about the actual extent of use in the community and report back to the group in a month. Make a list of potential sources of information and the type of information each might provide. If you could get all the information on your list, how close do you think you could come to making an estimate of how many current methamphetamine users there are in your community? Do you think it would be above or below the national average?

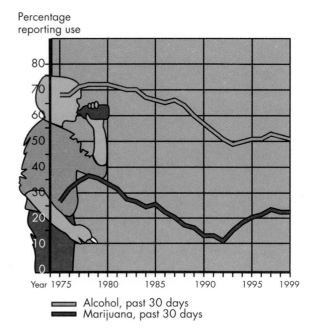

Percentage reporting use

— Alcohol, past 30 days
— Marijuana, past 30 days

Figure 1.1   Drug use by high school seniors, 1975 to 1999.

30 days for alcohol and for marijuana, the most commonly used illicit drug.[3] From this we can see that both the number of students reporting current alcohol use and the number reporting current marijuana use reached a peak in approximately 1978 to 1980, and both declined until 1992. From 1992 to 1999, alcohol use remained relatively constant, while marijuana use increased significantly. This decline and subsequent increase in marijuana use has been the subject of many news articles and political debates, but for now it's mainly important for us to realize the dramatic nature of this change over time. From the peak rate of self-reported use in 1978, marijuana use declined by almost 70 percent according to this measure. From its low point in 1992, marijuana use had doubled by 1999. It will be interesting for us all to observe whether this statistic will again climb back to the levels of the 1970s or whether it will

level off or begin to decline without reaching such high rates.

Another way to get broad-based self-report information is with house-to-house surveys. With proper sampling techniques, these studies can estimate the drug use in most of the population, not just among students. This technique is much more time consuming and expensive, it has a greater rate of refusal to participate, and we must suspect that individuals engaged in illegal drug use would be reluctant to reveal that fact to a stranger on their doorstep. Table 1.2 presents recent data from the National Household Survey on Drug Abuse,[4] obtained from more than 30,000 randomly selected individuals in carefully sampled households across the country. Data on current use are presented for three age groups: 12 to 17, 18 to 25, and 26 and older. You may notice that the data for the 18-to-25 group are similar to the comparable

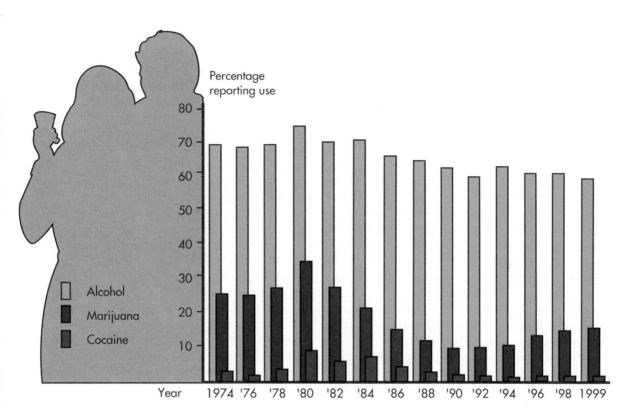

Figure 1-2 Trends in reported drug use within 30 days for young adults ages 18 to 25.

TABLE 1-2

Most Commonly Used Drugs Among Different Age Groups, 1999 NIDA Household Survey— Percentage Reporting Use in the Past 30 Days

Drug	Age 12–17	Age 18–25	Age 26+
Alcohol	19.0	61.0	49.0
Cigarettes	15.0	35.0	30.0
Marijuana	8.0	15.0	3.0
Cocaine	0.5	1.7	0.5

techniques produce similar results. Notice that, for all age groups, alcohol and cigarettes are the most commonly used of these substances. Although most of the data are not presented in this table, typically the highest rates of illicit drug use are in the 18-to-25 age group. Figure 1.2 shows trends in the *30-day* figures for this age group for alcohol, marijuana, and cocaine since 1974. Again, we see that the peak of reported use of all these substances was in 1980.

Correlates of Drug Use

Once we know that a drug is used by some percentage of a group of people, the next logical step is to ask about the characteristics of those who use the drug, as compared with those who

data from the high school survey. This kind of cross-checking gives us some additional confidence in the numbers, since different sampling

don't. Often the same questionnaires that ask each person which drugs they have used also include several questions about the persons completing the questionnaires. The researchers might then send their computers "prospecting" through the data to see if certain personal characteristics can be correlated with drug use. An important point to remember about these studies is that they rarely reveal much about either very unusual or very common types or amounts of drug use. For example, if we send a computer combing through the data from 1,000 questionnaires, looking for characteristics correlated with heroin use, only one or two people in that sample might report heroin use, and you can't correlate much based on one or two people. Likewise, it would be difficult to identify the distinguishing characteristics of the people who have "ever tried" alcohol, because that group usually represents over 90 percent of the sample.

Much of the research on **correlates** of drug use has used marijuana smoking as an indicator, partly because marijuana use has been a matter of some concern and partly because enough people have tried it so that meaningful correlations can be done. Other researchers focus on early drinking or on the amount of drinking, and others have developed composite "drug use" scores based on the use of alcohol and marijuana and experimentation with other substances. We have already seen that age is one factor that relates to drug use; another that shows up consistently is gender. Males of all ages are somewhat more likely to use alcohol or illicit drugs.[4]

You may be surprised at some of the factors that generally do *not* correlate well with alcohol or drug use. One of these is the *socioeconomic status (SES)* of the family. Whether reporting on illicit drug use or level of drinking, most studies find little correlation to the parents' fields of employment (professional, clerical, or blue-collar, for example). These results surprise people who think it's the kids with all the money who use drugs, as well as other people who believe

that it's the poor kids who use drugs. In fact, most of these studies do not gather enough data on the most economically disadvantaged youth, and when those groups are studied there is a higher rate of drug use.[5] So very low SES does play a role in drug and alcohol use, but, for the vast majority of the population, SES is not a significant factor. Another surprise for most people is the consistent finding that *personality problems* are such poor predictors of drug use. In spite of the fact that many theories of drug use assume that people use alcohol or drugs because of low self-esteem, depression, or anxiety, study after study have found that measures of these characteristics are only weakly correlated with drug use. People often report that they drink or use drugs when they're depressed or anxious, but they are probably referring to a temporary *state* of depression or anxiety, as opposed to a long-term personality *trait*.[5] Self-esteem apparently has complicated relationships to drug use because there is evidence that young people sometimes enhance their self-esteem by becoming involved with a drug- or alcohol-using group.[6] Also, please remember that these surveys are examining the overall range of drug or alcohol use as found in the population at large, as opposed to looking selectively at that small fraction of people who are addicts or alcoholics.

These studies are also fairly consistent in finding a collection of psychosocial factors that are related to drug use. Those students who are religious, attend school regularly and get good grades, have good relationships with their parents, and do not break the law are the students who report the least drinking and drug use. At the other end of the scale, the picture is that of general *nonconformity* to society, and drug use is one part of that overall picture. This doesn't account for every instance of drug use, but it is the most consistent overall finding. The nonconforming individual often has closer associations with peers than with his or her parents, and the peers are likely to be nonconforming. In other

Exploring Your Spirituality

Turning to Spiritual Resources Instead of Drugs

Do you, like most people, sometimes wonder about the meaning of life? ponder why bad things happen? wish you had a resource for lessening personal stress? When you feel anxious or down, it's sometimes tempting to have a drink or take a pill. What are some things you can do to improve your outlook on life without using drugs?

- *Develop your spirituality.* Your total well-being is influenced by your spiritual side, as well as by the other dimensions of health. Cultivating your spiritual health can help you discover how you fit into the universe. Although you can include affiliation with an organized religion if you hold such beliefs, your spirituality also encompasses your relationship to other living things, the role of a spiritual direction in your life, the nature of human behavior, and your willingness to serve others. Open yourself to new experiences with art, nature, music, and body movement. Meditate, reflect, or renew your faith.
- *Talk with a trusted friend.* Supportive friends can help provide the emotional resilience to deal with life's challenges. Confide your feelings to a close, trusted friend or family member. By opening up to another person, you'll gain insights into how to get beyond negative feelings without resorting to drug use.
- *Volunteer.* One way to feel good is to help others. Be a tutor, become a Big Brother or Big Sister, or work in an animal shelter or 24-hour crisis intervention center.
- *Get moving.* Join an aerobics class. Ride a bike. Take the stairs instead of the elevator. Physical activity is a natural mood enhancer, and you may find a connection with nature in a walk outdoors or a sense of community in a dance class. You'll return to your responsibilities with renewed enthusiasm.
- *Seek professional help.* If you've tried these strategies but still feel you're having trouble coping, consider talking with people trained to help you. Visit your college health center or counseling center. The important first step is up to you.

words, drug-using youngsters are often part of a *deviant subculture.*

Some researchers have looked for specific *risk factors*—that is, factors in the child's life that may be associated with a greater risk of substance abuse. One study of this type surveyed about 3,000 students in 7th, 9th, and 11th grades, asking about relationships with parents, peers, school, and religious institutions, as well as about personal factors.[7] They then correlated these answers with the students' self-reported use of various drugs to determine which factors were significantly associated with increased risk of drug abuse. Other researchers have looked at the issue the other way around. Instead of trying to predict which students will abuse drugs, they have tried to determine the factors that appear to protect some youth from becoming involved with drugs. One study followed a group of more than 1,000 students beginning in 7th and 8th grades.[8] The students were considered to be at risk by having an unemployed head of the household, family members with drug problems or previous arrests, or an official record of child abuse or maltreatment prior to their 12th birthday. The students were then surveyed each year to determine which were able to remain free of delinquency or regular drug use. Table 1.3 lists the risk factors from one study conducted on the West Coast and the protective factors derived from the other study conducted on the East Coast of the United States. These have been

correlate: (*core a let*) a variable that is statistically related to some other variable, such as drug use.

TABLE 1-3

Factors Associated with Substance Abuse

	Risk factors	Protective factors
Family factors	Parents acceptance of drug use Distrust of parent drug knowledge	Parental supervision Child's attachment to parent Parent's attachment to child
Educational factors	Absence from school (other than illness) Poor academic achievement Distrust of teacher drug knowledge	Reading percentile Mathematics percentile Commitment to school Attachment to teachers Parents expectation that child will go to college
Peer factors	Perceived peer approval of drug use	Peers' conventional values Parents' positive evaluation of peers
Other factors	Early alcohol intoxication (before age 13) Knowledge of adults who use drugs Emotional distress Dissatisfaction with life	Close relationship with adult outside the family Involvement in religious activities Involvement in prosocial activities High self-esteem

organized into categories for comparison purposes, and it is interesting to see that these two studies, done on different samples of students and looking at the question from opposite perspectives, have produced results consistent with one another. For example, one study found that frequent absence from school is a risk factor, and the other study found that commitment to school is a protective factor. Overall, these studies are consistent with the idea that students who get along well with their parents, are interested in school, and in general conform to conventional social norms are less likely to become regular users of illicit drugs, alcohol, or cigarettes. Figure 1.3 shows how important these risk and protective factors are: students with 7 or more risk factors were more than 10 times as likely as students with few risk factors to be abusing at least 1 substance (defined as daily use of alcohol, tobacco, or marijuana or weekly use of cocaine or other "hard" drugs). Likewise, in the at-risk population from the East Coast,

students with 6 or more protective factors were about 3 times as likely to remain "drug-free" (not initiating regular use) as students with a few protective factors.

The other side of this picture is that the same individuals who are at risk for drug abuse are also at risk for other deviant behaviors; fighting, stealing, vandalism, and early sexual activity are correlated with drug use and heavier alcohol use. Therefore, the pattern of deviance-prone activity might have both a variety of causes and a variety of behavioral expressions, one of which is drug use.

Antecedents of Drug Use

Finding characteristics that tend to be associated with drug use doesn't help us understand causal relationships very well. For example, do adolescents first become involved with a deviant peer group and then use drugs, or do they first use drugs and then begin to hang around with

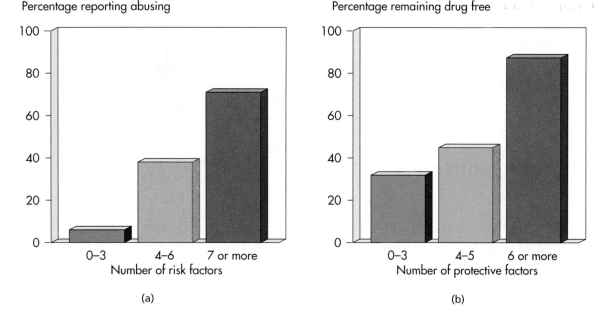

Figure 1-3 Risk and Protective Factors Related to Drug Use (a) relationship of risk factors to percentage of students reporting abuse of at least one substance (b) relationship of protective factors to percentage of students remaining drug-free for one year.

others who do the same? Does drug use cause them to become poor students and to fight and steal? To answer such questions, it is necessary to interview the same individuals at different times and look for **antecedents,** characteristics that predict later initiation of drug use. For example, one study started with seventh-graders who had not yet tried alcohol and then followed up 3 months and 12 months later.[9] At 3 months, those who had begun heavy alcohol use (more than 3 drinks per occasion) were most strongly predicted by their earlier association with peers who used marijuana and by their own expectancy that they might also use marijuana. Frequency of heavy drinking at 12 months was best predicted by their drinking behavior at 3 months and by peer approval of cigarette use.

A few scientists have been able to follow the same group of young people at annual intervals for several years in what is known as a **longitudinal study,** and those results have been quite informative. To answer our first question about the deviant peer group, the research results are consistent in reporting that other indicators of deviant behavior generally appear before drug use. For example, children often will be getting poor grades or getting into trouble for fighting or stealing before they first experiment with alcohol, cigarettes, or other substances.[10] This is important because it means that in most cases the conduct problems and

antecedent: (ant eh *see* dent) a variable that occurs before some event such as the initiation of drug use.

longitudinal study: (lon jeh *too* di nul) a study done over a period of time (months or years).

grade problems are not caused by drug use. We might not know what the ultimate causes of all these behaviors are, but it is both too simple and obviously illogical to conclude that all of the problems these kids have are a consequence of their using drugs, because the drug use usually comes later.

Gateway Substances

One very important study done in the 1970s[11] pointed out that there was a typical sequence of involvement with drugs. Most of the high school students in that group started their drug involvement with beer or wine. The second stage involved hard liquor, cigarettes, or both; the third stage was marijuana use; and only after going through those stages did they try other illicit substances. Not everyone followed the same pattern, but it is interesting that only 1 percent of the students began their substance use with marijuana or another illicit drug. It is as though they first had to go through the **gateway** of using alcohol and, in many cases, cigarettes. Let's keep our logic in order here: most of the illicit drug users had probably also eaten hamburgers before they smoked marijuana. The point is that the students who had not used beer or wine at the beginning of the study were much less likely to be marijuana smokers at the end of the study than the students who had used these substances. The cigarette smokers were about twice as likely as the nonsmokers to move on to smoking marijuana. There is evidence that the gateway function of cigarettes continues to be important: in the senior class of 1994, those who were daily smokers of a pack or more of cigarettes were about 15 times as likely as nonsmokers to have used cocaine and about 4 times as likely to have smoked marijuana.[12] From the Household Survey[13] among youth aged 12 to 17, just over one-third had ever tried cigarettes, but those who had tried cigarettes were more than 10 times as likely to have also tried marijuana. From the self-reported age at which each person first tried cigarettes or marijuana, it was found

that 75 percent smoked cigarettes before smoking marijuana.

One possible interpretation of the gateway phenomenon is that young people are exposed to alcohol and tobacco and that these substances themselves somehow make the person more likely to go on to use other drugs. Because most people who use these gateway substances do not go on to become cocaine users, we should be cautious about jumping to that conclusion. What seems more likely is that early alcohol use and cigarette smoking are common indicators of the general deviance-prone pattern of behavior that also includes an increased likelihood of smoking marijuana or trying cocaine. For example, in the senior class of 1994, a student with a D average was about 14 times as likely as a student with an A average to be a pack-a-day smoker.[12]

Because beer and cigarettes are more widely available to a deviance-prone young person than marijuana or cocaine, it is logical that beer and cigarettes would most often be tried first. The socially conforming students are less likely to try even these relatively available substances until they are older, and they are less likely ever to try the illicit substances. Let's ask the question another way: what if we managed to develop a prevention program that stopped all young people from smoking cigarettes? Would that cut down on marijuana smoking? Most of us think it might, because people who don't want to suck tobacco smoke into their lungs probably won't want to inhale marijuana smoke either. Would such a program keep people from getting D averages or getting into trouble of other kinds? Probably not. In other words, we think of the use of gateway substances not as the *cause* of later illicit drug use but, instead, as an early indicator of the basic pattern of deviant behavior resulting from a variety of psychosocial risk factors.

Parent and Peer Influences

It is generally true that adolescents are more influenced by their parents when it comes to long-term goals and plans, but their peers have more

Try It!

Do Your Goals and Behaviors Match?

One of the interesting things about young people who get into trouble with drugs or other types of deviant behavior is that they often express long-term goals for themselves that are pretty conventional. In other words, they want or perhaps even expect to be successful in life, but then do things that interfere with that success. One way to look at this is that their long-term goals don't match up with their short-term behavior. Everyone does this sort of thing to some extent—you want to get a good grade on the first exam, but then someone talks you into going out instead of studying for the next one. Or perhaps you hope to lose five pounds but just can't pass up that extra slice of pizza.

Make yourself a chart that lists your long-term goals down one side and has a space for short-term behaviors down the other side, like the one that follows:

	Goals (Long-Term)	Behaviors (Short-Term)
Educational		
Physical health and fitness		
Occupational		
Spiritual		
Physical		
Relationships		

Relationships

Write in your goal under each category as best you can. Then think about some things you do occasionally that tend to interfere with your achieving that goal and put a minus sign next to each of those behaviors. After you have gone through all the goals, go back and write down some short-term behaviors that you could practice to assist you in achieving each goal, and put a plus sign beside each of those behaviors.

How does it stack up? Are there some important goals for which you have too many minuses and not enough plusses? If study skills and habits, relationship problems, or substance abuse appear to be serious roadblocks for your success, consider visiting a counselor or therapist to get help in overcoming them.

influence over their immediate lifestyle and day-to-day activities.[14] Also, in early adolescence, parental influences are relatively strong; as adolescence progresses, peer influences become stronger. There is evidence from longitudinal research that both peers and parents influence adolescent drug-use behavior, but in general peer influences are more important. We can imagine situations in which peer and parental influences are in the same direction: a family that encourages school performance and long-term goals or a young person who does well in school and regularly attends religious services and is therefore surrounded by other young people who do well in school and hold similar values. Alternatively, we may have an environment in which one or more parents is an alcoholic, other drugs are used openly, success in school is not valued or encouraged, the family lives in a neighborhood with many such families, and many of the other young people have the same problems. More commonly, we think of a model in which there is a conflict—parents opposing drug or alcohol use and the peer group encouraging such behavior. Two longitudinal studies have tried to examine these influences over time. Although the results are complex, some of the major points can be summarized. As in previous research, the best predictors of drug use were peer variables. In one of the studies, having peers with antisocial attitudes was the strongest predictor of drug use.[10] In the other study, having peers who used marijuana was the best predictor of marijuana use.[14] The use of alcohol by parents did have an impact on alcohol use, but it was not clear whether this was because of direct "modeling" effects. For example, in one study it appeared that adolescents whose parents drank were more likely to have friends who drank, and the drinking pattern of friends was a big influence.[14] In the other study, it was argued that heavy drinking by the parent might interfere with parental *monitoring* of the child's activities, and poor monitoring by parents was found to be a major factor in allowing the child to associate with a deviant peer group.[10]

What advice for parents can we draw from all this research? First, encourage and reinforce the value of school and school achievement and of long-term life goals. When day-to-day activities and behavior are incompatible with those long-term goals, point that out. Second, be on the alert for school practices, such as remedial "tracks" or after-school detention, which might group your child with deviance-prone peers. Third, realize that you do have some influence over the types of peers your child associates with, particularly during childhood and early adolescence. Your child might associate with children who behave the way your family behaves, so it might pay to examine your own behavior. You can encourage or provide support for after-school activities that will bring your child into contact with positive peer groups. Monitoring involves knowing what your child is doing and with whom, as well as showing interest in school activities and accomplishments. This advice comes with no guarantee of success, but it is based on consistent research findings.

Motives for Drug Use

To most of us, it doesn't seem necessary to find explanations for normative behavior; we don't often ask why someone takes a pain reliever when she has a headache. Our task is to try to explain the drug-taking behavior that frightens and infuriates—the deviant drug use. There is one fact about human conduct that we should keep in mind throughout this book: in spite of good, logical evidence telling us we "should" avoid certain things, we all do some of them, anyway. We know that we shouldn't eat that

---

gateway: one of the first drugs (e.g., alcohol or tobacco) used by a typical drug user.

Targeting Prevention

Preventing What?

Chapter 1 provides an overview of psychoactive drug use, primarily based on data from the United States. As we look forward to the topic of prevention, it's appropriate to think about what aspects of psychoactive drug use we would most like to reduce. Following are some perspectives:

- We should work to prevent any use of tobacco or alcohol by those under 21, as well as any use at all of drugs such as marijuana, cocaine, and LSD. These drugs are all illegal, and we know that early use of tobacco and alcohol is associated with a greatly increased risk of illicit drug use in the future.
- Focusing only on drug use ignores the fact that illicit drug use is usually part of a larger pattern of deviant or antisocial behavior. Therefore, our efforts would be more effective if we were to target younger people and work to prevent poor academic performance, fighting, shoplifting, and other early indicators of this lifestyle, in addition to early experimentation with tobacco and alcohol.
- Wait a minute! We're confusing what might be desirable with what might be possible. We can't prevent everyone from doing things we don't like. For example, as adults most people will drink alcohol at least once in a while, yet perhaps only 10 percent of drinkers have most of the problems. Trying to prevent all drug use and other undesirable behavior is just too big a job, and it violates our sense of individual freedom. We need to focus our efforts on preventing addiction and the crime that goes with it. That's a much smaller problem, and we have a better chance of success.

With which of these perspectives do you most agree at this point? Are there other possible perspectives not represented by these three?

second piece of pie or have that third drink on an empty stomach. Cool-headed logic tells us so. We would be hard pressed to find good, sensible reasons why we should smoke cigarettes, drive faster than the speed limit, go skydiving, sleep late when we have work to do, flirt with someone and risk an established relationship, or use cocaine. Whether one labels these behaviors sinful or just stupid, they don't seem to be designed to maximize our health or longevity.

But humans do not live by logic alone; we are social animals who like to impress each other, and we are pleasure-seeking animals. These factors help explain why people do some of the things they shouldn't, including drugs.

The research on correlates and antecedents points to a variety of personal and social variables that influence our drug taking, and many psychological and sociological theorists have proposed models for explaining illegal or excessive drug use. We have seen evidence for one common reason that some people begin to take certain illegal drugs: usually young, and more often male than female, they have chosen to identify with a deviant subculture. These groups frequently engage in a variety of behaviors not condoned by the larger society. Within that group, the use of a particular drug might not be deviant at all but might, in fact, be expected. Occasionally the use of a particular drug becomes such a fad among a large number of youth groups that it seems to be a nationwide problem. However, within any given community there will still be groups of people of the same age who don't use the drug.

Rebellious behavior, especially among young people, serves important functions not only for the developing individual but also for the evolving society. Adolescents often try very hard to impress other people and may find it especially difficult to impress their parents. An adolescent who is unable to gain respect from people or who is frustrated in efforts to "go his or her own way" might engage in a particularly dangerous or

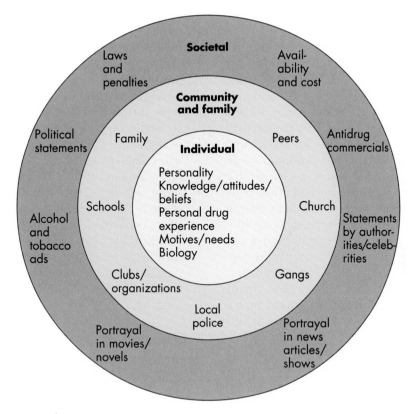

Figure 1-4 Influences on drug use.

disgusting behavior as a way of demanding that people be impressed or at least pay attention.

One source of excessive drug use may be found within the drugs themselves. Many of these drugs are capable of *reinforcing* the behavior that gets the drug into the system. **Reinforcement** means that, everything else being equal, each time you take the drug you increase slightly the probability that you will take it again. Thus, with many psychoactive drugs there is a constant tendency to increase the frequency or amount of use. Some drugs (such as intravenous heroin or cocaine) appear to be so reinforcing that this process occurs relatively rapidly in a large percentage of those who use them. For other drugs, such as alcohol, the process seems to be much slower. In many people, social factors, other reinforcers, or other activities prevent the increase from occurring at all. For some, however, the drug-taking behavior does increase and consumes an increasing share of their lives. These are the addicts and alcoholics we sometimes pity and sometimes fear but almost never respect.

reinforcement: a procedure in which a behavioral event is followed by a consequent event such that the behavior is then more likely to be repeated. The behavior of taking a drug may be reinforced by the effect of the drug.

Most drug users are seeking an altered state of consciousness, a different perception of the world than is provided by normal, day-to-day activities. It is usually impossible to separate this altered state from the reinforcing effect, because the altered state might be the psychological reflection of the reinforcing state. Many of the high school students in the nationwide surveys report that they take drugs "to see what it's like," or "to get high," or "because of boredom."[15] In other words, they are looking for a change, for something new and different in their lives. This aspect of drug use was particularly clear during the 1960s and 1970s, when lysergic acid diethylamide (LSD) and other perception-altering drugs were popular. We don't always recognize the altered states produced by other substances, but they do exist. A man drinking alcohol might have just a bit more of a perception that he's a tough guy, that he's influential, that he's well liked. A cocaine user might get the seductive feeling that everything is great and that she's doing a great job (even if she isn't). Many drug-abuse prevention programs have focused on efforts to show young people how to feel good about themselves and how to look for excitement in their lives without using drugs.

Another thing seems clear: although societal, community, and family factors (the outer areas of Figure 1.4) play an important role in determining whether an individual will first *try* a drug, with increasing use the individual's own experiences with the drug become increasingly important. For those who become seriously addicted, the drug and its actions on that individual become central, and social influences, availability, cost, and penalties play a less important role in the continuation of drug use.

SUMMARY

- Drug use is a form of behavior that has many things in common with other behaviors, as well as many of the same kinds of controlling variables.

- Any individual drug can have various effects, depending on who has taken it, how much has been taken, and how it has been taken.
- Drug use and problems caused by drug use are probably as old as humankind.
- Changes in American society since the 1950s have influenced fashion in many areas, and recreational drug use is no exception.
- Most of the information about current drug use comes from large-scale, nationwide surveys done in high schools or house-to-house.
- Drug use is greater among those who are more rebellious and who engage in other deviant behaviors, such as heavy drinking.
- Psychoactive drugs can be behaviorally reinforcing, produce altered states of consciousness, and help an individual make a social statement about what group he or she belongs to.

REVIEW QUESTIONS

1. Besides asking a person the question directly, what is one way a psychologist can try to determine why a person is taking a drug?
2. What two characteristics of a drug's effect might change when the dose is increased?
3. In what way might the development of oral contraceptives have changed people's views of drugs to make experimenting with psychoactive drugs more likely?
4. In about what year did drug use in the United States reach its peak?
5. What are the two types of large drug-use surveys sponsored by the federal government on a regular basis?
6. About what percentage of college students use marijuana?
7. What is the relationship between socioeconomic status and illicit drug use or heavy drinking?
8. Do parents or peers appear to have greater influences on adolescent drug use?

Web Watch

Activities to Assess Your Drug Knowledge

Take a General Assessment
Go to www.antibully.org.uk/drugsqui.htm and take the Drugs Quiz. This quiz gives you an overview of different kinds of drugs, their effects, their nicknames, and their misuses in social situations.

Do You Know Drug Slang?
Technical names for different kinds of drugs are often replaced with trendy nicknames or abbreviations. To discover how aware you are of slang terms for substances, take the quiz matching each drug with its nickname at broadcast.webpoint.com/wbzl/tedqz.htm.

Are You Educated About Drugs?
Take the Elks Drug Education Quiz at www.elks.org/drugs/quiz.cfm. The quiz asks questions about different kinds of drugs, their effects and uses, and societal trends. After answering each question, submit it and check out the answer to learn more.

9. In what sense is cigarette smoking a "gateway" to marijuana or cocaine use?

10. Why would a person purposefully act in ways that frighten and anger others?

REFERENCES

1. Sherman SP: America's new abstinence, *Fortune* pp. 20–23, Mar 18, 1985.
2. Johnston LD, O'Malley PM, Bachman JG: *National survey results on drug use from the Monitoring the Future Study, Volume II: College students and young adults.* Rockville, MD: National Institute on Drug Abuse, 2000.
3. Johnston LD, O'Malley PM, Bachman JG: *The monitoring the future national results on adolescent drug use: Overview of key findings, 1999.* Rockville, MD: National Institute on Drug Abuse, 2000.
4. *National household survey on drug abuse, 1999.* Bethesda, MD: SAMHSA Office of Applied Studies, 2000.
5. Oetting ER, Beauvais F: Common elements in youth drug abuse: Peer clusters and other psychosocial factors. In Peele S, editor: *Visions of addiction.* Lexington, MA: DC Heath, 1988.
6. Stein JA, Newcomb MD, Bentler PM: Personality and drug use: Reciprocal effects across four years, *Personality and Individual Differences* 8:419–430, 1987.
7. Newcomb MD and others: Substance abuse and psychosocial risk factors among teenagers: Associations with sex, age, ethnicity, and type of school, *American Journal of Drug and Alcohol Abuse* 13:413–433, 1987.
8. Smith C, Lizotte AJ, Thornberry TP, Krohn MD: Resilient youth: Identifying factors that prevent high-risk youth from engaging in delinquency and drug use. In Hagan J, editor: *Delinquency and disrepute in the life course.* Greenwich, CT: JAI Press, 1995.
9. Ellickson PL, Hays RD: Antecedents of drinking among young adolescents with different alcohol use histories, *Journal of Studies on Alcohol* 52:398–408, 1991.
10. Dishion TJ, Patterson GR, Reid JR: Parent and peer factors associated with drug sampling in early adolescence: Implications for treatment. In Rahdert ER, Grabowski J, editors: *Adolescent drug abuse: Analyses of treatment research,* NIDA Research Monograph, No 77, Washington, DC: U.S. Government Printing Office, 1988.
11. Kandel D, Faust R: Sequence and stages in patterns of adolescent drug use, *Archives of General Psychiatry* 32:923–932, 1975.
12. Bachman JG, Johnston LD, O'Malley PM: *Monitoring the future: A continuing study of the lifestyles and values of youth, 1994* [Computer file]. Conducted by University of Michigan, Survey Research Center. ICPSR ed. Ann Arbor, MI: Inter-University Consortium for Political and Social Research [producer and distributor], 1996.
13. Greenblatt J: Analysis shows correlation between smoking cigarettes and marijuana in adolescents. *SAMHSA News,* Substance Abuse and Mental Health Services Administration, Winter, 1997.
14. Kandel DB, Andrews K: Processes of adolescent socialization by parents and peers, *International Journal of the Addictions* 22:319–342, 1987.
15. Johnston LD, O'Malley PM: Why do the nation's students use drugs and alcohol? Self-reported reasons from nine national surveys, *Journal of Drug Issues* 16:29–66, 1986.

Chapter 2

Drug Use as a Social Problem

Online Learning Center Resources

www.mhhe.com/ray

Log on to our Online Learning Center (OLC) for access to these additional resources.

- Chapter key terms and definitions
- Learning objectives
- Additional behavior change objectives
- Student interactive questions and answer sites
- Self-scoring chapter quiz

The OLC also offers web links for study and exploration of health topics. Here are some examples of what you'll find:

www.appleby-solutions.com/

At this website, you can download assessment software for free. You can also find updated information and tips for health professionals and counselors who handle substance abuse.

washingtonpost.com/wp-srv/local/longterm/drugs/article.htm

This special report by the *Washington Post* investigates and provides evidence of the role of drugs on our streets and the effects on society. There are additional articles, links, and downloads available on this topic, as well as a quiz on local drug patterns.

www.drugsense.org/wodclock.htm

This website features a clock that displays the cost of the war on drugs up to the second.

Drugs in the Media
Counting Crack Babies

One toxicity issue that has received national media attention is the effect of crack cocaine use during pregnancy on the unborn child.

The image of the "crack baby" is a powerful one: born to a mother who was smoking crack during her pregnancy and up until the time of

Drugs in the Media Continued. . .

delivery, the infant is addicted at birth, suffers withdrawal agonies, and continues to suffer developmental abnormalities. In the early 1990s, politicians and news media attracted our attention by describing the plight of these innocent victims of drug abuse and by suggesting that large numbers of children were affected. While even one of these tragedies is too high a rate, just how many really occur? How can we find out?

The Partnership for a Drug-Free America in 1992 began running an ad showing crack in a baby bottle, claiming that "a crack baby is born every 5 minutes." This works out to about 100,000 infants a year. Are there that many crack babies?

The 1991 Household Survey data estimated that 280,000 women of all ages may have used crack at some time during the year. Perhaps most of these were of childbearing age, but most were not using the drug frequently and most were not pregnant,

so 100,000 crack babies would seem high. A call to the Partnership office revealed they had gotten the 100,000 figure from the 1989 National Drug Control Strategy published by the White House. The estimated 100,000 "cocaine babies" referred to in this document seems to be an estimate of the number of babies whose mothers used any form of cocaine, even once, at some time during their pregnancy.

We hear people use numbers ranging from 60,000 to more than 300,000 per year in referring to crack babies. If we mean only those babies who are born addicted because of recent heavy crack smoking by the mother, then all these numbers are probably too high. (Crack babies are discussed further in Chapter 8.) Why do you think politicians and the media tend to oversell the latest drug problem to the public?

Drugs are widely used, some legally and some illegally. If you hear someone talking about the "drug problem," the reference is probably to those situations in which groups or individuals are using drugs in such a way as to attract the disapproval of the rest of society (in other words, the type of deviant or excessive drug use described at the end of Chapter 1). One possible way to look at the "drug problem" is as a social conflict between drug-using or drug-selling individuals and the majority social group.

LAISSEZ-FAIRE

In the 1800s, the U.S. government had virtually no laws governing the sale or use of most drugs. The idea seemed to be that, if the seller wanted to sell it and the buyer wanted to buy it, let them do it—**laissez-faire**, in French. This term has been used to characterize the general nature of the U.S. government of that era. Some current thinkers have advocated a return to that attitude.[1] After all, buying and selling marijuana or cocaine can be called, like prostitution, a "victimless" crime. Both parties get what they want from the transaction, and neither party complains. Because that is often true, the only way society, through its enforcement agencies, can make many arrests for these crimes is to go looking for trouble, by pretending to be either buyer or seller. Instead, why not just look the other way?

---

laissez-faire: (lay say fair) a hands-off approach to government.

Exploring Your Spirituality

Having a Social Life Without Drug and Alcohol Use

When was the last time you went to a party where alcohol wasn't served? Drinking and socializing have many connections in our society. For example, we meet friends for happy hour or toast a special occasion; a bottle of wine is usually a welcome gift. Many people, including college students, associate alcohol with fun and relaxation, but it can easily become a crutch. Have you ever had a drink because it loosens you up and makes it easier to talk to people?

According to college and university drug counselors, students who undergo drug and alcohol counseling often say they started (or continue) to use drugs or alcohol because they feel inadequate in social situations. These students believe they aren't attractive, talented, wealthy, or socially skilled enough to start and maintain relationships. In dating situations, drugs or alcohol allows them to be more relaxed and less conscious of their perceived shortcomings. And if they do something embarrassing they have an excuse: the drug or alcohol has made them act inappropriately.

What drug-free strategies might enhance your social life? Plan fun around people and activities that don't involve drinking or drugs. Meet friends at a coffee or juice bar. Do something active such as backpacking, playing a team sport, or taking an exercise class. Order soda instead of beer with your pizza. Be open to new people and ideas. Be willing to laugh at yourself. Flexibility and humor can be great social assets.

How can you go to a party and feel comfortable not using alcohol or drugs? Choose a nonalcoholic drink, such as soda, juice, or water. (You probably won't be the only one.) If someone hassles you about your choice, be firm and just say pleasantly that that's what you want. You don't need to explain yourself.

How would you start a conversation without a substance to relax you? When you meet someone new, look for common interests. Think about how you can talk easily and naturally with your roommate or people in your cycling group. Show the other person you're interested in him or her by listening more than you talk. You'll soon get over any self-consciousness, because you'll be involved in the conversation.

In fact, state and federal laws controlling drug sales were passed because it was believed that there were victims in some of these transactions. Three main concerns aroused public interest: (1) *toxicity:* some drug sellers were considered to be endangering the public health and victimizing individuals because they were selling dangerous, toxic chemicals, often without labeling them or putting appropriate warnings on them; (2) *addiction:* some sellers were seen as victimizing individuals and endangering their health by selling them habit-forming drugs, again often without appropriate labels or warnings; and (3) *crime:* the drug user came to be seen as a threat to public safety—the attitude became widespread that drug-crazed individuals would often commit horrible, violent crimes. In Chapter 4, we will look at the roots of these concerns and how our current legal structures grew from

them. For now, let's look at each issue and develop some ground rules for the discussion of toxicity, addiction, and drug-induced criminality.

TOXICITY

Categories of Toxicity

The word **toxic** means "poisonous, deadly, or dangerous." All the drugs we discuss in this text can be toxic if misused or abused. We will use the term to refer to those effects of drugs that interfere with normal functioning in such a way as to produce dangerous or potentially dangerous consequences. Seen in this way, for example, alcohol can be toxic in high doses because it suppresses respiration—this can be dangerous if breathing stops long enough to induce brain damage or death. But we can also consider

TABLE 2.1		
Examples of Four Types of Drug-Induced Toxicity		
	Acute (immediate)	**Chronic (long-term)**
Behavioral	"Intoxication" from alcohol, marijuana, or other drugs that impair behavior and increase danger to the individual	Personality changes reported to occur in alcoholics and suspected by some to occur in marijuana users (amotivational syndrome)
Physiological	Usually results from taking too much of a drug, as in overdose	Heart disease, lung cancer, and other effects related to smoking; liver damage resulting from chronic alcohol exposure

alcohol to be toxic if it causes a person to be so disoriented that, for them, otherwise normal behaviors, such as driving a car or swimming, become dangerous. This is an example of something we refer to as **behavioral toxicity.** We make a somewhat arbitrary distinction, then, between behavioral toxicity and "physiological" toxicity—perhaps taking advantage of the widely assumed mind-body distinction, which is more convenient than real. The only reason for making this distinction is that it helps remind us of some important kinds of toxicity that are special to psychoactive drugs and that are sometimes overlooked.

Another distinction we make for the purpose of discussion is **acute** versus **chronic.** Most of the time when people use the word *acute,* they mean "sharp" or "intense." In medicine an acute condition is one that comes on suddenly, as opposed to a chronic or long-lasting condition. When talking about drug effects, we can think of the acute effects as those that result from a single administration of a drug or are a direct result of the actual presence of the drug in the system at the time. For example, taking an overdose of heroin can lead to acute toxicity. By contrast, the chronic effects of a drug are those that result from long-term exposure and can be present whether or not the substance is actually in the system at a given point in time. For example, smoking cigarettes can eventually lead to various types of lung disorders. If you have emphysema from years of smoking, that condition is

there when you wake up in the morning and when you go to bed at night, and whether your most recent cigarette was five minutes ago or five days ago doesn't make much difference.

Using these definitions, Table 2.1 can help give us an overall picture of the possible toxic consequences of a given type of drug. However, knowing what is *possible* is different from knowing what is *likely.* How can we get an idea of which drugs are most likely to produce adverse drug reactions?

Drug Abuse Warning Network

In an effort to monitor the toxicity of drugs other than alcohol, the federal government set up the Drug Abuse Warning Network (**DAWN**).

toxic: poisonous, dangerous.

behavioral toxicity: toxicity resulting from behavioral effects of a drug.

acute: referring to drugs, the short-term effects of a single dose.

chronic: referring to drugs, the long-term effects from repeated use.

DAWN: Drug Abuse Warning Network. System for collecting data on drug-related deaths or emergency room visits.

This system collects data on drug-related crises from several hundred hospital emergency rooms in metropolitan areas around the country. If an individual goes to the emergency room with any sort of problem that is determined to be related to drug abuse, then each drug involved (up to four) is recorded as "mentioned" in connection with a medical emergency. For DAWN's purposes, drug abuse includes improper uses of prescription or over-the-counter drugs and the use of any other substance for psychic effect, dependence, or suicide. Note that the recorded incident could arise because a person swallowed a bottle of aspirin in a suicide attempt or smoked marijuana and then suffered a panic reaction. In the latter case, probably no lasting harm would have occurred if the person had not gone to the emergency room, but each incident counts as one mention, anyway. You can imagine that doing the recordkeeping in any other way would require many subjective judgments on the part of the emergency room physicians. Was it really a serious medical emergency? Was that drug really responsible? This would probably result in systematic differences from one hospital or one city to another. Beginning in 1989, the sampling

procedure for including emergency rooms in the DAWN system was changed to better estimate the total number of episodes in the United States. The numbers for emergency room episodes given on the left-hand side of Table 2.2 are these national estimates for 1999.[2]

If a drug is involved in a person's death, the medical examiner (coroner) is expected to report in a consistent way to the DAWN system, and these drug-related deaths form a second set of statistics (with, of course, smaller numbers of mentions). Some of those death statistics are shown on the right-hand side of Table 2.2.[3]

Before looking at the specific DAWN results, it is important for us to remember a couple of important facts. First, alcohol is not counted if it is the only drug mentioned, but it is counted in the category "alcohol-in-combination" if it is mentioned along with other drugs. Second, more than one drug may be mentioned per incident, and each drug is counted as a separate "mention."

Now let's look again at Table 2.2, which lists the most frequently mentioned drugs in recent DAWN reports. Probably the most obvious thing is that alcohol-in-combination is near the top in both lists, a place it has held for several years. In

TABLE 2.2

Drug Mentions in the Drug Abuse Warning Network (DAWN)

	Emergency room episodes (1999)				Drug-related deaths (1998)		
Rank	Drug name	Number of mentions	Percentage of total episodes	Rank	Drug name	Number of mentions	Percentage of total episodes
1	Alcohol-in-combination	196,277	35	1	Cocaine	4,587	45
2	Cocaine	168,764	30	2	Heroin/morphine	4,330	43
3	Marijuana/hashish	87,150	16	3	Alcohol-in-combination	3,723	37
4	Heroin/morphine	84,408	15	4	Codeine	1,240	12
5	Acetaminophen	28,259	5	5	Diazepam (Valium)	781	8
6	Alprazolam (Xanax)	20,484	4	6	Marijuana/hashish	598	6
7	Clonazepam	16,585	3	7	Methadone	560	6
8	Hydrocodone	14,639	3	8	Diphenhydramine	504	5
9	Ibuprofen	14,400	3	9	Methamphetamine	501	5
10	Aspirin	12,815	2	10	d-Propoxyphene	423	4

Try It!

What's Your Risk of Drug Toxicity?

Any drug that has the ability to affect you in any way also has the potential to be toxic if used in too great a quantity or in the wrong combination with other drugs. If you use alcohol or other drugs, use the following assessment to estimate the risk of toxicity to which your drug use exposes you.

1. When you take over-the-counter medications, including headache remedies, do you read the instructions carefully and make sure not to exceed the recommended dose?
2. If you are already taking some sort of medication on a regular basis, do you always check with your doctor or pharmacist about the safety of taking any additional drug along with your regular medication?
3. Do you check the expiration dates of drugs in your medicine cabinet before using them?
4. If you drink alcohol, do you drink only in moderation and check to make sure the alcohol won't interact with a drug you are also taking?
5. Do you avoid taking drugs prescribed for someone else and avoid the use of street drugs of unknown strength and purity?

If you answered yes to all these questions, you are probably a responsible consumer of alcohol, prescription, and over-the-counter drugs, and it is unlikely that you will suffer from drug toxicity.

fact, if alcohol were counted alone and treated like other drugs in the system, its numbers would so overwhelm both sets of data that all the other drugs would appear to be unimportant beside it. This seems to indicate that alcohol is a pretty toxic substance. It is, but let us also remember that about half of all adult Americans drink alcohol at least once a month, whereas only a small number of people use cocaine, a drug that is also near the top of both DAWN lists. The DAWN system does not correct for frequency of use but, rather, gives us an idea of the total impact of a substance on medical emergencies and drug-related deaths. Cocaine has vied with alcohol-in-combination for the top spot on these lists since the mid-1980s. Methamphetamine moved into the top 10 during the 1990s.

You should notice that the three over-the-counter pain relievers acetaminophen, aspirin, and ibuprofen (see Chapter 14) would rank just below heroin in emergency room mentions if they were combined as a group. However, these drugs do not show up among the top 10 for drug-related deaths. They are often used in suicide attempts but usually do not result in death. Other suicide-related drugs include alprazolam (Xanax) and diazepam (Valium), which are widely prescribed sedatives (see Chapter 9). For these drugs, suicide was listed as the motive in about 70 percent of the emergency room episodes.

The importance of drug combinations, particularly combinations with alcohol, in contributing to these numbers cannot be overstressed. About half of the emergency room episodes were multiple-drug episodes, whereas three-fourths of the drug-related deaths mentioned multiple drugs. For both heroin and cocaine, alcohol was the most common "other" drug.

How Dangerous Is It?

Now that we have seen how complex the interpretation of these tables can become, let's see if we can use the information they present to ask some questions about the relative danger to a person of taking one drug versus another. We have seen that the DAWN data do not correct for incidence of use. Let's use the data presented in Table 1.2 (see Chapter 1, p. 13), obtained from home surveys, as a rough estimate of the relative proportions of use of these drugs in our society. The populations studied are not exactly the same, and there are other reasons that we would not want to use this approach to make fine distinctions among drugs. But we can easily see that marijuana, which was reported to be in current use by about 15 percent of the young adults, was associated with about 6 percent of drug-related deaths. About 2 percent of young adults reported using cocaine, but cocaine was

HealthQuest Activities

In Module 9 on *HealthQuest,* find the article "Substance Abuse Among Women" under *Our Changing World.* Read this article to learn about drug-abuse trends among women. Do you see evidence of these trends on your campus or in your city? What do you think are some of the strongest factors that motivate women to abuse drugs? Do you have any friends who are driven by these factors? Are you driven by these factors? Do you believe men are affected equally by these factors? Why or why not?

Go to Module 8 and look under *Our Changing World.* Find the article "Youth Behavior" and read about alcohol use among young people. Take a poll in class, around campus, or in your dormitory. How many people began drinking in high school, in middle school, or earlier? How many felt pressured by their peers to drink when they were first offered alcohol? How many are underage and drink in spite of being minors? How many feel that teenagers have the ability to be responsible drinkers? How many know a youth who was killed in a drunk driving crash?

more frequently associated with death than was any other substance in the DAWN report. From these statistics we can draw the obvious conclusion, even from imperfect data, that cocaine is many times more deadly than marijuana.

Heroin, which was reported in current use by many fewer people than was cocaine, was mentioned in almost as many drug-related deaths. Can we conclude from this that heroin use is more dangerous than cocaine use? Probably so, given the way each is typically used. Please keep in mind that the amount taken and how a drug is taken can greatly influence toxicity. Heroin was once sold in small doses in tablet form. If it were still available in that form as a prescription drug, many more people would be taking it, but almost none of those would die from it, and our estimates of heroin's relative toxicity would drop drastically. Cocaine is most often "snorted" into the nose, less often smoked as crack, and seldom injected, whereas heroin is often injected intravenously. An experiment indicated that rats allowed to intravenously self-inject as much cocaine as they wanted were more likely to die than rats allowed to self-inject as much heroin as they wanted,[4] so it might be that, if the two drugs were both taken intravenously by most of their human users, cocaine would cause many more deaths than heroin.

We cannot tell precisely from the DAWN data how many total deaths are related to the use of cocaine or heroin, because not all coroners are included in the system. Data are gathered from metropolitan areas that include about a third of the U.S. population, but they are areas that have higher than average use of illicit drugs. A rough estimate of the total annual number of deaths related to cocaine, for example, might be twice the reported DAWN figure, or about 9,000 per year. The total for all illicit drugs, including cocaine, heroin, marijuana, and methamphetamine, might be approximately 15,000. In a country in which more than two million people die each year, this is a relatively minor cause of death, a fact that is surprising to many people.

For comparison, it is estimated that alcohol is responsible for 100,000 deaths annually (see Chapter 12), and more than 400,000 annual deaths are attributed to cigarette smoking (see Chapter 13). Of course, many more people use those substances, and in terms of *relative* danger of toxicity, heroin and cocaine are probably more dangerous than alcohol or cigarettes. However, in looking at the *total* impact of these drug-related deaths on American society, if you were about to conclude that politicians and the news media have been paying a disproportionate amount of attention to cocaine and heroin-related toxicity, you would be right.

AIDS

There is a great deal of concern about the spread of acquired immunodeficiency syndrome (**AIDS**) among drug abusers. The human immunodeficiency virus (**HIV**) is a blood-borne agent capable of spreading the disease among addicts who share needles. The insidious thing about HIV is that a person can be infected for a year or two with no overt symptoms and during that time spread the disease to others. Both AIDS and hepatitis B, another blood-borne disease, have been responsible for hundreds of deaths among intravenous drug abusers. In large cities around the world, the proportion of intravenous drug users who test positive for HIV might be as high as 40 to 50 percent.[5] Because HIV also can be transmitted sexually, the public at large is at some risk of contracting HIV from intravenous drug users, especially considering that many female drug users earn money through prostitution.

It is important to point out that this type of drug-associated toxicity is not due to the action of the drug itself but is incidental to the sharing of needles, no matter which drug is injected or whether the injection is intravenous or intramuscular. A study of intravenous drug users in Baltimore found that about half the syringes and needles they used were obtained from street

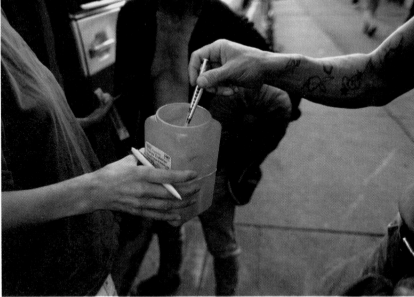

Collecting needles for an exchange program in an effort to prevent the spread of HIV among needle-using addicts.

dealers and that only about 30 percent came directly from a pharmacy. These needles were commonly used several times.[6] In a sense, the spread through needle sharing is due less to the drug addiction itself than to laws designed to prevent addiction—in particular, the laws restricting the sale of hypodermic equipment. Failing to use clean needles is the most significant risk factor leading to new HIV infections in cities with high infection rates.[7] Although the U.S. government does not support needle exchange programs, the number of such programs has grown rapidly. These programs vary from city to city in terms of how they are funded, where the needle exchanges take place, and other operating rules. Typically the programs require a one-for-one exchange of a used needle for a clean one, thus allowing for collection and proper disposal of potentially infected needles. In some communities the programs operate in violation of state laws or local ordinances, whereas in other communities specific legal exemptions have been passed for needle exchange programs. In many European countries and in Australia, needle exchange programs are an important component of government AIDS prevention programs. The primary concern in the United States is that providing clean needles appears to condone intravenous drug use or that new users would more readily begin intravenous drug use if the fear of AIDS were lessened. Small-scale studies conducted by needle exchange programs in some cities have not found any evidence for increased numbers of new users or of a decrease in the average age of users.

AIDS: acquired immunodeficiency syndrome.

HIV: human immunodeficiency virus.

Targeting Prevention

HIVS and AIDS

The spread of the human immunodeficiency virus (HIV) among drug users is associated primarily with the sharing of the needles used for injecting heroin and other drugs. Evidence from several studies indicates that HIV transmission can be reduced if clean syringes and needles are made readily available to injecting drug users. Do you know whether a user of illicit drugs in your community can get access to clean syringes and needles?

You might start learning about this by interviewing a local pharmacist to see what the rules are for purchasing these items, as well as how expensive they are. It will also be interesting to see how the pharmacist reacts to your questions about this topic. How do you react to the idea of possibly being looked at as a user of illegal drugs? You might want to take this book along to show that you do have an academic reason for asking!

Once you find out what the situation is with direct purchasing, see if you can find out if there is a needle exchange program in your community. This will be a little harder, but you can start by looking up "public health" in the phone book and calling that office.

Armed with those pieces of information, are there steps your community could take to make clean needles more readily available to users of illicit drugs? Do you believe that such programs might actually encourage or condone drug use? Would the program help prevent the spread of HIV in your community?

DRUG ADDICTION: PROBLEMS OF DEFINITION

In the early 1900s, the second major concern expressed by those urging passage of drug controls was for the victims of drug addiction. Those who unknowingly or carelessly took habit-forming drugs risked becoming enslaved by them. The unscrupulous sellers of these drugs were thus assured a steady market, whereas the addicts were forced to continue to endanger their own health and supposedly to undermine their own mental and moral strength. That is one major reason that the habit-forming drugs, such as cocaine and the opiates, were singled out for special taxation and recordkeeping in 1914 (see Chapter 5).

Chapter 3 deals in some detail with the concept of addiction, which has been defined in many ways over the years. As we will see, addiction to alcohol or another drug involves complex interactions among the individual, the substance, and the social environment. Therefore, questions such as "Is marijuana an addicting drug?" are too simple. Some people have developed what most professionals would agree is an addiction to marijuana, but most marijuana users have not. For most psychoactive drugs, the most accurate answer to the question of whether that drug "is addictive" is that addiction is possible. It does seem clear that some kinds of drug use are more likely to lead to addiction than are other kinds: intravenous use of heroin is more likely to become addicting than is marijuana smoking or LSD use. Thus, we might legitimately ask ourselves which drugs, or which methods of using those drugs, pose the greatest risk for addiction. One major study[8] reviewed 350 published articles to come up with relative ratings, then had the preliminary tables reviewed by a panel of psychopharmacologists for suggested changes. Based on that report, we can classify psychoactive drugs into seven categories of "dependence potential," from very high to very low (Table 2.3). Please remember, however, that such rankings ignore some very important biological, psychological, and social factors, which are also major contributors to the development of addiction (see Chapter 3).

CRIME AND VIOLENCE: DOES DRUG USE CAUSE CRIME?

It might seem obvious to a reader of today's newspapers or to a viewer of today's television that drugs and crime are linked. There are

TABLE 2.3		
Dependence Potential of Psychoactive Drugs		
Very high:	Heroin (IV)	
	Crack cocaine	
High:	Morphine	
	Opium (smoked)	
Moderate/high:	Cocaine powder	
	Tobacco cigarettes	
	PCP (smoked)	
Moderate:	Diazepam (Valium)	
	Alcohol	
	Amphetamines (oral)	
Moderate/low:	Caffeine	
	MDMA (Ecstasy)	
	Marijuana	
Low:	Ketamine (see Chapter 16)	
Very low:	LSD	
	Mescaline	
	Psilocybin	

LSD, lysergic acid diethylamide; MDMA, methylenedioxy methamphetamine

frequent reports of killings attributed to warring gangs of drug dealers. Our prisons house a large population of people convicted for drug-related crimes, and there have been several reports that a large fraction of arrestees for nondrug felonies have positive results from urine tests for illicit substances.

The belief that there is a causal relationship between many forms of drug use and criminality probably forms the basis for many of our laws concerning drug use and drug users. The relationship between crime and illegal drug use is complex, and only recently have data-based statements become possible. Facts are necessary because political actions are taken, and laws are enacted, on the basis of what we believe to be true.

The basis for concern was the belief that drug use *causes* crime. The fact that drug addicts engage in robberies or that car thieves are likely to also use illicit drugs does not say anything about causality. Both criminal activity and drug use could well be caused by other factors, producing both types of deviant behavior in the same individuals. There are several senses in which it might be said that drugs cause crime, but the most frightening possibility is that drug use somehow *changes the individual's personality in a lasting way,* making him or her into a "criminal type." For example, during the 1924 debate that led to a complete prohibition against heroin sales in the United States, a testifying physician asserted, regarding users, that heroin "dethrones their moral responsibility." Another physician testified that some types of individuals will have their mental equipment "permanently injured by the use of heroin, and those are the ones who will go out and commit crimes."[9] Similar beliefs are reflected in the introductory message in the 1937 film *Reefer Madness,* which referred to marijuana as "The Real Public Enemy Number One!" and described its "soul-destroying" effects as follows:

> emotional disturbances, the total inability to direct thought, the loss of all power to resist physical emotions, leading finally to acts of shocking violence . . . ending often in incurable insanity.

Such verbal excesses seem quaint and comical these days, but the underlying belief that drug use changes people into criminals still can be detected in much current political rhetoric. You should remember from Chapter 1 that longitudinal research on children and adolescents has led to the conclusion that indicators of criminal or antisocial behavior usually occur before the first use of an illicit drug. Several studies have concluded that criminal activity typically precedes drug use and "suggests that the relationship between drugs and crime is developmental rather than causal."[10]

A second sense in which drug use might *cause* criminal behavior is when the person is *under the influence* of the drug. Do the acute effects of a drug make a person *temporarily* more likely to engage in criminal behavior? There is little good evidence for this with most illicit substances. In most individuals, marijuana produces a state more akin to lethargy than to crazed violence (see Chapter 17), and heroin tends to make its users more passive and perhaps sexually impotent (see Chapter 15). Stimulants such as amphetamine and cocaine can make people paranoid and "jumpy," and this can indeed contribute to violent behavior in some cases (see Chapter 7). The hallucinogen PCP causes disorientation and blocks pain, so that users are sometimes hard to restrain (see Chapter 16). This has led to a considerable amount of folklore about the dangerousness of PCP users, although actual documented cases of excessive violence are either rare or nonexistent.

If there is some question as to whether the direct influence of illicit drugs produces a person more likely to engage in criminal or violent behavior, there has been less doubt about one commonly used substance: alcohol. A large number of studies indicate that alcohol is clearly linked with violent crime. In many assaults and sexual assaults, alcohol is present in both assailant and victim. You might not know that most homicides are among people who know each other—and alcohol use is associated with over three-fifths of all murders. Of all reported assaults, 40 percent involve alcohol, as do one-third of forcible rape and child-molestation cases.[11] A study of jail inmates found that almost half of those committing violent crimes reported being under the influence of alcohol or a combination of alcohol and other drugs at the time of the offense, whereas fewer than 10 percent reported being under the influence of only drugs other than alcohol.[12] However, the relationship between drinking and violence is complex, and it has recently been argued that alcohol might have been overestimated as a direct cause of violence.[13]

There is a third sense in which drug use may be said to cause crime, and that refers to *crimes carried out for the purpose of obtaining money* to purchase illicit drugs. It has long been noted that heroin addicts constitute a larger proportion of those arrested for robbery than of the general population. A survey of almost 400,000 jail inmates found that almost one-third of all

burglaries and robberies were committed to obtain money for drugs, as was almost one-fourth of all fraud. It is interesting that only about one-fifth of all drug-trafficking offenses were reported to be for the purpose of obtaining money to buy drugs.[14]

Although most addicts are criminals first and addicts second, a 1976 survey of heroin addicts found that most reported an increase in the amount of crime they committed, and many started committing new types of crime, after they became addicts. A 1981 report suggests just how much criminal activity increases during periods of addiction. When addicts were not dependent on heroin, their crime rate was 84 percent lower than when they were regularly using the drug.[15] Reducing heroin addiction will certainly result in lower crime rates.

Every year since 1987, the U.S. Justice Department has collected data on drug use from people arrested and booked into jails for serious crimes. The interviewers try not to sample too many people who are arrested for drug sale or possession, so that usually fewer than 20 percent of those in the study have been arrested on drug charges. All interviews and urine tests are anonymous; about 90 percent of arrestees who are asked agree to an interview, and about 80 percent of those agree to provide urine specimens. In 1999, in 34 sites around the country, a median figure of 64 percent of the adult male arrestees tested positive for the presence of at least one of the five drugs of interest (cocaine, marijuana, methamphetamine, opiates, and PCP). Among males, marijuana was the drug most frequently detected, followed by cocaine. Among female arrestees, 67 percent tested positive for at least one drug, with cocaine the most prevalent and marijuana second.[16] This level of drug use among those arrested for nondrug crimes is quite high; how can we account for it? First, those who adopt a deviant lifestyle might engage in both crime and drug use. Second, because most of these 1999 arrests were for crimes in which profit was the motive, the arrestees might have been burglarizing a house or stealing a car to get money to purchase drugs.

It would be remiss not to point out that the commission of crimes to obtain money for expensive illicit drugs is due, not primarily to a pharmacological effect of the drug, but to the artificially high cost of the drugs, which results from drug controls and enforcement. Both heroin and cocaine are inexpensive substances when obtained legally from a licensed manufacturer, and it has been estimated many times that if heroin were freely available it would cost no

more to be a regular heroin user than to be a regular drinker of alcohol. It is the black-market cost of these substances that makes the use of cocaine or heroin consume so much money.

There is a fourth and final sense in which drug use causes crime, and that is that *illicit drug use is a crime*. At first that may seem trivial, but there are two senses in which it is not. First, we are now making more than 1 million arrests for drug-law violations each year, and more than half of all federal prisoners are convicted on drug charges.[17] Thus, drug-law violations are one of the major types of crime in the United

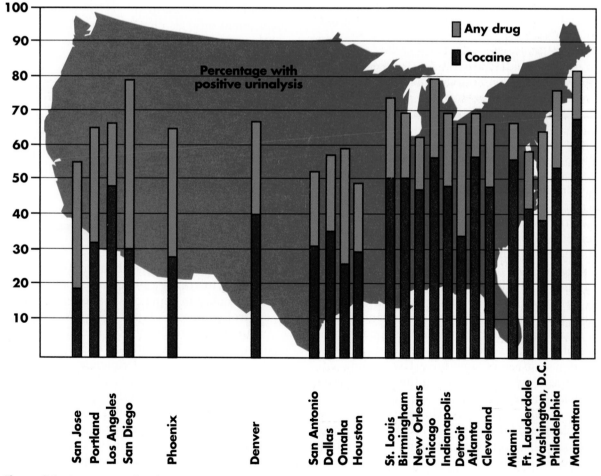

Figure 2.1 Percentage of male arrestees testing positive for drug use, January through December 1995.

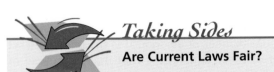

Taking Sides

Are Current Laws Fair?

There are things that people do all the time that are potentially dangerous for themselves and potentially messy and expensive for others. Driving faster than the speed limit, driving without a seat belt, and riding a motorcycle without a helmet are examples, some of which may not be illegal where you live. In what ways are these behaviors similar to a person "snorting" cocaine or injecting heroin into his or her veins? In what ways are they different? Do you feel that the laws as they currently exist in your area are appropriate and fair in dealing with these behaviors? If it were up to you, would you outlaw some things that are now legal, legalize some things that are now controlled, or some of each?

For more on this topic, log on to www.dushkin.com/online for current news and links to other popular and informative sites, as well as time-saving web search strategies and study tools.

States. Second, it is likely that the relationship between drug use and other forms of deviant behavior is strengthened by the fact that drug use is a crime. A person willing to commit one type of crime might be more willing than the average person to commit another type of crime. Some of the people who are actively trying to impress others by living dangerously and committing criminal acts might be drawn to illicit drug use as an obvious way to demonstrate their alienation from society. To better understand this relationship, imagine what might happen if the use of marijuana were legalized. Presumably, a greater number of otherwise law-abiding citizens might try using the drug, thus reducing the correlation between marijuana use and other forms of criminal activity. The concern over possibly increased drug use is, of course, one major argument in favor of maintaining legal controls on the illicit drugs.

WHY WE TRY TO REGULATE DRUGS

We can see that there are reasonable concerns about the potential toxicity and habit-forming nature of some drugs and even the criminality of some drug users. That does not mean that our current set of laws represents a rationally devised plan to counteract the most realistic of these concerns in the most effective manner. In point of fact, most legislation is passed in an atmosphere of emotionality, in response to a specific set of concerns. Often the problems have been there for a long time, but public attention and concern have been recently aroused and Congress must respond. Sometimes members of Congress or government officials play a major role in calling public attention to the problem for which they offer the solution: a new law, more restrictions, and a bigger budget for some agency. This is what is known in political circles as "starting a prairie fire." As we will see in Chapter 4, often the prairie fires include a lot of emotion-arousing rhetoric that borders on the irrational, and sometimes the results of the prairie fire and the ensuing legislation are unexpected and undesirable.

SUMMARY

- American society has changed from being one that tolerated a wide variety of individual drug use to being one that attempts strict control over some types of drugs. This has occurred in response to social concerns about drug toxicity, addiction potential, and drug-related crime and violence.

- *Toxicity* can refer either to physiological poisoning or to dangerous disruption of behavior. Also, we can distinguish acute toxicity, resulting from the presence of too much of a drug, from chronic toxicity, which results from long-term exposure to a drug.

- *Addiction* means different things to different people in different contexts. Although addiction does not depend solely on the drug itself, the use of some drugs is more likely to result in addiction than is the use of other drugs.
- The idea that narcotic drugs or marijuana can produce violent criminality in their users is an old and largely discredited idea. Narcotic addicts seem to engage in crimes mainly to obtain money, not because they are made more criminal by the drugs they take. One drug that is widely accepted as contributing to crimes and violence is alcohol.
- We can see that the laws that have been developed to control drug use have a legitimate social purpose, which is to protect the society from the dangers caused by some types of drug use. Whether these dangers have always been viewed rationally, and whether the laws have had their intended results, can be better judged after we have learned more about the drugs and the history of their regulation.

REVIEW QUESTIONS

1. The French term *laissez-faire* is used to describe what type of relationship between a government and its people?
2. What three major concerns about drugs led to the initial passage of laws controlling their availability?
3. Long-term, heavy drinking can lead to permanent impairment of memory. What type of toxicity is this (acute or chronic; physiological or behavioral)?
4. What two kinds of data are recorded by the DAWN system?
5. What drug other than alcohol is mentioned most often in both parts of the DAWN system?
6. Why has AIDS been of particular concern for users of illicit drugs?

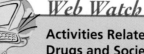

Web Watch

Activities Related to Drugs and Society

What are Your Experiences with Substance Abuse?

What are some experiences others have had with substance abuse? What wisdom can they share? How do your opinions compare with those of others? To answer these questions, join one of the discussion forums at www.wnet.org/cgi-bin/nf/closetohome/a/1. This site offers a variety of topics to choose from. If the forum is not open at the time you log on, you may submit a query or comment or view previous discussions.

Addiction's Effects in Your Society

Drugs and their effects play an integral role in today's society. Addiction may seem to affect only a single person or an immediate family, but the crimes related to drug abuse affect society as a whole. Take the quiz "Test Your Knowledge on Drugs and Society" on www.hazelden.org/quiz.dbm?ID=18 to discover statistics and other facts.

Can You Stand Your Ground?

Teens are often victims of peer pressure when it comes to drug use, but do we ever really grow up enough to be free from the influence of those around us? You may feel that, when you make a decision, you will remain steadfast in your opinion regardless of a trying situation. Take the quiz "Can You Stand Your Ground?" on www.antibully.org.uk/canyou.htm to discover if you can really stand up to peer pressure when you make decisions about drugs.

Testimonials About Substance Abuse

Read the real-life testimonies posted on www.antibully.org.uk/life.htm and www.antibully.org.uk/myfriend.htm. The first web page has comments and stories from young people who have had dangerous experiences with substance abuse. The second page is the story of one young person who decided to end his addiction when a friend with the same problem nearly died.

7. What drugs and methods of using them are considered to have very high dependence potential?

8. What is the apparent dependence potential of hallucinogenic drugs, such as LSD and mescaline?

9. What are four ways in which drug use might theoretically cause crime?

10. About how many arrests are made each year in the United States for violations of drug laws?

REFERENCES

1. Dennis RJ: The economics of legalizing drugs, *The Atlantic* Nov 1990.

2. *Year-end 1999 emergency department data from the Drug Abuse Warning Network.* Rockville, MD: SAMHSA, Office of Applied Studies, 2000.

3. *Drug Abuse Warning Network annual medical examiner data 1998.* Rockville, MD: SAMHSA, Office of Applied Studies, 2000.

4. Bozarth MA, Wise RA: Toxicity associated with long-term intravenous heroin and cocaine self-administration in the rat, *Journal of the American Medical Association* 254:81–83, 1985.

5. Des Jarlais DC and others: Maintaining a low HIV seroprevalence in populations of injecting drug users. *Journal of the American Medical Association* 274:1226–1231, 1995.

6. Gleghorn A and others: Acquisition and use of needles and syringes by injecting drug users in Baltimore, Maryland, *JAIDS* 10:97–103, 1995.

7. Friedman SR and others: Risk factors for human immunodeficiency virus seroconversion among out-of-treatment drug injectors in high and low seroprevalence cities, *American Journal of Epidemiology* 142:864–874, 1995.

8. Gable RS: Toward a comparative overview of dependence potential and acute toxicity of psychoactive substances used nonmedically, *American Journal of Drug and Alcohol Abuse* 19:263–281, 1993.

9. Prohibiting the importation of opium for the manufacture of heroin, Hearing before the Committee on Ways and Means, House of Representatives, *Congressional Record,* Apr 3, 1924.

10. Bureau of Justice Statistics: *Drugs, crime, and the justice system.* Washington, DC: U.S. Department of Justice, 1992.

11. *Alcohol and health: Fifth special report to the US Congress,* DHHS Pub No (ADM) 84–1291, Washington, DC: U.S. Government Printing Office, 1984.

12. *Drugs and Crime Data Center: Fact sheet: Drug data summary,* Bureau of Justice Statistics, Nov 1991, U.S. Department of Justice.

13. *Alcohol and health: Seventh special report to the US Congress,* DHHS Publication No. (ADM) 90–1656, Washington, DC: U.S. Government Printing Office, 1990.

14. Rouse BA (editor): *Substance abuse and mental health statistics sourcebook,* DHHS Publication No. (SMA) 95-3064, Washington, DC: Superintendent of Documents, U.S. Government Printing Office, 1995.

15. Ball JC and others: cited in Study stresses link between heroin dependence and incidence of crime, *New York Times* p 22, Mar 22, 1981.

16. *ADAM 1999 annual report on drug use among adult and juvenile arrestees.* U.S. Department of Justice, National Institute of Justice, 2000.

17. The White House Office of National Drug Control Policy: *National drug control strategy.* Washington, DC: 1994.

Chapter 3

Addictions: Theory and Treatment

KEY TERMS

tolerance

withdrawal syndrome

physical dependence

psychological dependence

reinforcement

catheters

Alcoholics Anonymous

biopsychosocial

DSM-IV

stages of change

abstinence

controlled drinking

detoxification

Online Learning Center Resources

www.mhhe.com/ray

Log on to our Online Learning Center (OLC) for access to these additional resources.

- Chapter key terms and definitions
- Learning objectives
- Additional behavior change objectives
- Student interactive questions and answer sites
- Self-scoring chapter quiz

The OLC also offers web links for study and exploration of health topics. Here are some examples of what you'll find:

www.casacolumbia.org/

The National Center on Addiction and Substance Abuse at Columbia University's website offers publications, a news-room, research and program information, resources, and links. Check out the FAQ page or subscribe to e-mail alerts.

www.ncadd.org/index.html

The National Council on Alcoholism and Drug Dependence, Inc., hosts a website with information on education, topics for parents and youth, campaigns for prevention, awareness activities, advocacy, treatment, and facts.

www.drugfreeamerica.org/

The Partnership for a Drug Free America home page offers information for parents and teens, the latest news, sources of help, updated facts, and statistics. You can also sign up to receive a newsletter.

Drugs in the Media

Hollywood Knows, and Shows, Hard Truth About Drugs

Hollywood stars and the talented creators in their orbit are hardly immune to the effects of substance abuse and addiction. The list of people who have battled drug, drink,

Drugs in the Media Continued. . .

and smoking-related problems includes some of the most famous names in show business: Robert Downey, Jr.; Drew Barrymore; Matthew Perry; Melanie Griffith; and others.

Many actors, directors, producers, and writers have recognized the media's responsibility to make others aware of how substance abuse destroys families, careers, health, and lives, and numerous luminaries attend the annual PRISM Awards, which honor creative achievement in accurate depictions of drug, alcohol, and tobacco use and addiction. The awards spotlight films, TV shows, comic books, community service efforts, and individual volunteerism, as well as special honors. They are presented jointly by the Entertainment Industries Council, the National Institute on Drug Abuse, and the Robert Wood Johnson Foundation, the nation's largest philanthropic organization dedicated exclusively to health and health care.

For decades Hollywood actors' personal nightmares with drugs have been kept under wraps by an industry mentality that tried to protect star and box-office receipts from scandal. And, oftentimes on screen, smoking, alcohol, and drugs have been portrayed as glamorous, fun, or cool. Many stars now realize they can use the power of their celebrity to help millions in their struggles against drugs. By giving an accurate depiction of the dangers of these substances, they believe they can prevent many others from taking that first step down a precarious path. To see recent PRISM Award honorees and video clips, go to www.prismawards.com.

Companion efforts to assist the creative community and complement the PRISM Awards include the publication of special drug abuse, alcohol, and tobacco volumes of "Spotlight on Depiction of Health and Social Issues," a resource encyclopedia; a technical assistance program called "First Draft"; and "PRISM Generation Next," a program to take the responsive depiction process to students enrolled in television and film schools.

Do you think the film industry can make a big impact on children and the general public by showing them the negative effects of drugs? Would hearing that a movie or TV show had received a PRISM award make you more interested in viewing it?

Thirty years ago, the term *addict* had a pretty narrow meaning for most people: someone who used heroin several times daily and who would suffer terrible withdrawal symptoms if he or she were late getting a "fix." Now it seems that addiction is everywhere: not only are alcoholics and cigarette smokers referred to as addicts, but we also hear about sex addicts, food addicts, gambling addicts, addictive relationships, and even addictive forms of politics.[1] What do we mean by addiction, and how have models of addiction become important for describing such a wide variety of human conduct?

DRUG ADDICTION

We begin by attempting to define drug addiction, both because this book is primarily about drugs and because that's where current concepts of addiction in general were formed. A leading addiction researcher has offered the following definition of drug addiction: "a behavioral

Exploring Your Spirituality

Hope Is the Way Out of Addiction

The subject of addiction has touched actor Martin Sheen more deeply than a mere movie role, emotionally and spiritually. He has seen firsthand the psychic pain and loss of independence that occur when someone's life deteriorates into looking for the next fix. Sheen's commitment to helping his son Charlie publicly battle substance-abuse problems has inspired many. Sheen — himself a recovering alcoholic — has also made appearances on behalf of supporting and improving the drug court system. At the March 2000 PRISM Awards, Sheen had the following compassionate words to offer to those desperately in need of perspective in their ordeals with substance abuse:

> Nearly everyone I've ever met or heard of who is involved in substance abuse is seeking some kind of transcendent experience because the pain of their lives is so very great. This goes across all the lines —

rich or poor, black or white, old or young, male or female. It appears that the necessity to be human brings with it such horrible pain to many of us that a drug or alcohol or some substance seems to be the only way we can deal with it.

It is in a way a spiritual journey. It's an effort to find God, the One or the Other, the higher power, however one thinks of the spiritual being. So it's important to remember that this is at the basis, the very start of addiction. And that's a very hopeful sign, because that will lead them out of the darkness and into the light. I want to offer that as an encouragement in your darkest hour when you're going with someone through this horrible, horrible pain and despair.

What do you think of the idea of addiction as a spiritual sickness or dysfunction?

---

pattern of drug use, characterized by overwhelming involvement with the use of a drug (compulsive use), the securing of its supply, and a high tendency to relapse after withdrawal."[2]

It is important to distinguish the defining component of addictive drug use (overwhelming involvement) from the proposed causes of that behavior. As we proceed, we will find that some people believe addiction to be a function of the drugs themselves and how they affect the user, whereas others believe the key to addiction lies in the individual's physiology and how the drug influences biological processes. Some believe that addiction grows out of early positive experiences with a drug, others believe that addiction is found in the personality of the user, and others find the key to addiction in social structures, such as the family, relationships with significant others, and even society itself. Finally, there are those for whom addiction reflects spiritual dysfunction: a mistaken seeking for understanding, peace, or bliss through drugs. There is value in

understanding each of these perspectives. However, the definition of addiction should not depend on its proposed causes but, rather, should be in terms of the behavior that causes us to call it addiction. Once the behavior is defined, we can explore possible causes of that behavior.

Three Basic Processes

There are three basic processes related to addiction that have been important in the history of drug addiction research. Defining these three concepts will help focus our discussion of drug addiction and will be useful in discussing each drug in more detail.

Tolerance

Tolerance refers to a phenomenon seen with many drugs, in which repeated exposure to the same dose of the drug results in a lesser effect. There are many ways this diminished effect can occur, and some examples are given in Chapter 7.

r now, it is enough for us to think of the body as developing ways to compensate for the chemical imbalance caused by introducing a drug into the system. As the individual experiences less and less of the desired effect, it is often possible to overcome the tolerance by increasing the dose of the drug. Some regular drug users might eventually build up to taking much more of the drug than it would take to kill a nontolerant individual. Tolerance has been proposed as a key component in some definitions of addiction or dependence.

Physical Dependence

Physical dependence is defined by the occurrence of a **withdrawal syndrome.** Suppose a person has begun to take a drug and a tolerance has developed. The person increases the amount of drug taken and continues to take these higher doses so regularly that the body is continuously exposed to the drug for days or weeks. With some drugs, when the person stops taking the drug abruptly, a set of symptoms begins to appear as the drug level in the system drops. For example, as the level of heroin drops in a heroin addict, that person's nose might run and he or she might begin to experience chills and fever, diarrhea, and other symptoms. When we have a drug that produces a consistent set of these symptoms in different individuals, we refer to the collection of symptoms as a withdrawal syndrome. These withdrawal syndromes vary from one class of drugs to another. Our model for why withdrawal symptoms appear is that the drug initially disrupts the body's normal physiological balances. These imbalances are detected by the nervous system, and over a period of repeated drug use the body's normal regulatory mechanisms compensate for the presence of the drug. When the drug is suddenly removed, these compensating mechanisms produce an imbalance. You can see that tolerance typically precedes physical dependence. To continue with the heroin example, when it is first used it slows intestinal movement and produces constipation.

After several days of constant heroin use, other mechanisms in the body counteract this effect and get the intestines moving again (tolerance). If the heroin use is suddenly stopped, the compensating mechanisms produce too much intestinal motility. Diarrhea is one of the most reliable and dramatic heroin withdrawal symptoms.

Because of the presumed involvement of these compensating mechanisms, the presence of a withdrawal syndrome is said to reflect **physical** (or physiological) **dependence** on the drug. In other words, the individual has come to depend on the presence of some amount of that drug to function normally; removing the drug leads to an imbalance, which is slowly corrected over a period of a few days.

Psychological Dependence

Psychological dependence (also called *behavioral dependence*) can be defined in terms of observable behavior. It is indicated by the frequency of using a drug or by the amount of time or effort an individual spends in drug-seeking behavior. Often it is accompanied by reports of *craving* the drug or its effects. A major contribution of behavioral psychology has been to point out the scientific value of the concept of **reinforcement** for understanding psychological dependence.

The term *reinforcement* is used in psychology to describe a process: a behavioral act is followed by a consequence, resulting in an increased tendency to repeat that behavioral act. The consequence may be described as pleasurable or as a "reward" in some cases (e.g., providing a tasty piece of food to someone who has not eaten for a while). In other cases, the consequence may be described in terms of escape from pain or discomfort. The behavior itself is said to be strengthened, or *reinforced,* by its consequences. The administration of certain drugs can reinforce the behaviors that led to the drug's administration. Laboratory rats and monkeys have been trained to press levers when the only consequence of lever pressing is a small intravenous injection of heroin, cocaine, or another drug. Because some drugs but not others are capable of serving this function, it is possible to refer to some drugs as having "reinforcing properties" and to note that there is a general correlation between those drugs and the ones to which people often develop psychological dependence.

Changing Views of Drug Addiction

Until the twentieth century, the most common view of alcoholism or dependence on opiates was probably that the addicted individuals were weak-willed, lazy, or immoral. Then medical and scientific studies began to be made of alcoholics, and later of narcotic addicts. It seemed as if something more powerful than mere self-indulgence was at work, and the predominant view began to be that addiction is a drug-induced illness.

Early Medical Models

If heroin addiction is induced by heroin, or alcoholism by alcohol, then why do some people become addicts and others not? An early guess was simply that some people, for whatever reasons, were exposed to large amounts of the substance for a long time. This could happen through medical treatment or self-indulgence. The most obvious changes resulting from long exposure to large doses are the withdrawal symptoms that occur when the drug is stopped. Both alcohol and the narcotics can produce rather dramatic withdrawal syndromes. Thus, addiction came to be defined by the presence of physical dependence (a withdrawal syndrome), and enlightened medically oriented researchers went looking for treatments based on reducing or eliminating withdrawal symptoms. According to the most narrow interpretation of this model, the medical addiction itself was cured when the person had successfully completed withdrawal and the symptoms disappeared, although, of course, there was concern that people often reacquired the addiction.

Pharmacologists and medical authorities continued into the 1970s to define "true" addiction as occurring only when physical dependence was seen. Based on this view, public policy decisions, medical treatment, and individual drug-use decisions could be influenced by the question "Is this an addicting drug?" If some drugs produce addiction but others do not, then legal restrictions on addicting drugs, care in the medical use of those drugs, and education in avoiding the recreational use of addicting drugs are appropriate. The determination of whether a drug is or is not "addicting" was therefore crucial.

It became a public issue in the 1960s that some drugs, particularly marijuana and amphetamine, were not considered to have well-defined, dramatic, physical withdrawal syndromes. The growing group of interested scientists began to refer to drugs such as marijuana, amphetamines, and cocaine as "merely" producing psychological dependence, whereas heroin produced a "true" addiction, which includes physical dependence. The idea seemed to be that psychological dependence was "all in the head," whereas with physical dependence actual bodily processes were involved, subject to physiological and biochemical analysis and possibly to improved medical treatments for addiction. This was the view held by most drug-abuse experts in the 1960s.

tolerance: reduced effect of a drug after repeated use.

withdrawal syndrome: a consistent set of symptoms that appears after discontinuing use of a drug.

physical dependence: drug dependence defined by the presence of a withdrawal syndrome, implying that the body has become adapted to the drug's presence.

Positive Reinforcement Model

In the 1960s a remarkable series of experiments began to appear in the scientific literature—experiments in which laboratory monkeys and rats were given intravenous **catheters** connected to motorized syringes and controlling equipment so that pressing a lever would produce a single brief injection of morphine, a narcotic very similar to heroin. In the initial experiments, monkeys were exposed for several days to large doses of morphine, allowed to experience the initial stages of withdrawal, and then connected to the apparatus to see if they would learn to press the lever, thereby avoiding the withdrawal symptoms. As you can see, these experiments were based on the predominant view of addiction as being driven by physical dependence. The monkeys did learn to press the levers. Later experiments sought to determine whether monkeys would make themselves "addicted," so the initial phase of drug exposure was dropped. Indeed, the monkeys began to press the lever to give themselves morphine, and, if doses were large enough and constant access was allowed, the monkeys would eventually display withdrawal symptoms when no longer allowed access to morphine. Thus, the monkeys had made "true" drug addicts of themselves.

This research next began to draw on the experience gained from many years of research with animals pressing levers to obtain food. It is not necessary to provide food for every lever press, because, once animals have learned to press the lever, they will continue if food is given for every other press, then for every third press, then every fifth press, every tenth, and so on. Some scientists began to ask how hard monkeys or rats would "work" to obtain their drug injections and how that compared with how hard they would work for food. With appropriate scheduling and training, it was possible to show that monkeys would press the lever hundreds of times for each drug injection. When food had been used in such experiments, the amount of food delivered each time was found to be important. A rat or monkey might press only 10 times for a small amount of food but be willing to press 30 times for a greater amount. Therefore, the drug-addiction researchers began to vary the amount of morphine given with each delivery, eventually finding that a great deal of lever pressing could be maintained with fairly small injections of drug. As these scientists began to publish their results and as more experiments like this were done, they pointed out some interesting facts. First, monkeys would begin pressing and maintain pressing without first being made physically dependent. Second, monkeys who had given themselves only fairly small doses and who had never experienced withdrawal symptoms could be trained to work very hard for their morphine. In fact, a history of physical dependence and withdrawal didn't seem to have much influence on response rates in the long run. Clearly, the small drug injections themselves were working as "positive reinforcers" of the lever-pressing behavior, just as food can be a positive reinforcer to a hungry rat or monkey. Thus, the idea spread that drugs can act as reinforcers of behavior and that this might be the basis of what had been called psychological dependence.[3] Drugs such as amphetamines and cocaine could easily be used as reinforcers in these experiments, and they were known to produce strong psychological dependence in humans.

Which Is More Important, Physical Dependence or Psychological Dependence?

The animal research that led to the positive reinforcement model implies that psychological dependence is more important than the development of physical dependence in narcotic addiction, and this has led people to examine the lives of heroin addicts from a different perspective. Stories were told of addicts who occasionally stopped taking heroin, voluntarily going through withdrawal so as to reduce their tolerance level and get back to the lower doses of drug they could more easily afford. When we examine the total daily heroin intake of many addicts, we see that they do not need a large amount and that the agonies of withdrawal they experience are probably more like a prolonged case of intestinal flu. We have known for a long time that heroin addicts who have already gone through withdrawal in treatment programs or in jail have a high probability of returning to active heroin use. In other words, if all we had to worry about was addicts' avoiding withdrawal symptoms, the problem would be much smaller than it actually is.

Psychological dependence, based on *reinforcement*, is increasingly accepted as the real driving force behind drug addiction, and tolerance and physical dependence are now seen as related phenomena that sometimes occur but probably are not critical to the development of addictive patterns of drug-using behavior.

Some scientists avoid using the term *addiction* altogether, because it has meant different things to different people and because the term also carries considerable emotional overtones. Instead, they prefer to talk about tolerance, physical dependence (withdrawal), and psychological dependence, because these terms are more clearly defined and less subject to misinterpretation. In this text, we will be less formal and will use the term *addiction*. When we do so, our intent is to refer to overwhelming involvement with a drug, very close to the definition of psychological dependence.

THE BROAD VIEWS OF ADDICTION

If we define drug addiction not in terms of withdrawal but in more behavioral or psychological terms, as an overwhelming involvement with getting and using the drug, then might this model also be used to describe other kinds of behavior? What about a man who visits prostitutes several times a day, someone who eats large amounts of food throughout the day, or someone who places bets on every football and basketball game, every horse race or automobile race, and who spends hours each day planning these bets and finding money to bet again? Shouldn't these also be considered addictions? Do the experiences of overeating, gambling, sex, and drugs have something in common—a common change in physiology or brain chemistry or a common personality trait that leads to any or many of these addictions? Are all of these filling an unmet social or spiritual need? More and more, addiction researchers are looking for these common threads and discussing "the addictions" as a varied set of behavioral manifestations of a common dependence process or disorder.

Is Addiction Caused by the Substance?

Especially with chemical dependence, many people speak as though the substance itself is the cause of the addiction. Certainly some drugs are more likely than others to result in addiction. For example, it is widely believed that heroin and crack cocaine are both extremely addicting, with most users becoming slaves to the habit. In contrast, most users of marijuana report occasional use and little difficulty in deciding when to use it and when not to.

---

psychological dependence: behavioral dependence; indicated by high rate of drug use, craving for the drug, and a tendency to relapse after stopping use.

catheters: (*cath* **a ters**) plastic or other tubing implanted into the body.

reinforcement: a procedure in which a behavioral event is followed by a consequent event such that the behavior is then more likely to be repeated. The behavior of taking a drug may be reinforced by the effect of the drug.

Self-administration studies with animals support this view: rats and monkeys readily learn to self-inject either heroin or cocaine, but no one has yet demonstrated reliable self-administration of marijuana in animal models. Can we then describe some drugs as "addicting," whereas others are not? We have already seen that this perspective was common in an earlier era, and it played a major role in the establishment of laws intended to limit access to those addicting drugs. Certainly alcohol prohibition in the 1920s was based on the view that alcohol itself was the main culprit in many of society's problems.

The problem is that, although some drugs are more likely than others to result in addiction, there is no clear distinction between substances that are addicting and those that are not. What about alcohol, perhaps the most common cause of serious chemical dependence? Most of its users avoid dependence, yet for perhaps one-tenth of drinkers alcohol use becomes an overwhelming habit. Contrary to popular opinion, many users of either heroin or crack cocaine use the drug only a few times a week or less, and not every user becomes overwhelmingly involved. And, contrary to the beliefs of some, there are quite a few marijuana users who become dependent, try to stop and cannot, and voluntarily seek treatment for their addiction. Any of these drugs can be "addicting" for some people, and some people can use any of them without becoming addicted. Thus, the drug itself cannot be the entire cause of addiction.

When we extend the concept of addiction to other activities, such as gambling, sex, or overeating, it seems harder to place the entire blame on the activity, again because many people do not exhibit addictive patterns of such behaviors. Some activities might be more addictive than others—few people become addicted to filling out income-tax forms, whereas a higher proportion of all those who gamble become overwhelmingly involved. Still, it is wrong to conclude that any activity is by its nature always "addicting."

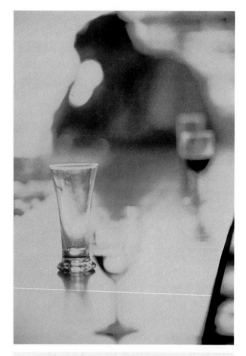

Alcohol causes serious chemical dependence in perhaps 1 of 10 drinkers.

When a chemical is seen as causing the dependence, there is a tendency to give that substance a personality and to ascribe motives to it. When we listen either to a practicing addict's loving description of his interaction with the drug or to a recovering addict describe her struggle against the drug's attempts to destroy her, the drug seems to take on almost human characteristics. We all realize that is going too far, yet the analogy is so powerful that it pervades our thinking. Alcoholics Anonymous (**AA**) members often describe alcohol as being "cunning, baffling, and powerful" and admit that they are powerless against such a foe. And those seeking the prohibition of alcohol, cocaine, marijuana, heroin, and other drugs have over the years tended to "demonize" those substances, making them into powerful forces of evil. The concept of a "war on

Try It!

Are You Addicted to an Activity?

Think of an activity other than substance use that you either really enjoy or find yourself doing quite a lot of. This can be a hobby, such as playing video games or watching movies; something more energetic, such as skiing or mountain biking; or something that involves spending money, such as buying books, CDs, or clothing or shopping on the Internet or TV shopping channels. It can be sexual behavior or gambling, or it can even be working longer hours than most people. Now, with the most "addictive" of those activities in mind, go through the *DSM-IV* diagnostic criteria one by one and ask whether your nondrug "addiction" meets each criterion, obviously substituting the behavior in question for the words *the substance* and *substance use*. Probably the most informative questions in this context are the following (note the words in italics):

- Have you *often* done more of the activity or for a longer period than was intended?
- Have you *persistently* tried to cut down or control the activity?
- Have you given up *important* social, occupational, or recreational activities because of this activity?
- Is the activity continuing despite recurrent physical or psychological problems likely to have been *caused or made worse* by the activity?

If you answered yes to all four questions, then whether or not you agree that you are "addicted" or "dependent," you should consider talking to a behavioral health professional to obtain some assistance in reducing the impact of this activity on your life.

drugs" reflects in part such a perspective—that some drugs are evil and war must be waged against the substances themselves.

Is Addiction Biological?

There has been increasing interest in recent years in the possibility that all addictive behaviors might have some common physiological or biochemical action in the brain. For example, many theorists have recently focused on dopamine, one of the brain's important neurotransmitters, which some believe to play a large role in the process of positive reinforcement. The idea is that any drug use or other activity that has pleasurable or rewarding properties releases dopamine in a particular part of the brain. This idea is discussed more fully in Chapter 6. Although this theory has been widely tested in animal models and there is much evidence that is consistent with it, there is also considerable evidence that this model is too simple and that other neurotransmitters and other brain regions are also important. A great deal of attention has been given to recent reports from various brain-scanning experiments done on cocaine users, showing that cocaine activates many areas that are widely separated in the brain, including some that are known to be dopamine-rich areas and some that are not.[4] Although these studies show some of the physiological *consequences* produced by cocaine or by even thinking about cocaine, they have not yet been useful in examining the possible biological *causes* of addiction. One important question that remains is whether the brains of people who have used cocaine and not become addicted to it show different responses, compared with the brains of cocaine addicts. Ultimately, the strongest demonstration of the power of such techniques would be if it were possible to know, based on looking at a brain scan, whether or not a person had become an addict or was on the way to becoming an addict. Many previous biological theories of addiction have failed this test:

so far, no genetic physiological or biochemical marker has been found that strongly predicts alcoholism or any other addiction.

Is There an Addictive Personality?

Perhaps the explanation for why some people become addicts but others do not lies in the personality—that complex set of attributes and attitudes that develops over time, partly as a result of particular experiences. Is there a common personality factor that is seen in addicts but not in others? This type of research has been conducted for decades, and its value is still controversial.[5] The problem with many studies on practicing or recovering addicts is that it is not possible to know whether the alcohol or other drug use has changed the person's personality. In retrospective studies of personality tests given to college students who later became alcoholics, the prealcoholic students showed what would be considered a "normal" overall personality profile. However, they also tended to be more independent, nonconformist, gregarious, and impulsive. Please note the word *tended*. In all of these studies, although there are statistical differences between the alcoholic and nonalcoholic groups, there is considerable overlap. Once again, personality factors might make some contribution, but they are not the sole cause of alcoholism, or of any other addictive behavior.

Is Addiction a Family Disorder?

Although few scientific studies have been done, examination of the lives of individual addicts— again, primarily alcoholics—reveals some typical patterns of family adaptation to the addiction. A common example in a home with an alcoholic father is that the mother enables this behavior, by calling her husband's boss to say he is ill or by making excuses to family and friends for failures to appear at dinners or parties and generally by caring for her incapacitated husband. The children might also compensate in various ways, and all conspire to keep the family secret. Thus, it is said that alcoholism often exists within a dysfunctional family—the functions of individual members adjust to the needs created by the presence of alcoholism. This new arrangement can make it difficult for the alcoholic alone to change his or her behavior, because doing so would disrupt the family system. Some people suspect that certain family structures actually enhance the likelihood of alcoholism developing. For example, the "codependent" needs of other family members to take care of someone who is dependent on them might facilitate drunkenness.

Much has been written about the effects on children who grow up in an "alcoholic family," and there is some indication that even as adults these individuals tend to exhibit certain personality characteristics. The "adult children of alcoholics" are then perhaps more likely to become involved in dysfunctional relationships that increase the likelihood of alcoholism, either in themselves or in another family member. Again, the evidence indicates that such influences are statistical tendencies and are not all-powerful. It is perhaps unfortunate that some people with alcoholic parents have adopted the role of "adult children" and try to explain their entire personalities and all their difficulties in terms of that status.

Is Addiction a Disease?

The most important reason for adopting a disease model for addiction is based on the experiences of the founders of Alcoholics Anonymous (AA) and is discussed in Chapter 12. Briefly, psychiatrists had commonly assumed that alcoholism was secondary to another disorder, such as anxiety or depression, and often attempted to treat the presumed underlying disorder while encouraging the drinker to try to "cut down." The founders of AA believed that alcoholism itself was the primary problem and needed to be recognized as such and treated directly. This is the reason for the continued insistence that alcoholism is a disease—that it is often the

primary disturbance and deserves to stand in its own right as a recognized disorder requiring treatment.

On the other hand, Peele[6] and others have argued that alcoholism does not have many of the characteristics of some classic medical diseases, such as tuberculosis or syphilis: we can't use an X ray or blood test to reveal the underlying cause, and we don't have a way to treat the underlying cause and cure the symptoms—we don't really know that there is an underlying cause, because all we have are the symptoms of excessive involvement. Furthermore, if addiction itself is a disease, then gambling, excessive sexual involvement, and overeating should also be seen as diseases and the addicts as victims of the disease. This in turn weakens our normal understanding of the concept of disease. Marlatt and Fromme[7] have pointed out that the disease model is perhaps best seen as an analogy—addictions are *like* diseases in many ways, but that is different from insisting that they *are* a disease. One reason for the conflict over the disease model of addiction may be differences in how we think of the term *disease.* For example, many would agree that high blood pressure is considered a disease—it's certainly viewed as a medical disorder. We know that high blood pressure can be produced by genetic factors, cigarette smoking, diet, lack of exercise, or by other medical conditions. In that context, the idea that alcohol or drug dependence is like a disease doesn't seem so far-fetched. This is taking a broad, **biopsychosocial** perspective that addiction might be related to dysfunctions of biology, personality, social interactions, or a combination of these factors.

ASSESSMENT OF ADDICTIVE DISORDERS: DIAGNOSIS

How do we know whether someone's drinking, marijuana smoking, or coffee consumption indicates an addiction to that substance? The notion of "overwhelming involvement" is somewhat subjective—do we mean that the person does

DSM-IV   PSYCHIATRIC DIAGNOSIS OF SUBSTANCE DISORDERS

Diagnostic Criteria for Substance Dependence

A maladaptive pattern of substance use, leading to clinically significant impairment or distress, as manifested by three (or more) of the following, occurring at any time in the same 12-month period:

1. Tolerance, as defined by either of the following:
   a. A need for markedly increased amounts of the substance to achieve intoxication or desired effect
   b. Markedly diminished effect with continued use of the same amount of the substance
2. Withdrawal, as manifested by either of the following:
   a. The characteristic withdrawal syndrome for the substance
   b. The same (or a closely related) substance is taken to relieve or avoid withdrawal symptoms.
3. The substance is often taken in larger amounts or over a longer period than was intended.
4. There is a persistent desire or unsuccessful efforts to cut down or control substance use.
5. A great deal of time is spent in activities necessary to obtain the substance.
6. Important social, occupational, or recreational activities are given up or reduced because of substance use.

7. The substance use is continued despite knowledge of having a persistent or recurrent physical or psychological problem that is likely to have been caused or exacerbated by the substance.

Diagnostic Criteria for Substance Abuse

A. A maladaptive pattern of substance use leading to clinically significant impairment or distress, as manifested by one (or more) of the following, occurring within a 12-month period:
   1. Recurrent substance use resulting in failure to fulfill major role obligations at work, school, or home
   2. Recurrent substance use in situations in which it is physically hazardous
   3. Recurrent substance-related legal problems
   4. Continued substance use despite having persistent or recurrent social or interpersonal problems caused or exacerbated by the effects of the substance
B. The symptoms have never met the criteria for substance dependence for this class of substance.

---

almost nothing else but get and use the drug and deal with the drug's effects, or that it is the predominant thing the person does, or just that the person does it much more than the average user of that substance? How do we distinguish the wine connoisseur, who reads and talks about wines, spends time and lots of money shopping for them, and tastes wines frequently, from the alcoholic who becomes intoxicated on a daily basis? Let us begin by examining the closest thing to an official method of diagnosis, which comes from the American Psychiatric Association's *Diagnostic and Statistical Manual,* fourth edition (**DSM-IV**).[8] Because of the controversy surrounding the definition of such terms as *alcoholism* and *addiction,* this manual describes "substance dependence," which includes tolerance and physical dependence among its criteria, and "substance abuse," which is based principally on

behavioral symptoms (see the *DSM-IV* box). The same basic criteria are used, whether the substance is alcohol, heroin, cocaine, tobacco, a

Alcoholics Anonymous: a worldwide organization of self-help groups based on helping each other stop drinking.

biopsychosocial: a theory or perspective that relies on the interaction of biological, individual psychological, and social variables.

DSM-IV: the *Diagnostic and Statistical Manual* of the American Psychiatric Association, fourth edition. Lists criteria for diagnosing psychiatric disorders, including substance dependence and substance abuse.

medication, or an inhaled solvent. The manual also describes criteria for substance intoxication and substance withdrawal.

ADDICTION TREATMENT

Every year, hundreds of thousands of Americans undergo treatment for alcoholism or addiction to other substances. The word *treatment* conjures up an image of hospitals, nurses, and physicians, but traditional medical approaches form only a small part of the overall treatment picture. As we will see, the variety of treatment approaches reflects the variety of substance-abuse problems, as well as the variety of theories about substance abuse.

Deciding to Quit

For many years, the predominant theories on why people seek treatment for addiction were based on the anecdotal experiences of alcoholics. According to the conventional wisdom, most addicts use the defense mechanism of *denial* and are obstinately unwilling to admit either that their drinking or drug use is unusual or that it has serious consequences for themselves or others. In this context, only when the addict "hits bottom"—that is, suffers sufficient consequences that the reality of the problem finally sinks in—will he or she be ready to seek help. If family and friends want to cause this reality to sink in sooner, then they may attempt an *intervention*—a meeting between the addict and several significant friends or family members who describe in specific terms the problems caused by the person's drinking or drug use and mutually and firmly insist that he or she recognize that the addiction is a problem that needs to be addressed. Certainly this approach has been used many times, and in many cases the result has been that the addict has sought treatment.

Studies on smokers who quit smoking without formal intervention led to descriptions of the cognitive stages they went through in making the decision to change their behavior. These **stages of change** have since been described more generally for alcohol and other drug use, as well as for other problem behaviors that might be addressed in psychotherapy.[9] In the *precontemplation* stage, the individual does not recognize that a problem exists. In the *contemplation* stage, the individual believes that a problem might exist and gives some consideration to the possibility of changing his or her behavior. In the *preparation* stage, the person decides to change and makes plans to do so. In the *action* stage, the individual takes active steps toward change, such as entering treatment. Finally, the *maintenance* stage involves activities intended to maintain the change. According to this model, in order to help someone move from one stage to another, you need to know where he or she is in the decision-making process.

Miller and his colleagues believe that aggressively confrontational approaches (intervention) may actually increase denial and resistance to change. They have developed a method called *Motivational Interviewing*, which uses a thorough assessment of the drinking or drug-using behavior and its consequences, and builds on the client's own concerns about possible problems. The results of the assessment are shared with the client, who then interprets them in light of his or her own concerns. The motivational interviewer listens and helps the client focus on the concerns and the problem behavior but does not directly tell the client what to do. Ideally, if the therapist knows which stage of change the client is in, the discussion can be guided appropriately to help move the client to the next stage. This approach is relatively new, and research on its effectiveness is now being carried out.[10]

Defining Treatment Goals

The particular theoretical view one has of alcoholism, narcotic addiction, or substance abuse in general influences not only the treatment approaches one is likely to take but even the goals of treatment. For example, if one accepts the increasingly predominant view of alcoholism as a disease, which someone either "has" or does not have and which has an inevitable progression to more and more drinking, then the only acceptable treatment goal is total **abstinence.** Other experts view alcoholism as representing one end of a continuum of drinking, with no clear dividing line. For some of these theorists, a possible beneficial outcome of treatment is **controlled** social **drinking.** Likewise, if one views narcotic addiction as inherently evil, undermining the physical and mental health of its victims (a common view until fairly recently), then abstinence from narcotics is the only acceptable goal. Americans seem to have come around to accepting addiction to the legal narcotic methadone as preferable to heroin addiction, so the goal has changed from eliminating narcotic use to eliminating heroin use. The case with cigarette smoking is similar; some programs have focused on cutting down on smoking or switching to cigarettes that are lower in tar and nicotine, whereas most programs aim for complete abstinence.

When we look for indicators of a treatment program's success, if we find that some people are still using, but using less, should we claim any benefit? Or should we assume, as some do, that any decreases will be temporary and that, unless the person quits entirely, there has been no real improvement? The answer depends on your goals. Recently researchers have begun to estimate the cost savings resulting from increased employment and decreased crime after treatment, and to compare these savings with the cost of treatment itself, to develop a cost-benefit analysis of the effectiveness of treatment.

Treatment Stages

To understand how most treatment programs work, it is helpful to think in terms of three stages: *detoxification, active treatment,* and *aftercare.*

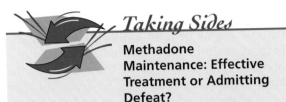

Taking Sides

Methadone Maintenance: Effective Treatment or Admitting Defeat?

One of the most common treatments for heroin addiction involves providing heroin users with a substitute narcotic called methadone. In these programs, the addict must show up daily at a clinic to be given his or her dose of methadone, which is taken by mouth. The addict often remains physically dependent on opiates, in the sense that the typical opiate withdrawal symptoms occur if he or she misses a dose of methadone. This treatment may be continued for months, even years in some cases. Supporters of the approach point out that offering methadone keeps addicts in treatment longer, reduces crime, and reduces relapse to heroin use, which is more dangerous, expensive, and illegal, and which may expose the addict to needles tainted with HIV, hepatitis, or other blood-borne diseases. Treatment clients are often able to work or attend school while taking oral methadone once a day. Critics argue that the addiction remains untreated, that it may be considered immoral to provide addicts with the means to continue their addictions, and that all we have done is trade one type of dependence for another. What do you think?

For more on this topic, log onto www.dushkin.com/online for current news and links to other popular and informative sites, as well as time-saving web search strategies and study tools.

Detoxification

If the addict is heavily intoxicated and the last dose has been recent, as might occur in an emergency room admission, then the first concern is the possibility of death from drug overdose. Various measures, such as clearing the

stages of change: a model for decision making consisting of precontemplation, contemplation, preparation, action, and maintenance.

stomach and giving diuretic drugs to increase urine flow, may be used to lower the blood levels quickly. In the case of a narcotic overdose, narcotic antagonists may be used to block the drug's immediate effects (see Chapter 16). The most common cause of drug overdose death is the depression of respiration (breathing), so it is important to monitor respiration rate, as well as blood pressure and heart rate. Breathing may need to be supported by artificial respiration. Once the person's respiration has stabilized, it is time to deal with the possibility of withdrawal.

Remember that the early medical model of addiction was based on the development of physical dependence and that withdrawal symptoms are the indicator of physical dependence. As the addict's body begins to metabolize the alcohol, heroin, or other drug and the blood levels drop, withdrawal symptoms might occur. Withdrawal from many kinds of drugs can be exceedingly uncomfortable, but withdrawal from alcohol or depressants is in many cases life threatening. Therefore, it might be necessary to give the addict small doses of a depressant drug to limit the severity of the withdrawal.

The word **detoxification** refers to the process of removing the offending substance (the "toxin") from the body, either by allowing the body to clear the drug by normal metabolism and excretion (see Chapter 7), or by more active methods, while preventing medical complications due to overdose or withdrawal. During this initial stage of treatment, there might be other medical issues of immediate concern, such as malnutrition, liver dysfunction in an alcoholic, or hepatitis or AIDS in an intravenous drug user. Also, because the addict might be either intoxicated or preoccupied with withdrawal during this first stage, not much in the way of addiction treatment is usually accomplished.

Detoxification is not always necessary, because the client might have been using a type of drug or using small enough quantities that neither overdose nor physical dependence is of much concern. Some clients will have already stopped using the substance days or weeks before entering the treatment program, and thus those immediate concerns will have passed.

Active Treatment

Early theories of addiction were based primarily on studying alcoholics and narcotic addicts, so it should come as no surprise that the history of treatment approaches also began with the treatment of alcoholism and narcotic addiction. Some of the specifics of treatment for those problems are described in Chapters 12 and 16. In addition to various approaches to treating alcoholism and narcotic addiction, there has been quite a lot of recent research on the treatment of cigarette smokers (see Chapter 12) and cocaine addicts (see Chapter 7). Most treatment programs today are not designed for a particular substance, but treat a variety of types of substance dependence.

Aftercare (Relapse Prevention)

After the period of active treatment has ended, the long-term issue then becomes avoiding use of the substance on a day-to-day basis. Many treatment programs rely on self-help approaches, such as AA and the similarly structured groups Cocaine Anonymous (CA) and Narcotics Anonymous (NA). The treatment program typically ensures that each client is referred to a local group for continued discussion of the recovery process. Some programs host such meetings themselves for clients who live in the area, and residential programs often invite their clients to return on a regular basis for weekend sessions.

Medically assisted treatment is, in a sense, aimed at relapse prevention from the start. Methadone maintenance, the most common type of substitution program for heroin addicts, may continue for months or years. Nicotine gum or patches are typically used only during treatment and are not given as long-term maintenance aids. Both narcotic antagonists and disulfiram (Antabuse) for alcoholics are

Targeting Prevention
Avoiding Relapse

One important type of substance-abuse prevention involves those who have been in treatment and are trying to avoid relapsing, or going back to their previously abusive behavior. Think about the messages these people receive each day from public media (such as television, movies, newspapers, and the web) and from other individuals. Which of these messages support relapse prevention and which tend to encourage relapse? Try to have a conversation with a friend, relative, or classmate who has been in treatment for substance abuse and has had to deal with the problem of relapse prevention. Ask what sorts of things were helpful for him or her and what sorts of things made it more difficult to avoid substance abuse.

often used for weeks or months, but indefinite maintenance for years is unusual with these approaches.

Treatment Approaches

Treatment programs can be divided into two major categories, *residential* and *outpatient*. This distinction is based on whether the client checks in to a hospital, group home, or other facility, where he or she eats and sleeps during the treatment phase, or whether the client lives elsewhere and goes to the treatment facility only to attend counseling or group meetings or to obtain medication. A further basic distinction is whether the treatment is *drug-free* or medication-assisted.

Residential Treatment

Although it is an oversimplification, we can think of residential programs as having two historical roots. The first was medical hospitalization, which was a common early approach to alcoholism and narcotic addiction. This was partly due to the importance of detoxification and partly because no other type of treatment facility was available. The second root was the *therapeutic community.*

Synanon. In 1958 Charles Dederick, a recovering alcoholic, felt that an organization similar to AA should be able to help narcotic addicts who wanted to be rehabilitated. However, instead of voluntarily attending meetings, the addicts would live in this supportive environment as residents. Just as AA literature asserts that an alcoholic is never "cured" of alcoholism, the philosophy that a narcotic addict is never cured led Synanon to conclude that addicts needed to stay closely connected to Synanon—so closely that many would remain Synanon residents for life. Thus, Synanon became a growing communal living organization during the 1960s and 1970s, staffed by former addicts.

Because of a belief that addicts have difficulty expressing emotions and identifying others' emotions, Dederick established the use of "seminars," or group encounters, several times a week. These encounters were often psychologically quite violent. The positive view of them is that they helped break through the residents' denial and teach them to see themselves and others more clearly. A less charitable view is that these sessions threatened or cajoled the new members into accepting life at Synanon.

Early reports of Synanon's high rate of success should be examined carefully. The program was not research oriented, and Dederick himself pointed out that thousands left the program.[11] Most of those returned to addiction, but no precise records were kept of the quitters. Thus, the high rates of nonaddiction related only to those who stayed with the program.

abstinence: no alcohol or drug use at all.

controlled drinking: the idea that alcohol abusers may be able to drink under control.

detoxification: an initial phase of treatment during which the alcohol or other drug clears out of the system.

As the use of various drugs increased in the 1960s, Synanon grew rapidly and began to include a much greater variety of members. For example, youngsters who were caught smoking marijuana were sometimes sent by their families to be rehabilitated at Synanon. Arrestees, whether for marijuana, LSD, amphetamine, or other drug use, sometimes volunteered to go to Synanon at the urging of their attorneys to avoid a jail sentence. The businesses Synanon started to provide employment for the residents became large and profitable, and Synanon became a $30 million organization. Dederick declared Synanon a religion in 1974, perhaps to avoid taxation. Investigative reports of Synanon's profits and of Dederick's cultlike control led to threats and to the attempted murder of a reporter. Dederick was forced to give up control in 1980 after pleading no contest to conspiracy to commit murder. Synanon has practically disappeared in the United States, except for a website maintained by former residents (www.synanon.org), but an active offshoot in Germany continues to welcome addicts and recovering addicts.

Other Therapeutic Communities. Other residential treatment communities were established in the 1960s, including Daytop Village, Phoenix House, Odyssey House, and Gateway Foundation. Because of the reported successes of such programs (although, again, such reports were not based on scientific evaluations), their number grew through the 1970s and 1980s. There are now many residential facilities across the country, serving narcotic addicts, alcoholics, and abusers of other substances. One major difference between these therapeutic communities and Synanon is the goal of returning their clients to society. Most of their staff usually consists of recovering alcoholics, former addicts, or abusers of other drugs, and there is still a focus on group sessions and on keeping the clients busy. Relatively high success rates reported for these therapeutic communities are based on those who stick with the program for the full

course of the treatment, which typically lasts for several months.

The Drug Abuse Reporting Program (DARP), financed by the National Institute on Drug Abuse (NIDA), followed the success of a large number of clients admitted to drug-abuse treatment programs from the years 1969 to 1973. In a 1982 follow-up, more than 4,000 of the original sample were contacted and interviewed about their drug use.[12] The data indicate that therapeutic communities did reduce drug use relative to untreated clients or to those who were detoxified and then released. For example, narcotic addicts who had been treated with either methadone maintenance or a therapeutic community approach had about a 20 percent chance of engaging in daily narcotic use during the last follow-up year, compared with about 30 percent for the untreated or detoxified groups. If clients had been treated for less than 90 days in the therapeutic community, their outcome measures were not more positive than for untreated groups, thus indicating that the length of treatment is an important variable for therapeutic communities. Other variables, such as treatment philosophy or types of services available in the program, did not influence the outcome.

Chemical Dependency Residential Programs. This refers to various short-term (three to eight weeks) private residential programs that combine some features of hospitalization with some features of therapeutic communities. Before the 1980s, these programs dealt almost exclusively with alcohol dependence. The majority of the staff in these programs consist of "chemical-dependency" counselors who typically are recovering alcoholics with limited formal training. They provided medical support for detoxification and relied for treatment mostly on the 12-step model of AA (see Drugs in Depth box). Patients who could afford to go away to "dry out," using either personal finances or medical insurance, kept these facilities in operation. The Betty Ford Clinic, which attracts many wealthy

Drugs in Depth

The 12 Steps of Alcoholics Anonymous

1. We admitted we were powerless over alcohol—that our lives had become unmanageable.
2. Came to believe that a Power greater than ourselves could restore us to sanity.
3. Made a decision to turn our will and our lives over to the care of God *as we understood Him.*
4. Made a searching and fearless moral inventory of ourselves.
5. Admitted to God, to ourselves, and to another human being the exact nature of our wrongs.
6. Were entirely ready to have God remove all these defects of character.
7. Humbly asked Him to remove our shortcomings.
8. Made a list of all persons we had harmed and became willing to make amends to them all.
9. Made direct amends to such people wherever possible, except when to do so would injure them or others.
10. Continued to take moral inventory and when we were wrong promptly admitted it.
11. Sought through prayer and meditation to improve our conscious contact with God *as we understood Him,* praying only for knowledge of His will for us and the power to carry that out.
12. Having had a spiritual awakening as the result of these steps, we tried to carry this message to alcoholics, and to practice these principles in all our affairs.

celebrities as clients, is an example of such a facility, although many are less expensive. In the 1980s, the increased use of medical insurance to pay for treatment of chemical dependence made this type of program a growth industry. Besides the traditional residential alcohol programs, which expanded to accept cocaine and other drug users, new private psychiatric hospitals sprang up all over the country, with adolescent drug-abuse clients as their primary market.[13] The potential for high profits led to many abuses, including active recruitment of clients who might not have been addicted. Inevitably, insurance companies began to be much more restrictive, and large numbers of these private-pay programs went out of business in the 1990s. Although reduced in number, these short-term programs remain the most common form of residential treatment. The Sandra Bullock film "28 Days" depicts a program of this type.

Medication-Assisted Treatment

Medical approaches have been a small part of the overall treatment picture, but they produce beneficial effects for many addicts, and with the development of new drugs they might play an increasingly important role. Especially with outpatient treatment, drugs might be used to assist the client in maintaining abstinence. There are three basic approaches to using medications for addiction treatment: *antagonism,* or blockade, of the abused substance; *substitution,* or provision of a drug that reduces the craving for the abused substance; and provision of a drug that is *medically incompatible* with the abused substance. The only example of the last approach is a drug called *Antabuse,* which is given to alcoholics (see Chapter 12). Antabuse blocks the normal metabolism of alcohol, so, if a client who is taking Antabuse drinks alcohol, he or she will become very ill. Both narcotic antagonists and the substitute narcotic methadone have been used with heroin addicts (see Chapter 16), and nicotine gum or patches have been used to reduce cravings in those quitting the use of tobacco (see Chapter 13). There is some evidence that the experimental drug buprenorphine can reduce cravings in both heroin and cocaine addicts, leading to hopes of developing a general-purpose drug for treating a variety of drug addictions.[14] Naltrexone, a narcotic antagonist, was shown to reduce craving in alcoholics and has been approved for such use (Chapter 12). And attention has recently focused on a drug once considered a hallucinogen: *ibogaine* has been described by some as useful in reducing addictive cravings from a wide variety of drugs. Although animal research is exploring possible mechanisms of ibogaine action,[15] controlled human trials have not been approved.

Outpatient Drug-Free Programs

Outpatient drug-free programs grew from two major sources. In the 1960s, because of a large number of panic reactions to LSD and other illicit drugs, "crisis clinics" were set up in most large communities. These clinics provided alternatives to the emergency room for a person who was frightened and needed someone to talk to until the drug wore off. These facilities ranged from telephone hot lines, to emergency room– associated clinics with medical support available, to "crash pads" where people could sleep off a drug's effects and receive some nonjudgmental advice and counseling. Another major source of outpatient services has been the community mental health centers that have been established all over the nation since the early 1960s. Treatment choices of a third kind are affiliated with hospitals, correctional facilities, or large employers and might be available only to specific populations.

Because of the large number of outpatient drug-free programs and their ready availability, they constitute the most popular form of drug-abuse treatment. Services often include individual psychotherapy, group counseling, vocational counseling, and other professional services. In contrast to therapeutic communities, the counselors in these programs are more likely to be professional psychologists, social workers, or trained vocational rehabilitation counselors. Perhaps because contacting one of these programs does not seem to be as big a step as entering a residential center, outpatient programs might be more likely to contact drug users earlier in their drug-abuse career, which might help their success rates.

Treatment: The Big Picture in the United States

In each state, the agency that has primary responsibility for public funding of substance-

abuse treatment submits annual reports to the U.S. Substance Abuse and Mental Health Services Administration (SAMHSA). Between 1993 and 1998, the data from more than 1.5 million admissions each year for substance abuse were compiled into the Treatment Episode Data Set.[16] In 1998, four substances accounted for 90 percent of these admissions: alcohol (47%), opiates (15%), cocaine (15%), and marijuana (13%). Most of those who reported opiates as their primary drug of abuse were heroin users, and most of those who reported cocaine as the primary drug were crack smokers. About half of those admitted with marijuana as the primary drug were under 20 years of age. In 1998, 88 percent of substance-abuse clients were treated as outpatients, 10 percent in a residential setting, and fewer than 2 percent as hospital inpatients.[17]

Is Treatment Effective?

There is a widespread belief that addiction treatment is often ineffective. We've all heard of well-known athletes who have been in treatment programs and are later found to be using illegal drugs, and we might know an alcoholic who had treatment and began drinking again. What we know is that treatment doesn't work for every client every time, especially if our expectation is that one treatment exposure will eliminate the use of the substance for the rest of the person's life. A more meaningful question is whether treatment programs have any effect at all—and, if they do, if their effects are worth their cost. A 1990 report from the Institute of Medicine[18] reviewed the evidence gathered to that point, which was based mainly on studies of heroin addicts. The report concluded (1) methadone maintenance pays for itself (in reduced crime and increased employment) during the time it is administered, and posttreatment effects are an economic bonus; (2) although therapeutic communities cost more than methadone maintenance, they result in better employment status after treatment; and (3) outpatient drug-free programs attract more clients without a criminal background and therefore do not reduce criminal activity as much as the other two approaches; they are inexpensive, however, and do produce a net benefit because of increased employment. A 1994 report by the California Department of Alcohol and Drug Programs[19] concluded that, on the average, seven dollars are saved for every dollar invested in the treatment of alcohol and other drug abuse. Alcohol and other drug use was reduced by about two-fifths after treatment; treatment for crack, powdered cocaine, and methamphetamine use was just as effective as for alcohol; and criminal activity declined by about two-thirds after treatment.

A recent report reviewed 53 studies of the effectiveness of adolescent substance-abuse treatment programs. Overall, most of the treated adolescents had significant reductions in substance use and problems in other life areas in the year following treatment, and an average of 32 percent remained abstinent at the end of a year. Successful program completion, involve-

ment in aftercare, and the inclusion of family therapy as one treatment component all appeared to predict success.[20]

Overall, substance abuse treatment does work. It saves lives and saves money and is a worthwhile investment.

SUMMARY

- The view of addiction has changed over the past 30 years and is now based on a behavioral definition; it is also applied to a wider variety of drugs and other activities.
- There is evidence that addiction may be influenced by genetics, biochemistry, personality, experience, and social context, but none of these factors can be called the sole cause of addiction. This idea is referred to as a biopsychosocial perspective on addiction.
- The *DSM-IV* diagnosis of substance dependence relies partly on tolerance and physical dependence, whereas the diagnosis of substance abuse uses behavioral indicators of excessive involvement.
- The addict's decision to seek treatment may involve a series of cognitive stages of change.
- Treatment is often divided into the three stages of detoxification, active treatment, and aftercare.
- Therapeutic communities are usually staffed by former substance abusers, and clients generally remain in them for several months.
- Outpatient drug-free programs are often associated with community mental health centers and employ trained counselors, psychologists, or social workers.
- Chemical-dependence residential programs also tend to employ former substance abusers, but treatment is usually limited to three to eight weeks.
- A variety of new medical approaches are being developed to treat addicts.

Web Watch

Activities Related to Addiction

Do You Abuse Substances?
Take the quiz "Do You Have a Substance Abuse Problem?" at www.health.cybear.com/atoz/teen/tsproblem.asp If you have completed the quiz and find you are at risk, click on the link to discover sources you can go to for assistance.

Learning About Addiction and Recovery
Take the "Addiction and Recovery Quiz" at library.thinkquest.org/29500/addictions/anr.quiz.shtml. You'll be tested on your knowledge of the signs of addiction and discover ways to recover.

Can You Talk About Drugs?
One of the first steps in dealing with a substance-abuse problem is talking about it. It's also a good idea to talk to a knowledgeable person about drugs before you develop an addiction or are even presented with an opportunity to use drugs. Go to www.antibully.org.uk/talking.htm. This page offers a brief overview of the effects of some types of drugs and the stages of addiction. Below this overview, find and read the tips on talking to someone about drugs.

Learn to Recognize Addiction
Can you recognize an addict? Read the article posted on www.indianhealthzone.com/drug/drug_recognise. asp. This article lists the signs of addiction specific to certain drugs. It also gives advice on how to help a person with an addiction.

4. Why does it make sense to discuss gambling, overeating, and other behaviors in the context of addiction? What problems result from such a broad definition of addiction?
5. Why do we sometimes speak about drugs as being able to cause addiction? What are the pitfalls of carrying the concept too far?
6. What personality variables tend to be stronger in prealcoholic students?
7. Why do some people say that addiction is a disease of the family?
8. Which types of diseases provide poor analogies, and which might provide better analogies, for addiction?
9. How does motivational interviewing relate to stages of change?
10. What kind of evidence do we have that treatment for substance abuse works?

REFERENCES

1. Forbes D: *False fixes.* Albany, NY: State University of New York Press, 1994.
2. Goldstein A: *Molecular and cellular aspects of the drug addictions.* New York: Springer-Verlag, 1989.
3. Kelleher RT, Goldberg SR: Control of drug taking behavior by schedules of reinforcement, *Pharmacol Review* 27:291, 1976.
4. Maas LC and others: Functional MRI of human brain activation during cue-induced cocaine craving, *American Journal of Psychiatry,* 155:124-126, 1998.
5. Kerr JS: Two myths of addiction: The addictive personality and the issues of free choice. *Human Psychopharmacology* 11:suppl, 1996.
6. Peele S, Brodsky A, Arnold M: *The truth about addiction and recovery.* New York: Fireside Press, 1992.
7. Marlatt GA, Fromme K: Metaphors for addiction. In S Peele, editor: *Visions of addiction.* Lexington, MA: DC Heath, 1988.
8. American Psychiatric Association: *Diagnostic and statistical manual of mental disorders,* 4th ed. Washington, DC: Author, 1994.
9. Belding MA and others: Stages and processes of change among polydrug users in methadone maintenance treatment, *Drug and Alcohol Dependence* 39:45, 1995.
10. Miller W: Motivational interviewing: Research, practice, and puzzles, *Addictive Behaviors* 21:835, 1996.

REVIEW QUESTIONS

1. How does physical dependence relate to tolerance?
2. What do we mean when we say that a drug has the ability to serve as a positive reinforcer of behavior?
3. Which is more important to our current understanding of addiction, physical dependence or psychological dependence? Why?

11. Brecher EM: *Licit and illicit drugs.* Boston: Little, Brown, 1972.

12. Simpson DD, Sells SB: *Evaluation of drug abuse treatment effectiveness: Summary of the DARP follow-up research,* DHHS Pub No (ADM)82–1194, Washington, DC: U.S. Government Printing Office, 1982.

13. Cowley G and others: Money madness, *Newsweek,* Nov 4, 1991.

14. Schottenfeld RS and others: Buprenorphine dose-related effects on cocaine and opioid use on cocaine-abusing opioid-dependent humans, *Biological Psychiatry* 34:66, 1993.

15. Sershen H, Hashim A, Lajta A: Ibogaine and cocaine abuse: Pharmacological interactions at dopamine and serotonin receptors. *Brain Research Bulletin* 42:161, 1997.

16. *Treatment episode data set (TEDS) 1993–1998.* SAMHSA Office of Applied Studies, U.S. Department of Health and Human Services, Sept 2000.

17. *1998 uniform facility data set (UFDS).* SAMHSA Office of Applied Studies, U.S. Department of Health and Human Services, Aug 2000.

18. Gerstein DR, Harwood HJ, editors: *Treating drug problems.* Washington, DC: National Academy Press, 1990.

19. Lewis DC: More evidence that treatment works, *The Brown University Digest of Addiction Theory and Application* 13:12, 1994.

20. Williams RJ, Chang SY: A comprehensive and comparative review of adolescent substance abuse treatment outcome, *Clinical Psychology, Science and Practice* 7:138–166, 2000.

Chapter 4

Preventing Substance Abuse

Online Learning Center Resources

www.mhhe.com/ray

Log on to our Online Learning Center (OLC) for access to these additional resources.

- Chapter key terms and definitions
- Learning objectives
- Additional behavior change objectives
- Student interactive questions and answer sites
- Self-scoring chapter quiz

The OLC also offers web links for study and exploration of health topics. Here are some examples of what you'll find:

www.nida.nih.gov/NIDA_Notes/NNVol15n4/Boys.html

At this website, see the NIDA's article "Boys and Girls Encounter Different Drug Offers, Use Different Refusal Strategies." The article points out the different sources that are more likely to offer drugs to boys or girls and common reactions according to gender.

www.naadac.org/

Check out the home page for the National Association of Alcoholism and Drug Abuse Counselors.

www.washingtonpost.com/wp-srv/local/longterm/drugs/article.htm

This special report by the *Washington Post* investigates and provides evidence for the role of drugs on our streets and the effects on society. There are additional articles, links, and downloads available on this topic as well as a quiz on local drug patterns.

Drugs in the Media

Prime-Time Drug-Prevention Programming

In late 1997, the U.S. Congress approved the expenditure of $1 billion over a five-year period for antidrug advertising on television networks. This was a lot of

Drugs in the Media Continued...

revenue for the networks, but the catch was that they had to broadcast the messages at half the normal market price. After industry protests, the White House Office of National Drug Control Policy struck deals to discharge networks from the half-cost advertising time requirements if they would incorporate drug-abuse prevention messages into the content of television shows. For example, the program *E.R.*, about a hospital emergency room, has included several episodes dramatizing the consequences of illicit drug use. The agreement was brought to light in early 2000 by the online news magazine salon.com, which raised concerns about hidden government "propaganda."

See if you can get a few people to keep an eye out for such integrated antidrug content for one week. Did you find some obvious examples? Have you been aware of this type of integrated content before? What is the danger involved in having the federal government influence the content of television programming in this subtle way?

Why can't we *do* something to keep young people from ruining their lives with drugs? As our society seeks to prevent drug abuse by limiting the availability of such drugs as heroin and cocaine, we are forced to recognize several other facts. First, as long as there is a sizable market for these substances, there will be people to supply them. Thus, only if we can teach people not to want the drugs can we attack the source of the problem. Second, these substances will never disappear entirely, so we should try to teach people to live in a world that includes them. Third, our society has accepted

the continued existence of tobacco and alcohol, yet some people are harmed by them. Can we teach people to coexist with both legal and illegal substances and to live in such a way that their lives and health are not impaired by them?

DEFINING GOALS AND EVALUATING OUTCOMES

Think about the process you are engaged in while reading and studying this book. The text is aimed at teaching its readers about drugs: their effects, how they are used, and how they relate to society. The goal of the authors is *education*. A person who understands all this information about all these drugs will perhaps be better prepared to make decisions about personal drug use, more able to understand drug use by others, and better prepared to participate in social discussions about drug use and abuse. We hope that a person who knew all this would be in a position to act more rationally, neither glorifying a drug and expecting miraculous changes from using it nor condemning it as the essence of evil. But our ultimate goal is not to change the reader's behavior in a particular direction. For example, the chapter on alcohol, although pointing out the dangers of its use and the problems it can cause, does not attempt to influence the readers to avoid all alcohol use. In a purely educational program, the primary goal is not to alter a person's drug-taking behavior. The success of this book is measured by how much a person knows about alcohol, tobacco, or marijuana, not by whether he or she is convinced never to drink or smoke.

On the other hand, there exists a tradition, going back to the "demon rum" programs of the late 1800s, of presenting negative information about alcohol and other drugs in the public schools with the clear goal of *prevention* of use. Some of these early programs presented information that was so clearly one-sided that they could have been classified as propaganda rather than education. We would not measure the success of such a program by how much objective information the students gained about the pharmacology of the narcotics, for example. A more appropriate index might be how many of the students did subsequently experiment with the drugs against which the program was aimed. Until the early 1970s, it was simply assumed that these programs would have the desired effect, and few attempts were made to evaluate them.

TYPES OF PREVENTION

The goals and methods of a prevention program also depend on the drug-using status of those served by the program. The programs designed to prevent young people from starting smoking might be different from those used to try to prevent relapse in smokers who have quit, for example. Until recently, drug-abuse prevention programs have been classified according to a public health model:

- **Primary prevention** programs are those aimed mainly at young people who have not yet tried the substances in question or who may have tried tobacco or alcohol a few times. As discussed in the section "Defining Goals and Evaluating Outcomes," such programs might encourage complete abstinence from specific drugs or might have the broader goal of teaching people how to view drugs and the potential influences of drugs on their lives, emotions, and social relationships. Because those programs are presented to people with little personal experience with drugs, they might be expected to be especially effective. On the other hand, there is the danger of introducing large numbers of children to information about a number of drugs that they might otherwise never have heard of, thus arousing their curiosity about them.
- **Secondary prevention** programs can be thought of as designed for people who have

tried the drug in question or a variety of other substances. The goals of such programs are usually the prevention of the use of other, more dangerous substances and the prevention of the development of more dangerous forms of use of the substances they are already experimenting with. We might describe the clientele here as more "sophisticated" substance users who have not suffered seriously from their drug experiences and who are not obvious candidates for treatment. Many college students fall into this category, and programs aimed at encouraging responsible use of alcohol among college students are good examples of this stage of prevention.

- **Tertiary prevention,** in our scheme, is relapse prevention, or follow-up programs. For alcoholics or cocaine or heroin addicts, treatment programs are the first order of priority. However, once a person has been treated or has stopped the substance use without assistance, we enter another stage of prevention. (Relapse prevention was discussed under the concept of *aftercare* in Chapter 3.)

Recently, the Institute of Medicine has proposed a new classification of the "continuum of care," which includes prevention, treatment, and maintenance.[1] Prevention efforts are categorized according to the intended target population, but the targets are not defined only by prior drug use:

- **Universal prevention** programs are designed for delivery to an entire population—for example, all schoolchildren or an entire community.
- **Selective prevention** strategies are designed for groups within the general population that are deemed to be at high risk—for example, students who are not doing well academically or the poorest neighborhoods in a community.
- **Indicated prevention** strategies are targeted at individuals who show signs of developing problems, such as a child who

Targeting Prevention

Preventing Inhalant Abuse

The abuse by children of spray paints and other products containing solvents appears to have increased somewhat in recent years (see Chapter 8). Several characteristics of this type of abuse make it an interesting problem for prevention workers. First, the variety of available products and their ready availability in stores, the home, and even in schools make preventing access to the inhalants a virtual impossibility. Second, most of the kids who use these substances probably know it's unhealthy and dangerous to do so, so further information of that sort may not add much in the way of preventing their use. Third, this use is very "faddish"—a group of eighth-graders in one school might start inhaling cleaning fluid; a group of sixth-graders in another neighborhood might be into gold paint (in distinct preference to black, yellow, or white).

Given these characteristics, where does a school-based prevention education program begin to attack the problem? Does it focus on a particular product and try to talk kids out of using gold paint? Does it talk about a whole variety of products and thereby perhaps introduce the kids to new things they hadn't thought of? One good videotape (*Inhalants: Kids in Danger, Adults in the Dark*) took the approach of attempting to inform parents and teachers of the varieties of paints, perfumes, solvents, and other spray products used by abusers and to inform them of some of the subterfuges used by some of the kids (carrying a small cologne vial to school, spraying paint into empty soft drink cans, etc.). However, this video is *not* meant to be shown to children, because it describes exactly what to do and how to do it. Probably the best idea in prevention classes is to reinforce to children in general terms the dangers of inhalants without describing a particular substance or method of use.

began smoking cigarettes at a young age or an adult arrested for a first offense of driving under the influence of alcohol.

PREVENTION PROGRAMS IN THE SCHOOLS

The Knowledge-Attitudes-Behavior Model

After the increase in the use of illicit drugs by young middle-class people in the 1960s, there was a general sense that society was not doing an adequate job of drug education, and most school systems increased their efforts. However, there was confusion over the methods to be used. Traditional antidrug programs had relied heavily on representatives of the local police, who went into schools and told a few horror stories, describing the legal trouble due anyone who got caught with illicit drugs. Sometimes the officers showed what the drugs looked like or demonstrated the smell of burning marijuana, so that the kids would know what to avoid. Sometimes, especially in larger cities, a former addict went and described how easy it was to get "hooked," the horrible life of the junkie, and the horror of withdrawal symptoms. The 1960s saw more of that, plus the production of a large number of scary antidrug films.

There was also the awareness that teachers and counselors knew little about these substances, and many teachers attended courses taught by experts in the field. Some of the experts were enforcement-oriented and presented the traditional scare-tactics information, whereas others were pharmacologists who presented the "dry facts" about the classification and effects of various drugs. The teachers then brought many of these facts into their classrooms. It was later pointed out that the programs of this era were based on an assumed model: that providing information about drugs would increase the students' *knowledge* of drugs and their effects, that this increased knowledge would lead to changes in *attitudes* about drug use, and that these changed attitudes would be reflected in decreased drug-using *behavior*.[2]

In the early 1970s, this model began to be questioned. A 1971 study indicated that students who had more knowledge about drugs tended to have a more positive attitude toward drug use.[3] Of course, it may have been that prodrug students were more interested in learning about drugs, so this was not an actual assessment of the value of drug education programs. A 1973 report by the same group indicated that four different types of drug education programs were equally effective in producing increased knowledge about drugs and equally ineffective in altering attitudes or behavior.[4] Nationwide, <u>drug use had increased even with the increased emphasis on drug education.</u> There began to be concern about the possibility that drug education may even have contributed to increased drug use. After all, before the 1960s, the use of marijuana and LSD was rare among school-age youngsters. Most of them didn't know much about these things, had given them little thought, and had probably never considered using them. Telling them over and over not to use drugs was a bit like telling a young boy not to put beans in his nose. He probably hadn't thought of it before, and your warning gives him the idea. At least one study in 1972 found that junior high school students who were exposed to a "fact-oriented" course actually increased their experimentation with drugs.[5] These concerns led the federal government in 1973 to stop supporting the production of drug-abuse films and educational materials until it could determine what kinds of approaches would be effective.

At this point it seemed clear that the question of effectiveness depended greatly on the goals of the program. Did we want all students *never to experiment* with cigarettes, alcohol, marijuana, or other drugs? Or did we want students to be prepared to *make rational decisions* about drugs? For example, a 1976 report indicated that students in drug education programs did increase their use of drugs over the two years after the program, but they were less likely to show drastic escalation of the amount or type of drug use over that period, when compared with a control group.[6] Perhaps by giving the students information about drugs, we make them more likely to try them, but we also make them more aware of the dangers of excessive use. For a time in the 1970s, it seemed as though teaching students to make rational decisions about their own drug use with the goal of reducing the overall harm produced by misuse and abuse could be a possible goal of prevention programs.

Affective Education

Educators have been talking for several years about education as including both a "cognitive domain" and an "*affective* domain," the domain of emotions and attitudes. One reason that young people might use psychoactive drugs is to produce certain feelings: of excitement, of relaxation, of power, of being in control. Or perhaps a child might not really want to take drugs but does so after being influenced by others. Helping children know their own feelings and express them, helping them achieve altered emotional states without drugs, and teaching them to feel valued, accepted, and wanted are all presumed to be ways of reducing drug use.

Values Clarification

The values clarification approach makes the assumption that what is lacking in drug-using adolescents is not factual information about drugs but, rather, the ability to make appropriate decisions based on that information.[7] Perhaps drug use should not be "flagged" for the students by having special curricula designed just for drugs but, instead, emphasis should be placed on teaching generic decision-making skills. Teaching students to analyze and clarify their own values in life is accomplished by having them discuss their reactions to various situations that pose moral and ethical dilemmas. It should be pointed out that groups of parents or other citizens who are concerned about drug abuse sometimes have great difficulty understanding and accepting these approaches because they do not take a direct antidrug approach. In the 1970s, when these programs were first developed, it seemed important that the schools not try to impose a particular set of values but, rather, to allow for differences in religion, family background, and so on. For this reason, the programs were often said to be *value-free*. To many parents, the purpose of **values clarification** training is not immediately clear, and teaching young children to decide moral issues for themselves may run contrary to the particular set of values the parents want their children to learn.

Alternatives to Drugs

Along with values clarification, another aspect of affective education involves the teaching of **alternatives** to drug use (Table 4.1). Under the assumption that students might take drugs for the experience, for the altered states of consciousness that a drug might produce, students

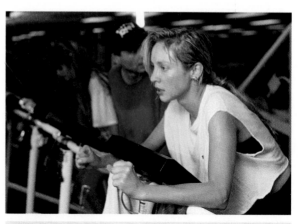

Adrenaline from exercise supplies a nondrug high.

are taught so-called natural highs, or altered states, that can be produced through relaxation exercises, meditation, vigorous exercise, or an exciting sport. Students are encouraged to try these things and to focus on the psychological changes that occur. These alternatives should be discussed with some degree of sensitivity to the audience; for example, it would make little sense to suggest to many inner-city 13-year-olds that such activities as scuba diving and snow skiing would be good alternatives to drugs.

Personal and Social Skills

Several studies indicate that adolescents who smoke, drink, or use marijuana also get lower grades and are less involved in organized sports or school clubs. One view of this is that students might take up substance use in response to personal or social failure. Therefore, teaching students how to communicate with others and

TABLE 4-1

Some Suggested Alternatives to Drug Use

Level of experience	Motives	Possible alternatives
Physical	Relaxation	Relaxation exercises
	Increased energy	Athletics, dancing
Sensory	Stimulation	Skydiving
	Magnify senses	Sensory awareness training
Interpersonal	Gain acceptance	Instruction in social customs
Spiritual/ mystical	Develop spiritual insight	Meditation

values clarification: teaching students to recognize and express their own feelings and beliefs.

alternatives: alternative nondrug activities, such as relaxation or dancing.

Taking Sides

Are "Alternatives to Drugs" Really Alternatives?

As one part of many drug education programs, students are taught that they can produce natural highs—that is, altered states of consciousness similar to those produced by drugs, but without using drugs.

One such alternative that has been mentioned in these programs is skydiving. Obviously an activity of that sort has all the glamour, danger, and excitement most of us would want. Maybe if the kids could do this whenever they wanted, they wouldn't want to try cocaine or marijuana. But let's examine this as an alternative for a bunch of junior high school kids. First, there's the matter of cost and availability. How realistic is it to think that most of these kids would have access to skydiving? Second, there's the issue of convenience. Even if you were a rich kid, with your own airplane, parachute, and pilot, it's unlikely that you'd be able to go skydiving every afternoon after school. Drugs and alcohol may not provide the best highs in the world, but often they are easy to get and use, compared with activities, such as skydiving.

Maybe skydiving isn't a *practical* alternative to drugs for a lot of people. Still, it seems more wholesome and desirable. Let's become social philosophers and ask ourselves why the image of a person skydiving is more positive than the image of a person snorting cocaine. After all, skydiving doesn't make any obvious contributions to society. Let's play devil's advocate and propose that skydiving is not preferable to taking cocaine. Either way, the person is engaged in dangerous, expensive, self-indulgent activity. Contrast skydiving with cocaine, and see if you can answer for yourself why skydiving has a more positive image than cocaine use. You may have to talk about this with several people before you get a consistent feeling for why our society respects one of these activities so much more than the other. What about skiing? bungee-cord jumping?

For more on this topic, log onto www.dushkin.com/online for current news and links to other popular and informative sites, as well as time-saving web search strategies and study tools.

---

giving them success experiences is another component of affective education approaches. For example, one exercise that has been used is having the students operate a school store. This is done as a group effort with frequent group meetings. The involved students are expected to develop a sense of social and personal competence without using drugs. Another approach is to have older students tutor younger students, which is designed to give the older students a sense of competence. An experiment carried out between 1978 and 1983 in Napa, California, combined these approaches with a drug education course, small-group discussions led by teachers, and classroom management techniques designed to teach discipline and communication skills and to enhance the students' self-concepts.[8] Although a small effect on alcohol, marijuana, and cigarette use was found among the girls, the effects were gone by the one-year follow-up.

"Just Say No!"

A 1984 review[9] of prevention studies concluded that

(1) most substance abuse prevention programs have not contained adequate evaluation components; (2) increased knowledge has virtually no impact on substance abuse or on intentions to smoke, drink, or use drugs; (3) affective education approaches appear to be experiential in their orientation and to place too little emphasis on the acquisition of skills necessary to increase personal and social competence, particularly those skills needed to enable students to resist the various interpersonal pressures to begin using drugs; and (4) few studies have demonstrated

any degree of success in terms of actual substance abuse prevention.

This last point is not entirely a criticism of the programs themselves but reflects the difficulty of demonstrating statistically significant changes in behavior over a period of time after the programs.

In response to the third point, that affective education approaches have been too general and experiential, the next efforts at preventing drug use focused on teaching students to recognize peer pressure to use drugs and on teaching specific ways to respond to such pressures without using drugs. This is sometimes referred to as psychological inoculation. In addition to the focus on substance use, "refusal skills" and "pressure resistance" strategies are taught in a broader context of self-assertion and social skills training. The first successful application of this technique was a film in which young actors acted out situations in which one person was being pressured to smoke cigarettes. The film then demonstrated effective ways of responding to the pressure gracefully without smoking. After the film, students discuss alternative strategies and practice the coping techniques presented in the film. This approach has been demonstrated to be successful in reducing cigarette smoking in adolescent populations. It has been adapted for use with groups of various ages and for a wider variety of drugs and other behaviors, and students are taught from kindergarten on to "just say no" when someone is trying to get them to do something they know is wrong.

Drug-Free Schools

In 1986, under the direction of then Secretary of Education William J. Bennett, the federal government launched a massive program to support "drug-free schools and communities." Among other things, the government provided millions of dollars' worth of direct aid to local school districts to implement or enhance drug-prevention activities. Along with this, the Department of Education produced a small book called *What Works: Schools Without Drugs,*[10] which made specific recommendations for schools to follow. This book did not recommend a specific curriculum, and in fact its most significant feature was the emphasis on factors other than curriculum, such as school policies on drug and alcohol use. There were suggestions for policies regarding locker searches, suspension, and expulsion of students. The purpose was not so much to take a punitive approach to alcohol or drug use as to point out through example and official policy that the school and community were opposed to drug and alcohol use by minors. Following this general drug-free lead, schools adopted "tobacco-free" policies, stating that not only the students but also teachers and other staff people were not to use tobacco products at school or on school-sponsored trips or activities.

According to this approach, the curriculum should include teaching about the laws against drugs, as well as about the school policies. In other words, as opposed to the 1970s values clarification approach of teaching students how to make responsible decisions for themselves, this approach wants to make it clear to the students that the society at large, the community in which they live, and the school in which they study have already made the decision not to condone drug use or underage alcohol use. This seems to be part of a more general educational trend away from "value-free" schools toward teaching values that are generally accepted in our society. For schools to be eligible for federal Drug-Free Schools funding, they must certify that their program teaches that "illicit drug use is wrong and harmful."

Peer Counseling

Several formalized programs have been developed for the selection and training of respected student leaders to be made available as "peer counselors" to discuss problems other students may be having. Usually the students are selected for such programs after being nominated by other students or by teachers or counselors. It is best to try to recruit respected students from various social groups in the school (i.e., they shouldn't all be "jocks" or student council leaders). The students are then given training in listening skills, in ways to limit the advice or suggestions they provide, and in the resources available for referral of serious problems.

Development of the Social Influence Model

Some of the most sophisticated prevention research in recent years has been focused directly on cigarette smoking in adolescents. This problem has two major advantages over other types of drug use, as far as prevention research is concerned. First, a large enough fraction of adolescents do smoke cigarettes so that measurable behavior change is possible in a group of subjects of reasonable size. In contrast, one would have to perform an intervention with tens of thousands of people before significant alterations in the proportion of heroin users would be statistically evident. Second, the health consequences of smoking are so clear with respect to cancer and heart disease that there is a fairly good consensus over goals: we'd like to prevent adolescents from becoming smokers at all. One research advantage is that there is a relatively simple verification available for self-reported use of tobacco: saliva samples can be measured for cotinine, a nicotine metabolite.

Virtually all the various approaches to drug-abuse prevention have been tried with smoking behavior; in fact, Evans's 1976 smoking prevention paper introduced the use of the psychological inoculation approach based on the **social influence model.**[11] Out of all this research, certain consistencies appear. The most important of these is that it *is* possible to design smoking prevention programs that are effective in reducing the number of adolescents who begin smoking.

Some practical lessons about the components of those programs have also emerged.[12] For example, presenting information about the delayed consequences of smoking (possible lung cancer many years later) is relatively ineffective. Information about the immediate physiological effects (increased heart rate, shortness of breath) is included instead. Some of the most important key elements that were shown to be effective were the following:

1. *Training refusal skills* (for example, eight ways to say no). This was originally based on films demonstrating the kinds of social pressures that peers might use to encourage smoking and modeling a variety of appropriate responses. Then the students engage in role-playing exercises in which they practice these refusal skills. By using such techniques as changing the subject or having a good excuse handy, students learn to refuse to "cooperate" without being negative. When all else fails, however, they are taught to be assertive and insist on their right to refuse.

2. *Public commitment.* Researchers found that having each child stand before his or her peers and promise not to start smoking and sign a pledge not to smoke are effective prevention techniques.

3. *Countering advertising.* Students are shown examples of cigarette advertising, and then the "hidden messages" are discussed (young, attractive, healthy, active models are typically used; cigarette smoking might be associated with dating or with sports). Then the logical inconsistencies between these hidden messages and the actual effects of cigarette smoking (e.g., bad breath, yellow teeth, shortness of breath) are pointed out. The purpose of this is to "inoculate" the children against cigarette advertising by teaching them to question its messages.

4. *Normative education.* Adolescents tend to overestimate the proportion of their peers who smoke. Presenting factual information about

the smoking practices of adolescents provides students with a more realistic picture of the true social norms regarding smoking and reduces the "everybody is doing it" attitude. When possible, statistics on smoking from the specific school or community should be used in presenting this information.

5
• *Use of teen leaders.* Presenting dry facts about the actual proportion of smokers should ideally be reinforced by example. If you're presenting the program to junior high students, it's one thing to *say* that fewer than one-fifth of the high school students in that community smoke, but it's another to bring a few high school students into the room and have them discuss the fact that neither they nor their friends smoke, their attitudes about smokers, and ways they have dealt with others' attempts to get them to smoke.

Possible improvements to those approaches are offered by the *cognitive developmental* approach to smoking behavior. McCarthy[13] has criticized the social influence/social skills training model for assuming that all students should be taught social skills or refusal skills without regard to whether they need such training. The model "is that of a defenseless teenager who, for lack of general social skills or refusal skills, passively accedes to social pressures to smoke." An alternative model[14] has been proposed in which the individual makes active, conscious decisions about smoking as part of a process of defining herself or himself as a person experimenting with smoking, as a person becoming a smoker, or as a confirmed smoker. The decision-making processes, and thus the appropriate prevention strategy, might be different at each of these "stages of cognitive development" as a smoker. Furthermore, smokers who begin smoking very young behave differently than smokers who begin as older adolescents (e.g., those who start young show more unanimity in selecting the most popular brand).[13] Given what is known about cognitive and social development, per-

haps programs should be tailored for the age group being targeted and for various stages in the development of smoking behavior. This model would not replace the social influence methods, which have been shown to be effective, but would modify them to take into account individual differences in smoking-related attitudes and behavior.

DARE

Perhaps the most amazing educational phenomenon in a long time had fairly modest beginnings in 1983 as a joint project of the Los Angeles police department and school district. Those who are familiar with the Drug Abuse Resistance Education (**DARE**) program will have recognized its components described under the social influence model of smoking cessation. The difference here is that the educational program with DARE is delivered by police officers in fifth- and sixth-grade classrooms. By basing the curriculum on sound educational research, by maintaining strict training standards for the officers who were to present the curriculum, and by encouraging the classroom teacher to participate, some of the old barriers to having nonteachers responsible for curriculum were overcome. The officers are in uniform, and they use interactive techniques as described for the social influence model. Most of the components are there: refusal skills, teen leaders, and a public commitment not to use illicit drugs. In addition, some of the affective education components are included: self-esteem building, alternatives to drug use, and decision making. The component on consequences of drug abuse is, no doubt, enhanced by the presence of a uniformed officer who can serve as an information

social influence model: a prevention model adopted from successful smoking programs.

Drugs in Depth

How Much Do You Know About DARE?

1. Almost everyone in the United State has heard of DARE. What do the letters stand for?
2. One component of DARE is practicing how to refuse using drugs. Do you know the origin of DARE's eight ways to say no?
3. DARE has been implemented in more schools than any other substance-abuse prevention program. Does research on its effectiveness show that it's one of the best at preventing drug abuse?
4. Besides school-based programs, what other kinds of substance-abuse prevention programs have been developed?
5. The Institute of Medicine has a relatively new way of categorizing prevention programs into various types. Do you know what factor is used to differentiate among the types?

Answers
1. Drug Abuse Resistance Education
2. This and most components of DARE were adopted from smoking prevention programs developed in the 1970s.
3. Research on the effectiveness of DARE has not demonstrated a strong impact on preventing drug use. Other programs described in this chapter appear to be more effective.
4. Parent, family, and community programs and public media campaigns have also been developed to prevent drug abuse.
5. The target population (the entire population, at-risk populations, and individuals with early signs of problems)

source and symbol for concerns over gang activity and violence and can discuss arrest and incarceration. The 17-week program is capped by a commencement assembly at which certificates are awarded.

This program happened to be in place at just the right time, both financially and politically. With the assistance of drug-free schools money and with nationwide enthusiasm for new drug-prevention activities in the 1980s, the program spread rapidly across the United States. By 1988, there were more than 500 programs in 38 states, reaching 1.5 million students annually. By the early 1990s, DARE programs were found in every state, and the federal Drug-Free Schools and Communities reauthorization bill of 1991 mandated that 10 percent of each state's share of the funds be used to support DARE.

The interesting thing about this program is that it was accepted so quickly by so many schools, and it is endorsed enthusiastically by educators, students, parents, and police participants. All this has occurred in spite of the fact that DARE's effectiveness in preventing drug use was not evaluated extensively until 1994. A review of this phenomenon pointed out that the program's expansion was due to meeting the needs of the communities, agencies, school districts, and officials to conduct prevention activities rather than in demonstrating an impact on drug use.[15] In 1994, two important, large-scale studies of the effects of DARE were reported. One was based on a longitudinal study in rural, suburban, and urban schools in Illinois, comparing students exposed to DARE with students who were not.[16] Although the program had some effects on reported self-esteem, there was no evidence for long-term reductions in self-reported use of drugs. The other report was based on a review of eight smaller outcome evaluations of DARE, selected from 18 evaluations based on whether the reports had a control group, a pretest-posttest design, and reliable outcome measures.[17]

The overall impact of these eight programs was to increase drug knowledge and knowledge

Drugs in Depth

Effective Prevention Programs

The Center for Substance Abuse Prevention (CSAP), a branch of the Substance Abuse and Mental Health Administration in the U.S. Department of Health and Human Services, has been studying research on effective prevention programs. Now it is developing a list of successful programs. Some of those on the list are described within this chapter, and more information on the others can be obtained from the SAMHSA website. Also, as new programs are approved, they are being added to the list, so for the most current list it is best to check on the web at www.samhsa.gov/csap.

Model Programs

- Across Ages
- Athletes Training and Learning to Avoid Steroids (ATLAS)
- Child Development Project
- Communities Mobilizing for Change on Alcohol
- Creating Lasing Connections
- Dare to Be You
- Family Advocacy Network
- Keep a Clear Mind
- Life Skills Training
- Project ALERT
- Project Northland
- Project STAR
- Project Toward No Tobacco Use
- Reconnecting At-Risk Youth
- Residential Student Assistance Program
- SMART Leaders
- SMART Team
- Stop Teenage Addiction to Tobacco
- Strengthening Families Program

popularity. Communities have not abandoned the program. Instead, DARE America has encouraged additional programming outside the original fifth- or sixth-grade. "Booster" programs in junior high and high school, and introductions at earlier grades, are becoming more and more common.

Programs That Work

Several school-based drug-use prevention programs have been modeled after the successful social influence model and have components similar to those of DARE. A few of these programs have now been demonstrated to have beneficial effects on actual drug use:

Project ALERT was first tested in 30 junior high schools in California and Oregon.[18] The program targeted cigarette smoking, alcohol use, and marijuana use. Before the program, each student was surveyed and classified as a nonuser, an experimenter, or a user for each of the three substances. The curriculum was taught either by health educators or by educators with the assistance of trained teen leaders. Control schools simply continued whatever health or drug curriculum they had been using. The program was delivered in the seventh grade, and follow-up surveys were done 3, 12, and 15 months later. Three "booster" lessons were given in the eighth grade.

The program surprisingly had no measurable effect on initiation of smoking by nonusers. However, those who were cigarette experimenters before the program began were more likely to quit or to maintain low rates of smoking than the control group. The group with teen leader support showed the largest reduction: 50 percent fewer students were weekly smokers at the 15-month follow-up.

about social skills, but the effects on drug use were marginal at best. There was a very small but statistically significant reduction of tobacco use and no reliable effect on alcohol or marijuana use. The repeated failures to demonstrate an impact of the DARE program on drug use remain a dilemma in light of its widespread

DARE: Drug Abuse Resistance Education, the most popular prevention program in schools.

The experimental groups drank less alcohol soon after the program was presented, for previous alcohol nonusers, experimenters, and users. However, this effect diminished over time and disappeared by the end of the study.

The most consistent results were in reducing initiation of marijuana smoking and reducing levels of marijuana smoking. For example, among those who were marijuana nonusers at the beginning, about 12 percent of the control-group students had begun using marijuana by the 15-month follow-up. In the treatment groups, only 8 percent began using during that time period, representing a one-third decrease in initiation to marijuana use.

Another program, the Life Skills Training program, has been subjected to several tests and has shown long-term positive results. This three-year program is based on the social influence model and teaches resistance skills, normative education, and media influences. Self-management skills and general social skills are also included. One study of this program found significantly lower use of marijuana, alcohol, and tobacco after six years. A subsequent application of this program among ethnic minority youth (Latino and African American) in New York City found reduced use on a two-year follow-up.[19]

PEERS, PARENTS, AND THE COMMUNITY

Our nation's public schools clearly are the most convenient conduit for attempts to achieve widespread social changes among young people, and that is why most efforts at drug-abuse prevention have been carried out there. However, there has also been a recognition that peers, parents, and the community at large also exert powerful social influences on young people. Because these groups are less accessible than the schools, there have been fewer prevention programs based on using parent and community influences. Never-

theless, important efforts have been made in all these areas.

Peer Programs

Most peer programs have taken place in the school setting, but some have used youth-oriented community service programs (such as YMCA, YWCA, and recreation centers) or have focused on "street" youth by using them in group community service projects.

- *Peer influence* approaches start with the assumption that the opinions of an adolescent's peers are significant influences on the adolescent's behavior. Often using an adult group facilitator/coordinator, the program's emphasis is on open discussion among a group of children or adolescents. These discussions might focus on drugs, with the peer group discussing dangers and alternatives, or they might simply have the more general goal of building positive group cohesiveness, a sense of belonging, and communication skills.
- *Peer participation* programs often focus on groups of youth in high-risk areas. The idea here is that young people participate in making important decisions and in doing significant work, either as "peers" with cooperating adults or in programs managed almost entirely by the youth themselves. Sometimes participants are paid for community service work, in other cases they engage in money-making businesses, and sometimes they provide youth-oriented information services. These groups almost never focus on drug use in any significant way; rather, the idea is to help people become participating members of society.

The benefits of these "extracurricular" peer approaches are measurable in terms of acquired skills, improved academic success, higher self-esteem, and a more positive attitude toward

Try It!

Does Your Family Function Well?

If you are a parent, think about your own family for a moment. Several of the risk and protective factors mentioned in Chapter 2 are related to family, and some of the effective prevention strategies target family activities. Consider the following questions (they can be answered either from the perspective of a child or a parent).

1. Is the interaction between the parent(s) and child generally positive? *yeah*
2. Do the parents provide attention and praise to the child? *one does*
3. Is discipline consistent and usually effective and never involves physical punishment? *TRUE*
4. Is the child able to communicate his or her feelings to the parent(s)? *NO*
5. Does the child feel comfortable discussing rules and consequences, especially when it comes to the use of substances or other inappropriate behavior? *NO*
6. Does the family spend time together doing things every week? *yeah*
7. Is the family capable of planning and organizing family activities? *yeah*

If the answer to most of these questions is yes, then your family is probably functioning pretty well. If the answer to most of them is no, then think about what steps you can take to change this situation. That might include scheduling some time with a family therapist or counselor.

peers and school. As to whether they alter drug use significantly, the data either are not available or are inconclusive for the most part.

Parent and Family Programs

The various programs that have worked with parents have been described as taking at least one of four approaches.[20] Most of the programs include more than one of these approaches.

- *Informational* programs provide parents with basic information about alcohol and drugs, as well as information about their use and effects. Although the parents often want to know simply what to look for, how to tell if their child is using drugs, and what the consequences of drug abuse are, the best programs provide additional information. One important piece of information is the actual extent of the use of various types of drugs among young people. Another goal might be to make parents aware of their own alcohol and drug use to gain a broader perspective of the issue. A basic rationale is that well-informed parents will be able to teach appropriate attitudes about drugs, beginning when their child is young, and will be better able to recognize potential problems relating to drug or alcohol use.
- *Parenting skills* might be taught through practical training programs. Communication with children, decision-making skills, how to set goals and limits, and when and how to say no to your child can be learned in the abstract and then practiced in role-playing exercises. One risk factor for adolescent drug and alcohol use is poor family relationships, and improving family interaction and strengthening communication can help prevent alcohol and drug abuse.
- *Parent support groups* can be important adjuncts to skills training or in planning community efforts. Groups of parents meet regularly to discuss problem solving, parent-

ing skills, their perceptions of the problem, actions to be taken, and so on.
- *Family interaction* approaches call for families to work as a unit to examine, discuss, and confront issues relating to alcohol and drug use. Other exercises might include more general problem solving or response to emergencies. Not only do these programs attempt to improve family communication, but also the parents are placed in the roles of teacher of drug facts and coordinator of family action, thus strengthening their knowledge and skills.

One selective prevention program, called the Strengthening Families program, targets children of parents who are substance abusers. This program has been successfully implemented several times within diverse populations. It has three major goals: improving parenting skills, increasing children's skills, (such as communication skills, refusal skills, awareness of feelings, and emotion expression skills), and improving family relationships (decreasing conflict, improving communication, increasing parent-child time together, and increasing the planning and organizational skills of the family). Children and parents attend evening sessions weekly for 14 weeks to learn and practice these skills. Evaluations of this program indicate that it reduces tobacco and alcohol use in the children as well as reduces substance abuse and other problems in the parents.[21]

Community Programs

There are two basic reasons for trying to organize prevention programs at the community level. The first is that a coordinated approach using schools, parent and peer groups, civic organizations, police, newspapers, radio, and television can have a much greater impact than an isolated program that occurs only in the school, for example. Another reason is that drug-abuse prevention and drug education are controversial and emotional topics. Parents might question

Exploring Your Spirituality

Integrating Treatment and Prevention with Pregnancy Services

Does your community provide needed services and compassionate support for pregnant women who use alcohol and drugs? An emerging consensus views alcohol, tobacco, and other drug use during pregnancy as a community problem. During this period when women anticipate major life change, prevention initiatives can enhance their motivation to have a healthy baby. And, for women with substance-abuse problems, pregnancy provides a similarly strong motivation to seek help.

Fear of blame, legal intervention, and loss of child custody prevent many women from getting help. To counteract these barriers to services, prevention initiatives should promote services that are safe and confidential. Services should be not only physically accessible but also culturally accessible. Efforts that recognize the importance of relationships to women can call on the support of family members and others for alcohol-free and other drug-free pregnancies. Prevention strategies that combine information with options for change have shown promising results in reducing drug use during pregnancy.

Find out if women in your area have access to an integrated system of alcohol, tobacco, and other drug treatment and maternal and child health care. An example is the Women's and Infants Clinic at Boston City Hospital, which since 1989 has provided pediatric care, child development services, and drug-abuse treatment services in an integrated service system.

encourages cooperation between the police and the schools, as well as encourages parental involvement.

Community-based programs can bring other resources to bear. For example, the city council and local businesses can be involved in sponsoring alcohol-free parties, developing recreational facilities, and arranging field trips so that, when the school-based program talks about alternatives, the alternatives are available. The public media can be enlisted not only to publicize public meetings and programs but also to present drug- and alcohol-related information that reinforces what is learned in the other programs.

Project STAR (Students Taught Awareness and Resistance) began as a school-based prevention model in Kansas City, Missouri, and was later extended into the community at large. It includes teacher training and curriculum implementation in the schools, a parent program, a media program, organization of community agencies, and health policy changes (such as restricting smoking in public places, supporting drug-free workplace policies, requiring proof of age for purchase of tobacco or alcohol, and supporting neighborhood watch groups). The Kansas City program had measurable effects on reducing alcohol, tobacco, and marijuana use, and some of these effects extended for as long as five years following the beginning of the project. A replication of this school- and community-based program in Indianapolis, Indiana, produced similar positive results. STAR is now recognized as an effective program and has been implemented in other communities.

Prevention in the Workplace

As a part of its efforts to reduce the demand for drugs, the federal government has encouraged private employers, especially those who do business with the government, to adopt policies to prevent drug use by their employees. Increasingly, these policies include random urine screens. In

the need for or the methods used in drug education programs in the schools. Jealousy and mistrust about approaches can separate schools, police, church, and parent groups. A program that starts by involving all these groups in the planning stages is more likely to receive widespread community support. Clearly, the spread of the DARE program in the schools is based partly on the fact that it demonstrates and

1989, rules went into effect requiring all companies and organizations that obtain grants or contracts from the federal government to adopt a "drug-free workplace" plan. The exact nature of the plan is up to the company, but guidelines were produced by the Department of Labor. Modeled after the Education Department's "What Works" book, the Labor Department's is called *What Works: Workplaces Without Drugs.*[22] At a minimum, the Labor Department expects employers to state clearly that drug use on the job is unacceptable and to notify employees of the consequences of violating company policy regarding drug use. The ultimate goal is not to catch drug users and fire them but to prevent drug use by making it clear that it is not condoned.

WHAT SHOULD WE BE DOING?

By now you have picked up some ideas for things to do to reduce drug use, as well as some things to avoid doing. But the answer as to what needs to be done in a particular situation depends on the motivations for doing it. Most states require drug- and alcohol-abuse prevention education as part of a health curriculum, for example. If that is the primary motive for doing something, and if there doesn't seem to be a particular problem with substance abuse in the schools, then the best thing would be to adopt one of the modern school-based programs that have been developed for this purpose, to make sure the teachers and other participants are properly trained in it, and to go ahead. In selecting from among the curricula, a sensible, balanced approach that combines some factual information with social skills training, perhaps integrated into the more general themes of health, personal values, and decision making, would be appropriate. The two mentioned in the section "Programs That Work" fit this general description, and each deserves a careful look. Above all, avoid sensational scare stories, preachy approaches from the teacher to the student, and untrained personnel developing their

HealthQuest Activities

In Modules 8, 9. and 10, you will find the "Stages of Change." Complete all three modules. These activities will assess the level of your dependence on drugs, alcohol, and tobacco. Each assessment will also provide you with specific advice, according to your results. If you have a healthy approach to these substances, the assessment encourages you to maintain your healthy lifestyle. If you have an addiction or are near to having one, the assessment gives you advice on how to solve the problem.

own curricula. Another good thing to avoid is the inadvertent demonstration of how to do things you don't want students to do.

If, on the other hand, there is a public outcry about the "epidemic" of drugs and alcohol abuse in the community, speakers have inflamed passions, and there is a widespread fervor to do something about it," this presents both a danger and an opportunity. The danger is that this passionate group might attack and undermine the efforts already being made in the schools, substituting scary, preachy, negative approaches, which can have negative consequences. The opportunity lies in the possibility that this energy can be organized into a community planning effort, out of which could develop cooperation, increased parent understanding, a focus on family communication, interest in the lives of the community's young people, and increased recreational and creative opportunities.

The key to making this happen is convincing the aroused citizenry of the possibly negative consequences of doing what seems obvious and selling them on the idea of studying what needs to be done. A good place to start is by visiting the website of the Center for Substance Abuse Prevention (www.samhsa.gov/csap). This agency produces updated materials for groups interested in developing drug- and alcohol-abuse prevention programs, provides technical assistance and training to communities interested in developing programs, and offers Community Partnership Grants. (A list of CSAP model programs was shown in the Drugs in Depth box on p. 77.)

SUMMARY

- We can distinguish between education programs with the goal of imparting knowledge and prevention programs aimed at modifying drug-using behavior.
- Most of the research over the past 30 years has failed to demonstrate that prevention programs can produce clear, meaningful, long-lasting effects on drug-using behavior.
- The affective education programs of the 1970s have been criticized for being too value-free.
- Based on the success of the social influence model in reducing cigarette smoking, a variety of school-based prevention programs have used the same techniques with illicit drugs.
- The DARE program has been adopted rapidly and widely, in spite of limited research evaluating its impact on drug-using behavior.
- Current school-based approaches use refusal skills, countering advertising, public commitments, and teen leaders. Several of these programs have been demonstrated to be effective.
- Other nonschool programs are peer-based through after-school groups or activities, parent-based through parent and family training, or community-based.

REVIEW QUESTIONS

1. What is the distinction between secondary and tertiary prevention?

    follow up prog. fro previous users |*people who HAVE tried the drug*

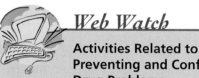

Web Watch

Activities Related to Preventing and Confronting Drug Problems

Find Out About Drug Abuse USA
Go to www.drug-abuse.com/. Read about the Drug Abuse USA organization, which seeks to educate, to prevent drug abuse, and to help those dealing with substance abuse. This Web Page has links, membership information, statistics on drug and alcohol abuse, and information on state-by-state assistance.

Can You Confront a Friend?
At www.mayohealth.org/mayo/9707/htm/alcohol.htm, read the articles "Alcoholism—Taking Off the Blinders," "Confronting an Alcoholic," and "Getting Treatment for Alcoholism or Alcohol Abuse." You'll discover characteristics of those struggling with an alcohol-related problem. You'll also find suggestions and processes for confronting and treating friends and family members who are dealing with alcohol abuse or alcoholism.

Deal with Your Drug Problem
Check out the Problem Page at www.antibully.org. uk/problem.htm. This is an advice page where young people send in queries about their drug-related problems. Advice is provided as a response. If you have any questions or are dealing with a specific drug-related problem and don't feel comfortable talking with someone in person, consider writing to an online advice page like this one for help.

2. What is the knowledge-attitudes-behavior model, and what information first called it into question? *70's kids knew more about drugs & had Pos. Att. toward them*
3. What were three of the training approaches used in values clarification programs?
4. Distinguish between student assistance programs and peer counseling.
5. What were the five successful components of the social influence model for smoking prevention? *pg 74*

6. In Project ALERT, what was the impact of using teen leaders to assist the instructors?

7. What distinguishes DARE from other similar programs based on the social influence model?

8. What do ALERT and Life Skills Training have in common, besides their effectiveness?

9. What are some of the "parenting" skills that might be taught and practiced in a prevention program?

10. What is the drug-free workplace plan?

REFERENCES

1. National Institute on Drug Abuse: *Drug abuse prevention for the general population.* Washington, DC: U.S. Department of Health and Human Services, 1997.

2. Goodstadt MS: Alcohol and drug education: Models and outcomes, *Health Education Monographs* 6:263–278, 1978.

3. Swisher JD and others: Drug education: Pushing or preventing? *Peabody Journal of Education* 49:68–75, 1971.

4. Swisher JD and others: A comparison of four approaches to drug abuse prevention at the college level, *Journal of College Student Personnel* 14:231–235, 1973.

5. Drug education is linked to use, *New York Times,* Dec 3, 1972.

6. Blum RH, Blum E, Garfield E: *Drug education: Results and recommendations,* Lexington, MA: D.C. Heath, 1976.

7. Swisher JD: Prevention issues. In DuPont RI, Goldstein A, O'Donnell J, editors: *Handbook on drug abuse.* Washington, DC: NIDA, U.S. Government Printing Office, 1979.

8. Schaps E and others: *The Napa drug abuse prevention project: Research findings.* Washington, DC: DHHS Pub No (ADM)84-1339, U.S. Government Printing Office, 1984.

9. Prevention research. In *Drug abuse and drug abuse research,* Washington, DC: DHHS Pub No (ADM)85-1372, U.S. Government Printing Office, 1984.

10. U.S. Department of Education: *What works: Schools without drugs,* Washington, DC: 1987.

11. Evans RI: Smoking in children: Developing a social psychological strategy of deterrence, *Preventive Medicine* 5:122–127, 1976.

12. Flay BR: What we know about the social influences approach to smoking prevention: Review and recommendations. In Bell CS, Battjes R, editors: *Prevention research: Deterring drug abuse among children and adolescents.* Washington, DC: NIDA Research Monograph 63, DHHS Pub No (ADM)85-1334, U.S. Government Printing Office, 1985.

13. McCarthy WJ: The cognitive developmental model and other alternatives to the social skills deficit model of smoking onset. In Bell CS, Battjes R, editors: *Prevention research: Deterring drug abuse among children and adolescents.* Washington, DC: NIDA Research Monograph 63, DHHS Pub No (ADM)85-1334, U.S. Government Printing Office, 1985.

14. Glynn K, Leventhal H, Hirschman R: A cognitive developmental approach to smoking prevention. In Bell CS, Battjes R, editors: *Prevention research: Deterring drug abuse among children and adolescents.* Washington, DC: NIDA Research Monograph 63, DHHS Pub No (ADM)85-1334, U.S. Government Printing Office, 1985.

15. Aniskiewicz R, Wysong E: Evaluating DARE: Drug education and the multiple meanings of success, *Policy Studies Review* 9:727–747, 1990.

16. Ennet ST and others: Long-term evaluation of Drug Abuse Resistance Education, *Addictive Behaviors* 19:113, 1994.

17. Ennett ST and others: How effective is Drug Abuse Resistance Education? A meta-analysis of Project DARE outcome evaluations, *American Journal of Public Health* 84:1394, 1994.

18. Ellickson PL, Bell RM: Drug prevention in junior high: A multi-site longitudinal test, *Science* 247:1299–1305, 1990.

19. Botvin GJ, Schinke SP: Effectiveness of culturally focused and generic skills training approaches to alcohol and drug abuse prevention among minority adolescents: Two-year follow-up results, *Psychology of Addictive Behaviors* 9:183, 1995.

20. Parent education. In *Prevention plus: Involving schools, parents, and the community in alcohol and drug education.* Washington, DC: DHHS Pub No (ADM)84-1256, U.S. Government Printing Office, 1984.

21. National Institute on Drug Abuse: *Drug abuse prevention for at-risk groups.* U.S. Department of Health and Human Services, 1997.

22. U.S. Department of Labor: *What works: Workplaces without drugs.* Washington, DC: 1989.

Chapter 5

Drug Regulations

Online Learning Center Resources

www.mhhe.com/ray

Log on to our Online Learning Center (OLC) for access to these additional resources.

- Chapter key terms and definitions
- Learning objectives
- Additional behavior change objectives
- Student interactive questions and answer sites
- Self-scoring chapter quiz

The OLC also offers web links for study and exploration of health topics. Here are some examples of what you'll find:

www.napra.org/ndsac/fedleg/ fdrindex.html

The *Food and Drug Regulations Index* includes information about administration, drugs, vitamins, amino acids, minerals, controlled and restricted drugs, public protection, pharmacies, pharmacists and practices, and federal legislation.

www.holistic-online.com/Herbal-Med/hol_herbalmed-drugreg.htm

At this site, you can read the article "Drug Regulation Today in the United States." This article addresses herbal products, food supplements, and FDA regulations. It compares U.S. regulations to the herbal markets in Europe and Asia.

Drugs in the Media

Is Media Coverage of New Prescription Drugs Too Rosy?

Until fairly recently, U.S. pharmaceutical companies weren't allowed to advertise prescription drugs directly to consumers, so the companies placed their advertising in medical journals. After all, these drugs cannot be obtained by the consumer unless prescribed by a physician. A

Drugs in the Media Continued. . .

few years ago, however, some companies began running ads that did not mention a drug but referred to certain medical conditions, such as baldness or erectile dysfunction, and suggested that consumers talk to their doctors. In 1997, the Federal Drug Administration began to allow commercials on radio and television to mention drugs by name. The ads must also mention the most important warnings and possible side effects associated with the drug. While such brief messages cannot provide complete information about the risks, costs, and benefits of new drugs, they may sway consumers' and physicians' demand for a drug.

In many ways, news coverage of new drugs has the same deficiencies as advertising. *A New England Journal of Medicine* study published in May 2000 found that most news stories do not fully convey the risks and cost of drugs. When a medical breakthrough is announced, fame for investigators and their institutions, future research grants, and corporate profits are often at stake, so reporters are barraged with daily news releases, expert testimonials, and public relations phone calls, which can cloud news judgment. Enthusiastic reporters may not be skeptical about what they read and may not put the benefits of a drug in context. For example they may paint a drug as providing a big breakthrough when in reality it decreases a disease's mortality rate by only a few percentage points. Overstating drug benefits can create demand among consumers, with the possible effect of physicians writing prescriptions for expensive drugs with potentially harmful side effects.

Watch for drug advertisements and news stories for several days, and check for answers to these questions: Does the ad make it clear what disease or condition the drug treats? What kinds of conditions seem to be most common among advertised prescription drugs? Does the ad's list of side effects and warnings sound potentially worse than the disorder being treated? In a news story, do you think the reporter gave a balance picture of the benefits and risks of the medication covered? How do you think your physician would react to your suggesting that he or she prescribe a specific drug?

Once upon a time in the United States, there weren't any regulations about drug use—at least there weren't any federal regulations. That lasted for about two years. In 1791, Congress passed an excise tax on whiskey, which resulted in a disagreement that historians call the Whiskey Rebellion. West of the Appalachian Mountains, where most whiskey was made, the farmers refused to pay the tax and tarred and feathered revenue officers who tried to collect it. In 1794, President George Washington called in the militia, which occupied counties in western Pennsylvania and sent prisoners to Philadelphia for trial. The militia and the federal government carried the day. The Whiskey Rebellion was an important test for the new government because it clearly established that the federal government had the power to enforce federal laws within the states.

In Chapter 2, we saw that drug regulations are passed mainly for what is perceived to be the public good. As the story of the laws and regulations about drugs unfolds, it will become clear that most of the debate centers on the question "What is the public good?" Issues of fact, morality, health, personal choice, and social order are intertwined—and sometimes confused. It should surprise no one that our laws about drug use resemble a patchwork quilt reflecting the many social changes that have occurred in this country. If we want to understand our current drug laws, we must see how they have evolved over the years in response to one social crisis after another.

THE BEGINNINGS

Reformism

The current federal approaches to drug regulation can be traced to two pieces of legislation passed in 1906 and 1914. Any student of American history will remember that the nation was moving out of the gilded age of *laissez-faire* capitalism into the reform area, in which legislation was passed regulating business and labor practices, meat packing, and food production. We should also remember that this general movement toward improvement of our nation's moral character was to bring us, in 1919, a constitutional amendment prohibiting the sale of alcoholic beverages. Theodore Roosevelt was president from 1901 to 1909 and continued to be influential after that time; his role in involving the federal government in both foreign treaties and domestic regulations was crucial to the development of these early drug laws.

Problems Leading to Legislation

The trend toward reform was given direction and energy by the public discussion of several drug-related problems, and those first laws reflected the problems that fueled their passage. Opium smoking among the Chinese, morphinism, cocaine use, and the peddlers of patent medicines provided the basic fuel used by political figures and newspapers to fire public opinion.

Opium and the Chinese

The roots of the Chinese opium smoking and the history of the Opium Wars are discussed in Chapter 16. It is important, however, to say that

in the mid-1800s many British and some American merchants were engaged in the lucrative sale of opium to the Chinese, and many reformers and world leaders disapproved. In 1833, the United States signed its first treaty agreeing to control international trade in opium, and regulatory tax on crude opium imported into this country was legislated in 1842.

The United States imported Chinese workers after the Civil War, mainly to help build the rapidly expanding railroads, and some of these people brought with them the habit of smoking opium. As always happens when a new pleasure is introduced into a society, the practice of opium smoking spread rapidly. Also, as always happens, the new practice upset the status quo and caused society to react. A contemporary report in 1882 described both the spread of opium smoking in San Francisco and the reactions it elicited:

> The practice spread rapidly and quietly among this class of gamblers and prostitutes until the latter part of 1875, at which time the authorities became cognizant of the fact, and finding . . . that many women and young girls, as also young men of respectable family, were being induced to visit the dens, where they were ruined morally and otherwise, a city ordinance was passed forbidding the practice under the penalty of a heavy fine or imprisonment, or both. Many arrests were made, and the punishment was prompt and thorough.[1]

This 1875 San Francisco ordinance was the first U.S. law forbidding opium smoking. In 1882, New York State passed a similar law aimed at opium use in New York City's expanding Chinatown. An 1890 federal act permitted only American citizens to import opium or to manufacture smoking opium in the United States. Although this law is sometimes viewed as a racist policy, it was partly in response to an 1887 agreement with China, which also forbade American citizens from engaging in the Chinese opium trade.

As more states and municipalities outlawed opium dens, the cost of black-market opium increased, and many of the lower-class opium addicts took up morphine or heroin, which were readily available and inexpensive.

Morphinism

The *hypodermic syringe* was introduced to the United States in 1856 and used on a large scale during the Civil War. Injecting **morphine**, the primary active ingredient in opium, gave nearly immediate relief from pain. Morphine was used widely, but not always wisely, in the treatment of the two major afflictions in the Civil War—pain and dysentery. So many soldiers became addicted to morphine that morphinism was called the "soldier's disease" or the "army disease" in the years after the war. By the turn of the twentieth century, most physicians, especially those who were younger and better trained, had become aware of the danger of morphine addiction and were much more conservative in their use of this drug.

Cocaine

Pure **cocaine** also became available at about the same time as the hypodermic needle, and physicians experimented with its many uses. Cocaine was widely touted as a cure for morphine addiction, and many physicians prescribed cocaine injections for this purpose. Within a few years it was clear that cocaine was itself habit forming and that in high enough doses a dramatic **psychotic** state occurred. In the early 1900s, there was considerable medical reaction against the indiscriminate use of cocaine.

Patent Medicines

The broadest impact on drug use in this country came from the widespread legal distribution of **patent medicines**. Patent medicines were dispensed by traveling peddlers and were readily available at local stores for self-medication. Sales of patent medicines increased from $3.5 million in 1859 to $74 million in 1904.

Within the boundaries of the United States, there was increasing conflict between the steady progress of medical science and the therapeutic claims of the patent medicine hucksters. The alcohol and other habit-forming drug content of the patent medicines was also a matter of concern. One medicine, Hostetter's Bitters, was 44 percent alcohol, and another, Birney's Catarrh Cure, was 4 percent cocaine. In October 1905, *Collier's* magazine culminated a prolonged attack on patent medicines with a well-documented, aggressive series entitled "Great American Fraud."[2]

1906 Pure Food and Drugs Act

President Theodore Roosevelt recommended in 1905 "that a law be enacted to regulate interstate commerce in misbranded and adulterated foods, drinks, and drugs."[3] The 1906 publication of Upton Sinclair's *The Jungle*, exposing the horribly unsanitary conditions in the meat packing industry, shocked Congress and America. It provided the necessary heat, which five months later led to the passage of the Pure Food and Drugs Act. This 1906 act prohibited interstate commerce in adulterated or misbranded foods and drugs. This brought the federal government full force into the drug marketplace, and subsequent modifications have built on it. A drug was defined as "any substance or mixture of substances intended to be used for the cure, mitigation, or prevention of disease." Of particular

---

morphine: a narcotic, the primary active chemical in opium. Heroin is made from morphine.

cocaine: a stimulant; the primary active chemical in coca.

psychotic: (sigh *cot* ick) out of touch with reality.

patent medicines: medicines sold directly to the public.

importance was the phrasing of the law with respect to misbranding. Misbranding referred *only to the label, not to general advertising*, and covered "any statement, design, or device regarding . . . a drug, or the ingredients or substances contained therein, which shall be false or misleading in any particular."

The act specifically referred to alcohol, morphine, opium, cocaine, heroin, *Cannabis indica* (marijuana), and several other agents. Each package was required to state how much (or what proportion) of these drugs was included in the preparation. This meant, for example, that the widely sold "cures" for alcoholism or morphine addiction had to indicate that they contained another addicting drug. However, as long as the ingredients were clearly listed on the label, addicting drugs could be sold and bought with no federal restrictions. The goal was to protect people from unscrupulous merchants, not from themselves. The 1906 Pure Food and Drugs Act provided the rootstock on which all our modern laws regulating pharmaceuticals have been grafted.

Harrison Act of 1914

In the early 1900s, Dr. Hamilton Wright, the father of American narcotics laws, decided that the United States could gain favored trading status with China by leading international efforts to aid the Chinese in their efforts to reduce opium importation. At the request of the United States, an international conference met in 1912 to discuss controls on the opium trade. Great Britain, which was giving up a very lucrative business, wanted morphine, heroin, and cocaine included as well, because, as opium was being controlled, these German products were replacing it.[4] Eventually an agreement was reached in which several nations agreed to control both international trade and domestic sale and use of these substances. In response, Dr. Wright drafted a bill, which was submitted by Senator Harrison of New York, titled "An Act to provide

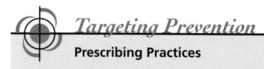

Targeting Prevention

Prescribing Practices

Some prescription drugs have the potential for patients to abuse them or to become dependent on them. According to the logic of the Controlled Substances Act, a drug that has such potential should be listed as a Schedule II–V controlled substance. This triggers laws limiting the way in which these drugs can be prescribed, in an effort to prevent them from being abused or creating dependence in users. These prescribing rules vary from state to state, but one of the most common limitations is that the prescriptions may not be automatically refilled. In other words, the physician must write a new prescription if the patient wants to get more of the drug. In spite of these rules, we do sometimes hear about people who develop dependence on a prescription drug. Do you think the current limitations are effective? Could changes be made that would effectively reduce the chances of patients' becoming dependent?

for the registration of, with collectors of internal revenue, and to impose a special tax upon all persons who produce, import, manufacture, compound, deal in, dispense, or give away opium or coca leaves, their salts, derivatives, or preparations, and for other purposes."[5] With a title like that, it's no wonder that this historic law is usually referred to as the Harrison Act.

For the first time, dealers and dispensers of the opiates and cocaine had to register annually, pay a small fee, and use special order forms provided by the Bureau of Internal Revenue. Physicians, dentists, and veterinary surgeons were named as potential lawful distributors if they registered. It is important for modern readers to realize that in 1914 there would have been no support and no constitutional rationale for a federal law prohibiting an individual from possessing or using these drugs. Congress would not have considered such a law; if it had, the Supreme Court would probably have declared it unconstitutional. The Harrison Act was a tax law, constitutionally similar to the whiskey tax.

It was not a punitive act, penalties for violation were not severe, and the measure contained no reference to users of "narcotics."

During congressional debate, some concern was expressed about the tax law's inconvenience to physicians and pharmacists, and it is doubtful that such a law would have been passed in the United States if its purpose had been merely to meet the rather weak treaty obligations of the 1912 Hague Conference. It was not meant to replace existing laws and, in fact, specifically supported the continuing legality of the 1906 Pure Food and Drugs Act and the 1909 Opium Exclusion Act. Dr. Wright had written and lectured extensively, waging an effective, emotional, and in some instances outright racist public campaign for additional controls over these drugs. For example, his claims about the practice of "snuffing" cocaine into the nose, which he said was popular among Southern blacks, caused a great deal of concern and fear.[6] Dr. Wright testified before Congress that this practice led to the raping of white women. Combining this depiction with the racially tinged fears about "those immoral Chinese opium dens" added the necessary heat to make the difference, and the Harrison Act passed and was signed into law in 1914. This law was the seed, which has since sprouted into all of our federal controlled-substance regulations.

Two Bureaus, Two Types of Regulation

By 1914 the basic federal laws had been passed that would influence our nation's drug regulations up to the current time. It might be significant that the Pure Food and Drugs Act was administered within the Department of Agriculture, whereas the Harrison Act was administered by the Treasury Department—two different federal departments administering two different laws. Many of the drugs regulated by the two laws were the same, but the political issues to which each agency responded were

different. The Agriculture Department was administering a law aimed at ensuring that drugs were pure and honestly labeled. On the other hand, the Treasury Department's experience was in taxing alcohol, and it would soon be responsible for enforcing Prohibition. The approach taken by each bureau was further shaped by court decisions, so that the actual effect of each law became something a bit different from what seems to have been intended.

REGULATION OF PHARMACEUTICALS

The 1906 law called for the government to regulate the purity of both foods and drugs, and evidence had been presented during the congressional debate that thousands of products in both categories were at fault. Where was the task of analyzing and prosecuting to begin? Dr. Harvey Wiley, chief chemist in the Department of Agriculture, had been a major proponent of the 1906 law and had drafted most of it. He was in charge of administering the law, and he influenced the direction its enforcement would take. His first concern was adulterated food, so most of the initial cases dealt with food products rather than drugs.

Purity

Most large drug manufacturers made efforts to comply with the new law, although they were not given specific recommendations as to how this should be accomplished. The manufacturer of Cuforhedake Brane-Fude modified its label to show that it contained 30 percent alcohol and 16 grains of a widely used headache remedy. The government took the manufacturer to trial in 1908 on several grounds: the alcohol content was a bit lower than that claimed on the label, and the label seemed to claim that the product was a "cure" and food for the brain, both misleading claims. After much arguing about different methods of describing alcohol content and about the label claims, the manufacturer was convicted by the jury, probably because of the "brane-fude" claim, and paid a fine of $700.[7]

Dr. Wiley went on vigorously testing products and pursuing any that were adulterated or didn't properly list important ingredients, but he also went after many companies on the basis of their therapeutic claims. In 1911, government action against a claimed cancer cure was overturned by arguing that the ingredients were accurately labeled and that the original law had not covered therapeutic claims, only claims about the nature of the ingredients. Congress rapidly passed the 1912 Sherley amendment, which outlawed "false and fraudulent" therapeutic claims on the label. Even so, it was still up to the government to prove that a claim was not only false but also fraudulent in that the manufacturer knew it to be false. In a 1922 case, the claim that "B&M External Remedy" could cure tuberculosis was ruled not to be fraudulent because its manufacturer, who had no scientific or medical training, truly believed that its ingredients (raw eggs, turpentine, ammonia, formaldehyde, and mustard and wintergreen oils) were effective.[7] This seems like an encouragement for the ignorant to become manufacturers of medicines!

From its beginning, the Food and Drug Administration (**FDA**) had adopted the approach of encouraging voluntary cooperation, which it could obtain from most of the manufacturers through educational and corrective actions rather than through punitive, forced compliance. As more and more cases were investigated, it became clear to the FDA officials that many of the violations of the 1906 law were unintentional and caused primarily by poor manufacturing techniques and an absence of quality control measures. The FDA began developing assay techniques for various chemicals and products and collaborated extensively with the pharmaceutical industry to improve standards.

In spite of these improvements, many smaller companies continued to bring forth quack medicines that were ineffective or even dangerous. The depression of the 1930s increased competition for business, and the Roosevelt administration took a more critical view of the pharmaceutical industry. FDA surveys in the mid-1930s showed that over 10 percent of the drug products studied did not meet the standards of the *United States Pharmacopeia* or *The National Formulary*. Several attempts were made during the early 1930s to enact major reforms, but opposition by the manufacturers of proprietary medicines prevented these changes from happening.

Safety

The 1930s had seen an expansion in the use of "sulfa" drugs, which are effective antibiotics. In searching for a form that could be given as a liquid, a chemist found that *sulfanilamide* would dissolve in diethylene glycol. The new concoction looked, tasted, and smelled fine, so it was bottled and marketed in 1937. Diethylene glycol causes kidney poisoning, and within a short time 107 people died from taking "Elixir Sulfanilamide." The federal government could not intervene simply because the mixture was toxic—there was no legal requirement that medicine be safe. The FDA seized the elixir on the grounds that a true elixir contains alcohol, and this did not. The chemist committed suicide, the company paid the largest fine ever under the 1906 law, and a public crisis arose, which led to passage of the 1938 Food, Drug, and Cosmetic Act.[7]

A critical change in the 1938 law was the requirement that *before* a new drug could be marketed its manufacturer must test it for toxicity. The company was to submit a "new drug application" (**NDA**) to the FDA. This NDA was to include "full reports of investigations which have been made to show whether or not such a drug is safe for use." If the submitted paperwork was satisfactory, the application was allowed to become effective. Between 1938 and 1962, about 13,000 NDAs were submitted and about 70 percent of the drugs were allowed to be marketed.

The new drug application provision was important in two ways: first, it changed the role of the FDA from testing and challenging some of the drugs already being sold to that of a gatekeeper, which must review every new drug before it is marketed. This increased power and responsibility led to a great expansion in the size of the FDA. Second, the requirement that companies conduct research before marketing a new drug, greatly reduced the likelihood of new drugs being introduced by small companies run by untrained people.

The 1938 act also stipulated that drug labels either give adequate directions for use or state that the drug is to be used only on the prescription of a physician. Thus, the federal law first recognized a difference between drugs that could be sold over the counter and prescription-only drugs.

Effectiveness

In the late 1950s, Senator Estes Kefauver began a series of hearings investigating high drug costs and marketing collaboration between drug companies. As the hearings progressed, manufacturers, physicians, and the FDA itself were criticized. One major concern was that some of the most widely advertised and sold over-the-counter medications were probably ineffective. For example, Carter's Little Liver Pills consisted of small bits of candy-coated dried liver. It was accurately labeled and made no unsubstantiated therapeutic claims on the label—if you jumped to the conclusion that it was supposed to help your liver, that wasn't the company's fault. And no law required the medicines to actually do anything. Amendments to the Food, Drug, and Cosmetic Act were written but were bottled up in committee. Again it took a disaster that raised public awareness and congressional concern before major reforms were implemented.

Thalidomide, a sedative and sleeping pill, was first marketed in West Germany in 1957.

The drug was widely used by pregnant women because it also reduced the nausea and vomiting associated with the morning sickness often experienced early in pregnancy. An American company submitted an NDA in 1960 to market thalidomide, but luckily the FDA physician in charge of the application did not approve it quickly. In 1961 and early 1962, it became clear that thalidomide had been responsible for birth defects. In West Germany, hundreds of children had been born with deformed limbs. The American company had released some thalidomide for clinical testing, but, because its NDA was not approved, a major disaster was avoided in the United States.[7]

The 1962 Kefauver-Harris amendments added several important provisions, including the requirement that companies submit plans for and seek approval of any testing to be done with humans before the clinical trials are conducted. Another provision required advertisements for prescription drugs (mostly in medical journals) to contain a summary of information about adverse reactions to the drug.

The most important change was one requiring that every new drug be demonstrated to be *effective* for the illnesses mentioned on the label. As with the details of safety testing required by the 1938 law, this research on effectiveness was to be submitted to the FDA. The FDA was also to begin a review of the thousands of products marketed between 1938 and 1962 to determine their effectiveness. Any that were found to be ineffective were to be removed from the market. In 1966, the FDA began the process of evaluating the formulations of prescription drugs. In

---

FDA: The United States Food and Drug Administration.

NDA: new drug application. Must be approved before a drug is sold.

the next eight years, the FDA took action to remove from the market 6,133 drugs manufactured by 2,732 companies.

Marketing a New Drug

To translate the 1962 law on the safety and effectiveness of a new drug, the FDA has established certain regular procedures and standards, which must be met by the pharmaceutical company that hopes to market a prescription drug. Developing a compound to the point where it can be marketed is a long and expensive procedure for the drug company, costing an average of $500 million.[8]

The FDA formally enters the picture only when a drug company is ready to study the effects of a compound on humans. At that time the company supplies to the FDA a "Notice of Claimed Investigational Exemption for a New Drug" (**IND**); it is also required to submit all information from preclinical (before human) investigations, including the effects of the drug on animals. The principal purpose of this preclinical work is to establish the safety of the compound.

As minimum evidence of safety, the animal studies must include acute, one-time administration of several dose levels of the drug to different groups of animals of at least two species. There must also be studies in which the drug is given regularly to animals for a period related to the proposed use of the drug in humans. For example, a drug to be used chronically requires two-year toxicology studies in animals. Again, two species are required. The method of drug administration and the form of the drug in these studies must be the same as that proposed for human use.

In addition to these research results, the company must submit a detailed description of the proposed clinical studies of the drug in humans. The company must also certify that the human subjects will be told they are receiving an investigational compound and that the sub-

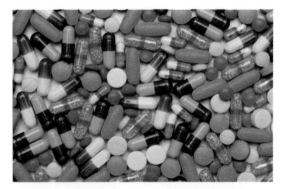

A new drug must move through three phases of clinical investigation before it reaches the market.

jects will sign a form, stating that they know they are to receive such a compound and that this is acceptable to them. Finally, the company must agree to forward annually a comprehensive report and to inform the FDA immediately if any adverse reactions arise in either animals or humans receiving the investigational drug.

If the FDA authorizes the use of the drug in humans, the company can move into the first of *three phases of clinical investigation:*

1. *Phase 1* encompasses studies with very small amounts of the drug on a limited number of healthy people—typically, 20 to 80 company employees, medical school personnel, prisoners, and others who volunteer for such trials. At this stage the researchers are primarily interested in learning how their drug is absorbed and excreted in healthy people, as well as the side effects it may trigger.
2. *Phase 2* of the human studies involves patients who have the condition the candidate drug is designed to treat. These studies involve about a few hundred patients who are chosen because the new agent might help them.
3. *Phase 3* is quite extensive and involves administering the drug to larger numbers of individuals than in phase 2 (typically, 1,000 to

5,000) with the disease or symptom for which the drug is intended. If the compound proves effective in phase 3, the FDA balances its possible dangers against the benefits for patients before releasing it for sale to the public.

There have been a few changes to this basic procedure since 1962. In 1983, Congress passed the Orphan Drug Act, offering tax incentives and exclusive sales rights for a guaranteed seven years for any company developing a drug for rare disorders afflicting no more than 200,000 people. Up to that time, companies had stayed away from much research on rare disorders because they couldn't earn enough to recover the enormous research costs. By 1999, almost 200 drugs developed under this act had received FDA approval.[8] On the "drug war" front, the Prescription Drug Marketing Act of 1988 tightened the procedures whereby drug company salespeople could provide free samples to physicians, after Congress had heard testimony about widespread diversion of samples. Also, because counterfeit and adulterated drugs had found their way into the U.S. market from abroad as shipments of "American goods returned," new regulations were added covering the transfer and reimportation of drugs.

There is one big, continually debated issue surrounding the FDA drug approval system: why does it take so long? The issue is not just one of concern for the individual who is sick. Pharmaceutical manufacturers have a 20-year patent on a new drug. They usually patent the chemical as soon as there is some evidence that it is marketable. The manufacturers claim that, by the time a drug is cleared for marketing, they have only a few years left on the patent. From the mid-1980s to the late 1990s, the average approval time was reduced from 32 months to 12 months—but the increased speed of the FDA's approval process has been more than offset by an increased amount of time spent by companies in clinical trials— an average of almost seven years.[8]

Health Quest Activities

Go to Module 9 and look under *Our Changing World*. Read "Buying Drugs Online." This article addresses the act of ordering prescriptions online and the necessity of regulations for online orders. Have you ever ordered prescriptions online? If so, did you feel the security regulations were adequate? Do you think stricter regulations are needed, or would they make the process of filling a prescription unnecessarily difficult?

In the same module, read "Over-the-Counter Drug Labels" in *Key Articles*. This article provides information on how to read OTC drug labels and why instructions are needed. Look around your own home for OTC drugs (such as cold and cough medicines, antacids, and aspirin). Compare the labels. Are the instructions about dosages (how many pills to take and when) clear enough? Do you ever take more than the recommended dosage? What kinds of warnings are listed? Have you ever experienced any of the side effects? Does the label include warnings about mixing this drug with others?

Certain classes of drugs, including drugs for AIDS, are considered for priority review by the FDA. In 1987, the first drug was approved for use in AIDS, and by 1997 there were 42 approved drugs and 122 in clinical trials.[8]

Dietary Supplements

Certain drug like products, such as vitamin pills, are not drugs but, rather, are considered dietary supplements and treated more as foods. This means that they don't need to be proved to be effective for a specific intended purpose. On the other hand, many questions arose about

IND: application to investigate a new drug in human clinical trials.

whether new products needed to be reviewed for safety prior to marketing them and whether some of the beneficial claims made by people selling them constituted mislabeling. The 1994 Dietary Supplement Health and Education Act cleared up many of those issues. For one thing, it broadened the definition of dietary supplements to include not only vitamins, minerals, and proteins but also herbs and herbal extracts. The labels are not allowed to make unsubstantiated direct claims, such as "cures cancer," but they are permitted to make general statements about the overall health and "well-being" that can be achieved by consuming the dietary ingredient. The label must then say, "This statement has not been evaluated by the Food and Drug Administration. This product is not intended to diagnose, treat, cure, or prevent any disease." Nevertheless, there has been an enormous growth in sales of herbal products and other dietary supplements, probably in large part because many consumers don't distinguish between the vague, general claims made by supplements and the specific, demonstrated effectiveness required of drugs.

NARCOTICS, DANGEROUS DRUGS, AND CONTROLLED SUBSTANCES

To most Americans the word *narcotics* means drugs that are manufactured and sold illegally. Pharmacologically, the term refers only to drugs having certain effects, with the prototype being the narcotic analgesics derived from opium, such as morphine and heroin. Although the Harrison Act controlled opiates, which are narcotics, and cocaine, which is not, the enforcement effort focused so much on the opiates that eventually the enforcement officers became known as narcotics officers, the office within the Treasury Department officially became the Narcotics Division, and people began to refer to the "Harrison Narcotics Act," though, as we have seen, the word *narcotics* was not in the original title. The meaning of the term changed so much in political use that later federal laws incorrectly classified cocaine and then marijuana as narcotics.

After the Harrison Act

In 1914, it was estimated that about 200,000 Americans—1 in 400—were addicted to opium or its derivatives. One way to administer the Harrison Act would have been to allow a continued legal supply of opiates to those addicted individuals through registered physicians and to focus enforcement efforts on the smugglers and remaining opium dens. After all, the Harrison Act stated that an unregistered person could purchase and possess any of the taxed drugs if they had been prescribed or administered by a physician "in the course of his professional practice and for legitimate medical purposes." Early enforcement efforts focused on smugglers and did not result in a large number of arrests. However, one very important arrest was to have later repercussions. It seems that a Dr. Webb was taking telephone orders for narcotics, including some from people he had never seen in person. Evidence was presented that this physician would prescribe whatever amount the caller requested. He was arrested, convicted, and appealed the conviction all the way to the U.S. Supreme Court, which in 1919 upheld his conviction on the grounds that his activity did not constitute a proper prescription in the course of the professional practice of medicine. It's interesting to speculate whether fears about unexpected uses for the telephone, which most people did not yet have in their homes, might have contributed to Dr. Webb's prosecution. In any event, there is a parallel with today's Internet pharmacies, some of which provide for medical consultation and prescription (although not for narcotics) through the home computer. Until the 1920s, most addicts continued to receive narcotics quietly through their private physicians, and in most large cities public clinics dispensed morphine to addicts who could not afford private care.

It is ironic that the single most important piece of legislation that has shaped the federal government's approach to controlled substances wasn't a "drug law" at all but, rather, the Eighteenth Amendment prohibiting alcohol. That law was also to be enforced by the Treasury Department, and a separate Prohibition unit was established in 1919. The Narcotics Division was placed within that unit, and Colonel Levi G. Nutt was appointed the first director, with 170 agents at his disposal.[4] Although the Harrison Act itself had not changed, the people enforcing it had. Just as with alcohol, these people believed that the cure for narcotic addiction was to prevent the addict from having access to the drug (in other words, narcotic "prohibition," at least for addicts). The new enforcers interpreted the Webb case to mean that any prescription of a habit-forming drug to an addict was not a "legitimate medical purpose," and they began to charge many physicians under the Harrison Act.

Arresting Physicians and Pharmacists

Because even cure programs were not exempt, the Internal Revenue Service (IRS) moved to close down municipal narcotics clinics in more than 30 cities from coast to coast. In the period from 1919 to 1929, the Narcotics Division arrested about 75,000 people, including 25,000 physicians and druggists.[4] The American Medical Association supported the view that reputable physicians would not prescribe narcotics to addicts. Because there was then no legal way for an addict to continue his or her habit, the addict was forced either to stop using narcotics or to look for drugs in the illegal market. Thus, this new method of enforcing the Harrison Act resulted in the growth of an illicit drug trade, which charged users up to 50 times more than the legal retail drug price. Narcotic addiction came increasingly to be viewed as a police, rather than a medical, problem.

Stiffer Penalties

Partly in response to the growing illicit market, in 1922 Congress passed the Jones-Miller Act, which more than doubled the maximum penalties for dealing in illegally imported narcotics to $5,000 and 10 years of imprisonment. This act was the first to mislabel cocaine as a narcotic, and it established the Federal Narcotics Control Board to initiate an active program against dealers. Included also was the stipulation that the mere possession of illegally obtained narcotics was sufficient basis for conviction, thus officially making the addict a criminal. Because illegal narcotics were so expensive, many addicts came to prefer the most potent type available, heroin. In 1924, another act entirely prohibited importing opium for the manufacture of heroin. Already by this time several important trends had been set: addicts were criminals at odds with the regulatory agency, the growth of the illicit market was responded to with greater penalties and more aggressive enforcement, and there was a focus on attempting to eliminate a substance (heroin) as though the drug itself were the problem. In the 1925 Linder case, the U.S. Supreme Court declared that it could be legal for a physician to prescribe narcotics for an addict if it were part of a curing program and did not transcend "the limits of that professional conduct with which Congress never intended to interfere."[5] However, the damage had been done, and most physicians would have nothing to do with addicts.

Prison vs. Treatment

By 1928, individuals sentenced for drug violations made up one-third of the total population in federal prisons. Even though the 1920s were the period of alcohol prohibition, during those years twice as many people were imprisoned for narcotics violations as for liquor violations.[9] In 1929, Congress viewed this enormous expenditure for narcotics offenders as an indicator that something was wrong and decided that addicts should be cured rather than repeatedly jailed. It voted to establish two narcotic farms for the treatment of persons addicted to habit-forming drugs (including marijuana and peyote) who had been convicted of violating a federal law. The farm in Lexington, Kentucky, opened in 1935 and generally held about a thousand patients, two-thirds of whom were prisoners.

The Bureau of Narcotics

Answering the call for new approaches to addiction, and in response to the end of Prohibition and to charges of corruption in the previous Narcotics Division, in 1930 Congress took several actions that culminated in the formation of a separate Bureau of Narcotics in the Treasury Department. Harry Anslinger became the first commissioner of that bureau in 1932 and took office with a pledge to stop arresting so many addicts and instead to go after the big dealers. Anslinger became the first "drug czar," although he wasn't called that at the time. To some extent, he followed the lead of J. Edgar Hoover, director of the Federal Bureau of Investigation (FBI). Each of these men was regularly reappointed by each new president, and each built up a position of considerable power and influence. Anslinger had almost total control of federal efforts in narcotics education, prevention, treatment, and enforcement for 30 years, from 1932 to 1962. No federal or state narcotics law was passed without his influencing it, and he also represented U.S. narcotics interests to international organizations, including the United Nations. He was tough-minded in the area of drug abuse and always opposed any form of ambulatory narcotic treatment (treatment outside a secure hospital environment).

The end of Prohibition, combined with depression-era cutbacks, had reduced the number of agents available for enforcement, but not for long. After some newspaper reports linked marijuana smoking with crime, Anslinger adopted this new cause and began writing, speaking, testifying, and making films depicting the evils of marijuana. This effort succeeded in bringing public attention to the fight his bureau was waging against drugs and resulted in the 1937 passage of the Marijuana Tax Act. Marijuana came under the same type of legal control as cocaine and the opiates, in that one was supposed to register and pay a tax to legally import, buy, or sell marijuana. From 1937 until 1970, marijuana was referred to in federal laws as a narcotic.

World War II caused a decrease in the importation of both legal and illegal drugs. With the end of the war and the resumption of easy international travel, the illegal narcotic trade resumed and increased every year, in spite of the 1951 Boggs amendment to the Harrison Act, which established mandatory minimum sentences for narcotics offenses. Testimony before a subcommittee of the Senate Judiciary Committee in 1955 included the statement that inducing drug addiction in U.S. citizens was one of the ways Communist China planned to demoralize the United States. Remember that this was the height of the McCarthy era, during which a mere hint by Senator Joseph McCarthy that someone associated with "known Communists" was enough to ruin that person's career. One interesting bit of history from that time was revealed years later. Anslinger and Hoover were aware that McCarthy, in addition to his widely known alcoholism, was addicted to morphine. Anslinger arranged for McCarthy to obtain a regular supply of his drug from a Washington, DC, pharmacy without interference from narcotics officers.[4] With both crime and communism to combat, Congress passed the 1956 Narcotic Drug Control Act, with the toughest penalties yet. Under this law, any offense except first-offense possession had to result in a jail term, and no suspension, probation, or parole was allowed. Anyone caught selling heroin to a person younger than 18 could receive the death penalty. Ansliger commented on that particular provision by saying, "I'd like to throw the switch myself on drug peddlers who sell their poisons to minors."[10]

Exploring Your Spirituality

Looking for More Humane Policies

If California is setting a trend, as it often does in fashion, entertainment, and politics, the United States may be having a change of heart in how it deals with drug addiction. In the November 7, 2000, election, more than 60 percent of California voters approved Proposition 36, requiring judges to sentence nonviolent first-time drug users to treatment instead of jail time.

It appears that Californians are prepared to give up "tough on crime" and "zero tolerance" policies for drug regulations they regard as more humane. Interestingly, the proposition was vigorously opposed by California law enforcement officials, many politicians in both parties, and the state's most influential newspapers, both conservative and liberal.

Opponents argue that giving a "free pass" to even first-time offenders will lead to more drug use, distribution, and crime. They say there's nothing in the proposition to encourage addicts to succeed in treatment.

Californians, who favor the measure however, don't think the war on drugs is working. They prefer to see more money spent on treatment. Proposition 36 calls for the state Department of Alcohol and Drugs to spend $120 million a year on treatment.

The disparity between being seen as a criminal and being viewed as a good person who has made mistakes and is worthy of help can affect a person's spiritual health—particularly among vulnerable adolescents and young adults. For those who believe that all people should love and respect themselves because they are uniquely valuable, the abuse that drug addicts inflict on themselves presents a spiritual dilemma also. Do you think a more tolerant attitude, veering away from incarceration toward treatment, is the best way to help drug addicts help themselves?

Drug Abuse Control Amendments of 1965

The early 1960s saw not only an increase in illegal drug use but also a shift in the type of drugs being used illegally. The trend was for the new drug users to be better educated and to emphasize drugs that alter mood and consciousness, such as amphetamines, barbiturates, and hallucinogens. Some hospitals in large cities reported that up to 15 percent of their emergency room calls involved individuals with adverse reactions to these drugs. Although amphetamines and barbiturates were legal prescription drugs, it was felt that they should be under the same types of controls as narcotics. The 1965 Drug Abuse Control amendments referred to these as dangerous drugs and included hallucinogens, such as LSD. The Bureau of Narcotics became the Bureau of Narcotics and Dangerous Drugs. Thus, the 1960s saw a number of major changes for

this agency. Anslinger had retired, the bureau had new classes of drugs to control, and it was facing widespread disregard of the drug laws by large numbers of young people who were not all members of the underprivileged and criminal classes.

Comprehensive Drug Abuse Prevention and Control Act of 1970

The Comprehensive Drug Abuse Prevention and Control Act of 1970, usually referred to as the *Controlled Substances Act,* almost lived up to its title. It was comprehensive, because it repealed and replaced or updated all previous laws concerned with both the narcotic and dangerous drugs. This basic law is still in effect, so it is important to understand its structure. The law specifically states that the drugs controlled by the act are under federal jurisdiction regardless of involvement in interstate commerce. The law did not eliminate state regulations; it just made clear that federal enforcement and prosecution are possible in any illegal activity involving controlled drugs.

Prevention and Treatment

The Controlled Substances Act dealt with the prevention and treatment of drug abuse by appropriating funds to expand the role of community mental health centers and Public Health Service hospitals in the treatment of those who misuse drugs. It authorized the development of educational material and drug education workshops for professional workers and in public schools.

Control Issues Resolved

The control aspects of the Controlled Substances Act were the most debated portions, and several basic philosophical, ethical, and legal issues were resolved by the law. First, this was a law to control drugs directly rather than through taxes. Enforcement authority was moved from the Treasury Department to the new Drug Enforcement Administration (**DEA**) in the Department of Justice. A second major issue was the separation of enforcement of the law from the scientific evaluation of the drugs considered for control. The attorney general is responsible for the administration of the control aspects of the law, but the secretary of the Department of Health and Human Services makes a binding recommendation about which drugs are to be controlled. This separation of enforcement from scientific and medical decisions about what should be controlled was a major victory for those arguing for a rational drug law.

Schedules

After specifically excluding "distilled spirits, wine, malt beverages, or tobacco," the law established five schedules of drugs that must be updated and published regularly. Table 5.1 summarizes the characteristics of drugs in each of the five schedules and gives a few examples.

Perhaps the most important distinction is between Schedule I and the others: Schedules II through V consist primarily of prescription drugs that are further controlled by these regulations, whereas the substances in Schedule I by definition "have no medical use" and are therefore not available by prescription. Notice that cocaine is on Schedule II and marijuana, which has no federally recognized medical uses, is on Schedule I.

Penalties for Possession

The penalties for simply possessing a drug is more lenient than before and do not depend on the schedule. Therefore, an individual is guilty of the same crime whether he or she has a Valium tablet prescribed for another person or a bag of heroin. A first offense of illegal possession of a controlled drug or "distributing a small amount of marijuana for no remuneration" can be punished by up to one year's imprisonment and/or a fine of $1,000 to $5,000. In lieu of this, the court can place the individual on probation for up to a year. If there is no violation of the conditions of probation, the charge is dismissed and the conviction is "erased," except that a nonpublic record of the action is kept to prevent a person from being a "first offender" more than once.

Penalties for Selling

The penalties for illegally making or selling controlled substances were not too complicated when the law passed in 1970, and the maximum first-offense penalty for distributing a Schedule I or II "narcotic" drug was 15 years and $25,000. In 1986, the penalties became much more complex, depending on the individual drug and the amount sold. Mandatory minimum penalties were again introduced, as they had been in the 1950s. First-offense sale of a large amount of heroin, cocaine, or several other drugs can, if the sale results in death or serious bodily injury, result in a life sentence and a fine of $4 million. First-offense sale of a small amount of mari-

TABLE 5-1

Summary of Controlled Substance Schedules

Schedule	Criteria	Examples
Schedule I	a. High potential for abuse b. <u>No currently acceptable</u> <u>medical use in treatment</u> in the United States c. Lack of accepted safety for use under medical supervision.	Heroin Marijuana LSD
Schedule II	a. High potential for abuse b. Currently accepted medical use c. Abuse may lead to severe psychological or physical dependence.	Morphine Cocaine Methamphetamine
Schedule III	a. Potential for abuse less than I and II b. Currently accepted medical use c. Abuse may lead to moderate physical dependence or high psychological dependence.	Amphetamine Most barbiturates PCP
Schedule IV	a. Low potential for abuse relative to III b. Currently accepted medical use c. Abuse may lead to limited physical or psychological dependence relative to III.	Barbital Chloral hydrate Paraldehyde
Schedule V	a. Low potential for abuse relative to IV b. Currently accepted medical use c. Abuse may lead to limited physical or psychological dependence relative to IV.	Mixtures having small amounts of codeine or opium

juana can result in imprisonment for up to five years and a fine of up to $250,000. No parole is allowed.[11]

Omnibus Drug Act

The 1988 Omnibus Drug Act made some interesting additions and adjustments to the Controlled Substances Act.[12] There were many components to this new law, involving the registration of airplanes, money laundering, firearms sales to felons, and chemicals used to manufacture drugs. One part allowed for the death penalty for anyone who murdered someone or orders the killing of someone in conjunction with a drug-related felony. Major sections of the law funded treatment and education programs as well. The most noteworthy change was a toughening of approaches toward drug users, aimed at reducing the *demand* for drugs (as opposed to

putting all federal efforts into reducing the *supply* of drugs). Before this law, there were few penalties and little interest in convicting users for possessing small (personal-use) amounts of controlled substances. Under the new law, here are some of the unpleasant possibilities if convicted of possession:

- A civil fine of up to $10,000
- Forfeiture of the car, boat, or plane conveying the substance
- Loss of all federal benefits, including student loans and grants, for up to one year after the

DEA: Drug Enforcement Administration, a branch of the Department of Justice.

first offense and up to five years after a second offense.

The 1988 law also removes from public housing the entire family of anyone who engages in criminal activity, including drug-related activity, on or near public-housing premises.

Office of National Drug Control Policy

To better coordinate all these federal efforts, the 1988 Omnibus Drug Act established the cabinet-level position of Director of National Drug Control Policy (commonly referred to as a "drug czar"). This individual is ordered by the legislation to prepare a national drug-control strategy

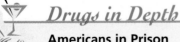

Drugs in Depth

Americans in Prison

Fueled largely by the increases in drug-law arrests, the number of people held in state and local prisons in the United States has reached record levels. From the 1920s through the mid-1970s, about 1 person was in prison for every 1,000 people in the U.S. population. There were peaks and valleys, with the highest peak in 1939 (the end of the Depression) at 1.39 per 1,000 population.

From 1974 to 1985, the rate doubled, from 1 to 2 per 1,000. By 1999, more than 3 million people were in U.S. prisons, a rate of more than 4.7 per 1,000 population. More than 3 million were on probation or parole, also record numbers and proportions.[21] The United States now has a greater proportion of its own citizens in prisons than does any other country.

Proportions of U.S. citizens in prison

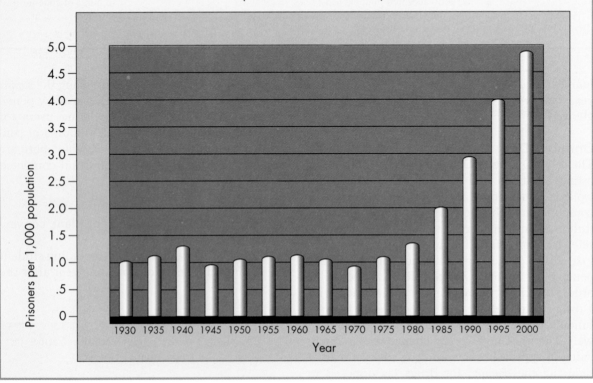

Try It!

Consider the Consequences

One of the most damaging things that can occur to a person who is working toward a successful and happy life is to get into trouble with the law and establish a criminal record. Many people have done a few things for which they could have been apprehended and either fined or arrested. Perhaps it is only parking illegally for a few minutes or driving a few miles over the speed limit. We all know that we don't get caught every time, or perhaps even most of the time, so there's a certain amount of luck involved. Also, of course, the seriousness of the violation and the ensuing consequence vary quite a bit. Most people can afford to pay a parking fine and it is not considered much of a blemish on their record. However, some people seem to tempt fate more often than others and for higher stakes—in other words, they do things that risk more serious consequences, and they do those things more often. Many of the risks that people take involve the use of substances, and often it seems they have not considered the possible consequences. Create a confidential list of such behaviors in the following table. For each behavior, indicate whether you have done it; whether you have been caught; if so, what the consequences were; and how the consequence or lack of consequence influenced your likelihood of doing it again.

	Behavior			
	Underage smoking	Underage drinking	Driving while intoxicated	Using an illegal drug
Done it? (Y/N)				
Caught? (Y/N)				
Consequence				
Influence on future behavior: +, −, none				

and an annual consolidated drug-control budget for all federal agencies involved, to advise the National Security Council, and to report directly to the president. The Office of National Drug Control Policy was reauthorized and given additional authority in 1998.

STATE AND LOCAL REGULATIONS

It is impossible to describe here all of the varied drug laws in the 50 states.[13] We should remember that most states and many local communities had laws regulating sales of drugs before the federal government got into the act in 1906. Some aspects of those old laws might still be in effect in some areas. Regarding the legal sales of prescription and over-the-counter drugs, there is considerable uniformity across the states, but some details do differ. For example, in some states licensed physician's assistants are allowed to prescribe many types of medication, and in a few states pharmacists are now allowed to prescribe a few types of drugs that had previously required prescription by a physician or dentist.

After the passage of the federal 1970 Controlled Substance Act, states began to adopt the *Uniform Controlled Substances Act*, a model state law recommended by the DEA. The same set of schedules is found in these state laws, and they generally follow a similar pattern of penalties, although a given penalty might be greater in one state than in another. This model act was meant to replace all previous drug legislation in each state, but sometimes vestiges of older laws remain. For example, some states define as a special crime the smuggling of intoxicating drugs into a jail or prison. Also, many states have modified the uniform laws since they were originally passed. Some states "decriminalized" possession of marijuana (see Chapter 17) by making it a civil offense punishable by a fine, and then later "recriminalized" it. The states have been pressured by the federal government to enact laws setting aside "drug-free school zones"— laws that make delivery penalties higher if the sale occurs near a school. Another federally encouraged action taken by most states is the removal of driver's license privileges for violations of controlled substance laws, even when driving is not involved in the offense.

In the mid-1970s a major industry grew up in the United States—the sale of legal items that were in some way related to the use of drugs. Sales of cigarette papers grew, whereas sales of loose cigarette tobacco declined. Water pipes and "bongs" (pipes for concentrating marijuana smoke) were big items, as were decorative "roach clips," sifters, and scales. These were mainly sold in "head shops," which catered to the drug-using subculture and in many cases were connected to music stores or other youth-oriented businesses. Although the items themselves were not illegal, their obvious relationship to illegal drug use and their visibility to young people raised concerns that drug use was being indirectly condoned and even advertised. Several communities passed ordinances aimed at controlling the sales of drug **paraphernalia**, and in 1977 Indiana passed the first statewide antiparaphernalia law.[14] In 1979, the DEA proposed, at the request of the White House, a model antiparaphernalia act, which states could adopt as an amendment to the Uniform Controlled Substances Act. Several have done so.

Interest in drug paraphernalia seemed to peak in about 1979 to 1980, with abundant television and newspaper reports, congressional hearings, and legal action. Concern was fueled by the sale of cocaine freebasing kits and other cocaine-related paraphernalia (straws, spoons, grinders, mirrors, and razors). Virtually every form of antiparaphernalia law has come under legal attack. We can best understand why by looking at the wording of a portion of the DEA's proposed model legislation, which bans

---

paraphernalia: (pare a fer *nail* ya)   equipment used in conjunction with any activity.

"blenders, bowls, containers, spoons, and mixing devices used, intended for use, or designed for use in compounding controlled substances."[15] Thus, a spoon or a bowl might or might not be considered drug paraphernalia, depending on its "intended use." An alligator clip sold as an electronic part would not be paraphernalia, but the same clip sold at a local "head shop" might be, depending on how it is displayed for sale and what the salesperson says about its use. Although some state laws have been thrown out by the courts, most of those based on the Model Act have been upheld. One consequence is that people selling the items have been careful to point out their legal intended use. There is now federal law prohibiting the use of the U.S. Postal Service to mail drug paraphernalia.

FEDERAL SUPPORT FOR URINE SCREENING

Military and Federal Employees

It wasn't until the 1970s that relatively inexpensive screening tests were invented that could detect a variety of abused substances or their metabolites in urine.[16] The navy, followed by the other armed forces, was the first to use random urine screening on a large scale. Soon to follow were people in various high-risk or high-profile positions, oil-field workers, air traffic controllers, and professional athletes. In 1986, President Reagan first declared that random urine tests should be performed on all federal employees in "sensitive" jobs. He also urged companies doing business with the federal government to begin testing their employees if they had not already done so.

Transportation Workers

In 1987, a collision between an Amtrak passenger train and a Conrail freight train near Baltimore, Maryland, resulted in the deaths of 16 people. The wreck was quickly blamed on drug use, because the Conrail engineer and brakeman had shared a marijuana joint shortly before the tragedy. The cause of the wreck can be argued: a warning indicator on the Conrail train was malfunctioning and the backup alarm had been silenced because it was too irritating. The marijuana use could be viewed as a symptom of a general "goofing off" attitude by the Conrail crew, who violated a number of safety procedures. Nevertheless, politicians and the news media saw this tragedy as a clear indication of the need for random urine testing. Transportation workers are now subject to surprise urine testing, and in 1992 this was expanded to interstate truck drivers. In addition, urine testing has become a common feature for prisoners, both while incarcerated and during probation or parole.

Private Employers

Private corporations, which may require urine testing before hiring a new employee and/or may periodically test employees, have two main reasons for adopting urine tests, but the bottom line in both cases is money. First, companies believe that drug-free workers will be absent less often, will make fewer mistakes, will have better safety records, and will produce more and better work. Second, by spending relatively few dollars on urine tests, they protect the company against negligence suits that might follow if a "stoned" employee hurt someone on the job or turned out a dangerously faulty product. Companies doing business with the federal government have an additional reason, in that they are required to have drug-free workplace rules in place.

Testing Methods

What is not widely discussed in the newspaper accounts of drug testing programs is which procedures will be used, which drugs will be looked for, and how well the tests work. Most drug screening programs test urine samples using a commercially available kit that is based on a method known as **EMIT** (enzyme multiplied

Taking Sides

Prescription Marijuana?

The Controlled Substances Act lists substances under Schedules II through V based on their abuse potential. However, all substances with "no medical use" fall under Schedule I. The active ingredient in marijuana, delta-9-tetrahydrocannabinol **(THC),** has recently caused some classification headaches for the DEA. For one thing, THC does now have a medical use—treating the nausea caused by cancer chemotherapy agents. Since 1986, under the generic name dronabinol, THC has been legally marketed as a prescription drug. The DEA's response to this has been to reschedule dronabinol *when dissolved in sesame oil and sealed in gelatin capsules,* as a Schedule II controlled substance. Any other preparation of THC is still Schedule I, as is marijuana itself. Marijuana is also being prescribed to some people for the treatment of glaucoma, and the government is even providing "official" marijuana cigarettes for this purpose. Marijuana has also been reported to provide some relief to multiple sclerosis patients. But marijuana cigarettes are not a generally available prescription drug. These prescriptions have been available only to about a dozen people under a "compassionate use" investigation of a new drug application. In 1992, the FDA stopped issuing new compassionate-use approvals for marijuana (see Chapter 17).

Since 1996, several states have passed citizen referenda allowing marijuana to be used for medical purposes. Because there are no legal sources of marijuana and because the federal government has actively opposed such measures, the referenda have not resulted in the widespread availability of legal medical marijuana in those states.

For more on this topic, log on to www.dushkin,com/online for current news and links to other popular and informative sites, as well as time-saving web search strategies and study tools.

---

immunoassay test). This method relies on the use of antibodies that react either to the drug in question or to a metabolite (breakdown product) of the drug. A problem with this type of assay is that it is possible for another drug or chemical to cross-react with the antibody and produce a false positive result.

Although the incidence of false positives is fairly low, they can occur; therefore, it is best to follow up the initial screen with another, more selective method, such as gas chromatography/mass spectrometry (GC/MS). This method is more specific and more sensitive but also more expensive: a typical EMIT test can be done for about $20 per sample, but GC/MS tests cost about $100.[17] An early problem with mass screening programs was sloppy handling of the samples, allowing for false reports based on mixups. However, the labs doing this type of work have improved their handling procedures and the companies making the test kits have improved their accuracy, so that it is theoretically possible for a company or government agency to obtain very accurate information. That is not always done in practice, however. For example, several over-the-counter drug products contain ingredients, such as ephedrine, that are chemically similar to amphetamine, and someone taking these legal substances might show up with an EMIT test positive for amphetamine. Until recently, products containing ibuprofen could cause a positive test for marijuana. These false positives can be ruled out if another portion of the same urine sample is subjected to GC/MS, because that test can distinguish between ephedrine and amphetamine and

EMIT: enzyme multiplied immunoassay test, a drug screening urine test.

THC: delta-9 tetrahydrocannabinol, the most important psychoactive chemical in marijuana.

between ibuprofen and marijuana metabolites. But the person paying for the testing has to want to spend the extra money.

EMIT kits can detect marijuana metabolites, the cocaine metabolite benzoylecgonine, PCP, and heroin. However, both the sensitivity and the duration over which the metabolites can be detected vary greatly among these substances. The cocaine metabolite clears within 1 or 2 days after a single use of a moderate amount, and it would probably be impossible to detect cocaine use after more than 3 or 4 days, even in someone chronically using high doses. The outside limit for PCP or heroin is about 4 days. After a single use of marijuana, metabolites can be reliably detected for 5 days or more, but, with chronic use of high doses, tests can be positive for 2 or 3 weeks or as long as 30 days. The point is that it is much easier for these tests to detect marijuana use for long periods of time than to detect other types of drug use. Combined with the much greater frequency of use of marijuana than of these other drugs, the odds are good that, if someone fails a drug screen, it is probably because of marijuana metabolites.

The U.S. Justice Department has conducted research on the use of hair samples to detect drug use.[18] This would theoretically allow detection of the use of a drug even weeks in the past, if the drug has been incorporated into the hair. Although not in widespread use yet, the possibility of such testing raises both practical and ethical concerns.

You should also be aware that all these drug screens can detect the presence of a drug or its metabolite, but they can't tell anything about the state of impairment of the individual at the time of the test. One person might show up at work Monday morning with a terrible hangover from drinking the night before, be unable to perform well on the job, and pass the drug screen easily. Another person might have smoked marijuana on Friday night, have experienced no effect for the past day and a half, and yet fail the screen. The general idea of the screens seems to be to discourage illicit drug use more than to detect impairment of performance.

THE IMPACT OF DRUG ENFORCEMENT

We can examine the current efforts at enforcing federal drug laws by asking ourselves three questions. What exactly are we doing to enforce drug laws? How much is it costing us? How effective is it? Although there had been previous "wars" on illicit drugs, the largest efforts to date began in 1982, when President Reagan announced a renewed and reorganized effort to combat drug trafficking and organized crime. For the first time, all federal agencies were to become involved, including the DEA; FBI; IRS; Alcohol, Tobacco and Firearms Bureau; Immigration and Naturalization; U.S. Marshals; U.S. Customs Service; and Coast Guard.[19] In some regions, Defense Department tracking and pursuit services were added. This last item had been legalized earlier in the Reagan administration and had signaled an important change in the role of the military. The idea of using our military forces to police our population had long been abhorrent to Americans, who had insisted that most police powers remain at the state and local levels. Because of the success of smugglers, we now use Air Force radar and aircraft and Navy patrol boats to detect and track aircraft and boats that might be bringing in drugs. These efforts have continued to expand, and in 1999 the Defense Department was spending almost $1 billion on drug interdiction activities.

Budget

A good overview of the widespread federal efforts can be obtained from the National Drug Control Strategy review and budget prepared each year by the White House.[20] The total requested for the 2001 budget was a record $19.2 billion. About $13 billion of that was for "supply

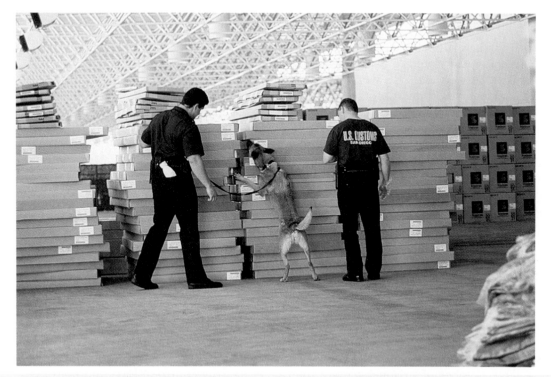

Customs officers use a trained dog to sniff for drugs in a warehouse.

reduction"—domestic enforcement, border control, and international efforts. This is a huge increase from less than $1 billion in 1980.

International Programs

International efforts aimed at reducing the drug supply include State Department programs that provide aid to individual countries to help them with narcotics controls, usually working in conjunction with the DEA. The DEA has agents in more than 40 countries, and they assist the local authorities in eradicating drug crops, locating and destroying illicit laboratories, and interfering with the transportation of drugs out of those countries. The State Department's International Narcotics Control Program budget for 2001 was $276 million. This included direct aid tied to drug enforcement and loans and support for South American countries to develop alternative crops and industries. The United States is providing increased military aid in the form of helicopters, "defensive" weapons, uniforms, and other supplies to be used in combating drug trafficking, plus military training to both army and police agencies. This program is restricted to countries that do not engage in a "consistent pattern of gross violations" of human rights. In addition, the State Department must make recommendations to the president, who must then report to Congress each year, regarding each country receiving *any* form of aid from the United States, on whether it can be certified to be cooperating with antinarcotics efforts. All foreign aid is to be suspended to any country that cannot be certified to be cooperating.

Other Federal Agencies

Efforts within the United States have broadened to include activities related to drug trafficking. The Customs Service and IRS were joined in 1990 by a Financial Crimes Enforcement Network to combat the "laundering" of drug profits through banks and other investments. The Federal Aviation Administration is involved not only in the urine testing of pilots and other airline workers but also in keeping track of private aircraft and small airports that might be used for transporting drug shipments. The Department of Agriculture Bureau of Land Management, and National Park Service are on the lookout for marijuana crops planted on federal land.

Other Costs

Besides the direct budget for drug control strategies, there are other costs, only some of which can be measured in dollars. We are paying to house a large number of prisoners: more than 230,000 drug-law violators in state prisons and local jails and more than 60,000 in federal prisons.[21] Add to this the cost of thousands on probation or parole, plus various forms of juvenile detention. We should also add the cost of crimes committed to purchase drugs at black-market prices and the incalculable price of placing so many of our state and local police, DEA, FBI, and other federal agents in danger of losing their lives to combat the drug trade, as some have done. A price that has been paid by many law enforcement agencies over the years is the corruption that is ever-present in drug enforcement. Because it is necessary for undercover officers to work closely with and to gain the trust of drug dealers, they must sometimes ignore an offense in hopes of gaining information about more and bigger deals in the future. They may even accept small favors from a drug dealer, and some officers have found it necessary to use drugs along with the suspects. Under those circumstances, and given the large amounts of money available to some drug dealers and the small salaries paid to most law officers, the possibility of accepting too large a gift and ignoring too many offenses is always there, and there might be no obvious "line" between doing one's job and becoming slightly corrupted.[22]

There are costs on the international level, also. The United States is put in an awkward position whenever one of our political allies becomes involved, even unwillingly, in drug trafficking. A great deal of heroin has been flowing through Pakistan, for example, and some might wonder why we haven't cut off aid to that country. First, Pakistan has been trying to control heroin with our help and its limited resources, but the problem is a large one. From the Pakistani point of view, perhaps the problem is caused more by our appetite for heroin than by Pakistan's need for money. Second, we cannot afford to lose Pakistan as an ally in that part of the world (it borders Iran and Afghanistan). So we must do the best we can to help Pakistan in its drug-control efforts and not to offend the Pakistanis with too many demands. Our drug-control efforts sometimes find us providing help to repressive governments, and it has been charged that some of our previous narcotics-control aid has been used for political repression, in both Latin America and Southeast Asia. Panama's General Noriega was indicted on drug-trafficking charges by a Florida grand jury before our invasion of that country, and his subsequent trial set a historical precedent: trying another country's deposed leader for violation of U.S. narcotics laws. To the extent that narcotics-control efforts place additional strains on our foreign policy needs in the East, the Caribbean, and Latin America, this also represents a significant cost to our country.

Finally, there is an unquantifiable cost in the loss of individual freedom that is inevitable when the government acquires increased powers. Because of increased drug-control efforts, American citizens are subjected to on-the-job urine tests; searches of homes, land, and vehicles;

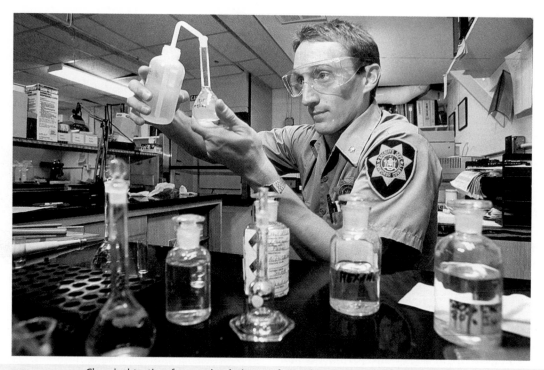

Chemical testing for cocaine being performed at a police Criminalistic Unit.

computer-coded passports that record each international visit; and increased government access to financial records. Americans are also threatened with seizure of their property and loss of federal benefits.

Given this effort and these costs, are our drug enforcement efforts effective? Do they work? Critics have pointed out that, despite escalating expenditures, more agents, and an increasing variety of supply-reduction efforts, the supplies of cocaine, heroin, and marijuana have not dried up; in fact, they may have increased. Although there have been record-breaking seizures of cocaine year after year, the price of cocaine has actually decreased since the 1980s. The United States government made a decision in 1924 to make heroin completely unavailable to addicts in this country, and after more than 75 years we can say only that it has been consistent in its

failure to accomplish that goal. Our efforts to eradicate illegal coca fields in South America have been described as a failure by the General Accounting Office, which has pointed out that many more new acres are being planted in coca each year than are being destroyed by our program.[23] A more recent economic analysis indicated that, even if eradication and interdiction efforts could result in massive disruption of a particular source country's production, it would take only about two years for the market to push production back to the previous levels.[24]

Effectiveness of Control

The laws do work at one level. It is estimated that 10 to 15 percent of the illegal drug supply is seized by federal agencies each year. In 1999, for example, U.S. government agencies seized a total of 132 tons of cocaine, 1.1 tons of heroin, and over 1,000 tons of cannabis.[22] These efforts have made it difficult and expensive to do business as a major importer. Evidence that supply is restricted can be found in the high prices charged on the streets. The price is many times more than the cost of the drug itself if sold legally. It is possible that the high cost is the only thing that regulates the amount taken by some of these addicts, many more of whom might die from overdoses. Local efforts make a difference, too. Small pushers forced to work out of sight are less able to contact purchasers, and both the buyer and the seller have a higher risk of being hurt or cheated in the transaction. This not only raises the cost of doing business, it also probably deters some people from trying the drugs. For example, suppose you were curious about heroin and wanted to try some. You might take some money to a rough part of one of our larger cities. If you are "lucky" enough to find a dealer, he might not be the sort of person you would trust. The transaction could take place in a nonpublic place, and if you were robbed, beaten, or just sold some worthless junk, you wouldn't be in a position to call the police!

Web Watch

Activities Related to Drug Regulations

Marketing Alcohol Among Students
Do you think there should be stricter government regulations against underage drinkers? Browse the article "Last Call for High-Risk Bar Promotions That Target College Students" at www.health.org/nongovpubs/lastcall. Explore the information about alcohol promotion among college students. Do you feel the information is accurate? Should we have stricter laws and higher standards to prohibit such marketing? Why or why not?

Do You Know the Drug Laws?
How much do you know about drug laws? Could you or someone you know unknowingly be running the risk of being charged or arrested? Read the points at www.antibully.org.uk/dgslaw.htm to find out.

Visit the FDA Online
The FDA home page includes the latest news on drugs, warnings, advisory committees, recalls, and the enforcement of drug regulations. You can also find information on how to petition the FDA at www.fda.gov.

SUMMARY

- In the early 1900s, two federal laws were passed on which our modern drug regulations are based.
- The 1906 Pure Food and Drugs Act, requiring accurate labeling, was amended in 1938 to require safety testing and in 1962 to require testing for effectiveness.
- A company wishing to market a new drug must first test it on animals, then file an IND. After a three-phase sequence of human testing, the company can file the NDA.
- The 1914 Harrison Act regulated the sale of opiates and cocaine.

- The Harrison Act was a tax law, but after 1919 it was enforced as a prohibition against providing narcotics to addicts.
- As narcotics became more scarce and their price rose on the illicit market, the illicit market grew. Harsher penalties and increased enforcement efforts, which were the primary strategies of Commissioner of Narcotics Harry Anslinger, failed to reverse the trend.
- Marijuana was added to the list of narcotics in 1937, and in 1965 amphetamines, barbiturates, and hallucinogens were also brought under federal control.
- The Controlled Substances Act of 1970 first provided for direct federal regulation of drugs, not through the pretense of taxing their sale.

- Controlled substances are placed on one of five schedules, depending on medical use and dependence potential.
- Amendments in 1988 were aimed at increasing pressure on users, as well as on criminal organizations and money laundering.
- Federal support for urine screening began in the military and has since spread to other federal agencies, nonfederal transportation workers, and many private employers.
- Current federal enforcement efforts involve thousands of federal employees and include activities in other countries, along our borders, and within the United States.
- Most states have adopted some version of the DEA's recommended Uniform Controlled Substances Act. Also, the federal government has mandated uniform minimum drinking age of 21 years in all states.
- Federal, state, and local enforcement limits the supply of drugs and keeps their prices high, but the high prices attract more smugglers and dealers. It will never be possible to completely eliminate illicit drugs.

REVIEW QUESTIONS

1. What four kinds of habit-forming drug use at the turn of the twentieth century caused social reactions leading to the passage of federal drug laws?
2. What were the two fundamental pieces of federal drug legislation passed in 1906 and 1914?
3. In about what year did it first become necessary for drug companies to demonstrate to the FDA that new drugs were effective for their intended use? *1962*
4. What three phases of clinical drug testing are required before a new drug application can be approved?
5. What historic piece of federal legislation did the most to shape our overall approach to

the control of habit-forming drugs in the United States? *18th Amd. prohibiting Alcohol*
6. Who was Harry Anslinger, and what was his role in marijuana regulation?
7. What is the important difference between a Schedule I and a Schedule II controlled substance?
8. What are drug paraphernalia laws, and why have they been subject to court challenges?
9. What are the limitations of the EMIT procedure used in urine screening?
10. Approximately how much is the United States spending per year on federal drug-control efforts?

REFERENCES

1. Kane HH: *Opium-smoking in America and China.* New York: G.P. Putnam's Sons, 1882.
2. Adams SH: The great American fraud, *Collier's,* six segments, Oct 1905 to Feb 1906.
3. *Congressional Record* 40:102 (Part 1), Dec 4, 1905 to Jan 12, 1906.
4. Latimer D, Goldberg J: *Flowers in the blood: The story of opium,* New York: Franklin Watts, 1981.
5. Terry CE, Pellens M: *The opium problem.* New York: Bureau of Social Hygiene, 1928.
6. Courtwright DT: *Dark paradise: Opiate addiction in America before 1940.* Cambridge, MA: Harvard University Press, 1982.
7. Young JH: *The medical messiahs: A social history of health quackery in twentieth-century America.* Princeton, NJ: Princeton University Press, 1967.
8. *Industry profile 2000,* Washington, DC: Pharmaceutical Manufacturers Association, 2000.
9. Schmeckebier LF: *The bureau of prohibition.* Service Monograph No 57, Institute for Government Research, 1929, Brookings Institute. Cited in King R: Narcotic drug laws and enforcement policies, *Law & Contemporary Problems* 22:122, 1957.
10. *U.S. News & World Report* 41:22, 1956.
11. *Controlled Substances Act as amended, with addenda.* Available from Drug Enforcement Administration, Washington, DC: U.S. Department of Justice.
12. Lawrence C: In its last act, Congress clears anti-drug bill, *Congressional Quarterly,* pp 3145–3151, Oct 29, 1988.
13. Bureau of Justice Statistics: *A guide to state controlled substances acts.* Washington, DC: U.S. Department of Justice, 1991.

14. *Community and legal responses to drug paraphernalia*, DHEW Pub No (ADM) 80-963, Washington, DC: U.S. Government Printing Office, 1980.

15. National Institute of Justice: *State and local experience with drug paraphernalia laws*. Washington, DC: U.S. Department of Justice, 1988.

16. *Employee drug screening: Detection of drug use by urinalysis*, DHHS Pub No (ADM) 86-1442, Washington, DC: U.S. Government Printing Office, 1986.

17. Drug testing: The state of the art, *American Scientist* 77:19–23, 1989.

18. *Hair analysis as a drug detector*. Washington, DC: U.S. Department of Justice, 1995.

19. Organized crime drug enforcement task forces: Goals and objectives, *Drug Enforcement*, pp 3-15, Summer 1984.

20. *National drug control strategy*. Washington, DC: The White House, 2000.

21. Beck AJ: *Prisoners in 1999*. Bureau of Justice Statistics Bulletin, U.S. Department of Justice, August 2000.

22. Why good cops go bad, *Newsweek*, Dec 19, 1994.

23. Culhane C: U.S. fails in South American drug war, *The U.S. Journal of Drug and Alcohol Dependence*, Jan 1989.

24. Riley KJ: *Snow job?* New Brunswick, NJ: Transaction, 1996.

Section II

How Drugs Work

A drug is nothing but a chemical substance until it comes into contact with a living organism. In fact, that's what defines the difference between drugs and other chemicals—drugs have specific effects on living tissue.

Because this book is about psychoactive drugs, the tissue we're most interested in is the brain. We want to understand how psychoactive drugs interact with brain tissue to produce effects on behavior, thoughts, and emotions.

Obviously, we don't put drugs directly into our brains; usually we swallow them, inhale them, or inject them. In Section II, we will find out how the drugs we take get to the brain, and what effects they might have on the other tissues of the body.

Chapter 6

The Nervous System

KEY TERMS

homeostasis

hormones

neurotransmitters

receptors

CNS

autonomic

sympathetic

parasympathetic

basal ganglia

Parkinson's disease

dopamine

nigrostriatal dopamine pathway

nucleus accumbens

mesolimbic dopamine pathway

acetylcholine

norepinephrine

serotonin

GABA

endorphin

precursors

uptake

(continued)

Online Learning Center Resources

www.mhhe.com/ray

Log on to our Online Learning Center (OLC) for access to these additional resources.

- Chapter key terms and definitions
- Learning objectives
- Additional behavior change objectives
- Student interactive questions and answer sites
- Self-scoring chapter quiz

The OLC also offers web links for study and exploration of health topics. Here are some examples of what you'll find:

www.nida.nih.gov/NIDA_Notes/NNVol15N4/Pursues.html

Check out this article: "NIDA Pursues Many Approaches to Reversing Methamphetamine's Neurotoxic Effects," which is posted on the NIDA website. The article discusses scientific research into blocking and reversing brain damage caused by methamphetamine abuse.

bjo.bmjjournals.com/cgi/collection/drugs%3Acentral_nervous_system

The *British Journal of Ophthalmology* posts various articles on its website, including articles that address the effects of drugs on the central nervous system.

pharmacology.about.com/health/pharmacology/cs/nervous_system/index.htm

This website, specially designed as a reference guide for pharmacists, offers information about drugs for several psychological disorders. It also includes links to news about treatments.

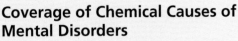

Drugs in the Media

Coverage of Chemical Causes of Mental Disorders

In the past, you may have been only vaguely aware of the number of reports that appear in newspapers and magazines

(continued)

| synthesis |
| enzymes |
| storage |
| release |
| binding |
| reuptake |
| metabolize |

Drugs in the Media Continued. . .

indicating a possible breakthrough in some type of mental illness. Because new brain chemicals are being discovered rapidly, it is inevitable that our hopes are high for new understanding and possible new treatments for schizophrenia, depression, and other major disorders. Chapter 10 presents the current state of our understanding and treatment of these problems.

In this chapter you will learn some things about the brain and its neurotransmitters and hormones, and you will probably pay more attention to such media coverage in the future. If you want to test and sharpen your knowledge of this important approach to understanding human behavior, go to your college library and look back over the last year's issues of current magazines, such as *Time, Newsweek,* or *Scientific American,* or search their websites. The publications will probably include quite a few brief news reports relating chemicals to mental disorders.

In current fashion and daily news, you'll find reports about researchers testing a drug called Celexa designed to cure shopaholics of "compulsive shopping disorder," which has only recently been nudged into the medical mainstream. The drug, similar to Prozac, is in the class of antidepressants known as selective serotonin reuptake inhibitors (SSRIs). Serotonin is thought to play a key role in mood and behavior.

Inclusion of health issues like these has not come about without careful consideration by magazine and newspaper editors. When surveyed, readers report that they want more coverage of health issues, and publishers have complied. Fortunately, the health editors and writers for major publications generally do an excellent job of preparing news reports. Most try to consult health researchers who are experts in their fields. But be inquisitive about whether there is more than one perspective on stories that interest you. You can find and read the original sources mentioned in the article. Many of these original sources are available at your library or on the Internet. If you have additional questions, ask professors, physicians, or someone else who is knowledgeable in the field. This way, magazines and newspapers can provide an ideal first step in your quest for new information concerning your health.

Drugs are psychoactive, for the most part, because they alter ongoing functions in the brain. To understand how drugs influence psychological processes, it is necessary to have some knowledge of the normal functioning of the brain and other parts of the nervous system and then to see how drugs can alter those normal functions. A person with little or no background in biology or chemistry can develop a good understanding of these topics at a conceptual level. Learning these concepts and some of the basic terminology will be very helpful in understanding the actions and effects of each of the major types of psychoactive drugs.

CHEMICAL MESSENGERS

Since the first multicellular organisms oozed about in their primordial tidal pools, some form of cell-to-cell communication has been necessary to ensure the organism's survival. Those first organisms probably needed to coordinate only a few functions, such as getting nutrients into the system, distributing them to all of the cells, and then eliminating wastes. At that level of organization, perhaps one cell excreting a chemical that could act on neighboring cells was all that was necessary. As more complex organisms evolved with multicellular systems for sensation, movement, reproduction, and temperature regulation, the sophistication of these communication mechanisms increased markedly. It became necessary for many types of communication to go on simultaneously and over greater distances. Although those early organisms were at the mercy of the sea environment in which they lived, we carry our own sea-water-like cellular environment around with us and must maintain that internal environment within certain limits. This process is known as **homeostasis.** This word can be loosely translated as "staying the same," and it describes the fact that many biological factors are maintained at or near certain levels. For example, most of the biochemical reactions basic to the maintenance of life are temperature dependent, in that these reactions occur optimally at temperatures near 37°C (98.6°F). Because we cannot live at temperatures too much above or below this level, our bodies have many mechanisms they can use to either raise or lower temperature: perspiring, shivering, altering blood flow to the skin, and others. Similar homeostatic mechanisms regulate the acidity, water content, and sodium content of the blood; glucose concentrations; and other physical and chemical factors that are important for biological functioning. In humans and other mammals, we find a variety of sophisticated systems for chemical communication within the body; presumably these evolved at different times, forming layers of communication and control, which interact with one another at many levels. These chemical messengers can be divided into two broad classes: hormones and neurotransmitters.

Hormones

Hormones are chemicals that are released from specialized groups of secretory cells (often called glands) and that affect other cells, which we think of as "target" cells (Figure 6.1). For example, the male sex hormone testosterone is released from the testes into the bloodstream. It then circulates throughout the body, influencing muscular and neural development, sexual and aggressive behavior, and other functions. Another gland, the pituitary, releases several hormones that circulate through the bloodstream, each having specific effects on the appropriate target cells. Many of these target tissues are themselves glands, and the pituitary therefore controls the release of other hormones. Some pituitary hormones have more direct actions. For example, when blood pressure drops, the pituitary releases vasopressin, which signals the kidneys to release less fluid into the urine. Drinking alcohol inhibits the release of vasopressin, so the kidney releases more fluid into the urine.

Neurotransmitters

In the nervous system, more discrete signals are found (Figure 6.2). Neurons act as secretory cells, target cells, and conductors of electrical signals. Each neuron releases one or a few specialized

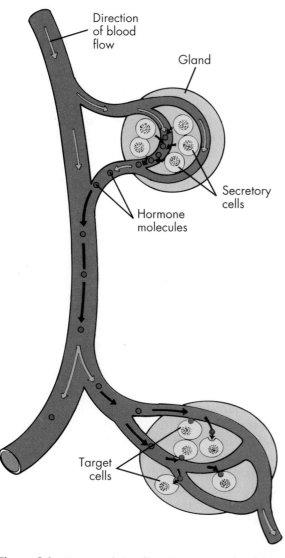

Figure 6.1　Hormonal signaling. Hormone molecules are released by secretory cells in a gland. The molecules are carried by the blood to distant target cells, where they exert their signaling effect.

signaling chemicals, called **neurotransmitters.** There are about 50 chemicals believed to act as neurotransmitters, and each neuron is sensitive to one or a few of them.[1]

What makes the action of neurotransmitters more discrete than that of hormones is that they are not released into the blood but, rather, are released into a small space, called a synapse, between two neurons. The chemical released into that synapse affects only one neuron, rather than a whole group of target cells, at once. Because only a small amount of neurotransmitter chemical is released into this small synapse, it can be removed quickly once it has sent its signal. Therefore, the signal is discrete in time, as well as in space. This allows the sending of detailed information from one specific place to another in the nervous system. To give some idea of scale, the synaptic space is less than 1/10,000th of an inch across. Several thousand neurotransmitter molecules are released at once, and it takes only microseconds for these molecules to diffuse across the synapse.

Although many neurotransmitters have been identified, we are concerned mostly with those few that we believe to be associated with the actions of the psychoactive drugs we are studying. Those neurotransmitters include *acetylcholine, norepinephrine, dopamine, serotonin, γ-aminobutyric acid (GABA),* and the endorphins.

Chemical signals are useful only if the target cells are able to detect the presence of the signal

homeostasis: maintenance of an environment of body functions within a certain range (e.g., temperature, blood pressure).

hormones: chemical messengers that send signals over a fairly wide area.

neurotransmitters: chemical messengers released from neurons and having brief, local effects.

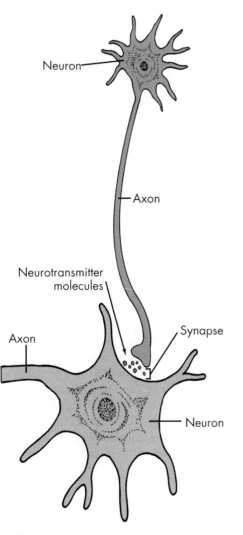

Figure 6.2 Chemical signaling in the nervous system. When an electrical signal reaches the terminal end of an axon, it causes release of neurotransmitter molecules into the synapse, a small space between the terminal and another neuron. The second neuron is affected by the transmitter molecules, which influences electrical activity in the second neuron.

molecules and then perform an action on the basis of having received that signal. The specialized structures that perform these functions are called **receptors**—subcellular structures that are part of the target-cell membrane.[2] These receptors play an important role in the actions of

many of the drugs we discuss in this book, and it is therefore important for you to have a feeling for how they work in the nervous system.

Each of the neurotransmitter chemicals has a unique three-dimensional structure that is characteristic of each of its molecules and is different from the molecules of other neurotransmitters. Some parts of the molecule are electrically more positive or negative than other parts, and the locations of these electrical charges also help make the molecule unique. One analogy that has been used to describe the interaction between the neurotransmitter and its receptor is that of a lock and key: the neurotransmitter fits into a receptor as a key fits into a lock. That model is useful for pointing out the specificity of the interaction based on the three-dimensional structure of the neurotransmitter, but it is difficult to explain the dynamic properties of the interaction using the lock-and-key analogy. In fact, a given molecule might be more or less attracted to a receptor, depending on its degree of fit and the locations of electrical charges on both the molecule and the receptor. This means that molecules vary widely in their *affinity* for a receptor, whereas we generally think of a key as either fitting or not fitting a lock. Figure 6.3 shows a schematic diagram of a portion of a synapse and depicts neurotransmitter molecules being released from the terminal of one neuron and binding to receptors of another neuron. The schematic diagram indicates that, in the process of binding, the receptor structure has to change its shape slightly in order to match up with the neurotransmitter molecule. This change in shape is the trigger that sets off changes in the electrical activity of the receiving neuron.

In neurons, the effect of a neurotransmitter's binding to its receptor might be to allow an electrical current to flow across the membrane. Because neurons conduct electrical signals along their membranes, the effect of a particular type of receptor is either to *excite* this electrical activity or to *inhibit* it. Figure 6.4 describes information flow in the nervous system. Electrical

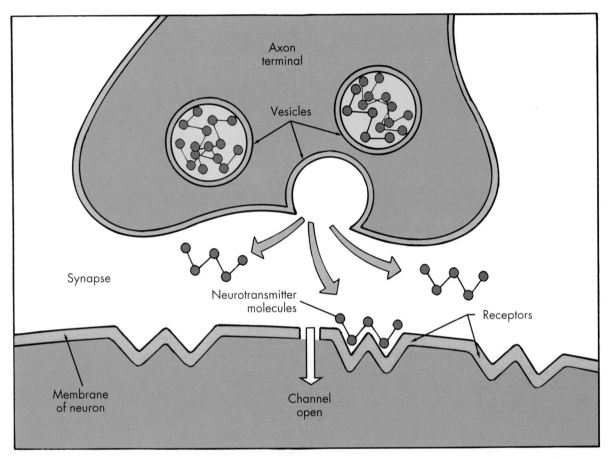

Figure 6.3 Schematic representation of the release of neurotransmitter molecules from synaptic vesicles in the axon terminal of one neuron and the passage of those molecules across the synapse to receptors in the membrane of another neuron. A neurotransmitter molecule has bound to the center receptor and has distorted it so as to open a channel through the membrane of the second cell. This channel allows the flow of electrically charged ions through the membrane, thus altering the electrical charge on the membrane of the second cell.

activity along the nerve membrane conducts information from one place to another, and, once that activity arrives at the nerve terminal, it results in the release of a neurotransmitter chemical, which influences the electrical activity of the next neuron. The electrical signal traveling along the membrane is brief—if it is amplified and sent to a loudspeaker, one hears a pop as the signal travels past the recording electrode. Neurons "fire" these signals several times a second under normal conditions, and excitatory or inhibitory influences can be seen as increasing or decreasing the firing rate of the neuron.

Whether the effect of a neurotransmitter is excitatory or inhibitory depends on the type of receptor. One of the neurotransmitters, GABA, seems to act at only inhibitory receptors.

receptors: recognition mechanisms that respond to specific chemical signals.

Electrical   Electrical   Chemicals   Chemicals attach   Chemicals in   Initiates
pulse in   →   pulse in   →   released   →   to receptor   →   receptor sites →   electrical
axon   terminals   from terminals   site   cause changes   impulse in
                                                                                in electrical   axon
                                                                                activity of
                                                                                dendrite

Figure 6.4   Sequence and mode of information movement in the nervous system.

Therefore, GABA is often called an inhibitory neurotransmitter. But acetylcholine acts at three or four types of receptors in the brain, and its action can be either excitatory or inhibitory, depending on the receptor. Most other neurotransmitters also have several types of receptors—some excitatory, some inhibitory.

THE NERVOUS SYSTEM(S)

Although we often speak of the nervous system, it is perhaps more appropriate to remember that there are several communication and control systems that are based on neurons and neurotransmitters. Some important distinctions among these systems will help us understand drug actions.

Central Nervous System

The central nervous system (**CNS**) consists of the brain and spinal cord. These two structures form a central mass of nervous tissue, with sensory nerves coming in and motor nerves going out. This is where most of the integration of information, learning and memory, and coordination of activity occur.

Somatic Nervous System

The nerve cells that are on the "front lines," interacting with the external environment, are referred to as the *somatic* system. These peripheral nerves carry sensory information into the CNS and carry motor (movement) information back out. The cranial nerves that relate to vision, hearing, taste, smell, chewing, and movements of the tongue and face are included, as are spinal nerves carrying information from the skin and joints and controlling movements of the arms and legs. We think of this system as serving voluntary actions. For example, a decision to move your leg results in activity in large cells in the motor cortex of your brain. These cells have long axons, which extend down to the spinal motor neurons. These neurons also have long axons, which are bundled together to form nerves, which travel out directly to the muscles. The neurotransmitter at neuromuscular junctions in the somatic system is acetylcholine, which acts on receptors that excite the muscle.

Autonomic Nervous System

Your body's internal environment is monitored and controlled by the **autonomic** nervous system (ANS), which regulates the visceral, or involuntary, functions of the body, such as heart rate and blood pressure. It is important for us to understand this system, because many psychoactive drugs have simultaneous effects in the brain and on the ANS. The ANS is also of interest because it is where chemical neurotransmission was first studied. If the vagus nerve in a frog is electrically stimulated, its heart slows. If the fluid surrounding that heart is then withdrawn and placed around a second frog's heart, it, too, will slow. This is an indication that elec-

TABLE 6.1		
Sympathetic and Parasympathetic Effects on Selected Structures		
Structure or function	**Sympathetic reaction**	**Parasympathetic reaction**
Pupil	Dilation	Constriction
Heart rate	Increase	Decrease
Breathing rate	Fast and shallow	Slow and deep
Stomach and intestinal glands	Inhibition	Activation
Stomach and intestinal wall	No motility	Motility
Sweat glands	Secretion	No effect
Skin blood vessels	Constriction	Dilation
Bronchi	Relaxation	Constriction

trical activity in the vagus nerve causes a chemical to be released onto the frog's heart muscle. When Otto von Loewi first demonstrated this phenomenon in 1921, he named the unknown chemical "vagusstoffe." We now know that this is acetylcholine, the same chemical that stimulates muscle contraction in our arms and legs. Because a different type of receptor is found in the heart, acetylcholine inhibits heart muscle contraction.

The ANS is divided into **sympathetic** and **parasympathetic** branches. The inhibition of heart rate by the vagus nerve is an example of the parasympathetic branch; acetylcholine is the neurotransmitter at the end organ. In the sympathetic branch, norepinephrine is the neurotransmitter at the end organ. Table 6.1 gives some examples of parasympathetic and sympathetic influences on various systems. Note that often, but not always, the two systems oppose each other.

Because the sympathetic system is interconnected, it tends to act more as a unit, to open the bronchi, reduce blood supply to the skin, increase the heart rate, and reduce stomach motility. This has been called the "fight or flight" response and is elicited in many emotion-arousing circumstances in humans and other animals. Amphetamines, because they have a chemical structure that resembles norepinephrine,

stimulate these functions in addition to their effects on the brain. Those drugs that activate the sympathetic branch are referred to as sympathomimetic drugs.

THE BRAIN

The Whole Brain

Although most of us don't think about it very often, the brain is obviously the most complex organ in our bodies. In fact, it is still the most amazing functional system in the world. We carry around in that small package a machine

---

CNS: brain and spinal cord.

autonomic: the part of the nervous system that controls "involuntary" functions, such as heart rate.

sympathetic: the branch of the autonomic system involved in flight or fight reactions.

parasympathetic: the branch of the autonomic system that stimulates digestion, slows the heart, and has other effects associated with a relaxed physiological state.

capable of storing and analyzing more information than the most powerful supercomputers. It might not be as fast at repetitive calculations, but it is able to deal simultaneously with thousands of kinds of input, select the important from the unimportant, and process images in ways unmatched by the most complex video devices. We might humbly remember that it is this fantastically complex machine that we are tinkering with when we take psychoactive drugs.

The brain has a rich supply of blood from four major arteries, so that drugs circulating in the blood have rapid access to the brain. However, the capillaries in the brain are different from those in the rest of the body—the cells are tightly joined, so that some molecules cannot pass freely out of the blood and into the brain. This specialization is part of the blood-brain barrier, which keeps many drugs from reaching the brain. Of course, for a drug to be psychoactive, its molecules must be capable of passing the blood-brain barrier.

The brain contains billions of neurons, and each can influence or be influenced by hundreds of other neurons. If these neurons all looked alike and were connected in random ways, it would be difficult for us to begin to understand anything about the organization of brain activity and function. Therefore, it would be impossible to understand psychoactive drug action by studying the brain. Luckily, study of the brain has revealed both structural and chemical organization, which helps us understand many of the functional effects of psychoactive drugs.

Major Structures

Knowing about a few of the major brain structures makes it easier to understand some of the effects of psychoactive drugs. When looking at the brain of most mammals, and especially of a human, much of what one can see consists of *cerebral cortex,* a layer of tissue that covers the top and sides of the upper parts of the brain (Figure 6.5). Some areas of the cortex are known to be involved in processing visual information; other areas are involved in processing auditory or somatosensory information. Relatively smaller cortical areas are involved in the control of muscles (motor cortex), and large areas are referred to as association areas. Higher mental processes, such as reasoning and language, take place in the cerebral cortex. In an alert, awake individual, arousal mechanisms keep the cerebral cortex active. When a person is asleep or under the influence of sedating drugs, the cerebral cortex is much less active, whereas other parts of the brain might be equally active whether a person is awake or asleep.

Underneath the cerebral cortex on each side of the brain and hidden from external view are the basal ganglia. The **basal ganglia** are important for the maintenance of proper muscle tone. For example, when you are standing still in a relaxed posture, your leg muscles are not totally relaxed. If they were, you would fall down in a slump. Instead, you remain standing, partly because of a certain level of muscular tension, or tone, that is maintained by the output of the basal ganglia. Too much output from these structures results in muscular rigidity in the arms, legs, and facial muscles. This can occur as a side effect of some psychoactive drugs that act on the basal ganglia, or it can occur if the basal ganglia are damaged by **Parkinson's disease.**

The *hypothalamus* is a small structure near the base of the brain just above the pituitary gland (Figure 6.6). The hypothalamus is an important link between the brain and the hormonal output of the pituitary and is thus involved in feeding, drinking, temperature regulation, and sexual behavior.

The *limbic system* consists of a number of connected structures that are involved in emotion, memory for location, and level of physical activity. Together with the hypothalamus, the limbic system involves important mechanisms for behavioral control at a more primitive level than that of the cerebral cortex.

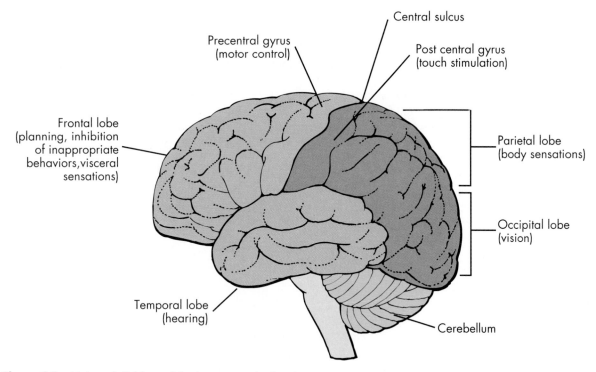

Figure 6.5   Major subdivisions of the human cerebral cortex.

The midbrain, pons, and medulla are the parts of the brain stem that connect the larger structures of the brain to the spinal cord. Within these brain-stem structures are many groups of cell bodies (nuclei) that play important roles in sensory and motor reflexes as well as coordinated control of complex movements. Within these brain-stem structures also lie the nuclei that contain most of the cell bodies for the neurons that produce and release the neurotransmitters dopamine, norepinephrine, and serotonin. Virtually all of the brain's supply of these important neurotransmitters is produced by a relatively small number of neurons (a few thousand for each neurotransmitter) located in these brain-stem regions.

In the lower *brain stem,* a couple of small areas of major importance are found. One area is the vomiting center. Often when the brain detects foreign substances in the blood, such as alcohol, this center is activated, and vomiting results. It is easy to see the survival value of such a system to animals, including humans, that have it. Another brain-stem center regulates the rate of breathing. This respiratory center can be suppressed by various drugs, resulting in respiratory depression, which can lead to death.

These structures and their functions have been understood in general terms for many years. Knowledge about such things comes

basal ganglia: subcortical brain structures controlling muscle tone.

Parkinson's disease: degenerative neurological disease involving damage to dopamine neurons.

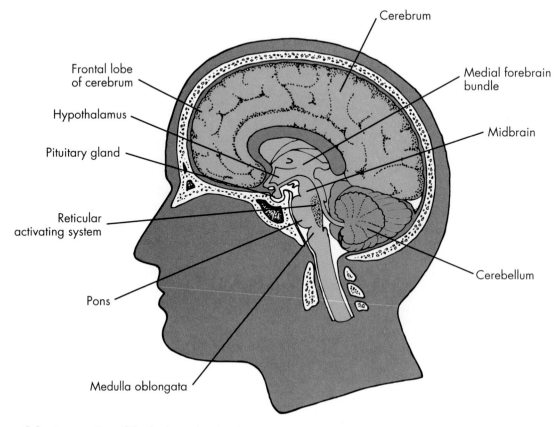

Figure 6.6   Cross section of the brain: major structures.

partly from people who have suffered accidental brain damage and partly from experiments using animals. These basic structures exist in mammals other than humans, with functions and connections that are basically the same, so it is possible to learn a great deal about human brain function from animal experiments.

Chemical Pathways

Dopamine

In some cases, groups of cells in a particular brain region contain a particular neurotransmitter chemical, and axons from these cells are found grouped together and terminating in another brain region. We think of many psychoactive drug actions in terms of a drug's effect on one of these chemical pathways. For example, we know that cells in the basal ganglia receive input from **dopamine** fibers that arise in the substantia nigra in the midbrain, course together past the hypothalamus, and end in the corpus striatum (part of the basal ganglia). This **nigrostriatal dopamine pathway** is what is damaged in Parkinson's disease and what is affected by the tranquilizers that produce muscular rigidity as a side effect (see Chapter 10).

Another important dopamine pathway also begins in the midbrain but projects to the **nucleus accumbens,** which is part of the limbic system. This **mesolimbic dopamine pathway** has been proposed to play a role in some types of psychotic behavior. Also, the most widely studied neurochemical theory of drug dependence is based on the idea that all addictive drugs, from alcohol to nicotine, stimulate dopamine neurons in the mesolimbic system. The mesolimbic system is proposed to be the main component responsible for the "reward" properties of electrical stimulation of the midbrain or limbic system. Thus, according to this theory, drugs lead to psychological dependence because they stimulate this reward system, which is responsible for telling the rest of the brain "that's good—do that again."[3]

Acetylcholine

Pathways containing **acetylcholine** arise from cell bodies in the *nucleus basalis* in the lower part of the basal ganglia and project to much of the cerebral cortex. In patients who have died from *Alzheimer's disease,* these cells are damaged and the cortex contains much less acetylcholine than normal. This degenerative disease affects millions of older Americans, causing personality changes, memory loss, and widespread mental deterioration. Because this link with an acetylcholine pathway was only recently discovered, much research activity is currently focused on finding chemical means to diagnose and treat Alzheimer's disease. Acetylcholine has also been one of the main neurotransmitters studied with regard to the initiation of REM (rapid eye movement) sleep, during which most dreaming occurs.

Norepinephrine

Pathways arising from the *locus ceruleus* in the brain stem have numerous branches and project both up and down in the brain, releasing **norepinephrine** and influencing the level of arousal and attentiveness. It is perhaps through these pathways that stimulant drugs induce wakefulness. Norepinephrine pathways play an important role in the initiation of food intake, although other transmitter systems are also involved in the very important and therefore very complex processes of controlling energy balance and body weight.

Serotonin

Serotonin-containing pathways arise from the brain-stem *raphe nuclei* and have projections both upward into the brain and downward into the spinal cord. Animal research has suggested one or more roles for serotonin in the complex control of food intake and the regulation of body weight. The diet drug fenfluramine, one half of the notorious "fen-phen" combination that became so popular in the 1990s, might cause its (limited) weight-reducing effects in humans by releasing and blocking the reuptake of serotonin.[4] Research on aggressiveness and impulsivity has also focused on serotonin. In studies with monkeys, low levels of serotonin metabolites in the blood have been associated with impulsive aggression, as well as with excessive alcohol consumption. And some humans who commit suicide or who make serious attempts show low levels of serotonin metabolites in the blood.[5] The success of selective serotonin reuptake inhibitors, such as Prozac, in treating major

---

dopamine: (*dope* **ah meen**) neurotransmitter found in the basal ganglia and other regions.

nigrostriatal dopamine pathway: one of two major dopamine pathways; damaged in Parkinson's disease.

mesolimbic dopamine pathway: (**meh zo** *lim* **bick**) one of two major dopamine pathways; may be involved in psychotic reactions and in drug dependence.

acetylcholine: (**eh see till** *co* **leen**) neurotransmitter found in the parasympathetic branch in the cerebral cortex.

norepinephrine: neurotransmitter that may be important for regulating waking and appetite.

serotonin: (**sehr o** *tone* **in**) neurotransmitter found in the raphe nuclei; may be important for impulsivity, depression.

Exploring Your Spirituality

Harnessing the Mind and Spirit

Powers of the mind and spirit can help us be resilient in the face of adverse conditions, such as extreme physical hardship. Take the case of American cyclist Lance Armstrong. Armstrong, now free of testicular cancer, which had spread to his abdomen, lungs, and brain, giving him a 50 percent chance of survival at best, won the grueling Tour de France bicycle race not once, but twice.

In October 1996, Armstrong was diagnosed with advanced testicular cancer. After his diagnosis, but before he started aggressive therapy, Armstrong called himself "a cancer survivor, not a cancer victim." He convinced himself, his family, and his medical team that he could beat the odds against him. He battled through his therapy without giving up hope that the disease would be defeated.

Miraculously, Armstrong's cancer disappeared. He then stunned the cycling world by training to make a comeback and competing in the 1999 Tour de France. As his physical condition improved, fans believed that he might be able to compete in—but not win—the famous bike race. But Armstrong's mental and spiritual resilience helped give him the strength to win the race. He won the race again in 2000, securing his place as one of the most amazing athletes of all time.

Lance Armstrong's success has undoubtedly inspired many others to take charge of their lives, overcome seemingly insurmountable obstacles, and bounce back to pursue their dreams. Do you think this kind of resilience can be learned? What role might the neurotransmitters play in the mind's influences over the body?

depressive disorder has also led to theories linking serotonin to depression. In all these cases (food intake and weight control, aggression and impulsivity, alcohol use, and depression), it is clear that environmental influences play important roles, and other drugs that work through different neurotransmitter systems can also influence these behaviors. Therefore, it is much too simple to attribute these behavioral problems to low serotonin levels alone. Hallucinogenic drugs, such as LSD, are believed to work by influencing serotonin pathways.

GABA

GABA is one neurotransmitter that is *not* neatly organized into discrete pathways or bundles. GABA is found in most areas of the CNS and exerts generalized inhibitory functions. Many sedative drugs act by enhancing GABA inhibition (see Chapter 9). The club drug GHB is a close chemical relative of the neurotransmitter GABA. Interfering with normal GABA inhibition, such as with the GABA-receptor-blocking drug strychnine, can lead to seizures resembling those seen in epilepsy.

Endorphins

Several chemicals in the brain produce effects similar to those of morphine and other drugs derived from opium. The term **endorphin** was coined in reference to endogenous (coming from within) morphinelike substances. These substances are known to play a role in pain relief, but they are found in several places in the brain as well as circulating in the blood, and not all their functions are known. Although it is tempting to theorize about the role of endorphins in addictions to drug use or other activities, the actual evidence linking addiction to endorphins has not been strong, and other neurotransmitter systems (particularly dopamine and serotonin systems) have also been shown to influence behaviors related to addiction.

DRUGS AND THE BRAIN

A drug is carried to the brain by the blood supply. How does each drug know where to go once it gets into the brain? The answer is that the drug doesn't know; it goes everywhere. But, because the drug molecules of LSD, for example,

Try It!

What's Your Body's Natural Cycle?

Can your behavior affect your brain chemistry? You bet! One of the more interesting aspects of brain biochemistry being studied is the daily changes in serotonin and other brain chemicals that follow a regular pattern, known as a circadian rhythm. The term *circadian* means "approximately daily" and reflects the fact that humans deprived of any information about time of day tend to follow a pattern of waking, sleeping, and eating that varies somewhat from day to day but usually averages out to a cycle just a bit more than 24 hours. Most people under normal circumstances report that they have certain peak times of the day when they feel most energetic and mentally sharper, and people are more likely to be hungry around their normal mealtimes and sleepy at their normal bedtimes. We also know that people whose jobs keep them on irregular schedules of sleeping and waking (repeated shift changes) and people who have recently flown across several time zones (jet lag) do not perform at their best. Also, most people who suffer from major depressive disorder show some disruption of normal patterns of sleeping, waking, and eating.

Thus, one thing you can do to help your brain chemistry maintain its natural cycles is to keep a fairly consistent schedule. Following is a checklist to help you:

1. On most days of the week, do you wake up at approximately the same time each day (within 30 minutes or so)?   Yes   No
2. Do you spend at least a few minutes out of doors in the morning every day? Even on a cloudy day, sunlight is usually brighter than most indoor lighting, and light is an important stimulus to your brain's circadian rhythms.   Yes   No
3. Do you eat breakfast every morning, at about the same time each day?   Yes   No
4. Do you get some physical exercise on most days, and is it usually at about the same time of day?   Yes   No
5. On most days of the week, do you usually go to sleep at about the same time each night? The timing of when you go to sleep is apparently somewhat less important than consistency in when you wake up.   Yes   No

If your own pattern is quite variable from day to day, try being more consistent and see if it helps you feel more energetic and able to focus your attention. If your pattern is fairly consistent from day to day, try to determine when you feel the most mentally alert, and see if you can schedule your most challenging mental activities close to that time of day.

Targeting Prevention

Sexual Dysfunction in Chronic Drug Users

One common problem faced by chronic users of alcohol, opiates, stimulants, and other psychoactive drugs is some form of sexual dysfunction. It may range from decreased interest in sex, to a man's inability to maintain an erection, to disruptions in a woman's menstrual cycle, to decreased sperm count. There are a variety of potential causes of these disruptive effects, mostly linked to the influence of these drugs on brain neurotransmitters. For example, although many of these drugs produce increased dopamine activity, dopamine release often decreases in the pituitary, leading to an excessive production of prolactin in both men and women. Prolactin, which is associated with milk production, also regulates other reproductive functions. Chronic drug use also alters thyroid and adrenal functions, leading to a state similar to chronic stress and possibly interfering with reproductive biology and behavior.[6]

Do you think that most people are aware of the link between chronic drug use and sexual dysfunction in both men and women? Could better publicity about these effects be an effective prevention message?

have their effect by acting on serotonin systems, LSD affects the brain systems that depend on serotonin. The LSD molecules that reach other types of receptors appear to have no particular effect. Because the brain is so well supplied with blood, an equilibrium develops quickly for most drugs, so that the drug's concentration in the brain is about equal to that in the blood and the number of molecules leaving the blood is equal to the number leaving the brain to enter the blood. As the drug is removed from the blood (by the liver or kidneys) and the concentration in the blood decreases, more molecules leave the brain than enter it, and the brain levels begin to decrease.

We are currently able to explain the mechanisms by which many psychoactive drugs act on the brain. In most of these cases, the drug has its effects because the molecular structure of the drug is similar to the molecular structure of one of the neurotransmitter chemicals. Because of this structural similarity, the drug molecules interact with one or more of the stages in the life cycle of that neurotransmitter chemical. We can therefore understand some of the ways drugs can act on the brain by looking at the life cycle of a typical neurotransmitter molecule.

Life Cycle of a Neurotransmitter

Neurotransmitter molecules are made inside the cell from which they are to be released. This makes sense, because, if they were just floating around everywhere in the brain, then the release of a tiny amount from a nerve ending wouldn't have much information value. However, the raw materials, or **precursors,** from which the neurotransmitter will be made are found circulating in the blood supply and generally in the brain. A cell that is going to make a particular neurotransmitter needs to bring in the right precursor in a greater concentration than exists outside the cell, so machinery is built into that cell's membrane for active **uptake** of the precursor. In this process, the cell expends energy to bring the precursor into the cell, even though the concentration inside the cell is

---

GABA: inhibitory neurotransmitter found in most regions of the brain.

endorphin: opiate-like chemical that occurs naturally in the brain of humans and other animals.

precursors: chemicals that are acted on by enzymes to form neurotransmitters.

uptake: energy-requiring mechanism by which selected molecules are taken into cells.

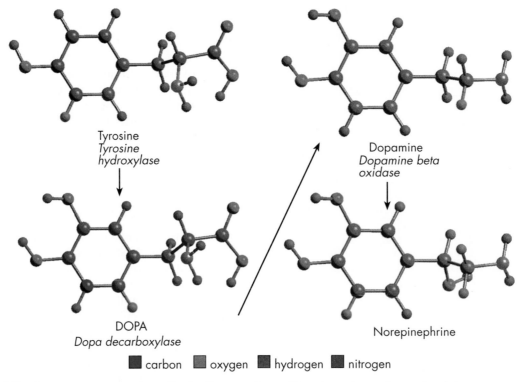

Tyrosine
*Tyrosine
hydroxylase*

Dopamine
*Dopamine beta
oxidase*

DOPA
Dopa decarboxylase

Norepinephrine

■ carbon   ■ oxygen   ■ hydrogen   ■ nitrogen

Figure 6.7   Neurons use enzymes to synthesize the neurotransmitters dopamine and norepinephrine.

already higher than that outside the cell. Obviously, this uptake mechanism must be selective and must recognize the precursor molecules as they float by. Many of the precursors themselves are amino acids that are derived from proteins in the diet, and these amino acids are used in the body for many things besides making neurotransmitters. In the example diagram of the life cycle of the neurotransmitter norepinephrine in Figure 6.7, the amino acid tyrosine is recognized by the norepinephrine neuron, which expends energy to take it in.

After the precursor molecule has been taken up into the neuron, it must be changed, through one or more chemical reactions, into the neurotransmitter molecule. This process is called **synthesis.** At each step in the synthetic chemical reactions, the reactions are helped along by

enzymes. These enzymes are themselves large molecules that recognize the precursor molecule, attach to it briefly, and hold it in such a way as to make the synthetic chemical reaction occur. Figure 6.8 provides a schematic representation of such a synthetic enzyme in action. In our example diagram of the life cycle of the catecholamine neurotransmitters dopamine and norepinephrine (Figure 6.7), the precursor tyrosine is acted on first by one enzyme to make DOPA and then by another enzyme to make dopamine. In dopamine cells the process stops there, but in our norepinephrine neuron, a third enzyme is present to change dopamine into norepinephrine.

After the neurotransmitter molecules have been synthesized, they are stored in small, round packages, called *vesicles,* near the terminal

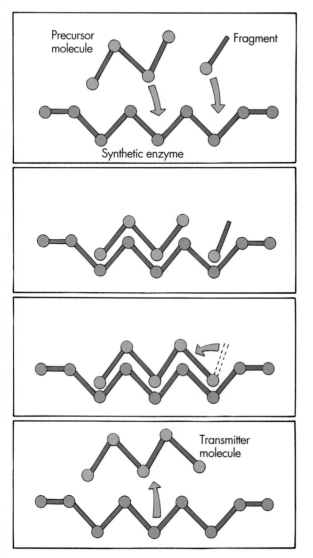

Figure 6.8 Schematic representation of the action of a synthetic enzyme. A precursor molecule and another chemical fragment both bind to the enzyme. The fragment has a tendency to connect with the precursor, but the connection is made much more likely because of the way the enzyme lines up the two parts. After the connection is made, the new transmitter molecule separates from the enzyme.

from which they will be released. This **storage** process also calls for recognizing the transmitter molecules and concentrating them inside the vesicles.

As an electrical signal arrives at the axon terminal, some of the vesicles fuse with the cell membrane and then open, releasing several thousand neurotransmitter molecules at once. This process of neurotransmitter **release** takes place within a few thousandths of a second after the electrical signal reaches the terminal.

Once the neurotransmitter molecules are released into the small synaptic space between neurons, a particular molecule might just float around briefly, or it might be one of the ones **binding** to the receptor on the membrane of the other neuron (Figure 6.3). This receptor is the most important recognition site in the entire process, and it is one of the most important places for drugs to interact with the natural neurotransmitter. With thousands of neurotransmitter molecules floating freely in the synapse, some will come near these receptors, bind to them briefly, then float away again. In the process of binding, the neurotransmitter distorts the receptor, so that a tiny passage is opened through the membrane, allowing an electrical current in the form of charged ions moving through the membrane (Figure 6.3). This opening does not last long, however, and within a

synthesis: the forming of a neurotransmitter by the action of enzymes on precursors.

enzyme: large molecule that assists in either the synthesis or metabolism of another molecule.

reuptake: the taking back of recently released neurotransmitter molecules into a neuron.

metabolize: to break down or inactivate a neurotransmitter (or a drug) through enzymatic action.

few thousandths of a second the neurotransmitter molecule has left the receptor and the ion channel is closed.

The small, localized electrical current found at a single receptor might not have much effect all by itself. However, these electrical currents spread, and, if enough receptors are activated at about the same time, then an electrical signal will be sent all the way down the axon to the terminal and a transmitter will be released there. The actual mechanisms by which this electrical current flows and moves along the membrane are too complicated to go into here. For our purposes, we need remember only that electrical signals carry information within a neuron and cause the release of chemical signals that carry information between neurons. These chemical signals, in turn, cause electrical signals in the next neuron, and so on (Figure 6.4).

Because signaling in the nervous system occurs at a high rate, once a signal has been sent in the form of neurotransmitter release, it is important to terminate that signal, so that the next signal can be transmitted. Thus, the thousands of neurotransmitter molecules released by a single electrical signal must be removed from the synapse. Two methods are used for this. In some cells, there is a process of **reuptake,** in which the neurotransmitter is recognized by a part of the membrane on the neuron from which it was released, and the releasing neuron then expends energy to recapture its released neurotransmitter molecules. With other neurotransmitters, enzymes in the synapse **metabolize,** or break down, the molecules (Figure 6.9). In either case, as soon as neurotransmitter molecules are released into the synapse, some of them are being removed or metabolized and never get to bind to the receptors on the other neuron. All neurotransmitter molecules might be removed in less than one-hundredth of a second from the time they are released. In the case of our example neurotransmitter, norepinephrine, those molecules are rapidly taken back up into the neuron from which they were released. Once inside the

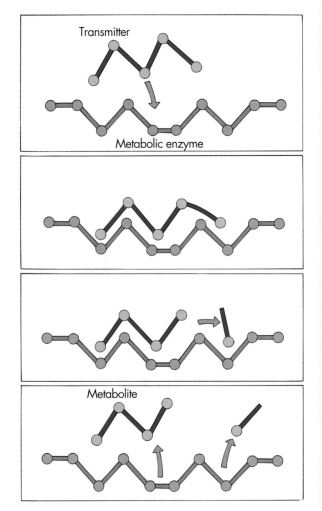

Figure 6.9 Schematic representation of the action of a metabolic enzyme. The transmitter molecule binds to the enzyme in such a way that the transmitter molecule is distorted and "pulled apart." The fragments then separate from the enzyme.

neuron, the norepinephrine molecules are metabolized by an enzyme found in the cell.

Examples of Drug Actions

It is possible to divide the actions of drugs on neurotransmitter systems into two main types. Through actions on synthesis, storage, release, reuptake, or metabolism, drugs can alter the *availability of the neurotransmitter in the synapse.* Either the amount of transmitter in the synapse, when it is released, or how long it remains before being cleared from the synapse will be affected. The second main type of drug effect is *directly on the receptors.* A drug can mimic the action of the neurotransmitter and thus directly activate the receptor (an *agonistic* action), or it can occupy the receptor and prevent the neurotransmitter from activating it (an *antagonistic* action).

Drug Effects on Neurotransmitter Availability

The drug L-dopa, which is used in the treatment of the CNS disorder Parkinson's disease, is actually the normal precursor for dopamine and is converted into dopamine by synthetic enzymes inside the neurons. This makes more dopamine available for release each time the neuron fires.

Perhaps one of the most interesting mechanisms is interference with the reuptake "pumps" that clear neurotransmitters, such as norepinephrine, serotonin, and dopamine, from the synapse by bringing them back into the neuron from which they were just released. Both the stimulant drug cocaine and most of the antidepressant drugs block one or more of these reuptake pumps and cause the normally released neurotransmitter to remain in the synapse longer than normal. One of the most exciting research areas in the neurosciences is the search for greater understanding of how altering these reuptake processes can produce either cocaine-like or antidepressant effects, depending perhaps on the neurotransmitter systems affected and the time course of the drug's action.

Drug Effects on Neurotransmitter Receptors

One method by which a drug can influence a receptor is to mimic the action of the neurotransmitter molecules. For example, the stimulant drug amphetamine is structurally similar to norepinephrine and dopamine, and one of its effects is to mimic these neurotransmitters at their receptors. Nicotine has effects very similar to the effects of the neurotransmitter acetylcholine (ACh) at some types of cholinergic receptors (they are called *nicotinic* acetylcholine receptors for this reason).

You may remember from Figure 6.3 the idea that, when the neurotransmitter binds to its receptor, in the process of matching up the structure of the transmitter molecule with the structure of the receptor, the receptor has to bend or stretch slightly, thus opening a small pore in the membrane. Suppose a drug molecule matched up so well with the receptor that the receptor didn't have to bend or stretch during the binding process. That drug molecule would fit the receptor better than the natural neurotransmitter. However, because the receptor doesn't have to change, there would be no effect on the electrical activity of the cell. Such agents are called antagonists, or "blockers," because by occupying the site they prevent the normal neurotransmitters from having a postsynaptic effect. The antipsychotic (also called neuroleptic or major tranquilizer) drugs, such as haloperidol (Haldol), block receptors for dopamine. Please remember that, when we refer to *blocking receptors,* only enough drug is given to block some of the receptors some of the time, so the net effect is to modulate, or alter, the activity in an ongoing system. Generally, if enough drug were given to block most of the receptors most of the time, the result would be highly toxic or even lethal.

Let's see if we can use our understanding of these mechanisms to predict what would happen if we tried to treat a psychotic patient who has Parkinson's disease with both L-dopa and haloperidol. The L-dopa is used to counteract damage to the dopamine systems in Parkinson's disease by making more dopamine available at the synapses. Haloperidol is used to control psychotic behavior, and it acts by blocking dopamine receptors. Thus, the drugs seem to have opposing actions. In fact, haloperidol often produces side effects that resemble Parkinson's disease, and L-dopa often produces hallucinations in its users. The two drugs are not used in the same patient because each tends to reduce the effectiveness of the other.

CHEMICAL THEORIES OF BEHAVIOR

Drugs that affect existing biochemical processes in the brain often affect behavior, and this has led to many attempts to explain normal (not drug-induced) variations in behavior in terms of changes in brain chemistry. For example, differences in personality between two people might be explained by a difference in the chemical makeup of their brains, or changes in an individual's reactions from one day to the next might be explained in terms of shifting tides of chemicals. Ancient Greek physician Hippocrates believed that behavior patterns reflected the relative balances of four *humors:* blood (hot and wet, resulting in a sanguine or passionate nature); phlegm (cold and wet, resulting in a phlegmatic or calm nature); yellow bile (hot and dry, resulting in a choleric, bilious, or bad-tempered nature); and black bile (cold and dry, resulting in a melancholic or gloomy nature). The Chinese made do with only two basic dispositions: *yin,* the moon, representing the cool, passive, "feminine" nature; and *yang,* the sun, representing the warm, active, "masculine" nature. Thus, any personality could be seen as a relative mixture of these two opposing forces. Unfortunately, most of the chemical-balance theories that have been proposed based on relative influences of different transmitters have not really been more sophisticated than these yin-yang and humoral notions of ancient times. Searches for differences in the amounts of norepinephrine, dopamine, serotonin, or other transmitters have not found evidence to relate the levels of these substances to personality differences, psychopathology, or mood swings. It is particularly tempting to speculate that alcoholics and drug addicts differ from "normal"

HealthQuest Activities

In Module 9, take some time alone to complete the assessment *Drugs: Are You at Risk?* How do you feel about your overall performance and the advice provided on the CD? Is it accurate and helpful? Think about the characteristics in your lifestyle, health, approach to drugs, and family influences that could put you more or less at risk.

In Module 8, read "Substance Abuse and Mental Illness," found under *Key Articles.* The article discusses possible links between substance abuse and mental illness. Based on what you have read in this chapter and what you've encountered in your life, what are some other physical ailments that may result from substance abuse?

Find the article "Emphysema Advances" in Module under *Key Articles.* This article addresses a specific illness resulting from tobacco abuse. If you smoke regularly, does the risk of emphysema concern you? If you do not smoke, are there some health factors, such as emphysema, that prevent you from doing so?

people in the function of an enzyme or neurotransmitter receptor, but, as mentioned in Chapter 3, no single biochemical theory of addiction has yet obtained sufficient experimental support to be considered an explanation.

One biochemical theory that still seems to have a lot of merit continues to guide people's thinking about major alterations in moods, such as those seen in clinical depression. Drugs that interfere with the catecholamines (norepinephrine and dopamine) are able to bring on a depressed mood, and drugs such as cocaine and amphetamines that stimulate activity in these catecholamine systems produce a temporary mood elevation. Thus, the *catecholamine theory of mood* is that too little activity in these systems can cause depression and too much can cause an excited or manic state (seen with high doses of amphetamines and cocaine). Although there

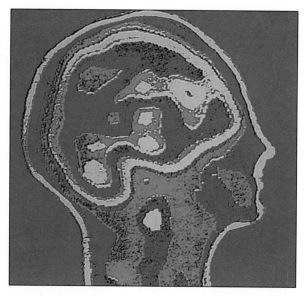

Figure 6.10   PET scan.

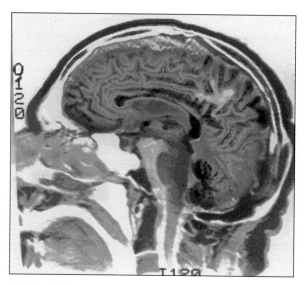

Figure 6.11   MRI scan.

is clear evidence that other neurotransmitter systems also play a role in the normal modulation of mood, the catecholamine theory is able to account for many of the basic drug effects on mood.

BRAIN IMAGING TECHNIQUES

Two techniques were developed during the 1980s for obtaining chemical maps of the brains of living humans. These techniques offer exciting possibilities for furthering our understanding of brain chemistry, abnormal behavior, and drug effects.

One of the techniques is positron emission tomography (PET) (Figure 6.10). In this technique, a radioactively labeled chemical is injected into the bloodstream, and a computerized scanning device then maps out the relative amounts of the chemical in various brain regions. Because all neurons in the brain rely on blood glucose for their energy, a labeled form of glucose can be used to see which parts of the brain are most active, and these vary depending

on what the person is doing. Similarly, blood flow to a particular brain region reflects the activity there, and labeled oxygen or other gases can map regional cerebral blood flow, which also changes depending on what the person is doing. More recently, labeled drugs that bind to dopamine, serotonin, or opiate receptors have been used, and it is therefore possible to see where the binding of those chemicals takes place in a living human brain. There is no doubt that our understanding of normal and abnormal brain function and of psychoactive drug effects will be advanced rapidly by these techniques over the next few years. Because these systems are very expensive to operate, they are found in only a few research hospitals.

Magnetic resonance imaging (MRI) is another brain imaging technique (Figure 6.11). Rather than using radioactive labels, the technique relies on applying a strong magnetic field and then measuring the energy released by various molecules as the field is collapsed. The signals are complex, but with the aid of computers it is possible to detect certain chemical "fingerprints" in the signals. This technique gives a high-resolution image and does not require the administration of expensive radiochemicals; because it can provide much information not attainable with simple X-ray studies, it has been rapidly adopted by the medical community. MRI systems have been installed in most major hospitals. A refinement of this technique (functional MRI), using higher-energy magnetic fields and more complex computational techniques, is beginning to be used to study apparent changes in metabolic activity in specific brain regions.[7]

SUMMARY

- Chemical signals in the body are important for maintaining homeostatis. The two types of chemical signals are hormones and neurotransmitters.
- Neurotransmitters act over brief time periods and very small distances because they are released into the synapse between neurons and are then rapidly cleared from the synapse.
- Receptors are specialized structures that recognize neurotransmitter molecules and, when activated, cause a change in the electrical activity of the neuron.
- The nervous system can be roughly divided into the central nervous system, the somatic system, and the autonomic system.
- The autonomic system, with its sympathetic and parasympathetic branches, is important because so many psychoactive drugs also have autonomic influences on heart rate, blood pressure, and so on.
- Specialized chemical pathways contain the important neurotransmitters dopamine, acetylcholine, norepinephrine, and serotonin.
- The nigrostriatal dopamine system is damaged in Parkinson's disease, leading to muscular rigidity and tremors.
- The mesolimbic dopamine system is thought by many to be a critical pathway for the dependence produced by many drugs.

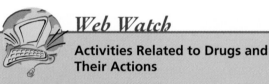

Web Watch

Activities Related to Drugs and Their Actions

The Effects of Illegal Drugs
Take the "Illegal Drugs Quiz" at library.thinkquest.org/29500/addictions/drugs.quiz.shtml and discover how familiar you are with the actions of illegal drugs on the body.

Drug Reactions and Interactions
Take the true-or-false quiz on illegal drugs at www.outerhebyouth.com/drugquiz.htm. Learn about some of the reactions first-time users have to certain drugs. Also take note of the amount of chemicals ingested and the effects of mixing certain drugs.

Drugs and Their Actions
Go to www.bulgpharmgroup.com/sopharma/categories/i_cns.html. This site offers an extensive pharmacological index of drugs and their effects on the nervous system. Click on a drug name and read the description of the drug and its actions.

- The neurotransmitter GABA is inhibitory and is found in most parts of the brain.
- The life cycle of a typical neurotransmitter chemical involves uptake of precursors, synthesis of the transmitter, storage in vesicles, release into the synapse, interaction with the receptor, reuptake into the releasing neuron, and metabolism by enzymes.
- Psychoactive drugs act either by altering the availability of a neurotransmitter at the synapse or by directly interacting with a neurotransmitter receptor.

REVIEW QUESTIONS

1. What are some examples of homeostatis in the human body?
2. What are the similarities and differences between hormones and neurotransmitters?

blood   *synapses*

lock → key

3. Describe the process of neurotransmitter release and receptor interaction.

4. Give some examples of the opposing actions of the sympathetic and parasympathetic branches of the autonomic nervous system. What is the neurotransmitter for each branch?

5. What is the function of the basal ganglia, *muscle tone* and which neurotransmitter is involved? *dopamine*

6. What is the proposed role of the mesolimbic dopamine system in drug dependence?

7. Alzheimer's disease produces a loss of which neurotransmitter from which brain structure?

8. What neurotransmitter seems to have only inhibitory receptors?

9. After a neurotransmitter is synthesized, where is it stored while awaiting release?

10. What are the two main ways in which drugs can interact with neurotransmitter systems?

11. PET and MRI are two examples of what technology?

REFERENCES

1. Feldman RS, Meyer JS, Quenzer LF: *Principles of neuropsychopharmacology.* Sunderland, MA: Sinauer, 1997.

2. Cooper JR, Bloom FE, Roth RH: *The biochemical basis of neuropharmacology.* 7th ed. New York: Oxford University Press, 1996.

3. Koob GF, LeMoal M: Drug abuse: Hedonic hemostatic dysregulation, *Science* 278:52–58, 1997.

   Weintraub M: Long-term weight control study: Conclusions, *Clinical Pharmacology and Therapeutics* 51: 586–594, 1992.

5. Azar B: Environment is key to serotonin levels, *Monitor,* American Psychological Association, Apr 1997.

6. Sexual dysfunction and addiction treatment. *Addiction Treatment Forum* 9: 1–8, 2000.

7. Maas LC and others: Functional MRI of human brain activation during cue-induced cocaine craving, *American Journal of Psychiatry,* 155:124-126, 1998.

Chapter 7

The Actions of Drugs

Online Learning Center Resources

www.mhhe.com/ray

Log on to our Online Learning Center (OLC) for access to these additional resources.

- Chapter definitions
- Learning objectives
- Student interactive questions-and-answer sites
- Self-scoring chapter quiz

The OLC also offers web links for study and exploration of health topics. Here are some examples of what you'll find:

pharmacology.about.com/health/
pharmacologylibrary/weekly/
aa970430.htm

At this site, read the article "Are Drugs Safe In Pregnancy?" It addresses the effects of illicit, prescription, and OTC drug use during pregnancy.

www.rush.edu/worldbook/articles/
004000a/004000148.html

The article posted here, "Effects of Drug Abuse," reports the habit-forming effects of amphetamines, cocaine, nicotine, LSD, and inhalants.

medstat.med.utah.edu/WebPath/
TUTORIAL/DRUG/DRUG.html

This website is a tutorial on the results of, diseases caused by, and actions of drug abuse. It offers specifics on tobacco, alcohol, cocaine, intravenous drugs, methamphetamine, and anabolic steroids.

Drugs in the Media

The Grapefruit-Juice Effect

Reports about the "grapefruit-juice effect"—the observation that grapefruit juice may boost the absorption of some commonly prescribed drugs—recently resurfaced in the news, leaving some citrus fans wondering if it's okay to

KEY TERMS (continued)

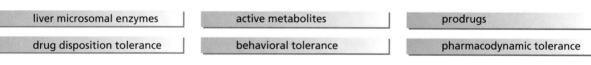

liver microsomal enzymes	active metabolites	prodrugs
drug disposition tolerance	behavioral tolerance	pharmacodynamic tolerance

Drugs in the Media Continued...

pop pills with their morning glass of juice. Drinking grapefruit juice to wash down some prescription medications may be dangerous because the juice can raise blood concentrations of the drug beyond what the dosage calls for.

Unlike other citrus juices, grapefruit juice inhibits one of the body's intestinal enzyme systems and can result in marked increases in serum levels of some prescription drugs, such as calcium-channel blockers used to control blood pressure and protease inhibitors given to treat HIV. An unknown chemical in grapefruit juice lowers the levels of a specific intestinal enzyme, allowing more of the drug to be absorbed. This enzyme normally breaks down drug molecules before they reach the bloodstream.

Researchers say grapefruit juice enhances the absorption of the cancer drug Vinblastine; the allergy medication Fexofenadine; the drug Digoxin, which is used to treat congestive heart failure; the blood pressure drug Losartan; and the drug Cyclosporine, an immunosuppressant medication used by organ transplant recipients. Interactions between grapefruit juice and certain drugs—which have been known but not extensively

studied—are particularly worrisome for elderly people, who are more likely to take medications and may drink calcium-fortified grapefruit juice.

Although some drugs are prescribed with others to enhance their effects, grapefruit juice should not be used for this purpose because its effects can be unpredictable and potentially dangerous. Only about 1 in 10 people are affected, but in those who are, the juice has boosted a drug's potency as much as 40 percent.

Researchers are working to identify exactly what gives grapefruit juice this unusual property. There is hope that better understanding of this phenomenon will lead to improvement in the effectiveness of some kinds of drugs, potentially lowering the amount of drug needed. It may also lead to more consistency in doses from patient to patient, because individual variations in the activity of this intestinal enzyme account for big differences in the effective dose from one person to another.

For more information, log on to the Grapefruit Juice–Drug Interactions website at *powernetdesign.com/grapefruit.*

SOURCES AND NAMES OF DRUGS

Sources of Drugs

You're probably already aware that most of the drugs in use 50 years ago originally came from plants. Even now, most of our drugs either come from plants or are chemically derived from plant substances. Have you ever wondered why the plants of this world produce so many drugs? Suppose a genetic mutation occurred in a plant so that one of its normal biochemical processes was changed and a new chemical was produced.

If that new chemical had an effect on an animal's biochemistry, when the animal ate the plant the animal might become ill or die. In either case, that plant would be less likely to be eaten and more likely to reproduce others of its own kind. Such a selection process must have taken place many thousands of times in various places all over the earth. Many of those plant-produced chemicals have effects on the intestines or muscles; others alter brain biochemistry. In large doses the effect is virtually always unpleasant or dangerous, but in controlled doses those chemicals might alter the biochemistry just enough to produce interesting or even useful effects. In primitive cultures the people who learned about these plants and how to use them safely were important figures in their communities. Those medicine men and women were the forerunners of today's pharmacists and physicians, as well as being important religious figures in their tribes.

Today the legal pharmaceutical industry is one of the largest and most profitable industries in the United States, with sales well over $100 billion a year.[1] With pharmaceutical sales in the billions of dollars, many people expect that there are zillions of drugs. Not so. Over half of all prescriptions are filled with only 200 drugs.

Names of Drugs

Commercially available compounds have several kinds of names: *brand, generic,* and *chemical.* The *chemical* name of a compound gives a complete chemical description of the molecule and is derived from the rules of organic chemistry for naming any compound. Chemical names of drugs are rarely used except in a laboratory situation where biochemists or pharmacologists are developing and testing new drugs.

Generic names are the official (i.e., legal) names of drugs and are listed in the *United States Pharmacopeia (USP).* Although a **generic** name refers to a specific chemical, it is usually shorter and simpler than the complete chemical name. Generic names are in the public domain, meaning they cannot be trademarked.

The *brand* name of a drug specifies a particular formulation and manufacturer, and the trademark belongs to that manufacturer. A brand name is usually quite simple and as meaningful (in terms of the indicated therapeutic use) as the company can make it. For example, the name *Elavil* was chosen for an antidepressant drug to indicate that it would elevate mood. However, brand names are controlled by the FDA, and overly suggestive ones are not approved.

When a new chemical structure, a new way of manufacturing a chemical, or a new use for a chemical is discovered, it can be patented. Patent laws in the United States now protect drugs for 20 years, and after that time the finding is available for use by anyone. Therefore, for 20 years a company that has discovered and patented a drug can manufacture and sell it without direct competition. After that, other companies can apply to the FDA to sell the "same" drug. Brand names, however, are copyrighted and protected by trademark laws. Therefore, the other companies have to use the drug's generic name or their own brand name. The FDA requires these companies to submit samples to demonstrate that their version is chemically equivalent and to do studies to demonstrate that the tablets or capsules they are making will dissolve appropriately and result in blood levels similar to those of the active drug. When a drug "goes generic," the original manufacturer might reduce the price of the brand name product in order to remain competitive.

CATEGORIES OF DRUGS

Physicians, pharmacologists, chemists, lawyers, psychologists, and users all have drug classification schemes that best serve their own purposes. A drug such as amphetamine might be categorized as a weight-control aid by a physician, because it reduces food intake for a period of time.

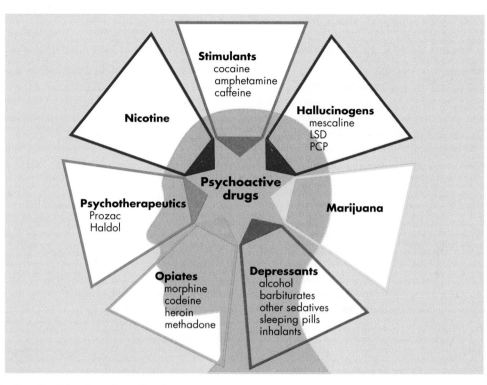

Figure 7-1　Classification of psychoactive drugs.

It might be classed as a phenylethylamine by a pharmacologist, because its basic structure is a phenyl ring with an ethyl group and an amine attached. The chemist says that amphetamine is 2-amino-1-phenylpropane. To the lawyer, amphetamine might be only a controlled substance falling in Schedule III of the federal drug law, whereas the psychologist might say simply that it is a stimulant. The user might call it a diet pill or an upper. The important thing to remember is that any scheme for categorizing drugs has meaning only if it serves the purpose for which the classification is being made.

The scheme presented here organizes the drugs according to their effects on the user, with first consideration given to the psychological effects. The basic organization and examples of each type are given in Figure 7.1, but it is worthwhile to point out some of the defining characteristics of each major grouping.

At moderate doses, *stimulant drugs* produce wakefulness and a sense of energy and well-being. The more powerful stimulants, such as cocaine and amphetamines, can at high doses produce a manic state of excitement combined with paranoia and hallucinations.

If you know about the behavioral effects of alcohol, then you know about the *depressant drugs.* At low doses they appear to depress inhibitory parts of the brain, leading to disinhibition or relaxation and talkativeness that can give

generic: (juh *ner* ic) a name that specifies a particular chemical but not a particular brand.

Exploring Your Spirituality

Taking Good Care of Yourself

Average life expectancy in the United States has increased dramatically from just a few generations ago: it's now 80 years for women and 76 years for men. Thanks to advances in medical science and technology, many people are enjoying healthy, happy, and spiritually fulfilling lives well into their later years.

This longevity means that making healthful choices every day—including exercise, a balanced diet, adequate rest, and opportunities for emotional and spiritual expression—takes on new significance. If you're going to live an "extra" 10 years, how can you make the best use of that time? Taking charge of your health when you're young and healthy can be one of the most empowering things you can do. By consciously choosing a healthy lifestyle—limiting your alcohol intake, avoiding drugs and cigarette smoking, and limiting your sexual partners—you are building a solid foundation for good health in your old age.

By becoming more responsible for your own health, you'll be better equipped to handle a serious medical problem, should that ever be necessary. Many people interested in self-care even develop the expertise to prevent or manage many kinds of illness and injury. They learn to assess their health status and treat, monitor, and rehabilitate themselves, when appropriate, in a way that was once considered possible only with the direct help of a physician or another health-care specialist. For example, many people are now administering injections for allergies and migraine headaches and are continuing physical therapy programs at home. Diabetes, asthma, and hypertension are other conditions that can be managed or monitored through self-care, with periodic consultation with a doctor.

Knowing you're doing everything you can to take care of yourself—being an informed health-care consumer, choosing a healthy lifestyle, fostering a positive outlook—brings a sense of peace. You're enhancing the quality of your life today and preparing for an active and rewarding tomorrow.

---

way to recklessness. As the dose is increased, other neural functions become depressed, leading to slowed reaction times, uncoordinated movements, and unconsciousness. It should be pointed out that stimulants and depressants do not really counteract one another. Although it may be possible to keep a drunk awake with cocaine, he or she would still be reckless, uncoordinated, and so on. Regular use of depressant drugs can lead to a withdrawal syndrome characterized by restlessness, shakiness, hallucinations, and sometimes convulsions.

Opiates are a group of analgesic (painkilling) drugs that produce a relaxed, dreamlike state; moderately high doses often induce sleep. Pharmacologically, this group is also known as the narcotics, and it is important to distinguish them from the "downers," or depressants. With opiates there is a clouding of consciousness without

the reckless abandon, staggering, and slurred speech produced by alcohol and other depressants. Regular use of any of the narcotics can lead to a withdrawal syndrome different from that of depressants and characterized by diarrhea, cramps, chills, and profuse sweating.

The *hallucinogens* produce altered perceptions, including unusual visual sensations and quite often changes in the perception of one's own body.

The *psychotherapeutic drugs* include a variety of drugs prescribed by psychiatrists and other physicians for the control of mental problems. The *antipsychotics,* such as haloperidol, are also called neuroleptics. They can calm psychotic patients and over time help them control hallucinations and illogical thoughts. The *antidepressants,* such as fluoxetine (Prozac), help some people recover more rapidly from seriously depressed mood states. Lithium is used to control manic episodes and to prevent mood swings in manic depressives.

As with any system of classification, there are some things that don't seem to fit into the classes. Nicotine and marijuana are two such drugs. Nicotine is often thought of as being a mild stimulant, but it also seems to have some of the relaxant properties of a low dose of a depressant. Marijuana is often thought of as a relaxant, depressive type of drug, but it doesn't share most of the features of that class. It is sometimes listed among the hallucinogens because at high doses it can produce altered perceptions, but that classification doesn't seem entirely appropriate for the way most people use it.

DRUG IDENTIFICATION

There are many reasons to identify exactly what drug is represented by a tablet, capsule, or plant substance. For example, the *Physician's Desk Reference (PDR)* has for many years published color photographs of many of the legally manufactured pharmaceuticals.[2] In this way a physician can determine from the pills themselves what drugs a new patient has been taking and in what doses. More critically, in emergency rooms it is possible to determine what drugs a person has just taken, if some of the pills are available for viewing. Police chemistry labs also use the *PDR* to get a preliminary indication of the nature of seized tablets and capsules.

Even illicit drugs can sometimes be identified by visual appearance. Often the makers of illicit tablets containing amphetamines or LSD mark them, however crudely, in a consistent way, so that they can be recognized by their buyers. Such visual identification is far from perfect, of course. Cocaine or heroin powder can also be wrapped and labeled in a consistent way by street dealers. Some plant materials, such as psilocybin mushrooms, peyote cactus, or coca or marijuana leaves, can be fairly easy to identify visually, although again not with perfect accuracy.

If a case involving illicit drugs is to be prosecuted in court, the prosecution will usually be expected to present the testimony of a chemist indicating that the drug had been tested and identified using specific chemical analyses.

DRUG EFFECTS

No matter what the drug or how much of it there is, it can't have an effect until it is taken. For there to be a drug effect, the drug must be brought together with a living organism. After a discussion of the basic concepts of drug movement in the body, you will be better able to understand such important issues as blood alcohol level, the dependence potential of crack cocaine, and urine testing for marijuana use.

Nonspecific (Placebo) Effects

The effects of a drug do not depend solely on chemical interactions with the body's tissues. With psychoactive drugs in particular, the influences of expectancy, experience, and setting are also important determinants of the drug's effect. For example, a good "trip" or a bad trip on LSD seems to be more dependent on the personality and mood of the user before taking the drug than on the amount or quality of drug taken. Even the effect of alcohol depends on what the user expects to experience. *Nonspecific* effects are those that derive from the user's unique background and particular perception of the world. In brief, the nonspecific effects can include anything except the chemical activity of the drug and the direct effects of this activity. Nonspecific effects are also sometimes called **placebo** effects, because they can often be produced by an inactive chemical (placebo) that the user believes to be a drug. The effects of a drug that depend on the presence of the chemical at certain concentrations in the target tissue are called *specific* effects. One important task for psychopharmacologists is to separate the specific effects of a drug from the nonspecific effects.

Suppose you design an experiment with two conditions: one group of people receives the drug you're interested in testing, in a dose that you have reason to believe should work. Each person in the control group receives a capsule that looks identical to the drug but contains no active drug molecules (a placebo). It is very important that the people be randomly assigned to the groups and that they be treated and evaluated identically except for the active drug molecules in the capsules of the experimental group. For this reason, tests for the effectiveness of a new drug must be done using a **double-blind procedure.** Neither the experimental subject nor the person evaluating the drug's effect knows whether a particular individual is receiving a placebo or an experimental drug. Only after the experiment is over and the data have all been collected is the code broken, so that the results can be analyzed.

The double-blind procedure can also be used to compare the effectiveness of two different drugs. One investigator[3] studied the differential effects of two sedatives on anxiety in a group of patients of general practitioners. Neither the patient nor the physician knew which drug was being used, and before the start of medication, both the physician and patient had to indicate whether they were optimistic, indifferent, or pessimistic about the outcome of treatment. After two months, regardless of the drug used, patients for whom the doctors had been optimistic showed a 50 percent reduction in symptoms, whereas the patients for whom the physician had been pessimistic showed only a 20 percent decrease. Optimistic patients showed a 45 percent reduction in their anxiety symptoms, while the patients pessimistic about outcome showed a symptom drop of 35 percent. This experiment demonstrates the strength of nonspecific factors and how the physician's expectations might be even more influential than the patient's expectations.

Nonspecific effects are not caused by the chemicals in drugs, but they are still "real" effects that in some cases might have a chemical basis. In a dental study,[4] some patients receiving a placebo reported a reduction of pain. When they were given a drug whose only effect is to block the opiate receptor in the brain, pain increased (just as it would have if the pain reduction were the result of morphine rather than a placebo). We know (see Chapter 16) that the body manufactures chemicals—*endorphins*—very similar to morphine and that these endorphins play an important role in the normal control of pain. The results of the dental study suggest that the placebo (i.e., the belief that the individual was taking a drug that would reduce pain) resulted in an increase in production of endorphins and thus a decrease in pain. However, not all placebo effects on pain are mediated by endorphins. Some of the effect may be on the perception of the pain's severity.

Dose-Response Relationships

Perhaps the strongest demonstration of the specific effects of a drug is obtained when the dose of the drug is varied and the size of the effect changes directly with the drug dose. A graph showing the relationship between the dose and the effect is called a **dose-response curve.** Typically, at very low doses no effect is seen. At some low dose there is an observable effect on the response system being monitored. This dose is the *threshold,* and as the dose of the drug is increased, there are more molecular interactions and a greater effect on the response system. At the point where the system shows maximal response, further additions of the drug have no effect.

In some drug-response interactions, the effect of the drug is all-or-none, so that when the system does respond, it responds maximally. There might, however, be variability in the dosage at which individual organisms respond, and as the dose increases, there is an increase in the percentage of individuals who show the response.

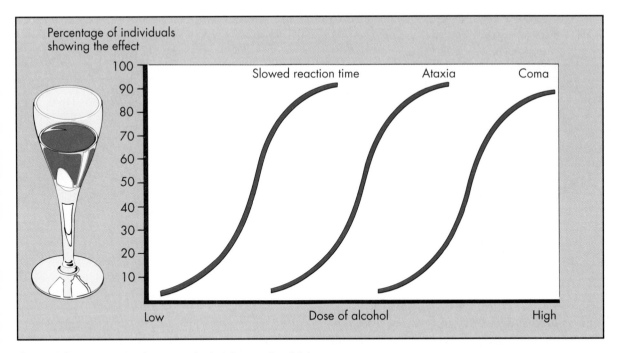

Figure 7.2   Relationship between alcohol dose and multiple responses.

As the drug dose increases, sometimes new response systems are affected by the drug. This fact suggests that some response systems have higher drug thresholds than others. Figure 7.2 shows a series of dose-response curves for three different effects of alcohol. As the dose increases from the low end, first a few and then more and more of the individuals show a slowing of their reaction times. If we also have a test for **ataxia** (staggering or inability to walk straight), we see that, as the alcohol dose reaches the level at which most individuals are showing slowed reaction times, a few are also beginning to show ataxia. As the dose increases further, more people show ataxia, and some become **comatose** (they pass out and cannot be aroused). At the highest dose indicated, all of the individuals would be comatose. Note that we could draw curves for other effects of alcohol on such a figure; for example, at the high end we would begin to see some deaths from

overdose, and a curve for lethality could be placed to the right of the coma curve.

In the rational use of drugs, there are four questions about drug dosage that must be answered. First, what is the effective dose of the drug for a desired goal? For example, what dose

placebo: (pluh _see_ bo) an inactive drug.

double-blind procedure: experiment in which neither the doctor nor the patient knows which drug is being used.

dose-response curve: a graph comparing the size of response to the amount of drug.

ataxia: (ay _tax_ ee ah) uncoordinated walking.

comatose: (_co_ mah tose) unconscious and unable to be aroused.

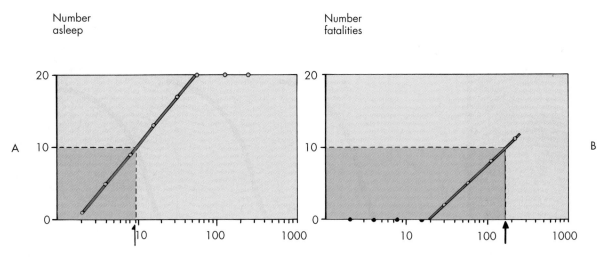

Figure 7-3   Calculation of **A,** effective dose, and **B,** lethal dose.

of morphine is necessary to reduce pain? What amount of marijuana is necessary for an individual to feel euphoric? How much aspirin will make the headache go away? The second question is what dose of the drug will be toxic to the individual? Combining those two, the third question is what is the safety margin—how different are the effective dose and the toxic dose? Finally, at the effective dose level, what other effects, particularly adverse reactions, might develop? Leaving aside for now this last question, a discussion of the first three deals with basic concepts in understanding drug actions.

Estimating the safety margin is an important part of the preclinical (animal) testing that is done on any new drug before it is tried in humans. In order to determine an *effective dose (ED),* it is necessary to define an effect in animals that is meaningful in terms of the desired human use. Although in some cases this is difficult, let us use the example of a new sleeping pill (hypnotic), and use several groups of 20 mice each. Each group will receive a different dose of our new hypnotic agent, and an hour later we will check to see how many mice in each group are sleeping. Let us assume that at the lowest

dose we tested, only 1 of the 20 mice was asleep, and at the highest doses all were asleep, with other values in between as shown in Figure 7.3. By drawing a line through these points, we can estimate the dose required to put any percentage of the mice to sleep. Even if we don't have a dose in our experiment that results in exactly 10 of the 20 mice sleeping, it is customary to calculate the **ED$_{50}$** (effective dose for 50 percent of the animals—in this case, mice—tested).

Toxicity is usually measured in at least one early animal study by determining how many mice die as a result of the drug. Let's say we check each cage the next day to see how many mice in each group died. From such a study we can estimate the **LD$_{50}$** (lethal dose for 50 percent of the mice; see Figure 7.3). The **therapeutic index (TI)** is defined as LD$_{50}$/ED$_{50}$. Since the *lethal dose* should be larger than the *effective dose,* the TI should always be greater than 1. The question is, how large should the TI be if the company is going to go forward with expensive clinical trials? The answer is that it depends partly on the TIs of the drugs already available for the same purpose. Also, it should be obvious that the TI will depend on what effect was used

Taking Sides

Animal Toxicity Tests

There has been increasing interest in the welfare of laboratory animals, and this has resulted in improved standards for housing, veterinary care, and anesthesia. Some animal rights groups have suggested that most types of animal research should be stopped altogether because the experiments are claimed to be either unnecessary or even misleading. The use of the LD_{50} test by drug companies, in which the researchers estimate the dose of a drug required to kill half the animals (usually mice), has been a particular target. The groups have claimed that these tests are outmoded and that toxicity could be predicted from computer models or work on isolated cell cultures.

A pamphlet published by People for the Ethical Treatment of Animals (PETA), one of the most well-known animal rights groups, claims on the one hand that the laboratory animals are sensitive beings with "distinct personalities. Just like you and me . . . ," but on the other hand that toxicity tests on animals are not relevant to humans because of basic biological differences. In reality, most basic biological functions are quite similar among all mammals, whereas the greatest differences between laboratory mice and humans would probably be found in the areas of thoughts, emotions, and "personality."

A specific case cited by PETA was thalidomide testing (see Chapter 5), which it claims "passed animal safety tests with flying colors" and later caused thousands of human deformities. Some critical points in that argument were, however, omitted. Thalidomide caused birth defects when taken during pregnancy. Otherwise, its human toxicity was quite low. Thalidomide was not tested on pregnant animals. If it had been, the birth defects would have been detected. And because of thalidomide, the laws were changed 30 years ago to *require* that drugs to be used by humans during pregnancy first undergo testing in pregnant animals.

Admittedly, giving drugs to pregnant animals to see if they produce birth defects or spontaneous abortions may seem cruel. Would you volunteer to be the first living animal to take a new drug whose toxicity had been estimated by a computer model? Which pregnant humans should be the first?

to define the effective doses. If the same drug is to be used for surgical anesthesia, a deeper sleep will be required (one from which the mice will not awake when they are poked and prodded). Higher doses would be required for such an effect; thus, the ED_{50} would be larger and the TI would be smaller.

This approach of estimating the dose to affect 50 percent of the mice is used in early animal tests because it is statistically more reliable to estimate the 50 percent point using a small number of mice per group than it is to estimate the 1 percent or 99 percent points. However, with humans we don't do LD_{50} experiments. Also, with some disorders, perhaps the best drugs we have can help only half of the people. What we ultimately want is to estimate the dose that will produce a desired effect in some fraction of the patients (ED_{99}? ED_{60}?) and a dose that

might be the lowest lethal dose (LD_1), or the lowest dose producing some other unacceptable toxic reaction. The difference between these doses would be called the **safety margin.**

Most of the psychoactive compounds have an LD_1 well above the ED_{95} level, so the practical

---

ED_{50}: effective dose for half of the animals tested.

LD_{50}: lethal dose for half of the animals tested.

therapeutic index (TI): ratio of LD_{50} to ED_{50}.

safety margin: dosage difference between an acceptable level of effectiveness and the lowest toxic dose.

Targeting Prevention

Avoiding Withdrawal Symptoms

Withdrawal symptoms may appear after ceasing the use of many psychoactive drugs if the user has been taking high doses for a prolonged period of time. When a hospital patient needs to be treated with narcotics for pain control (analgesia), how can the drug be given in such a way as to reduce the chances of developing physical dependence, as evidenced by withdrawal symptoms? Obviously, keeping doses as low as possible and giving the drug for as short a time as possible are two important keys. Ironically, one way to keep the dose as low as necessary while still obtaining adequate pain control is the use of a "PCA" (patient-controlled anesthesia or analgesia) pump. Within limits, each patient is allowed to administer just the amount of narcotic needed to control his or her pain. This prevents two problems: (1) giving more of the drug than is necessary just to make sure the pain is controlled, and (2) not giving quite enough of the drug, so that the patient experiences pain and has to request and wait for more of the drug before the pain is relieved. Dependence may actually be less of a problem when the patient is allowed to take the drug as needed.

limitation on whether or not, or at what dose, a drug is used is the occurrence of **side effects.** With increasing doses there is usually an increase in the number and severity of side effects—the effects of the drug that are not relevant to the treatment. If the number of side effects becomes too great and the individual begins to suffer from them, the use of the drug will be discontinued or the dose lowered, even though the drug may be very effective in controlling the original symptoms. The selection of a drug for therapeutic use should be made on the basis of effectiveness in treating the symptoms with minimal side effects.

Potency

The **potency** of a drug is one of the most misunderstood concepts in the area of drug use. Potency refers only to the *amount of drug* that must be given to obtain a particular response. The smaller the amount needed to get a particular effect, the more potent the drug. Potency does not necessarily relate to how effective a drug is or to how large an effect the drug can produce. *Potency* refers only to relative effective dose; the ED_{50} of a potent drug is lower than the ED_{50} of a less potent drug. For example, it has been said that LSD is one of the most potent psychoactive drugs known. This is true in that hallucinogenic effects can be obtained with 50 micrograms (μg), compared with several milligrams (mg) required with other hallucinogens (a μg is 1/1000 of a mg, which is 1/1000 of a gram [g]). However, the effects of LSD are relatively limited—it doesn't lead to overdose deaths the way heroin and alcohol do. Alcohol has a greater variety of more powerful effects than LSD, even though in terms of the *dose* required to produce a psychological effect LSD is thousands of times more *potent*.

Time-Dependent Factors in Drug Actions

In the mouse experiment, we picked 1 hour after administering the drug to check for the sleeping effect. Obviously, we would have had to learn a bit about the **time course** of the drug's effect before picking 1 hour. Some very rapidly acting drug might have put the mice to sleep within 10 minutes and be wearing off by 1 hour, and we would pick a 20- or 30-minute time to check the effect of that drug. The time course of a drug's action depends on many things, including how the drug is administered, how rapidly it is absorbed, and how it is eliminated from the body.

Figure 7.4 describes one type of relationship between administration of a drug and its effect

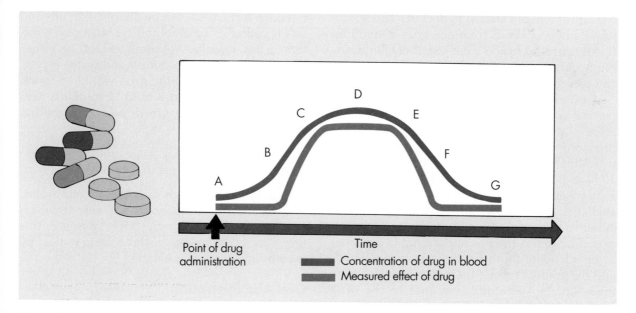

Figure 7-4   Possible relationship between drug concentration in the body and measured effect of the drug.

over time. Between points *A* and *B* there is no observed effect, although the concentration of drug in the blood is increasing. At point *B* the threshold concentration is reached, and from *B* to *C* the observed drug effect increases as drug concentration increases. At point *C* the maximal effect of the drug is reached, but its concentration continues increasing to point *D*. Although deactivation of the drug probably begins as soon as the drug enters the body, from *A* to *D* the rate of absorption is greater than the rate of deactivation. Beginning at point *D* the deactivation proceeds more rapidly than absorption, and the concentration of the drug decreases. When the amount of drug in the body reaches *E,* the maximal effect is over. The action diminishes from *E* to *F,* at which point the level of the drug is below the threshold for effect, although there is still drug in the body up to point *G*.

It should be clear that, if the relationship described in Figure 7.4 is true for a particular drug, then increasing the dose of the drug will not increase the magnitude of its effect. Aspirin and other headache remedies are probably the most misused drugs in this respect—if two are good, four should be better, and six will really stop this headache. No way! When the maximum possible therapeutic effect has been reached, increasing the dose primarily adds to the number of side effects.

The usual way to obtain a prolonged effect is to take an additional dose at some time after the first dose has reached its maximum

side effects: unintended effects that accompany therapeutic effects.

potency: measured by the amount of drug required to produce an effect.

time course: timing of the onset, duration, and termination of a drug's effect.

concentration and started to decline. The appropriate interval varies from one drug to another. If doses are taken too close together, the maximum blood level will increase with each dose and can result in **cumulative effects.**

One of the important changes in the manufacture of drugs is the development of time-release preparations. These compounds are prepared so that after oral ingestion the active ingredient is released into the body over a 6- to 10-hour period. With a preparation of this type, a large amount of the drug is initially made available for absorption, and then smaller amounts are released continuously for a long period. The initial amount of the drug is expected to be adequate to obtain the response desired, and the gradual release thereafter is designed to maintain the same effective dose of the drug even though the drug is being continually deactivated. In terms of Figure 7.4, a time-release preparation would aim at eliminating the unnecessarily high drug level at C–D–E while lengthening the C–E time interval.

GETTING THE DRUG TO THE BRAIN

A Little "Chemistry"

Obviously, if some drugs act quickly and others more slowly, it must be something related to the chemistry of the drug molecules that determines this. One of the most important considerations is the **lipid solubility** of the molecules. You've seen the demonstration that oil and water don't mix: shake up some salad oil with some water, let it stand, and the oil ends up floating on top. When other chemicals are added, sometimes they "prefer" to be concentrated more in the water or in the oil. For example, if you put sodium chloride (table salt) in with the oil and water and shake it all up, most of the salt will stay with the water. If you crush a garlic clove and add it to the mix, most of the chemicals that give garlic its flavor will remain in the oil. The extent

to which a chemical can be dissolved in oils and fats is called its lipid solubility. Most psychoactive drugs dissolve to some extent in either water or lipids, and in our oil-and-water experiment some fraction of the drug would be found in each. The importance of lipid solubility will become clear as we see how molecules get into the brain.

Routes of Administration

We rarely put chemicals directly into our brains. All psychoactive drugs reach the brain tissue by way of the bloodstream. Most psychoactive drugs are taken by one of three basic routes: by mouth, injection, or inhalation.

Oral Administration

Most drugs begin their grand adventure in the body by entering through the mouth. Even though oral intake might be the simplest way to take a drug, absorption from the gastrointestinal tract is the most complicated way to enter the bloodstream. A chemical in the digestive tract must withstand the actions of stomach acid and digestive enzymes and not be deactivated by food before it is absorbed. The antibiotic tetracycline provides a good example of the dangers in the gut for a drug. This antibiotic readily combines with calcium ions to form a compound that is poorly absorbed. If tetracycline is taken with milk (calcium ions), blood levels will never be as high as if it were taken with a different beverage.

The drug molecules must next get through the cells lining the wall of the gastrointestinal tract and into the blood capillaries. If taken in capsule or tablet form, the drug must first dissolve and then, as a liquid, mix into the contents of the stomach and intestines. However, the more other material there is in the stomach, the greater the dilution of the drug and the slower it will be absorbed. The drug must be water soluble for the molecules to spread throughout the stomach. However, only lipid-soluble and very small water-soluble molecules are readily absorbed into the capillaries surrounding the small intestine, where most absorption into the bloodstream occurs.

Once in the bloodstream, the dangers of entering through the oral route are not over. The veins from the gut go first to the liver (see Figure 7.5). If the drug is the type that is metabolized rapidly by the liver (nicotine is one example), very little may get into the general circulation. Thus, nicotine is much more effective when inhaled than when swallowed.

Injection

Chemicals can be delivered with a hypodermic syringe directly into the bloodstream or deposited in a muscle mass or under the upper layers of skin. With the **intravenous (IV)** injection, the drug is put directly into the bloodstream, so the onset of action is much more rapid than with oral administration or with other means of injection. Another advantage is that irritating material can be injected this way, because blood vessel walls are relatively insensitive. Also, it is possible to deliver very high concentrations of drugs intravenously, which can be both an advantage and a danger. A major disadvantage of IV injections is that the vein wall loses some of its strength and elasticity in the area around the injection site. If there are many injections into a small segment of a vein, as with an addict who must inject where he or she can see, the wall of that vein eventually collapses, and blood no longer moves through it, necessitating the use of another injection site. The greatest concern about IV drug use is the danger of introducing infections directly into the bloodstream, either from bacteria picked up on the skin as the needle is being inserted or from contaminated needles and syringes containing traces of blood. This risk is especially great if syringes and needles are shared among users, and this has been an important means by which AIDS and other blood-borne diseases have been spread (see Chapter 2).

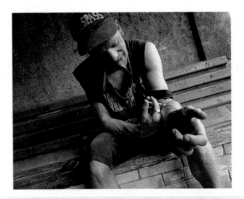

For many heroin users, the preferred route of administration is by intravenous injection.

Subcutaneous and **intramuscular** injections have similar characteristics, except that absorption is more rapid from intramuscular injection. Muscles have a better blood supply than the underlying layers of the skin and thus more area over which absorption can occur. Absorption is most rapid when the injection is into the deltoid muscle of the arm and least rapid when the injection is in the buttock. Intermediate between these two areas in speed of drug absorption is injection into the thigh. There is less chance of irritation if the injection is intramuscular because of the better blood supply and

cumulative effects: effects of giving multiple doses of the same drug.

lipid solubility: tendency of a chemical to dissolve in oil, as opposed to in water.

intravenous (IV): (in trah *vee* nuss) injection directly into a vein.

subcutaneous: (sub cue *tay* nee us) injection under the skin.

intramuscular: injection into a muscle.

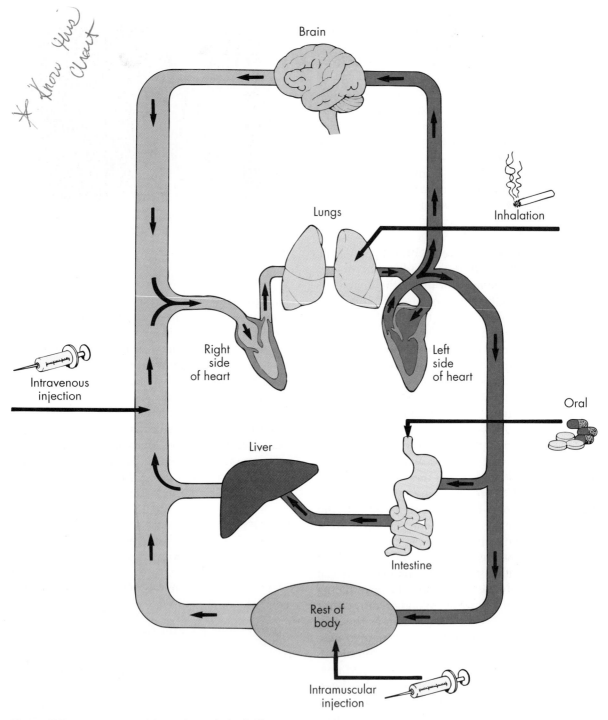

Brain

Lungs

Inhalation

Intravenous
injection

Right
side
of heart

Left
side
of heart

Oral

Liver

Intestine

Rest of
body

Intramuscular
injection

Figure 7-5   Distribution of drugs through the body.

faster absorption. Another advantage is that larger volumes of material can be deposited in a muscle than can be injected subcutaneously. Sometimes it is desirable to have a drug absorbed very slowly (over a period of several days or even weeks). A form of the drug that dissolves only very slowly in water might be injected into a muscle, or the drug might be microencapsulated (tiny bits of drug coated with something to slow its absorption).

One disadvantage of subcutaneous injection is that, if the material injected is extremely irritating to the tissue, the skin around the site of injection might die and be shed. This method of injection is not very common in medical practice but has long been the kind of injection used by beginning narcotic users. This is commonly called "skin popping."

Inhalation

Inhalation is the drug delivery system used for smoking nicotine, marijuana, and crack cocaine, and for "huffing" gasoline, paints, and other inhalants; it is used medically with various anesthetics. It is a very efficient way to deliver a drug. Onset of drug effects is quite rapid because the capillary walls are very accessible in the lungs, and the drug thus enters the blood quickly. For psychoactive drugs, inhalation can produce more rapid effects than even intravenous administration. This is because of the patterns of blood circulation in the body (review Figure 7.5). The blood leaving the lungs moves fairly directly to the brain, taking only 5 to 8 seconds to do so. By contrast, blood from the veins in the arm must return to the heart, then be pumped through the lungs before moving on to the brain, and this takes 10 to 15 seconds. Aerosol dispensers have been used to deliver some drugs via the lungs, but three considerations make inhalation of limited value for medical purposes. First, the material must not be irritating to the mucous membranes and lungs. Second, control of the dose is more difficult than with the other drug delivery systems. Last, and

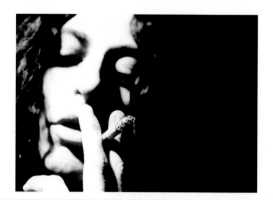

Inhalation is a very effective means of delivering a drug to the brain.

perhaps the prime advantage for some drugs and disadvantage for others, there is no depot of drug in the body. This means that the drug must be given as long as the effect is desired and that, when drug administration is stopped, the effect rapidly decreases.

Other Routes

Topical application of a drug to the skin is not widely used because most drugs are not absorbed well through the skin. However, for some drugs this method can provide a slow, steady absorption over many hours. For example, a skin patch results in the slow absorption of nicotine over an entire day. This patch has been found to help prevent relapse in people who have quit smoking. Application to mucous membranes results in more rapid absorption than through the skin because these membranes are moist and have a rich blood supply. Both rectal and vaginal suppositories take advantage of these characteristics, although suppositories are used only rarely. The mucous membranes of the nose are used by most cocaine users, who "snort" or "sniff" cocaine powder into the nose, where it dissolves and is absorbed through the membranes. Also, the mucosa of the oral cavity provide for the absorption of nicotine from chewing tobacco directly into the bloodstream without going through the stomach, intestines, and liver.

Transport in the Blood

When a drug enters the bloodstream, often its molecules will attach to one of the protein molecules in the blood, albumin being the most common protein involved. The degree to which there is binding of drug molecules to plasma proteins is important in determining drug effects. As long as there is a protein-drug complex, the drug is inactive and cannot leave the blood. In this condition, the drug is protected from inactivation by enzymes.

An equilibrium is established between the free (unbound) drug and the protein-bound forms of the drug in the bloodstream. As the unbound drug moves across capillary walls to sites of action, there is a release of protein-bound drug to maintain the proportion of bound to free molecules. Considerable variation exists among drugs in the affinity that the drug molecules have for binding with plasma proteins. Alcohol has a low affinity and thus exists in the bloodstream primarily as the unbound form. In contrast, most of the molecules of THC, the active ingredient in marijuana, are bound to blood proteins, with only a small fraction free to enter the brain or other tissues. If there were two drugs identical in every respect except protein binding, the one with greater affinity for blood proteins would require a higher dose to reach an effective tissue concentration. On the other hand, the duration of that drug's effect would be longer because of the "storage" of molecules on blood proteins.

Because different drugs have different affinities for the plasma proteins, one might expect that drugs with high affinity would displace drugs with weak protein bonds, and they do. This fact is important because it forms the basis for one kind of drug interaction. When a high-affinity drug is added to blood in which there is a weak-affinity drug already largely bound to the plasma proteins, the weak-affinity drug is displaced and exists primarily as the unbound form. The increase in the unbound drug concentration helps move the drug out of the bloodstream to the sites of action faster and can be an important influence on the effect the drug has. At the very least, there is a shortening of the duration of action.

Blood-Brain Barrier

The brain is very different from the other parts of the body in terms of drugs' ability to leave the blood and move to sites of action. A barrier keeps certain classes of compounds in the blood and away from brain cells. Thus, some drugs act only on neurons outside the central nervous system—that is, only on those in the peripheral nervous system, whereas others may affect all neurons.

The **blood-brain barrier** is not well developed in infants; it reaches complete development only after one or two years of age in humans. Although the nature of this barrier is not well understood, several factors are known to contribute to the blood-brain barrier. One is the makeup of the capillaries in the brain. They are different from other capillaries in the body, because they contain no pores. Even small water-soluble molecules cannot leave the capillaries in the brain; only lipid-soluble substances can pass the lipid capillary wall.

If a substance can move through the capillary wall, another barrier unique to the brain is met. About 85 percent of the capillaries are completely covered with glial cells; there is little extracellular space next to the blood vessel walls. With no pores and close contact between capillary walls and glial cells, almost certainly an active transport system is needed to move chemicals in and out of the brain. In fact, known transport systems exist for some naturally occurring agents.

Drugs in Depth

Drug Interactions

It should be clear that there are many ways in which various drugs can interact with one another: they may have similar actions and thus have additive effects, one may displace another from protein binding and thus one drug may enhance the effect of another even though they have different actions, one drug may stimulate liver enzymes and thus reduce the effect of another, and so on.

Even restricting ourselves to psychoactive drugs, we find that there is such a variety of possible interactions that it would not make sense to try to catalog them all here. Instead, a few of the most important interactions will be described.

Respiratory Depression (Alcohol, Other Depressants, Opiates)
There is no doubt that the single most important type of drug interaction for psychoactive drugs is the effect on respiration rate. All depressant drugs (sedatives such as Valium and Xanax, barbiturates, sleeping pills), alcohol, and all narcotics tend to slow down the rate at which people breathe in and out, because of effects in the brainstem. Combining any of these drugs can produce effects that are additive and in some cases may be more than additive. Respiratory depression is the most common type of drug overdose death: people simply stop breathing.

Stimulants and Antidepressants
Although antidepressant drugs such as amitriptyline (Elavil) and Prozac are not in themselves stimulants, they can potentiate the effects of stimulant drugs, such as cocaine and amphetamine, possibly leading to manic overexcitement, irregular heartbeat, high blood pressure, or other effects.

Stimulants and Depressants
It might seem that the "uppers" and "downers" would counteract one another, but that's generally not the case when it comes to behavior. Drugs such as Valium, Xanax, and alcohol may lead to disinhibition and recklessness. When combined with the effects of stimulants, explosive and dangerous behaviors are possible.

Cocaine + Alcohol = Cocaethylene
Although this may sound like a special case of combining a depressant and a stimulant (it is), there is another possible interaction in that cocaine can combine chemically with ethyl alcohol to produce a substance called cocaethylene—a potent stimulant that animal studies indicate may be 20 times as toxic as cocaine. The ramifications of this recent discovery are not yet clear (see Chapter 8).

A final note on the mystery of the blood-brain barrier is that cerebral trauma can disrupt the barrier and permit agents to enter that normally would be excluded. Concussions and cerebral infections frequently cause enough trauma to impair the effectiveness of this screen, which normally permits only selected chemicals to enter the brain.

Possible Mechanisms of Drug Actions

Many types of actions are suggested in chapters 8-18 as ways in which specific drugs can affect physiochemical processes, neuron functioning, and ultimately thoughts, feelings, and other behaviors. It is possible for drugs to affect all neurons, but many exert actions only on very specific presynaptic or postsynaptic processes.

Effects on All Neurons

Chemicals that have an effect on all neurons must do it by influencing some characteristic common to all neurons. One general character-

blood-brain barrier: structure that prevents many drugs from entering the brain.

istic of all neurons is the cell membrane. It is semipermeable, meaning that some agents can readily move in and out of the cell, but other chemicals are held inside or kept out under normal conditions. The semipermeable characteristic of the cell membrane is essential for the maintenance of an electric potential across the membrane. It is on this membrane that some drugs seem to act and, by influencing the permeability, alter the electrical characteristics of the neuron.

Most of the general anesthetics have their effects on the central nervous system by a general influence on the cell membrane. Note that the agents that act in this way are depressants and that there are no drugs that increase the cell's activity level by affecting general membrane characteristics. The classical view of alcohol's action on the nervous system is that it has effects similar to the general anesthetics through an influence on the neural membrane. However, recent evidence has pointed to a more specific possible mechanism for alcohol's effects,[5] and even the gaseous anesthetics might be more selective in their action than was previously thought. Thus, the entire notion that some drugs act nonspecifically through altering the nerve membrane's electrical properties is in dispute.[6]

Effects on Specific Neurotransmitter Systems

The various types of psychoactive drugs (e.g., narcotics, stimulants, depressants) produce different types of effects primarily because each type interacts in a different way with the various neurotransmitter systems in the brain. In Chapter 6, it was pointed out that the brain's natural neurotransmitters are released from one neuron into a small space called a *synapse,* where they interact with receptors on the surface of another neuron. Psychoactive drugs can alter the *availability* of a neurotransmitter by increasing or decreasing the transmitter chemical's rate of synthesis, metabolism, release from storage

vesicles, or reuptake into the releasing neuron. Or the drug might act directly on the *receptor,* either to activate it or to prevent the neurotransmitter chemical from activating it. With the existence of more than 50 known neurotransmitters, and considering that different drugs can interact with several of these in different combinations, and given the variety of mechanisms by which each drug can interact with the life cycle of a natural neurotransmitter, the potential exists for an endless variety of drugs with an endless variety of actions. However, all of these actions are nothing more mysterious than a modification of the ongoing (and quite complex) functions of the brain.

DRUG DEACTIVATION

Before a drug can cease to have an effect, one of two things must happen to it. It may be excreted unchanged from the body (usually in the urine), or it may be chemically changed so that it no longer has the same effect on the body. Although different drugs vary in how they are deactivated, the most common way is for enzymes in the liver to act on the drug molecules to change their chemical structure. This usually has two effects: one, the **metabolite** no longer has the same action as the drug molecule; two, the metabolite is more likely to be excreted by the kidneys.

The kidneys operate in a two-stage process. In the first step, water and most of the small and water-soluble molecules are filtered out. Second, most of the water is reabsorbed, along with some of the dissolved chemicals. The more lipid-soluble molecules are more likely to be reabsorbed, so one way in which the liver enzymes can increase the elimination of a drug is by changing its molecules to a more water-soluble and less lipid-soluble form.

The enzymes of the liver that metabolize drugs are quite different from the enzymes in the rest of the body. These **liver microsomal enzymes** do not normally have much to do, since there are no naturally occurring chemicals within the body for them to act on. They seem to be specialized for inactivating various general kinds of foreign chemicals that the organism might ingest. This is not like the immune system, in which foreign proteins stimulate the production of antibodies for that protein—the enzymes already exist in the liver and are waiting for the introduction of certain types of chemicals. Various plants have evolved the ability to produce chemicals that do nothing directly for the plant but kill or make ill any animals that eat the plant. In defense, apparently many animals have evolved mechanisms for eliminating these toxic chemicals once they are eaten.

Although the enzymes are already present, the introduction of a drug may stimulate an increased production of the enzymes and an increase in their activity. More than 200 drugs have been shown to increase the activity of these drug-metabolizing enzymes: phenobarbital and DDT have this effect in common. When the enzymes are stimulated, drug metabolism speeds up, and the duration of action of that drug and other drugs in the body is decreased.

Not all of the metabolites of drugs are inactive. Both diazepam (Valium) and marijuana have **active metabolites** that produce effects similar to those of the original (parent) drug and prolong the effect considerably. In fact, so-called **prodrugs** are being developed that are inactive in the original form and become active only after they are altered by the liver enzymes.

MECHANISMS OF TOLERANCE AND PHYSICAL DEPENDENCE

You should remember that the phenomena of tolerance and physical dependence have historically been associated with drug addiction. *Tolerance* refers to a situation in which repeated administration of the same dose of a drug

---

metabolite: (muh *tab* oh lite) product of enzyme action on a drug.

liver microsomal enzymes: (my cro *zhome* al) enzymes that metabolize drugs.

active metabolites: metabolites that have drug actions of their own.

prodrugs: drugs that are inactive until acted on by enzymes in the body.

results in gradually diminishing effects. There are at least three mechanisms by which a reduced drug response can come about: drug disposition tolerance, behavioral tolerance, and pharmacodynamic tolerance.

Drug Disposition Tolerance

Sometimes the use of a drug increases the drug's rate of metabolism or excretion. This is referred to as **drug disposition tolerance**, or pharmacokinetic tolerance. For example, phenobarbital induces increased activity of the liver microsomal enzymes that metabolize the drug. Increased metabolism reduces the effect of subsequent doses, perhaps leading to increased dosage. But additional amounts of the drug increase the activity of the enzymes even further, and the circle continues. Another possible mechanism for increased elimination has to do with the pH (acidity) of the urine. Amphetamine is excreted unchanged in the urine, and the rate of excretion can be increased by making the urine more acidic. Both amphetamine itself and the decreased food intake that often accompanies heavy amphetamine use tend to make the urine more acidic. Amphetamine is excreted 20 times as rapidly in urine with a pH of 5 as in urine with a pH of 8.

Behavioral Tolerance

Particularly when the use of a drug interferes with normal behavioral functions, individuals may learn to adapt to the altered state of their nervous system and therefore compensate somewhat for the impairment. In some ways, this is analogous to a person who breaks a wrist and learns to write with the nonpreferred hand—the handwriting probably won't be as good that way, but with practice the disruptive effect on writing will be reduced. A person who regularly drives a car after drinking alcohol will never be as good a driver as he or she would be sober, but with experience the impairment may be reduced. In this type of tolerance, called **behavioral tolerance,** the drug may continue to have the same biochemical effect but with a reduced effect on behavior.

Pharmacodynamic Tolerance

In many cases the amount of drug reaching the brain doesn't change, but the sensitivity of the neurons to the drug's effect does change. This is best viewed as an attempt by the brain to maintain its level of functioning within normal limits (an example of homeostasis). There are many possible mechanisms for this. For example, if the CNS is constantly held in a depressed state through the regular use of alcohol or another depressant drug, the brain might compensate by reducing the amount of the inhibitor neurotransmitter GABA that is released, or by reducing the number of inhibitory GABA receptors (many studies show that the brain does regulate the numbers of specific types of receptors). This adjustment might take several days, and after it occurs the depressant drug doesn't produce as much CNS depression as it did before. If more drug is taken, the homeostatic mechanisms might further decrease the release of GABA or the number of GABA receptors. If the drug is abruptly stopped, the brain now does not have the proper level of GABA inhibition, and the CNS becomes overexcited, leading to wakefulness, nervousness, possibly hallucinations, and the sensation that something is crawling on the skin. In severe cases, brain activity becomes uncontrolled and seizures can occur. These withdrawal symptoms are the defining characteristic of physical dependence. Thus, **pharmacodynamic tolerance** leads not only to a reduced effectiveness of the drug but also to these withdrawal reactions which indicate physical dependence. After several days the compensating homeostatic mechanisms return to a

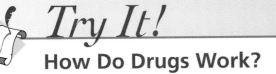

Try It!

How Do Drugs Work?

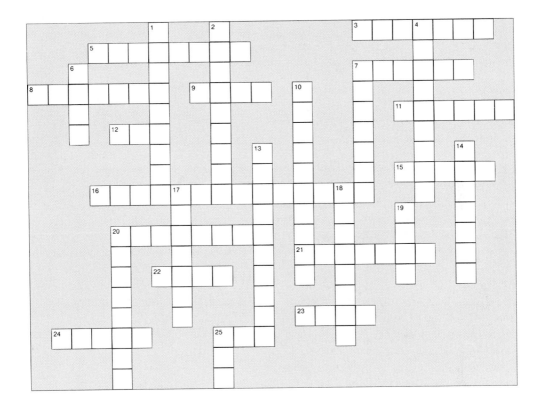

ACROSS

3. Space between two neurons
5. Cause for tobacco dependence
7. Brain part for integration of information, planning
8. Chemical signal carried through the blood
9. Amount of drug given
11. Fastest way to get a drug to the brain
12. Agency responsible for regulating pharmaceuticals
15. Where most drugs are broken down
16. Transmitter in the sympathetic branch
20. Transmitter in the mesolimbic system
21. Most widely used depressant
22. Axons, dendrites are part of the nerve _____.
23. Most rapid method of injection is into a _____.
24. Potent CNS drugs must be _____ soluble.
25. Type of modern brain scan using radioactive chemicals

DOWN

1. Reduced effect of a drug after repeated use
2. Opiate-like substance found in the brain
4. Nervous system controlling heart, pupils of the eye, etc.
6. Chemical that affects a living organism
7. Powerful stimulant derived from a South American plant
10. An _____ signal travels along the axon.
13. Drug that makes you drowsy, drunk, uncoordinated
14. Drug name used by several companies
17. Inactive or "fake" drug
18. Opium, morphine, heroin, etc.
19. Neuron part that carries electrical signals to the terminals
20. Neuron part that picks up signals from other neurons
25. Hallucinogen sometimes smoked on marijuana

normal state, the withdrawal symptoms cease, and the individual is no longer as tolerant to the drug's effect.

SUMMARY

- Most drugs are derived directly or indirectly from plants.
- The legal pharmaceutical industry is one of the largest and most profitable industries in the United States.
- Brand names belong to one company; the generic name for a chemical may be used by many companies.
- Most psychoactive drugs can be categorized as stimulants, depressants, opiates, hallucinogens, or a psychotherapeutic agent.
- Drugs can be identified by the appearance of commercial tablets or capsules, in some cases by the packaging or appearance of illicit drugs, or by a variety of chemical assays.
- Specific drug effects are related to the concentration of the chemical; nonspecific effects can also be called placebo effects.
- Because each drug is capable of producing many effects, many dose-effect relationships can be studied for any given drug.
- The ratio of LD_{50} to ED_{50} is called the therapeutic index and is one indication of the relative safety of a drug for a particular use or effect.
- The potency of a drug is the amount needed to produce an effect, not the importance of the effect.
- The time course of a drug's effect is influenced by many factors, including route of administration, protein binding in the blood, and rate of elimination.
- The blood-brain barrier prevents many drugs from reaching effective concentrations in the brain.
- Virtually all psychoactive drugs have relatively specific effects on one neurotransmitter

system or more, either through altering availability of the transmitter or by interacting with its receptor.
- The liver microsomal enzyme system is important for drug deactivation and for some types of drug interactions.
- Drug tolerance can result from changes in distribution and elimination, from behavioral adaptations, or from changes in the responsiveness of the nervous system caused by compensatory (homeostatic) mechanisms. Physical dependence (withdrawal) can be a consequence of this last type of tolerance.

REVIEW QUESTIONS

1. Morton's makes table salt, also known as sodium chloride. What is the chemical name, what is the generic name, and what is the brand name?
2. Into which major category does each of these drugs fall: heroin, cocaine, alcohol, LSD, Prozac? _Opiates   Stimulant   depressent   Hallucinogen   phycotharapoetics_
3. Why might nonspecific factors influence psychoactive drug effects more than the effect of an antibiotic?
4. Why should LD_{50} always be greater than ED_{50}?
5. Why do people say that LSD is one of the most potent psychoactive drugs?
6. Which route of administration gets a drug to the brain most quickly?

---

drug disposition tolerance: tolerance caused by more rapid elimination of the drug.

behavioral tolerance: tolerance caused by learned adaptation to the drug.

pharmacodynamic tolerance: tolerance caused by altered nervous system sensitivity.

Web Watch

Activities Related to Drugs and Their Actions

How Much Do You Know About the Effects of Illegal Drugs?
You already know about the effects of using illegal drugs, but perhaps there is a great deal more to learn. Take the Quick Quiz: Illegal Drugs and Health at www.sybercuse.com/shared/health/special/drugquiz.html and discover more about the effects of drug use.

Learn How to React in a Drug-Related Emergency
If you found yourself in a situation in which someone was suffering from the effects of drug abuse, would you know how to react and help him or her? Read "Would You Know What to Do?" at www.antibully.org.uk/would you.htm. This page simulates an emergency situation and provides a list of actions to take. It also suggests learning first aid to provide further help.

Classifications and Actions of Drugs
Drugs are often classified by their effects on the human body. Take the quiz at www.bayfront.org/cgi-bin/bayquiz98.cgi/ask/9801bfquiz_questions.html to assess your knowledge of drug classifications and actions.

7. If an elderly person has less protein in the blood than a younger person, how would you adjust the dose of a drug that has high protein binding?
8. How might two drugs interact with each other through actions on the liver microsomal enzyme system?
9. Which type of tolerance is related to physical dependence, and why?

REFERENCES

1. *Industry profile 2000.* Washington, DC: Pharmaceutical Research and Manufacturing Association.
2. *Physician's desk reference.* Oradell, NJ: Medical Economics Company.
3. Wheatley D: Effects of doctors' and patients' attitudes and other factors on response to drugs. In Rickels K, editor: *Nonspecific factors in drug therapy.* Springfield, IL: Charles C Thomas, 1968.
4. Fields HL, Levine JD: Biology of placebo analgesia, *American Journal of Medicine* 70:745, 1981.
5. Kolata G: New drug counters alcohol intoxication, *Science* 234:1198, 1986.
6. Franks NP, Lieb WR: Stereospecific effects of inhalational general anesthetic optical isomers on nerve ion channels, *Science* 254:427, 1991.

Section III

Uppers and Downers

We start our review of drugs by studying two types that have straight-forward actions on behavior. Stimulants generally excite the central nervous system, whereas depressants generally inhibit it. In Section III, we find that most drugs used in treating mental disorders are not simply uppers or downers—their action is more complicated. However, this can best be appreciated by comparing them with the stimulants and depressants. Antidepressant drugs, used in treating psychological depression, are not stimulants. When taken for several weeks they can help raise a depressed mood into the normal range, but they don't produce excited, sleepless effects as stimulants do. Likewise, the tranquilizers used in treating psychotic behavior are not depressants and do not always produce the drowsiness that sedatives and sleeping pills do.

Chapter 8

Stimulants

Online Learning Center Resources

www.mhhe.com/ray

Log on to our Online Learning Center (OLC) for access to these additional resources.

- Chapter definitions
- Learning objectives
- Student interactive question-and-answer sites
- Self-scoring chapter quiz

The OLC also offers web links for study and exploration of health topics. Here are some examples of what you'll find:

www.schick-shadel.com/cocaine.html

The Schick-Shadel Hospital's website provides an online overview of cocaine addiction treatment. You can also take its drug addiction quiz (find the link to it on the left sidebar).

thriveonline.oxygen.com/weight/drugs/

On this homepage, you can find topics about diet drugs. You can find out whether you qualify to use diet drugs, and you can chat online, check out the FAQs page, read about the benefits and risks of diet aids, and post a message.

www.usnews.com/usnews/issue/001002/suit.htm

The U.S. News website recently posted an article on lawsuits against conspiracies to sell Ritalin. Doctors as well as teachers were accused of putting pressure on parents whose children are diagnosed as having ADHD. Read the article here.

Drugs in the Media

Should Herbal Supplements Be Regulated?

Fans of the herb ephedra say that it decreases appetite, speeds metabolism, burns body fat, improves

Drugs in the Media Continued...

concentration, and even enhances sexual performance. In postings on the Internet, thousands of users give testimonials claiming that ephedra has raised their energy, increased their muscle tone, and helped them lose weight.

Critics, however, say that ephedra is a dangerous substance that requires more study and regulation. They maintain that its active ingredient, ephedrine, is a central nervous system stimulant similar to amphetamine and that reactions to it can vary widely.

Sold in health food stores and on the Internet, ephedra—also known as *ma huang*—is an herb commonly grown in Asia. It is found in many diet supplements, drinks, and diet bars. According to the *The New York Times* (October 12, 1999), ephedrine has been used in over-the-counter cold and asthma medications since the 1920s, and the ephedra plant has been in use for thousands of years in Chinese medicine. Recent studies, however, suggest that ephedra can produce a wide array of side effects, including anxiety, hypertension, insomnia, tachycardia (rapid heart beat), kidney damage, dependence, psychosis, heart attack, and stroke. The drug can even be fatal. The Food and Drug Administration (FDA) says it has received hundreds of reports from doctors, government health authorities, and others about adverse reactions to ephedrine-based products. Whereas over-the-counter drugs are subject to FDA regulation, herbal supplements are essentially unregulated; the assumption is that they are safe unless proved otherwise.

In the late 1990s, ephedrine-based products figured prominently in two widely publicized deaths. Julia Campagna, a 28-year-old woman from Kirkland, Washington, was found not criminally responsible for the deaths of two teenage girls in a car crash in British Columbia in 1998. Psychiatrists testified that Campagna had been in a state of psychosis, a reaction to the ephedrine-based supplement Xendrine, which she had taken for five days. In another case, 37-year-old Anne Marie Capati, who had high blood pressure, died of a stroke at a Manhattan health club in 1998. Her husband sued the manufacturer of Thermadrene, an ephedra supplement she had been taking for five days. Many brands of ephedrine-based products, including Thermadrene, have warning labels making clear that they should not be taken by people with certain medical conditions, such as high blood pressure.

Despite critics, ephedrine-based products, such as the pill Metabolife 356, produced by Metabolife International, Inc., of San Diego, are flying off the shelves. The use of ephedrine-based products among athletes is said to be rampant, even though such products have been banned by the National Collegiate Athletic Association and the U.S. Olympic Committee. Critics say that the public has a blind spot about herbal supplements. They point out that a drug is a drug, whether it's from a natural source or made in a laboratory.

Do you think the ephedrine debate raises serious questions about the effectiveness and safety of herbal supplements? Would you recommend that herbal supplements be regulated by the government?

Stimulants are the drugs that can keep you going, both mentally and physically, when you should be tired. There have been lots of claims about the other things these drugs can do for (and to) people. Do they really make you smarter, faster, or stronger? Can they sober you up? improve your sex life? Do they produce dependence?

We can divide the stimulants somewhat arbitrarily: the mild stimulants nicotine and caffeine are discussed in Chapters 14 and 15; *cocaine* and the amphetamines are covered in this chapter. These two powerful stimulants produce effects that were virtually unknown to most humans until just over a hundred years ago. Since the widespread introduction of cocaine into western Europe and the United States in the 19th century, there has always been a fair-sized minority of individuals committed to the regular recreational use of the stimulants, but neither cocaine nor the amphetamines have ever achieved widespread social acceptance as recreational drugs.

COCAINE

History

The origin of the earliest civilization in the Americas, the beginning around 5000 B.C. of what was to become the Inca Empire in Peru, has recently been traced to the use of **coca**. Natives of the Andes mountains in Bolivia and Peru today still use coca as their ancestors did: chewing the leaves and holding a ball of coca leaf almost continually in the mouth. The freedom from fatigue provided by the drug is legendary in allowing these natives to run or to carry large bundles great distances over high mountain trails. The psychoactive effects can be made stronger by adding some calcified lime to raise the alkalinity inside the mouth—we now know that this increases the extraction of **cocaine** and allows greater absorption into the blood supplying the inside of the mouth. It

appears that humans in the Andes first settled down and formed communities around places where this calcified lime could be mined.[1] Eventually they took up the planting and harvesting of crops in the nearby fields—and one of those important crops was, of course, coca.

The terrain of the Andes in Bolivia and Peru is poorly suited for growing almost everything. *Erythroxylon coca,* however, seems to thrive at elevations of 2,000 to 8,000 feet (600 to 2,400 meters) on the Amazon slope of the mountains, where over 100 inches (254 centimeters) of rain fall annually. The shrub is pruned to prevent it from reaching the normal height of 6 to 8 feet (1.8 to 2.4 meters), so that the picking, which is done three or four times a year, is easier to accomplish. The shrubs are grown in small, 2- to 3-acre patches called cocals, some of which are known to have been under cultivation for over 800 years.

Before the sixteenth-century invasion by Pizarro, the Incas had built a well-developed civilization in Peru. The coca leaf was an important part of the culture, and although earlier use was primarily in religious ceremonies, coca was treated as money by the time the conquistadors arrived. The Spanish adopted this custom and paid coca leaves to the native laborers for mining and transporting gold and silver. Even then the leaf was recognized as increasing strength and endurance while decreasing the need for food.

Early European chroniclers of the Inca civilization reported on the unique qualities of this plant, but it never interested Europeans until the last half of the nineteenth century. At that time the coca leaf contributed to the economic well-being and fame of three individuals. They, in turn, brought the Peruvian shrub to the notice of the world.

The first of the men was Angelo Mariani, a French chemist. His contribution was to introduce the coca leaf indirectly to the general public. Mariani imported tons of coca leaves and used an extract from them in many products.

You could suck on a coca lozenge, drink coca tea, or obtain the coca leaf extract in any of a large number of other products. It was Mariani's coca wine, though, that made him rich and famous. Assuredly, it had to be the coca leaf extract in the wine that prompted the pope to present a medal of appreciation to Mariani. Not only the pope but royalty and the general public benefited from the Andean plant. For them, as it had for the Incas for a thousand years and was to do for Americans who drank early versions of Coca-Cola (see Chapter 14), the extract of the coca leaf lifted their spirits, freed them from fatigue, and gave them a generally good feeling.

Local Anesthesia

Coca leaves contain, besides the oils that give them flavor, the active chemical cocaine (up to almost 2 percent). Cocaine was isolated before 1860, but there is still debate over who did it first and exactly when. Simple and inexpensive processing of 500 kilograms of coca leaves yields 1 kilogram of cocaine. An available supply of pure cocaine and the newly developed hypodermic syringe improved the drug delivery system, and in the 1880s physicians began to experiment with it. In the United States, the second of cocaine's proponents, Dr. W. S. Halsted, who was later referred to as "the father of modern surgery," experimented with the ability of cocaine to produce local anesthesia and to block sensation from a large area if the drug is injected near a nerve trunk.

Early Psychiatric Uses

The third famous man to encourage cocaine use was a young Viennese physician named Sigmund Freud, who studied the drug's psychological effects. In 1884, Freud wrote to his fiancée that he had been experimenting with "a magical drug." He had had dazzling success in treating a case of gastric catarrh, and he wrote, "If it goes well I will write an essay on it and I expect it will win its place in therapeutics by the side of morphium, and superior to it. . . . I take very small doses of it regularly against depression and against indigestion, and with the most brilliant success." He urged his fiancée, his sisters, his colleagues, and his friends to try it, extolling the drug as a safe exhilarant, which he himself used and recommended as a treatment for morphine addiction. For emphasis he wrote in italics, "*inebriate asylums can be entirely dispensed with.*"[2]

In an 1885 lecture before a group of psychiatrists, Freud commented on the use of cocaine as a stimulant, saying, "On the whole it must be said that the value of cocaine in psychiatric practice remains to be demonstrated, and it will probably be worthwhile to make a thorough trial as soon as the currently exorbitant price of the drug becomes more reasonable"—the first of the consumer advocates!

Freud was more convinced about another use of the drug, however, and in the same lecture said,

> We can speak more definitely about another use of cocaine by the psychiatrist. It was first discovered in America that cocaine is capable of alleviating the serious withdrawal symptoms observed in subjects who are abstaining from morphine and of suppressing their craving for morphine. . . . On the basis of my experiences with the effects of cocaine, I have no hesitation in recommending the administration of cocaine for such withdrawal cures in subcutaneous injections of 0.03–0.05 g per dose, without any fear of increasing the dose.

coca: a bush that grows in the Andes and produces cocaine.

cocaine: the active chemical in the coca plant.

On several occasions, I have even seen cocaine quickly eliminate the manifestations of intolerance that appeared after a rather large dose of morphine, as if it had a specific ability to counteract morphine.[3]

Even great men make mistakes. The realities of life were harshly brought home to Freud when he used cocaine to treat a close friend, Fleischl, to remove his addiction to morphine. Increasingly larger doses were needed, and eventually Freud spent a frightful night nursing Fleischl through an episode of cocaine psychosis. After that experience he generally opposed the use of drugs in the treatment of psychological problems.

Besides Mariani, Halsted, and Freud, one well-known fictional character revealed that the psychological effects of cocaine, both the initial stimulation and the later depression, had been well appreciated by 1890:

> Sherlock Holmes took his bottle from the corner of the mantelpiece, and his hypodermic syringe from its neat morocco case. With his long, white nervous fingers, he adjusted the delicate needle and rolled back his left shirtcuff. For some little time his eyes rested thoughtfully upon the sinewy forearm and wrist, all dotted and scarred with innumerable puncture-marks. Finally, he thrust the sharp point home, pressed down the tiny piston, and sank back into the velvet-lined armchair with a long sigh of satisfaction.
>
> Three times a day for many months I had witnessed this performance, but custom had not reconciled my mind to it. . . .
>
> "Which is it today," I asked, "Morphine or cocaine?"
>
> He raised his eyes languidly from the old black-letter volume which he had opened.
>
> "It is cocaine," he said, "a seven-per-cent solution. Would you care to try it?"
>
> "No, indeed," I answered brusquely. "My constitution has not got over the Afghan campaign yet. I cannot afford to throw any extra strain upon it."
>
> He smiled at my vehemence. "Perhaps you are right, Watson," he said. "I suppose that its

influence is physically a bad one. I find it, however, so transcendently stimulating and clarifying to the mind that its secondary action is a matter of small moment."

> "But consider!" I said earnestly. "Count the cost! Your brain may, as you say, be roused and excited, but it is a pathological and morbid process which involves increased tissue-change and may at least leave a permanent weakness. You know, too, what a black reaction comes upon you. Surely the game is hardly worth the candle. Why should you, for a mere passing pleasure, risk the loss of those great powers with which you have been endowed? Remember that I speak not only as one comrade to another but as a medical man to one for whose constitution he is to some extent answerable."
>
> He did not seem offended. On the contrary, he put his finger-tips together, and leaned his elbows on the arms of his chair, like one who has a relish for conversation.
>
> "My mind," he said, "rebels at stagnation. Give me problems, give me work, give me the most abstruse cryptogram, or the most intricate analysis, and I am in my own proper atmosphere. I can dispense then with artificial stimulants. But I abhor the dull routine of existence. I crave for mental exaltation."[4]

Although physicians were well aware of the dangers of using cocaine regularly, nonmedical and quasimedical use of cocaine was widespread in the United States around the turn of the twentieth century. It was one of the secret ingredients in many patent medicines and elixirs but was also openly advertised as having beneficial effects. The Parke-Davis Pharmaceutical Company noted in 1885 that cocaine "can supply the place of food, make the coward brave, and silent eloquent" and called it a "wonder drug."[5]

Legal Controls on Cocaine

With so much going for cocaine, and its availability in a large number of products for drinking, snorting, or injection, it may seem strange that, between 1887 and 1914, 46 states passed laws to regulate the use and distribution of cocaine. One historian provided extensive documentation and concluded

> All the elements needed to insure cocaine's outlaw status were present by the first years of the twentieth century: it had become widely used as a pleasure drug, and doctors warned of the dangers attendant on indiscriminate sale and use; it had become identified with despised or poorly regarded groups—blacks, lower-class whites, and criminals; it had not been long enough established in the culture to insure its survival; and it had not, though used by them, become identified with the elite, thus losing what little chance it had of weathering the storm of criticism.[6]

Cocaine was included in all sorts of nerve tonics, patent medicines, and home remedies, often without being mentioned on the label, until the 1906 Pure Food and Drugs Act was passed. As we saw in Chapter 5, coca and cocaine were included along with opium and its derivatives in the Harrison Act of 1914, which taxed its importation and sale. During the Prohibition era of the 1920s, when the Harrison Act was used by federal Treasury agents as a tool to suppress drug abuse, cocaine became less available and more expensive. Not that it went away: cocaine was sometimes mixed with heroin and injected intravenously (the combination was called a "speedball"), and some of the carefree and wealthy young people of the era dabbled in its use. "Cocaine Lil," a song written in the 1920s, included the line "Lil went to a 'snow' party one cold night, and the way she sniffed was sure a fright." Cole Porter's "I Get a Kick Out of You" in 1934 originally contained the verse:

> I get no kick from cocaine
> I'm sure that if
> I took even one sniff
> It would bore me terrifically too
> But I get a kick out of you.

With the introduction in the 1930s of inexpensive and easily available amphetamine, the use of cocaine declined among both occasional recreational users and serious drug addicts. Little concern was given to cocaine until, at the end of the 1960s when amphetamines became harder to obtain, cocaine use again began to increase. In 1970, it was reported that federal agents were becoming concerned; the amount of cocaine seized by U.S. Customs agents had increased from about 50 pounds in 1967 to almost 200 pounds in 1969.[7] America's second era of flirtation with cocaine grew during the next 30 years, with U.S. seizures reaching over 100 *tons* in 1996.[8]

Crack

Sometime in the 1970s it was discovered that mixing cocaine with some simple household chemicals, including baking soda, and then drying it resulted in a lump of cocaine in a smokable form. When smoked, a relatively small amount of cocaine can produce a rapid and short-lived high, and during the 1980s the street sales of **crack** or **rock** made this experience available to anyone with $10, a butane torch or lighter, a glass pipe, and access to a dealer. The practice spread rapidly during 1985 and 1986, at first in the ghetto areas of large cities. Cocaine, which had come to symbolize the rich and famous, was now available to the poor.[9]

Basic Pharmacology

Forms of Cocaine

As a part of the process of making illicit cocaine, the coca leaves are mixed with an organic solvent, such as kerosene or gasoline. After thorough soaking, mixing, and mashing, the excess liquid is filtered out to form a substance known

---

crack: a simple and stable preparation of cocaine base for smoking.

rock: another name for crack.

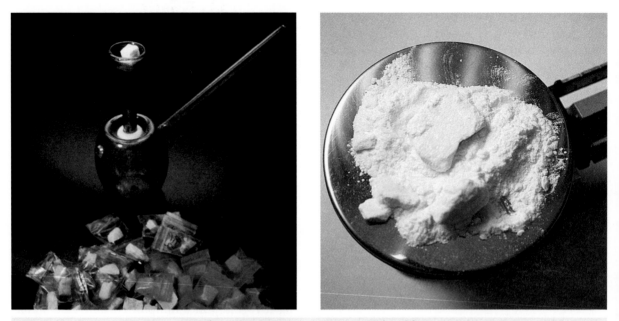

A crack cocaine pipe and cocaine in powdered form.

as **coca paste.** In South America this paste is often mixed with tobacco and smoked, but that practice has not caught on in the United States, perhaps because the lingering solvent gives the smoke a unique flavor. The paste can be made into **cocaine hydrochloride,** a salt that mixes easily in water and is so stable that it cannot be heated to form vapors for inhalation. Some U.S. users who want to smoke the cocaine convert it into **freebase** by extracting it into a volatile organic solvent, such as ether. The freebase can be heated and the vapors inhaled, but putting fire and ether fumes together can be an "enlightening" experience, because ether is so explosive. The popularity of this form of freebasing began to decline with the discovery that a different type of freebase cocaine could be made by mixing cocaine with baking soda and water. When a piece of this cocaine crack, or rock, is heated, cocaine vapors are produced and can be inhaled.

The chemical structure of cocaine is shown in Figure 8.1. This is a fairly complicated molecule, which doesn't resemble any of the known transmitters in an obvious way. In fact, the structure of cocaine doesn't give us much help at all in understanding how the drug works on the brain.

Mechanism of Action

The more we learn about cocaine's effects on brain chemistry, the more complex the drug's actions seem. Cocaine blocks the reuptake of dopamine, norepinephrine, and serotonin, causing a prolonged effect of these neurotransmitters. The observation that the blockage of dopamine receptors or the destruction of dopamine-containing neurons lessened the amount of cocaine that laboratory animals self-administered led many cocaine researchers to focus on dopamine neurons. After several years of intense scientific research, enthusiasm regarding dopamine's exclusive role in cocaine-related behaviors has been tempered, in part, because drugs that block only dopamine reuptake do not produce the same behavioral effects

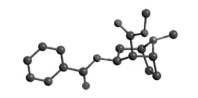

□ carbon □ oxygen ■ nitrogen (hydrogen omitted)

Figure 8-1   Cocaine.

as cocaine. Additionally, these drugs have been unsuccessful in treating cocaine dependence. Because cocaine is a "dirty" drug, affecting many neurotransmitters, the latest bet is that cocaine's behavioral effects depend on an interaction of multiple neurotransmitters, including dopamine, serotonin, GABA, and glutamate.[10]

Absorption and Elimination

People can, and do, use cocaine in many ways. Chewing and sucking the leaves allows the cocaine to be absorbed slowly through the mucous membranes. This results in a slower onset and much lower blood levels than are usually obtained by the most common recreational method of "snorting," or sniffing. In snorting, the intent is to get the very fine cocaine hydrochloride powder high into the nasal passages—right on the nasal mucosa. From there it is absorbed quite rapidly and, through circulatory mechanisms that are not completely understood, reaches the brain rather quickly.

The intravenous use of cocaine delivers a very high concentration to the brain, producing a rapid, powerful, and brief effect. For that reason, intravenous cocaine used to be a favorite among compulsive users, many of whom switched from intranasal to IV use. However, the smoking of crack is now preferred by most compulsive users because this route is less invasive (no needles) and the onset of its effects may be slightly faster than with IV use. Because the lungs provide a large surface area for absorption, and blood circulation from the lungs to the brain is quite rapid, smoking crack produces

more rapid dependence than even IV use (see Chapter 7).

The cocaine molecules are metabolized by enzymes in the blood and liver, and the activity of these enzymes is variable from one person to another. In any case, cocaine itself is rapidly removed, with a half-life of about one hour. The major metabolites, which are the basis of urine screening tests, have a longer half-life of about eight hours.

Beneficial Uses

Local Anesthesia

The local anesthetic properties of cocaine—that is, its ability to numb the area to which it is applied—were discovered in 1860 soon after its isolation from coca leaves. It was not until 1884 that this characteristic was used medically; the early applications were in eye surgery and dentistry. The use of cocaine spread rapidly because it apparently was a safe and effective

---

coca paste: a crude extract containing cocaine in a smokable form.

cocaine hydrochloride: the most common form of pure cocaine, it is stable and water soluble.

freebase: a method of preparing cocaine as a chemical base so that it can be smoked.

drug. The potential for misuse soon became clear, though, and a search began for synthetic agents with similar anesthetic characteristics but little or no potential for misuse. This work was rewarded in 1905 with the discovery of procaine (Novocain), which is still in wide use.

Local anesthetics probably block pain by preventing the generation and conduction of nerve impulses. They seem to act quite specifically on the nerve membrane. By disrupting the membrane processes necessary for the initiation and generation of electrical impulses, impulse conduction and information processing are stopped. Many drugs have been synthesized since 1905 that have local anesthetic properties similar to those of cocaine but have little or no ability to produce CNS stimulation. Those drugs have largely replaced cocaine for medical use. However, because cocaine is absorbed so well into mucous membranes, it remains in use for surgery in the nasal, laryngeal, and esophageal regions.

Other Claimed Benefits

Because cocaine produces a feeling of increased energy and well-being, it enjoyed an important status among achievers of the 1980s who self-prescribed it to overcome fatigue. It seemed that many athletes and entertainers felt that they could not consistently perform at their peak without the assistance of cocaine, and this resulted in widespread cocaine use among these groups. It should be remembered that cocaine has not been used medically for its CNS effects for many years because its effects are brief, there is a subsequent period of depressed mood, attempts to maintain the euphoria lead rapidly to tolerance and acceleration of the dose, and high doses result in unpleasant restlessness, paranoia, and other side effects. Thus, whereas the drug can provide a brief sense of increased energy, the long-term consequences are frequently disruptive. It seems that enough people experienced these disruptive effects during the 1980s that the drug's popularity has declined considerably since then.

Causes for Concern

Acute Toxicity

There is no evidence that occasional use of small amounts of cocaine is a threat to the individual's health. However, many people have increased the amount they use to the point of toxicity. Acute cocaine poisoning leads to profound CNS stimulation, progressing to convulsions, which can lead to respiratory or cardiac arrest. This is in some ways similar to amphetamine overdose, with the exception that there is much greater individual variation in the uptake and metabolism of cocaine, so that a lethal dose is much more difficult to estimate. In addition, there are very rare, severe, and unpredictable toxic reactions to cocaine and other local anesthetics, in which individuals die rapidly, apparently from cardiac failure. Cocaine can trigger the chaotic heart rhythm called ventricular fibrillation by somehow preventing the vagus nerve from controlling the heartbeat.[11] Intravenous cocaine users might also experience an allergic reaction either to the drug or to some additive in street cocaine. The lungs fill rapidly with fluid, and death can occur.

It was reported in 1992 that the combination of cocaine and alcohol (ethanol) in the body could result in the formation of a chemical called **cocaethylene,** which was subsequently shown to be more toxic than cocaine in mice. However, this finding is inconsistent with results from studies that have compared the effects of cocaine and cocaethylene in humans. These studies have shown that cocaethylene is less potent than cocaine with respect to its cardiovascular and subjective effects.[12]

Chronic Toxicity

Regularly snorting cocaine, and particularly cocaine that has been "cut" with other things, can irritate the nasal septum, leading to a chronically inflamed, runny nose. Because cocaine has a tendency to decrease food intake, many chronic cocaine users may be malnourished. Use of cocaine in a binge, during which the drug is taken repeatedly and at increasingly high doses, leads to a state of increasing irritability, restlessness, and paranoia. In severe cases, this can result in a full-blown paranoid psychosis, in which the individual loses touch with reality and experiences auditory hallucinations.[13] This experience is disruptive and quite frightening. However, most individuals seem to recover from the psychosis as the drug leaves the system.

There has been concern for several years about the effects of chronic cocaine use on the heart muscle. It appears that, in some users, frequent, brief disruption of the heart's function can damage the heart muscle itself.[14] It is not clear how often such damage occurs.

Dependence Potential

There is no doubt that cocaine can produce dependence in some users, particularly among those who inject it or inhale the vapors of crack. This phenomenon is substantiated by the fact that cocaine accounts for the largest proportion of admissions for drug treatment in most major U.S. cities. Additionally, in laboratory experiments, human research volunteers will perform rigorous tasks in order to receive a dose of cocaine.[15] Virtually every species of laboratory animal, when given the opportunity, will readily self-administer cocaine and if given unlimited access to cocaine they will self-administer the drug until their eventual death.[16] Thus, it appears that cocaine can be a powerfully reinforcing drug: take it and it will make you want to take it again.

Throughout the 1970s, the importance of this dependence potential went unrecognized, partly because cocaine was expensive and in short supply and largely because the only common method of using cocaine during this time was snorting it. The 1980s saw an increase in freebasing and then of the more convenient form of smokable cocaine, crack or rock. As large numbers of people began to smoke cocaine in the mid-1980s, the powerful dependence potential

of this form of use became clear to the American public and to the users themselves.

Because at one time addiction was linked to the presence of physical withdrawal symptoms (when the abused substance was removed), a number of experiments have studied whether physical withdrawal symptoms appear after repeated cocaine use. After prolonged daily cocaine administration in animals, there were no obvious withdrawal signs (for example, no diarrhea or convulsions), and many scientists concluded that cocaine produces no physical dependence and is therefore not a dependence-producing drug. The experiences of the 1980s led to a different way of looking at this issue. Abuse potential of a drug is no longer defined solely by the presence of physical withdrawal symptoms during drug abstinence. As was discussed in Chapter 3, a person may be diagnosed with a cocaine use disorder if he or she exhibits a set of maladaptive behaviors listed in the *DSM-IV,* which may or may not include physical withdrawal symptoms. Following several consecutive days of cocaine use (a binge), during which the user neither eats nor sleeps, a constellation of symptoms may be present, including depression, anxiety, agitation, cocaine craving, increased appetite, and exhaustion. The presence of these symptoms may vary greatly among individuals.

Reproductive Effects

Cocaine has been shown in animal studies to restrict blood flow to the placenta, and several human studies have reported that babies are of below-average size when born to women who reported using cocaine during pregnancy or whose urine tested positive for cocaine at the time of birth.[17] The earliest studies reporting

---

cocaethylene: (co cah *eth* eh leen) a chemical formed by mixing ethanol and cocaine.

this effect on birth weight and head circumference were not well controlled, in that most of the mothers had also used alcohol and tobacco, and both poor nutrition and lack of prenatal care also characterized the populations studied. These and other reports of babies being born under the influence of cocaine resulted in lurid media accounts of the "crack baby" phenomenon, which unfortunately overstated both the number of such children (see the Drugs in the Media box in Chapter 2) and the expected long-term effects. A follow-up study[18] reported that by 3 months of age the deficiencies in body weight and length were made up for in the cocaine-exposed infants. By 24 months there were no longer any significant differences between cocaine-exposed and control groups. Bayley Scales of Infant Development scores, which measure both mental and psychomotor development, also revealed no differences at 24 months. In addition to concerns about the long-term effects on the developing fetus, there are more immediate problems associated with cocaine use during pregnancy—there is increased risk for both spontaneous abortions (miscarriages) and a torn placenta.

Supplies of Illicit Cocaine

Cocaine is readily available on the illicit market in all major U.S. metropolitan areas. The U.S. Drug Enforcement Agency develops annual estimates of the prices of these illicit drugs and their purity, both indicators of supply. Theoretically, if supplies become scarce, street prices will increase and the purity of seized samples will decrease as the available drug is diluted by street traffickers. Both measures vary widely from one place to another, so what is important is the annual trend in estimated average price and purity. As the 1990s ended, it appeared that there had been no overall changes in the past decade in either of these measures. Gram quantities of cocaine remained just about 60 percent in average purity, and cost fluctuated

between $20 and $200 per gram. Thus, increased efforts to control the supply of cocaine appear to have been countered by changes in production and smuggling practices.[8]

Illicit cocaine comes to the United States primarily from three South American countries: Peru, Bolivia, and Colombia. In 1997, over 250,000 tons of coca leaf were produced in South America, enough to produce about 650 tons of cocaine hydrochloride. Bolivia typically produces about half as much coca as Peru, and Colombia somewhat less than Bolivia. In all of these countries, attempts to control production are complex: U.S. DEA agents assist local anti-narcotics police, who may be in conflict with army units fighting against local guerrillas. Often the price and availability of coca in these countries are determined more by local politics than by the DEA's eradication and interdiction efforts. Although we might pay some farmers to grow alternative crops, the high profits from growing illicit cocaine draw others to plant new fields. An economic analysis of the impact of eradication efforts indicates that even the most successful projects result in at best only temporary shortages.[19]

Large shipments of cocaine were traditionally routed by boat or plane to any of hundreds of islands in the Caribbean, and from there to Miami or other ports in the eastern United States, again by small boat or airplane. Although sea routes continue to be important, the pressure brought by Navy, Air Force, and Coast Guard interdiction efforts has shifted trafficking somewhat more to land routes through Central America and Mexico.

Current Patterns of Cocaine Use

Cocaine was the drug of abuse for the 1980s. Throughout the early 1980s, the national household survey conducted by National Institute on Drug Abuse (NIDA) (see Chapter 1) found that 7 to 9 percent of young adults reported use of cocaine within the past month. In 1998, the

Targeting Prevention

Cocaine and Friendship

Imagine you have a good friend, Terry, who has been using cocaine off and on for a year. However, in the past couple of months it seems that Terry's use has become more and more frequent. You have had to stop lending her money because she never pays it back. When you hinted that her cocaine use might be getting out of hand, she did not respond. When you tried direct confrontation, she angrily denied that she had a problem. You are still good friends. You certainly don't want to turn Terry in to the police, but you are getting pretty worried. What do you think you should do?

Obviously, there is no correct answer to this problem, but it might be interesting to discuss this hypothetical situation with a group of your friends. Find out how they would want to be treated under the circumstances. How would you want to be treated?

comparable figure was less than 2 percent, and the use of cocaine had dropped significantly in the general population. Recently concern has been raised, however, regarding the number of new cocaine users. Between 1990 and 1998, the number of first-time cocaine users rose by 37 percent, suggesting that cocaine use in the general population might be on the rise again. From 1985 to 1994, the annual high school senior survey (see Chapter 1) also showed a substantial decrease in current cocaine use (down by 80 percent), but during the mid- and late 1990s, cocaine use showed a gradual rise, consistent with National Household Survey data. The DAWN data on emergency-room mentions and cocaine-related deaths followed the same pattern, with cocaine-related emergencies and deaths continuing to rise during the late 1990s. The concern is that the type of drug use shifted in this period to a more dangerous form (crack), along with a shift to younger and poorer users, more of whom are unemployed and African American.

In a study of crack use among newly arrested individuals, contrary to the popular view

of crack users being slaves to their pipes all day every day, most of the users reported smoking fewer than three "rocks" per day on the average. The effect of each rock lasts only a few minutes, so most of these users were not high continuously. In fact, many crack users are occasional users. Crack's abuse potential might be higher than with other forms of cocaine, but that still doesn't mean that all users become dependent.[20]

Cocaine Treatment

The 1980s saw an enormous increase in the number of people seeking treatment for cocaine dependence. Although cocaine use declined in the general population in the 1990s, the shift to crack cocaine use ensured a steady demand for treatment in many areas of the country.

Cocaine overdose is potentially lethal, and medical treatments have been developed to deal with the acute emergencies resulting from excessive cocaine use. Beta-adrenergic blocking drugs, such as propranolol, can be used to treat rapid, irregular heart rate and high blood pressure. Psychotic symptoms can be controlled with haloperidol (Haldol). If seizures occur, they can be controlled with intravenous diazepam (Valium).

Regarding the search for a medication that helps initiate abstinence, lessen abstinence symptoms, or prevent relapse, no medication has received FDA approval for cocaine treatment, despite the large number of medications that have been intensively studied. However, recent studies have focused on developing cocaine treatment medications for subpopulations of cocaine users (e.g., users who are depressed). Early findings suggest that this approach might be more successful than treating cocaine abusers as a homogeneous group.[21] For example, during cocaine abstinence, some patients become depressed and feel sluggish and irritable. The antidepressant drug desipramine has been shown to be helpful for many of these depressed cocaine users, particularly for those who use the drug intranasally (administered with a nasal spray). Other medications, however, have not been effective.

As the 1990s ended, disappointed with the many unsuccessful medications investigated as potential cocaine therapies, many scientists began advocating alternative approaches. The following represents an increasingly popular perspective: "Pharmacotherapeutic interventions [drug treatments] likely will not cure a chronic, relapsing disorder such as stimulant abuse. Rather, given that the problem of stimulant abuse is a behavioral one, the hope is that pharmacotherapy will provide a window of opportunity during which behavioral and psychosocial interventions can be applied."[22]

Several behavioral approaches have been studied in the treatment of cocaine abuse. One such approach is contingency contracting.[23] In this approach, individuals receive immediate rewards (merchandise vouchers) for providing cocaine-free urine samples, and the value of the rewards is increased with consecutive cocaine-free urine samples. However, rewards are withheld if the patient's urine sample is positive for cocaine. In addition to receiving rewards, patients participate in counseling sessions weekly, where they learn a variety of skills to help them minimize drug use. In a series of experiments, several teams of researchers have reported significant reductions in cocaine use when employing contingency contracting methods.

Another behavioral strategy is called relapse prevention, an approach that uses cognitive-therapy techniques with behavioral-skills training. Individuals learn to identify and change behaviors that may lead to continued drug use. Relapse prevention has been shown to be more effective at decreasing cocaine use than general interpersonal psychotherapy, and these effects persist for at least one year following treatment.[24] Additionally, group therapy, support groups (groups calling themselves Cocaine Anonymous or Narcotics Anonymous are available in many areas), individual psychotherapy, job counseling, and family counseling are all

important components of many cocaine treatment programs. Promotion of exercise and general health consciousness fits in with current American trends and is felt to reduce the craving for cocaine.

As with other drugs, treatment is probably more effective than no treatment, but the failure rate is still high. It will be several years before the effectiveness of different approaches to cocaine dependence can be evaluated.

Cocaine's Future

In attempting to predict the future, we can learn from two writers who have made successful predictions about cocaine use in the past. The first, writing in the early 1970s, pointed out that historically, as cocaine use declined, amphetamine use increased. Looking at the decline in amphetamine use in the late 1960s, he predicted the increased use of cocaine that we saw in the 1970s and early 1980s.[7] The other writer[5] pointed out that at the height of cocaine use in 1986 we were reliving an earlier cycle of cocaine use that occurred around the turn of the twentieth century. As you know, when cocaine was first introduced in the 1880s, the experts had mostly positive opinions about its effects, and it was regarded as a fairly benign substance. In the second stage (1890s), more and more people used cocaine, and its dangers and side effects became well known. In the third stage, in the early 1900s, society turned against cocaine and passed laws to control it. After many years with little cocaine use, in the early 1970s the drug again had the reputation of being fairly benign and not truly addicting. In the 1980s, we were in the second stage, in which widespread use eventually made us all aware of the dangers. This comparison led to the prediction that Americans would again turn away from cocaine and would pass increased legal restrictions on it. This prediction certainly came true during the 1990s. As the rejection of cocaine continues, we would not expect substantial increases in cocaine use for several years in the future. But more than 30 years have passed since the peak of amphetamine's popularity and widespread concerns about it. We therefore made the prediction in the previous edition of this text that the next wave of illicit stimulant use would see increases in the use of amphetamine. Unfortunately, that prediction is now coming true, particularly in the western United States.

AMPHETAMINES

History

Development and Early Uses

For centuries the Chinese have made a medicinal tea from herbs they call *ma huang,* which American scientists classify in the genus *Ephedra.* The active ingredient in these herbs is called **ephedrine,** and it is used to dilate the bronchial passages in asthma patients. Bronchial dilation can be achieved by stimulating the sympathetic branch of the autonomic nervous system, and that is exactly what ephedrine does (it is referred to as a **sympathomimetic** drug). Of course, this drug also has other effects related to its sympathetic nervous system stimulation, such as elevating blood pressure (review the Drugs in the Media box at the beginning of this chapter). In the late 1920s, researchers synthesized and studied the effects of a new chemical that was similar in structure to ephedrine: **amphetamine** was patented in 1932.

All major effects of amphetamine were discovered in the 1930s, although some of the uses developed later. Amphetamine's first use was as a replacement for ephedrine in the treatment of asthma. Quite early it was shown that amphetamine was a potent dilator of the nasal and bronchial passages and could be efficiently delivered through inhalation. The Benzedrine (brand name) inhaler was introduced as an over-the-counter (OTC) product in 1932 for treating the stuffy noses caused by colds.

Some of the early work with amphetamine showed that the drug would awaken anesthetized dogs. As one writer put it, amphetamine is the drug that won't let sleeping dogs lie! This led to the testing of amphetamine for the treatment of **narcolepsy** in 1935. Narcolepsy is a condition in which the individual spontaneously falls asleep 5, 10, 50 times a day. Amphetamine enables these patients to remain awake and function almost normally. In 1938, however, two narcolepsy patients treated with amphetamine developed acute *paranoid psychotic* reactions. The paranoid reaction to amphetamine has reappeared regularly and has been studied (as is discussed in later chapters).

In 1937, amphetamine became available as a prescription tablet, and a report appeared in the literature suggesting that amphetamine, a stimulant, was effective in reducing activity in hyperactive children. Two years later, in 1939, notice was taken of a report by amphetamine-treated narcolepsy patients that they were not hungry when taking the drug. This *appetite-depressant* effect became the major clinical use of amphetamine. A group of psychology students at the University of Minnesota began experimenting with various drugs in 1937 and found that amphetamine was ideal for "cramming," because it allowed them to stay awake for long periods of time. Truck drivers also noted this effect, and they used "bennies" to stay awake during long hauls.

---

ephedrine: (eh *fed* rin) a sympathomimetic drug used in treating asthma.

sympathomimetic: (sim path o mih *met* ick) a drug that stimulates the sympathetic branch of the autonomic nervous system.

amphetamine: a synthetic CNS stimulant and sympathomimetic.

narcolepsy: a disease that causes people to fall asleep suddenly.

Wartime Uses

In 1939, amphetamine went to war. There were many reports that Germany was using stimulants to increase the efficiency of its soldiers. A 1944 report in the *Air Surgeon's Bulletin,* titled "Benzedrine Alert," stated, "This drug is the most satisfactory of any available in temporarily postponing sleep when desire to sleep endangers the security of a mission."[25] Some studies were reported, including one in which

> . . . one hundred Marines were kept active continuously for sixty hours in range firing, a twenty-five mile forced march, a field problem, calisthenics, close-order drill, games, fatigue detail and bivouac alerts. Fifty men received seven 10-milligram tablets of benzedrine at six hour intervals following the first day's activity. Meanwhile, the other fifty were given placebo (milk sugar) tablets. None knew what he was receiving. Participating officers concluded that the benzedrine definitely "pepped up" the subjects, improved their morale, reduced sleepiness and increased confidence in shooting ability. . . . It was observed that men receiving benzedrine tended to lead the march, tolerate their sore feet and blisters more cheerfully, and remain wide awake during "breaks," whereas members of the control group had to be shaken to keep them from sleeping.

Amphetamines were widely used in Japan during World War II to maintain production on the home front and to keep the fighting men going. To reduce large stockpiles of methamphetamine after the war, the drug was sold without prescription, and the drug companies advertised them for "elimination of drowsiness and repletion of the spirit." Such widespread use was accompanied by considerable overuse and abuse. In 1948 and again in 1955, strict controls on amphetamine were put into force, along with treatment and education programs. Although the Japanese government claimed to have "eliminated" the amphetamine-abuse problem before 1960, there were smaller Japanese "epidemics" of methamphetamine use in the 1970s and 1980s.

In 1944 in Sweden, because such a large number of people were using oral amphetamines, prescriptions became tightly controlled. This resulted in a significant decline in amphetamine sales and a decrease in the total number of individuals using the amphetamines. But those who were heavy abusers would not be denied, so there arose a black market in amphetamines and an amphetamine subculture similar to our American heroin subculture. To get the most value out of their expensive black-market amphetamine, some Swedes began injecting it intravenously. In 1968, Sweden banned virtually all prescriptions for amphetamines and related stimulants. The black market, of course, continued to flourish.

The "Speed Scene" of the 1960s

Most of the misuse of amphetamines until the 1960s was through the legally manufactured and legally purchased oral preparation. In 1963, the AMA Council on Drugs stated, "At this time, compulsive abuse of the amphetamines is a small problem."[26] But at exactly this time, trouble was brewing in California. It is difficult to pinpoint exactly when intravenous abuse of the amphetamines began in the United States, but it was probably among IV users of heroin and cocaine. In the 1920s and 1930s, when IV use of those drugs was spreading among the drug subculture, the combination of heroin and cocaine injected together was known as the "speedball," presumably because the cocaine rush or flash occurs rapidly after injection, thus speeding up the high. So, on the streets, one name for cocaine was "speed." When the amphetamines became so widely available after World War II, some of these enterprising individuals discovered that they could get an effect similar to that of cocaine if they injected amphetamine along with the heroin. Thus, slowly and out of the awareness of most Americans, the amphetamines came to be known as **speed** by that small drug underground that used heroin intravenously. By the 1960s, amphetamines had become so widely available at such a low price that more IV drug users were using them, either in combination with heroin or alone. Although they were prescription drugs, it was not difficult to obtain a prescription to treat depression or obesity.

The most desired drug on the streets was methamphetamine, which was available in liquid form in ampules for injection. Hospital emergency rooms sometimes used this drug to stimulate respiration in patients suffering from overdoses of sleeping pills (no longer considered an appropriate treatment), and physicians also used injectable amphetamines intramuscularly to treat obesity. In the San Francisco Bay area, reports appeared in the early 1960s of "fat doctors" who had large numbers of patients coming in regularly for no treatment other than an injection of methamphetamine.

Because some heroin addicts would inject amphetamines alone when they could not obtain heroin, some physicians also felt that methamphetamine could serve as a legal substitute for heroin and thus be a form of treatment. In those days, amphetamines were not considered to be addicting, so these physicians were quite free with their prescriptions.[7] Reports of those abuses led to legislation, including federal regulation of amphetamines within the new concept of dangerous drugs in the 1965 law. Unfortunately, all of the publicity associated with these revelations and the ensuing legislation fell on the ears of young people whose identity as a generation was defined largely by experimentation with drugs their parents and government told them were dangerous. To the Haight-Ashbury district of San Francisco came the flower children, to sit in Golden Gate Park, smoke marijuana, take LSD, and discuss peace, love, and the brotherhood of humanity. They moved in next door to the old, established drug subculture, in which IV drug use was endemic. That mixture resulted in the speed scene and young people who became dependent on IV amphetamines. Although in historical perspective

the speed scene of the late 1960s was relatively short-lived and only a small number of people were directly involved, it was the focus of a great deal of national concern, and it helped change the way the medical profession and society at large viewed these drugs, which had been so widely accepted.

As use of the amphetamines began to be considered abuse, physicians prescribed less and less of the drugs. Their new legal status as dangerous drugs put restrictions on prescriptions and refills, and in the 1970s there were limits placed on the total amount of these drugs that could be manufactured. Thus, within less than a decade, amphetamines went from being widely used and accepted pharmaceuticals to being less widely used, tightly restricted drugs associated in the public mind with drug-abusing "hippies."

As controls tightened on legally manufactured amphetamines, there were at least three reactions that continued to affect the drug scene. The first reaction was that a market began to develop for "look-alike" pills: legal, milder stimulants (usually caffeine or ephedrine) packaged in tablets and capsules that were virtually identical in color, shape, and markings to prescription amphetamines. Later the makers of look-alikes began to expand the variety of shapes and sizes to attract a wider market. Because these pills contained legally available, OTC ingredients, their sellers could not be prosecuted. By the early 1980s, these products were so popular that the odds were good that if someone bought "speed" pills from a street dealer they were actually getting look-alikes. The national high school survey had to apply a correction factor to its data to account for these look-alikes and get a more accurate measure of actual amphetamine use. The FDA began to crack down on manufacturers and distributors of pills containing large amounts of caffeine or mixtures of caffeine and

---

speed: street name for amphetamine.

other legal stimulants, and states passed regulations making it illegal to distribute any substance that is misrepresented to be a controlled substance.

The reduced availability of legally manufactured amphetamines had a second important effect. As the price went up and the quality of the available speed became more questionable, the drug subculture began, slowly and without fanfare, to rekindle its interest in a more "natural," reportedly less dangerous stimulant—cocaine. In 1970, federal agents in Miami reported that "the traffic in cocaine is growing by leaps and bounds."[7] And as we now know, they were seeing only the small beginnings of a cocaine trade that would swell to much greater size by the mid-1980s.

The Return of Methamphetamine

The third reaction to limited amphetamine availability was an increase in the number of illicit laboratories making methamphetamine, which acquired the name *crank*. Both the process for making methamphetamine and the name **crank** have been around on the streets since the 1960s, and illicit laboratories have been raided every year. By the late 1980s, the increasing number of confiscations by authorities led some to wonder if this would be the next drug fad.

In 1989, the media began to describe what many claimed would be America's next drug epidemic: the "smoking" of methamphetamine hydrochloride crystals, also known by the street names **ice** and **crystal meth.** The practice had been reported among youth in Hawaii and was said to be spreading into California. Along with the scare of a potential new menace came unsubstantiated reports that ice produced effects lasting for a day or more, compared with a few minutes for cocaine (such reports make no sense in terms of the half-life of methamphetamine). Concerns about methamphetamine use increased considerably in the 1990s when rates of methamphetamine seizures increased dramatically and the DAWN reports indicated large relative increases in methamphetamine-related emergency room admissions and deaths. Much of the concern has focused on the rural West, where small clandestine laboratories are making methamphetamine, supplemented by increasing importation of both raw materials and finished product from Mexico.[27]

Basic Pharmacology

Chemical Structures

Take a couple of minutes to look at Figure 8.2, to see some similarities in the structures of amphetamines and related drugs. First, note the similarity between the molecular structures of the catecholamine neurotransmitters (dopamine and norepinephrine) and the basic amphetamine molecule. It appears that amphetamine produces its effects because it is recognized as one of these catecholamines at many sites in both the central and the peripheral nervous systems. The amphetamine molecule has both "left-handed" and "right-handed" forms (*l* and *d* forms). The original Benzedrine was an equal mixture of both forms. The *d* form is several times more potent in its CNS effects, however, and in 1945 d-amphetamine was first marketed as Dexedrine for use as an appetite suppressant. Next, look at the methamphetamine molecule, which simply has a methyl group added to the basic amphetamine structure. This methyl group seems to make the molecule cross the blood-brain barrier more readily and thus further increase the CNS potency. (If more of the molecules get into the brain, then fewer total molecules have to be given.) However, the behavioral significance of this in humans has yet to be determined, as studies directly comparing the two compounds report no difference on many measures, including subjective drug-effect ratings and heart rate.[28] Next, look at the structures for ephedrine, the old Chinese remedy that is still used to treat asthma, and for phenylpropanolamine (PPA). Before the year 2000, PPA was an ingredient in OTC weight-control preparations (see Chapter 15) and in many of the look-alikes. Both of these molecules have a

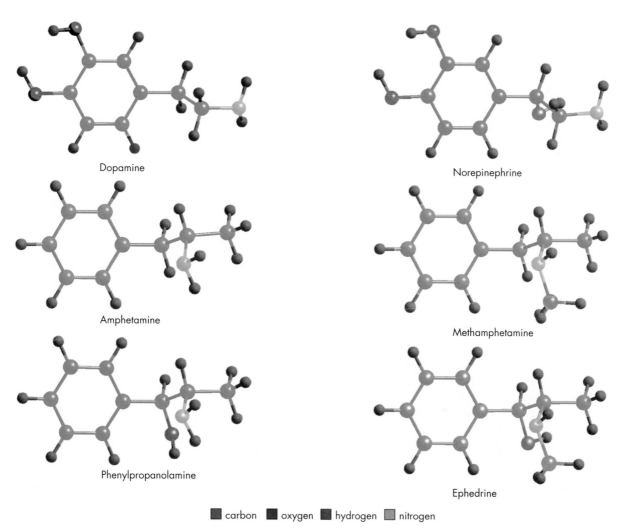

Dopamine

Norepinephrine

Amphetamine

Methamphetamine

Phenylpropanolamine

Ephedrine

■ carbon ■ oxygen ■ hydrogen ■ nitrogen

Figure 8-2 Molecular structures of stimulants.

structural addition that makes them not cross the blood-brain barrier as well; therefore, they produce peripheral effects without as much CNS effectiveness.

Mechanism of Action

The stimulant types of amphetamine have at least two effects on catecholamine (dopamine and norepinephrine) synapses. The presynaptic storage mechanism recognizes and tries to store amphetamine molecules, which results in the leakage of catecholamines into the synapse,

where they can interact with the receptor. Second and probably less important is the ability of amphetamine molecules to occupy the reuptake

crank: street name for illicitly manufactured methamphetamine.

crystal meth; ice: street names for crystals of methamphetamine hydrochloride.

mechanism, so that catecholamines released into the synapse are not taken back up as readily and therefore stay longer in the synapse. Both of these mechanisms produce increased stimulation of the dopamine and norepinephrine receptors.

Exactly which of amphetamine's effects are related to which neurotransmitter is controversial, but current theories can be summarized. Stimulation of the norepinephrine neurons arising from the locus ceruleus would produce the alerting and antifatigue effects, and stimulation of the mesolimbic dopamine pathway would produce euphoria and increased motor activity. Higher doses would activate the nigrostriatal dopamine pathway to produce stereotyped, repetitive movements. Too much activity in the mesolimbic system could be responsible

HealthQuest Activities

Go to Module 9 and find the section *Drug Interactions*. Under *OTC Drugs,* read "Stimulants." The article lists the reactions that stimulants have when mixed with other drugs. Go to your medicine cabinet or wherever you keep OTC drugs, and take out those you use often or have used before. Have you ever mixed these drugs with another on this list? You may not realize that they can react with something as simple as a cup of coffee or a soda. Have you ever experienced any of the side effects?

Now look under *Illicit Drugs* and read "Methamphetamine." Taking "meth" is a current trend in America. How common is it on your campus? Take an anonymous poll of those who have tried meth, use it regularly, and mix it with other drugs. Print out this article and provide copies for all those who take the poll.

In the same module, complete "Drug F/X Exploration." This activity lists several drugs. Click on cocaine, answer the questions, and assess your risk of abuse.

for the paranoid psychotic reaction seen with very high doses.

Absorption and Elimination

Amphetamines can be taken by a variety of routes. When taken orally, the peak effects occur about 1.5 hours after ingestion. The half-life of amphetamine is 10 to 12 hours, and the half-life for methamphetamine is 4 to 5 hours. A fairly stable blood level can be achieved with oral administration at 4- to 6-hour intervals, and virtually complete elimination of the drug occurs within 2 days of the last dose.

With IV injection, peak effects are much more rapid. With higher doses a tachyphylaxis (rapid tolerance) may be seen. Because amphetamine produces its effects largely by displacing the catecholamine transmitters from their storage sites, with large doses the catecholamines might be sufficiently depleted, so that another dose within a few hours may not be able to displace as much catecholamine, and a reduced effect will be obtained.

Beneficial Uses

Previous Use for Depression

During the 1950s and early 1960s, amphetamines were prescribed for depression and feelings of fatigue. If we look at an individual's mood as potentially ranging from very depressed, up through sadness into a normal range, and then into euphoria and finally the excited, manic range (Figure 8.3), we can better understand amphetamine's effects on mood. Note that the person who is seriously depressed is not just sad; he or she feels helpless and hopeless with no energy and might think of suicide. Amphetamines are capable of temporarily moving the mood up the scale, so that a depressed person might, for a few hours, move into a normal range. The problem is that, when the drug wears off, that person doesn't stay "up." The mood drops, often below the predrug level. To keep the mood up, one needs to keep taking

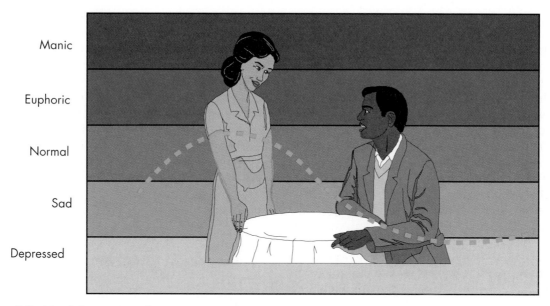

Figure 8-3 Mood changes over time.

amphetamine. Amphetamine does interfere with sleep, so some physicians prescribed sleeping pills for nighttime. These patients often go for a daily "ride" on an emotional roller coaster, waking up depressed and taking a pill to get going in the morning, and either coming off the drug or taking a "downer" at night. As we will see in Chapter 10, other treatments are now used for depression, and amphetamines are not recommended.

Weight Control

Probably the most common medical use for the amphetamines through the mid-1960s was for weight control. It is clear that amphetamines can reduce food intake and body weight. This is obvious in people of normal or below-average weight who take the drug for other reasons and especially obvious in those who take very large doses. Studies on rats show that amphetamine reduces food intake and body weight compared with rats given a placebo. With one-third of Americans overweight, there is a vast market for

a pill that would help us lose weight. For years the common medical response was some form of amphetamine or related sympathomimetic stimulant. Physicians dispensed prescriptions for pills and some gave injections, and a number of people did lose weight. But in the 1960s, when people began to view the amphetamines with greater concern, it was also clear that some people who took these stimulants regularly were still overweight.

To understand the role of stimulant drugs in weight control, let's imagine a typical experiment to test the value of amphetamine in treating obesity. Patients who meet some criterion for being overweight are recruited for the study. All are brought to a hospital or clinic, where they are weighed, interviewed, given physical examinations, and given a diet to follow. Half are given amphetamine and half a placebo in a double-blind design. Each week the patients return to the hospital, where they are interviewed, weighed, and given their supply of drug for the next week. After two months the drug code is broken and the amount of weight loss in each group is calculated. This type of study virtually always finds that both groups lose weight, mostly in the first two or three weeks. After that, the weight loss is much slower. This initial weight loss by both groups probably is a result of beginning a new diet and being involved in a medical study in which they know they will be weighed each week. Over the first two or three weeks the amphetamine group will lose a little more weight than the placebo group. The difference between the two groups after two or three weeks might be about two or three pounds, which is statistically significant but probably not medically or cosmetically important. The interesting thing is that, as the study goes on, the gap doesn't widen but stays about the same. In other words, in such studies the amphetamine effect is real but small and limited in duration. Even with moderate dose increases, four to six weeks seems to be the limit before tolerance occurs to this effect. Increasing to high doses might produce some further effect, but these experiments don't allow that, and it would be foolhardy as a treatment approach. The use of amphetamines for weight reduction came under attack from various sources, and the FDA in 1970 restricted the legal use of amphetamines to three types of conditions: narcolepsy, hyperkinetic (hyperactive) behavior, and "short-term" weight-reduction programs.

Amphetamine and several related stimulant drugs are still used for weight control. Preparations of *d*-amphetamine and methamphetamine are available by prescription for short-term weight loss, as are the other sympathomimetics diethylpropion, phentermine, phenmetrazine, phendimetrazine, and some related but slightly different drugs, fenfluramine and mazindol. The FDA allows the sale of all these drugs even though experts point out that the drugs make a clinically trivial contribution to the overall weight reduction seen in the experiments. The package insert for each of these drugs includes the following FDA mandated statements:

The natural history of obesity is measured in years, whereas most studies cited are restricted to a few weeks duration; thus, the total impact of drug induced weight loss over that of diet alone must be considered clinically limited. . . .[Drug name] is indicated in the management of exogenous obesity as a short-term (a few weeks) adjunct in a regimen of weight reduction based on caloric restriction. The limited usefulness of agents of this class must be weighed against possible risk factors inherent in their use.[29]

The introduction in 1992 of a new combination of two old drugs, fenfluramine and phentermine, as a more effective aid to weight loss[30] started the well-known "fen-phen" craze and renewed public interest in the use of prescription stimulants as appetite suppressants. This was followed in 1996 by the introduction of a new relative of fenfluramine, dexfenfluramine (Redux). However, in August 1997 the FDA began warning physicians and the public that the fen-phen combination had been associated with damage to heart valves and that several patients had also developed a serious lung disease. By September 1997, it was clear that the culprit was fenfluramine (Pondimin) and that its new relative, dexfenfluramine (Redux), might have the same effects. As warnings went out from the FDA to stop taking these medications, the manufacturer removed them from the market.

Then in November 1997, another new weight-control drug, sibutramine (Meridia), was introduced.[31] Intended for use only in those who are extremely overweight, this drug is believed to act by blocking reuptake of both norepinephrine and serotonin, which would make its mechanism more similar to some of the antidepressants (Chapter 10) than to the more traditional stimulants.

Narcolepsy

Narcolepsy is a sleep disorder in which individuals do not sleep normally at night and in the daytime experience uncontrollable episodes of muscular weakness and falling asleep. Although there has been increased interest in sleep disorders in general and sleep-disorder clinics are now associated with almost every major medical center in the United States, the best available treatment still seems to be to keep the patient awake during the day with amphetamine or methylphenidate, a related stimulant. There is no doubt that some individuals who receive stimulants from a general practitioner under the diagnosis of narcolepsy are actually suffering from some other sleep disorder or from depression, which often includes disruptions of normal sleep patterns. Accurate diagnosis of narcolepsy requires checking in to a sleep-disorder clinic for some sleep recordings on an electroencephalogram (EEG). However, for these recordings to be accurate, the programs usually require that the patient be drug-free for two to three weeks preceding the recordings.

Hyperactive Children

Even though it has been more than 50 years since the first report that amphetamine could reduce activity levels in hyperactive children, and even though hundreds of thousands of children are currently being treated with stimulant drugs for this problem, we still have controversy over the nature of the disorder being treated, we still don't understand what the drugs are doing to reduce hyperactivity, and we still don't have a widely accepted solution to the apparent paradox: what's a "stimulant" drug doing producing what appears to be a "calming" effect?

The disorder itself was referred to as childhood hyperactivity for many years, and the children who received that label were the ones who seemed absolutely incapable of sitting still and paying attention in class. Many of these children had normal or even above-average IQ scores yet were failing to learn. During the 1960s, it was proposed that lead toxicity or early oxygen deprivation might be the cause of a small amount of brain damage. Pointing out that many of these children exhibit "soft" neurological signs

(impairments in coordination or other tests that are not localizable to a particular brain area), the term *minimal brain dysfunction* (MBD) became popular. By 1980, there was a feeling that there had been too much focus on activity levels and that the basic disorder was a deficit in attention, which usually, but not always, was accompanied by hyperactivity. Thus, the *Diagnostic and Statistical Manual* of the American Psychiatric Association used the term *attention deficit disorder.* However, the 1994 revision of that manual, the *DSM-IV,* recognizes the strong relationship between attention deficit and hyperactive behavior by using the term *attention-deficit hyperactivity disorder* (**ADHD**).[32] The criteria used to diagnose this disorder are listed in the DSM-IV box above.

The cause or causes of the disorder are not known. One idea that attracted a lot of attention was that it is the additives in the foods we eat that are the basis for ADHD. Many studies were done, and in 1982 a blue-ribbon panel handed down the verdict on diets without food additives: "there is no firm evidence that the diets work. Claims that the diets produce dramatic effects simply did not hold up in well-designed clinical trials."

Some hyperactive children have histories of difficult births or encephalitis when very young. Some reports indicate a higher incidence of abnormal EEGs in these children than in children who do not have ADHD. There are as many children with ADHD, however, who do not show abnormal EEGs or medical histories, so the importance of these factors is not clear. There is also no evidence that a large percentage are mentally retarded, although school achievement is usually quite poor. Some believe that children with ADHD suffer only from a maturational lag: they are exhibiting behavior that is typical of children several years younger.

ADHD: attention-deficit hyperactivity disorder.

DSM-IV — Diagnostic Criteria for Attention-Deficit Hyperactivity Disorder

A. Either (1) or (2):
  (1) Six (or more) of the following symptoms of inattention have persisted for at least 6 months to a degree that is maladaptive and inconsistent with developmental level:

  Inattention
    a. Often fails to give close attention to details or makes careless mistakes
    b. Often has difficulty sustaining attention in tasks or play
    c. Often does not seem to listen when spoken to directly
    d. Often does not follow through on instructions and fails to finish schoolwork, chores, or duties
    e. Often has difficulty organizing tasks and activities
    h. Is often easily distracted by extraneous stimuli
    i. Is often forgetful in daily activities

  (2) Six (or more) of the following symptoms of hyperactivity-impulsivity have persisted for at least 6 months to a degree that is maladaptive and inconsistent with developmental level:

  Hyperactivity
    a. Often fidgets with hands or feet or squirms in seat
    b. Often leaves seat in classroom or in other situations in which remaining seated is expected
    c. Often runs about or climbs excessively in situations in which it is inappropriate
    d. Often has difficulty playing or engaging in leisure activities quietly
    e. Is often "on the go" or often acts as if "driven by a motor"
    f. Often talks excessively

  Impulsivity
    g. Often blurts out answers before questions have been completed
    h. Often has difficulty awaiting turn
    i. Often interrupts or intrudes on others

B. Some hyperactive-impulsive or inattentive symptoms that caused impairment were present before age 7 years.
C. Some impairment from the symptoms is present in two or more settings.
D. There must be clear evidence of clinically significant impairment in social, academic, or occupational functioning.
E. The symptoms do not occur exclusively during the course of a Pervasive Developmental Disorder or other disorder and are not better accounted for by another mental disorder.

It is interesting that the disorder is at least three times more common in boys than in girls, though that fact hasn't helped us understand its cause. Also, in many cases the problems seem to be reduced once the child reaches puberty. It was once thought that this was an absolute developmental change, but now we recognize that as many as one-third of the children continue to have hyperactivity problems even into adulthood, and there are arguments as to whether the disorder fades in the other children or just changes its character to something else, such as antisocial personality disorder.

Regardless of the cause, there is clear evidence of the beneficial effect of both amphetamine and **methylphenidate (Ritalin)**. Methylphenidate is now considered the drug of choice for treating ADHD. It is a milder stimulant than amphetamine, with a potency between that of the amphetamines and that of caffeine. Why either type of stimulant drug should work is still not known. One theory that has been around for years is worth considering, even if it has been difficult to test experimentally: assume that the child with ADHD is receiving inadequate sensory input to the CNS, and that his or

Exploring Your Spirituality

How Far Should We Go to Enhance Human Abilities?

New drugs, as well as increasing or innovative use of old drugs, are causing medical professionals to confront a spiritual and ethical question that has dogged the age of pharmacology: how far does our society want to go in its efforts to enhance human abilities?

One example is the popularity of the stimulant Ritalin, a common treatment for children with attention-deficit hyperactivity disorder (ADHD), who are impulsive, easily distracted, and unable to sit still and concentrate in school. After more than three decades of use, Ritalin's sales boomed throughout the 1990s, increasing by more than 500 percent, according to Drug Enforcement Administration reports. Physicians and others, such as former first lady Hillary Rodham Clinton, have expressed concern that Ritalin is being prescribed for children whose symptoms do not clearly meet the specific diagnostic criteria for ADHD but who have difficulty paying attention and for adults who find themselves easily distracted.

Pediatricians and psychiatrists say that Ritalin can help anyone concentrate, whether or not he or she has a neurological problem. Some people, though no one knows how many, are using the drug simply to improve their mental performance. Although it is clear that a learning disorder can disrupt one's life, some experts say it is too easy to see ADHD everywhere we look. Anxiety, stress, and depression can also cause kids to be inattentive or somewhat hyperactive. And some experts fear that the diagnosis of adult ADHD is becoming an excuse for any sort of psychological problem. Adults may want to believe that problems with their families or their jobs are caused by problems with impulsivity and attention. Is it more socially acceptable now to have ADHD than depression or anxiety?

There is no single definitive test for ADHD. A medical expert makes a diagnosis after evaluating the patient. Symptoms, including restlessness, a short attention span, distractability, and impulsiveness, must cause a significant impairment in school performance or home behavior and must have appeared by the age of seven. Not every person with ADHD has every symptom, and no one symptom leads to a diagnosis.

There are concerns that parents and others are misusing Ritalin as a Band-Aid approach to therapy and that, in doing so, they may be treating the symptoms, not the problem. But as consumer demand for choice allows market forces to take more and more control of the health-care industry, patients are redefining the purpose of "medicine." Rather than just being prevention or treatment oriented, we now want to enhance the average.

The spiritual and ethical dilemma centers on whether the ends justify the means. Is it appropriate to medicate children without a clear diagnosis in the hope that they will do better in school? Should the drug be prescribed for adults who are failing in their careers, who are procrastinators, or who are otherwise not living up to their potential? Is the current trend toward using drugs to enhance mental performance, sexual performance, and athletic performance really making us better human beings?

---

her noisiness, rocking movements, running, and crashing into things are an effort to obtain sensory stimulation. The stimulant drugs might arouse the CNS partly by allowing sensory information more direct access to the thalamus and cerebral cortex. Thus, children treated with stimulants could better attend to environmental stimuli and would have less need for hyperactivity and noisiness. Although this theory is plausible, please understand that there are other theories and none has yet been widely accepted.

One of the more disturbing side effects of stimulant therapy is a suppression of height and weight increases during drug treatment. Amphetamine produces a slightly greater effect in most studies than methylphenidate. If drug treatment is stopped over the summer vacation,

methylphenidate (Ritalin): (meth il *fen* ih date) a stimulant used in treating ADHD.

there is a rebound and a growth spurt that makes up for most of the suppressed height and weight gain.

The seemingly indiscriminate but medically prescribed use of stimulant drugs to influence the behavior of school-age children has evoked much social protest and commentary. After widespread publicity about the use of amphetamines for this purpose in the late 1960s, coinciding with public reaction against amphetamine use, there was a decline in stimulant prescriptions for children and a switch to methylphenidate. More recently there has been a considerable increase in the number of schoolchildren receiving stimulant medication for hyperactivity, and it is now estimated that over a million children are receiving such treatment in the United States.[33] What is not clear is whether this increase represents more awareness of the disorder and its proper treatment or whether more children are being given the medication inappropriately. Whenever drug therapy is used, it should be only one component of an effective treatment program.

"Smart Pills"

In the 1960s, a number of studies seemed to show that rats learned faster and performed better if they were given amphetamine or some other stimulant. Abbott Laboratories obtained a patent for the stimulant it named Cylert, which it was testing as a "smart pill." A great deal of animal and human research has since been done on the role of stimulants in improving mental performance, and it is now possible to summarize the ideas that have come from that work. One way to represent the effects of stimulants can be seen in Figure 8.4, which schematically relates degree of mental performance to the arousal level of the CNS. At low levels of arousal, such as when the individual is sleepy, performance suffers. Increasing the arousal level into the normal range with a stimulant can then improve performance. At the very high end of the arousal scale the person is so maniacal or

so involved in repetitive, stereotyped behavior that performance suffers, even on the simplest of tasks. In the region of the graph labeled "Excited," it can be seen that some simple tasks can be improved above normal levels, but complex or difficult tasks are disrupted because of difficulty in concentrating, controlling attention, and making careful decisions. Cylert never made it to the market as a smart pill, but the company later introduced it as an alternative to Ritalin in the treatment of ADHD.

In Figure 8.4, we can see that anyone trying to improve his or her mental performance level with amphetamines or other stimulants is taking a chance. Depending on the type of task, predrug performance level, and dose, one might obtain improvement or disruption. A small dose could be beneficial to a tired person driving alone at night on a deserted interstate highway but would probably only add to the confusion of a school bus driver trying to negotiate a Los Angeles freeway interchange at 7:30 A.M. with a load of noisy students. As for the students themselves, a small dose of a stimulant might help keep them awake to study when they should be sleeping, but a larger dose? There's an old piece of college folklore recounting something that probably never happened but has the ring of possible truth to it. It involves a student who stayed awake for days studying with the help of amphetamines, went into a final exam "wired up," wrote feverishly and eloquently for two hours, and only later when he received his exam back with an *F* saw that he had written the entire answer on one line, using the line over and over, so that it was solid black and the rest of the paper was blank.

Athletics

Under some conditions the use of amphetamine or other stimulants at an appropriate dose can produce slight improvements in athletic performance. The effects are so small as to be meaningless for most athletes, but at the highest levels of competition even a 1 percent improvement

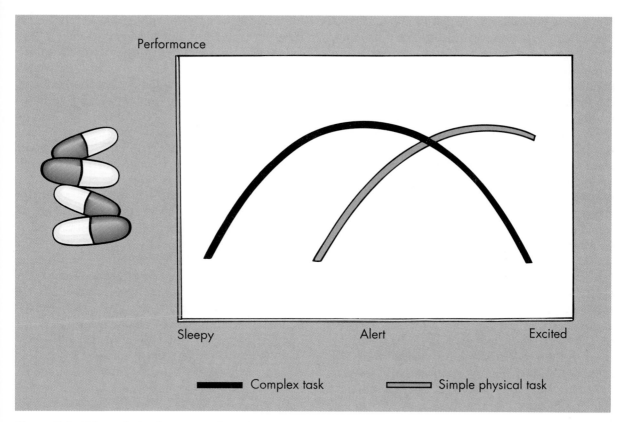

Figure 8-4   Effects of stimulants on performance

can mean the difference between winning a medal or coming in sixth. The temptation has been strong for athletes to use amphetamines and other stimulants to enhance their performances, and this topic is discussed in more detail in Chapter 19.

Causes for Concern

Acute Toxicity

During the period of amphetamine intoxication with above-normal doses, what dangers are caused by the altered behavior patterns (acute behavioral toxicity)? As we have seen, even at moderate doses complex decision making can be impaired. At higher doses there is a tendency

to be easily panicked and to become suspicious to the point of paranoia. Combine this with increased feelings of power and capability, and there is concern that incidents of violence may increase.

There were multiple reports of the association of amphetamine use and violence and aggression in the late 1960s and early 1970s. Those reports returned along with increased amphetamine use in the 1990s. Users of large amounts of amphetamine are good people to stay away from. The triad of paranoid ideas, impulsive behavior, and hypersensitivity is directly related to the pharmacological actions of the amphetamines and will occur no matter what the personality of the user. Although the amount of demonstrated violence due to amphetamine use cannot compare with that resulting from alcohol use, it is still a matter of concern, especially when the two are combined. Stimulants and alcohol do not counteract one another in most behavioral effects, and in the case of violence they combine to form an especially explosive mixture.

At one time there was concern that high doses of amphetamines would push the blood pressure so high that small strokes would occur and cause some slight brain damage, which would, of course, be cumulative for repeated high-dose users. However, no direct human evidence has been obtained indicating this to be a problem. More recently it was demonstrated in rats that high doses of methamphetamine result in the production in the brain of a chemical that selectively destroys catecholamine neurons.[34]

The possible long-term behavioral consequences for humans are unclear because the dosing regimens used in animal studies have been excessive and do not mimic self-administration by human amphetamine users. Nevertheless, some have expressed concern that, as abusers of amphetamine-like drugs age, they may be at a greater risk of developing movement disorders, such as Parkinson's disease (see Chapter 6).[35] Only time and better-controlled studies will tell.

Chronic Toxicity

The development of a paranoid psychosis has long been known to be one of the effects of sustained cocaine use. The first amphetamine psychosis was described in 1938, but little attention was given this syndrome until the late 1950s. There have been many suggestions as to the reason for the psychosis: that heavy methamphetamine users have schizoid personalities or that the psychosis is really caused by sleep deprivation, particularly dream-sleep deprivation. The question of the basis for the amphetamine psychosis was resolved by the demonstration that it could be elicited in the laboratory in individuals who clearly were not prepsychotic and who did not experience great sleep deprivation. It seems, then, that the paranoid psychosis after high-dose IV use of amphetamine is primarily the result of the drug and not the personality predisposition of the user. There is evidence that the paranoid psychosis results from dopaminergic stimulation, probably in the mesolimbic system. In some cases in which paranoid psychoses have been produced by amphetamines, the paranoid thinking and loss of touch with reality have been slow to return to normal, persisting for days or even weeks after the drug has left the system. There is no good evidence for permanent behavioral or personality disruption.

There is another behavior induced by high doses of amphetamine: compulsive and repetitive actions. The behavior might be acceptable (the individual might compulsively clean a room over and over) or it might be bizarre (one student spent a night counting corn flakes). There is a precedent for this stereotyped behavior in animal studies using high doses of amphetamine; it probably results from an effect of amphetamine on dopaminergic systems in the basal ganglia.

Dependence Potential

Theories about the abuse potential of amphetamines parallel the history of such theories regarding cocaine. For years experts argued about whether the amphetamines were truly "addicting." Because amphetamine withdrawal didn't produce the kinds of obvious physical symptoms seen with heroin or barbiturate withdrawal, most people decided that amphetamine did not produce physical dependence, yet there is evidence that repeated use of high doses of amphetamine produces a consistent set of withdrawal symptoms: several hours after the last dose the user "crashes." Mood and energy level drop dramatically, and the user might then sleep for 24 hours or more. On awakening, the user is in a depressed mood, which can last for days. During this time the individual feels helpless, worthless, and as though he or she could "just

TABLE 8-1

Dependence Liability of Stimulants

Drug and route	Tolerance	Physical dependence	Probability of behavioral dependence
Cocaine, snorted	Yes	At high doses	High
Cocaine, intravenous	Yes*	At high doses	Very high
Cocaine, freebase inhaled	Yes	At high doses	Very high
Amphetamines, oral	Yes, short- and long-term	At high doses	Moderate
Amphetamines, intravenous	Yes, long- and short-term	At high doses	Very high

sit there and die." Talk of death is common during this period. Of course, taking amphetamine again seems the most rapid way to overcome this mood and get high again. Because this set of symptoms occurs reliably after high-dose amphetamine use, and because it can, within limits, be reversed by taking amphetamine, it does fit our definition of a withdrawal syndrome. Therefore, use of high doses of amphetamine can lead to physical dependence (see Table 8.1).

It has been known for years that amphetamines could be habit forming—that is, produce behavioral dependence. Until a few years ago that was not considered very important. Amphetamine was even considered by some to be a so-called soft drug. It was available by prescription, and it produced only psychological dependence, which most users did not develop. The idea seemed to be that, although it could be habit forming in some individuals, its potential for abuse was limited. Now we realize that important factors such as dose and route of administration were not being taken into account. Small doses (5 or 10 mg) taken orally by people acting under their physician's orders for some purpose other than achieving a high rarely result in dependence. A larger dose injected intravenously for the purpose of getting high can result in a rapid development of dependence. Taken in this way, amphetamine is as potent a reinforcer as

any known drug. Animal studies reveal that rats and monkeys will quickly learn to press a lever that produces IV injections of amphetamine. If required to do so, an animal will press hundreds of times for a single injection.[36]

Supplies of Illicit Amphetamine

Illicit amphetamine for U.S. consumption is primarily produced in small "stovetop laboratories," which might exist for only a few days at a time in a remote area before moving on. Most of these labs produce methamphetamine, although some produce amphetamine itself. For the past several years, law enforcement officers have seized an increasing number of these small methamphetamine labs each year.[8] One reaction to this pressure has been an increase in the importation of "Mexican meth," made in larger laboratories in Mexico and shipped across the border, using the methods established for smuggling marijuana and cocaine.

Current Patterns of Amphetamine Abuse

These days there are many fewer people using prescription amphetamines, and the main concern of law enforcement and treatment officials is methamphetamine (crank) made in illicit laboratories. The drug of the 1960s urban hippie has become associated with biker gangs and with laboratories in rural areas of the West.[27] Methamphetamine can be smoked, snorted, or injected, but it is used by only a small fraction of the population.

While current use of amphetamine was reported by less than 1 percent of the population in the 1999 Household Survey, nearly 5 percent of those sampled in the 1999 High School Senior Survey reported current amphetamine use. Amphetamine use by seniors has steadily increased since the late 1980s. Additionally, according to DAWN data, amphetamine-related emergency department episodes increased by 361 percent between 1991 and 1994. The apparent renewed popularity of amphetamine led the National Institute on Drug Abuse, in 1996, to launch an initiative aimed at increasing scientific knowledge about the drug, including its abuse potential. Eastern states have not experienced amphetamine-related problems to the extent of those reported in states such as California, despite law enforcement officials' warnings of an impending eastward spread of amphetamine abuse.

SUMMARY

- The most effective CNS stimulants are cocaine and amphetamine.
- The stimulants can reverse the effects of fatigue, maintain wakefulness, and temporarily elevate the mood of the user.
- Cocaine is derived from the coca plant. Coca leaves have been chewed for centuries.
- Cocaine's earliest uses in the United States were as a local anesthetic and in psychiatry.
- Coca paste and crack are smokable forms of illicit cocaine.
- Cocaine appears to act by interacting with several neurotransmitters, including dopamine and serotonin.

- Excessive cocaine use can result in a paranoid psychotic reaction.
- Cocaine and amphetamine produce dependence.
- Use of cocaine has declined in the general population since 1985.
- Amphetamine is a synthetic sympathomimetic similar to ephedrine.
- The amphetamine-like drugs are similar in structure to dopamine and norepinephrine.
- Amphetamines are used in short-term weight reduction, narcolepsy, and ADHD (methylphenidate is preferred for ADHD, however).
- Illicit use of amphetamine has been associated with violent behavior.
- Illicit methamphetamine is primarily made in small laboratories or imported from Mexico.
- Amphetamine use is currently at a low level in the general population but has increased over the past several years.

REVIEW QUESTIONS

1. At about what periods in history did cocaine reach its first and second peaks of popularity, and when was amphetamine's popularity at its highest?
2. How did Mariani, Freud, and Halsted popularize the use of cocaine?
3. How are coca paste, freebase, crack, and ice similar?
4. What similarities and what differences are there in the toxic effects of cocaine and amphetamine?
5. What effect would there be on medical practice if both cocaine and amphetamine were placed on Schedule I?
6. Contrast the typical "speed freak" of the 1960s with the typical cocaine user of the early 1980s and with our stereotype of a modern crack smoker.

Web Watch

Activities Related to Stimulant Use

Check Out Publications on Stimulants

The National Clearinghouse for Drug and Alcohol Information offers a listing of publications about certain types of drugs. Go to the following sites to find and, if you wish, order brochures or other publications about the following stimulants, www.health.org/catalog/catalog.asp?key=14&detail=false; cocaine, www.health.org/catalog/catalog.asp?key=4&detail=false; crack cocaine, www.health.org/catalog/catalog.asp?key=21&detail=false; and methamphetamine, www.health.org/catalog/catalog.asp?key=10&detail=false.

Do You Know About Cocaine and Pregnancy?

How severely can cocaine hurt an unborn or newborn baby? What are the specific effects on a child whose mother used cocaine during pregnancy? At www.noah-health.org/english/pregnancy/march_of_dimes/substance/cocaine.html, you'll find the answers to these questions, as well as other information about cocaine use during pregnancy. You can also read about strategies the March of Dimes is using to address these issues.

Learn More About Cocaine Addiction

At www.cocaineaddiction.com you can find a variety of facts about cocaine, including the history of the drug, news articles, photos, stories, links, and research results. You can also read about the NARCON rehabilitation program.

Are You Addicted to Cocaine?

To assess your own or someone else's risk of cocaine addiction, go to www.cocaineaddiction.com/contact.html. This site provides a form to fill out and information about contacting NARCON's rehabilitation program.

---

7. How does the chemical difference between methamphetamine and amphetamine relate to the behavioral effects of the two drugs?
8. Compare the dependence potential of cocaine with that of amphetamine.

REFERENCES

1. Dillehay TD and others: The Nanchoc tradition: The beginnings of Andean civilization, *American Scientist* 85:46–55, 1997.
2. Taylor N: *Flight from reality,* New York: Duell, Sloan & Pearce,1949.
3. Freud S: *On the general effect of cocaine,* lecture before the Psychiatric Union on March 5, 1885. (Reprinted in *Drug Dependence* 5:17, 1970.)
4. Doyle AC: The sign of the four. In *The complete Sherlock Holmes.* New York: Garden City, 1938.
5. Musto DF: Opium, cocaine and marijuana in American history, *Scientific American,* p 40, July 1991.
6. Ashley R: *Cocaine: Its history, uses and effects.* New York: Warner Books, 1976.
7. Brecher EM: *Licit and illicit drugs.* Boston: Little, Brown, 1972.
8. U.S. Drug Enforcement Administration, National Narcotics Intelligence Consumers Committee: *The supply of illicit drugs to the United States.* Washington, DC: U.S. Government Printing Office, 1998.
9. Witkin G: The men who created crack, *U.S. News & World Report,* p 44, Aug 19, 1991.
10. Feldman RS, Meyer JS, Quenzer LF: *Principles of neuropsychopharmacology.* Sunderland, MA: Sinauer, 1997.
11. Williams S: Cocaine's harmful effects, *Science* 248:166, 1990.
12. Hart CL and others: Comparison of intravenous cocaethylene and cocaine in humans, *Psychopharmacology* 149:153, 2000.
13. Brady KT and others: Cocaine-induced psychosis, *Journal of Clinical Psychiatry* 52:509, 1991.
14. Bunn WH, Giannini AJ: Cardiovascular complications of cocaine abuse, *American Family Physician* 46:769, 1992.
15. Haney M and others: Effects of pergolide on intravenous cocaine self-administration in men and women, *Psychopharmacology* 137:15, 1998.
16. Johanson CE and others: Self-administration of psychomotor stimulant drugs: The effects of unlimited access, *Pharmacology Biochemistry & Behavior* 4:45, 1976.

17. Zuckerman B and others: Effects of maternal marijuana and cocaine use on fetal growth, *New England Journal of Medicine* 320:762, 1989.

18. Zuckerman B: "Crack kids": Not broken, *Pediatrics* 89: 337, 1992.

19. Riley KJ: *Snow job?* New Brunswick, NJ: Transaction, 1996.

20. Martz L: A dirty secret: Hyping instant addiction doesn't help, *Newsweek*, p 74, Feb 19, 1990.

21. Mendelson JH, Mello NK: Management of cocaine abuse and dependence, *New England Journal of Medicine* 334:965, 1996.

22. Fischman MW, Haney M: Neurobiology of stimulant abuse. In Galanter M, Kieber HD, editors: *The American Psychiatric Press textbook of substance abuse treatment* (2nd ed.). 1999.

23. Higgins ST and others: Incentives improve outcome in outpatient behavioral treatment of cocaine dependence. *Archives of General Psychiatry* 51:568, 1994.

24. Carroll K and others: One-year follow-up of psychotherapy and pharmacotherapy for cocaine dependence: Delayed emergence of psychotherapy effects. *Archives of General Psychiatry* 51:989, 1994.

25. Benzedrine alert, *Air Surgeon's Bulletin* 1(2):19–21, 1944.

26. *Journal of the American Medical Association* 183:363, 1963.

27. Bai M: White storm warning, *Newsweek*, Mar 30, 1997.

28. Martin WR and others: Physiologic, subjective, and behavioral effects of amphetamine, methamphetamine, ephedrine, phenmetrazine, and methylphenidate in man. *Clinical Pharmacology & Therapeutics* 12:245, 1971.

29. Physician's Desk Reference Medical Economics, Ordell, NJ. Annual.

30. Weintraub M: Long-term weight control, *Clinical Pharmacology & Therapeutics* 51:581–594, 1992.

31. *Weight loss drug receives FDA clearance*, press release, Nov 24, 1997.

32. American Psychiatric Association: *Diagnostic and statistical manual of mental disorders* (4th ed.). Washington, DC: Author, 1994.

33. O'Toole K and others: Effects of methylphenidate on attention and nonverbal learning in children with attention-deficit hyperactivity disorder, *Journal of the American Academy of Child and Adolescent Psychiatry* 36:531–537, 1996.

34. Marek GJ and others: Dopamine uptake inhibitors block long-term neurotoxic effects of methamphetamine upon dopaminergic neurons, *Brain Res* 513:274, 1990.

35. McCann UD and others: Reduced striatal dopamine transporter density in abstinent methamphetamine and methcathinone users: Evidence for positron emission tomography studies with [11C]WIN-35,428, *The Journal of Neuroscience* 18:8417, 1998.

36. Griffiths RR and others: Predicting the abuse liability of drugs with animal self-administration procedures: Psychomotor stimulants and hallucinogens. In Thompson T, Dews P, editors: *Advances in behavioral pharmacology* (Vol. 2). New York: Academic Press, 1979.

Try It!

Sensation-Seeking Scale

For each of the 13 items, select the choice that best describes your likes or dislikes, or the way that you feel. Select only one statement for each item.

Question 1:
   A. I would like a job that requires a lot of traveling.
   B. I would prefer a job in one location.

Question 2:
   A. I am invigorated by a brisk, cold day.
   B. I can't wait to get indoors on a cold day.

Question 3:
   A. I get bored seeing the same old faces.
   B. I like the comfortable familiary of everyday friends.

Question 4:
   A. I would prefer living in an ideal society in which everyone is safe, secure, and happy.
   B. I would have preferred living in the unsettled days of our history.

Question 5:
   A. I sometimes like to do things that are a little frightening.
   B. A sensible person avoids activities that are dangerous.

Question 6:
   A. I would not like to be hypnotized.
   B. I would like to have the experience of being hypnotized.

Question 7:
   A. The most important goal of life is to live it to the fullest and experience as much as possible.
   B. The most important goal of life is to find peace and happiness.

Question 8:
   A. I would like to try parachute jumping.
   B. I would never want to try jumping out of a plane, with or without a parachute.

Question 9:
   A. I enter cold water gradually, giving myself time to get used to it.
   B. I like to dive or jump right in to the ocean or a cold pool.

Question 10:
   A. When I go on vacation, I prefer the comfort of a good room and bed.
   B. When I go on vacation, I prefer the change of camping out.

Question 11:
   A. I prefer people who are emotionally expressive even if they are a bit unstable.
   B. I prefer people who are calm and even-tempered.

Question 12:
   A. A good painting should shock or jolt the senses.
   B. A good painting should give one a feeling of peace and security.

Question 13:
   A. People who ride motorcycles must have some kind of unconscious need to hurt themselves.
   B. I would like to drive or ride a motorcycle.

To Score::

Give yourself one point for each of the following items you circled: 1A, 2A, 3A, 4B, 5A, 6B, 7A, 8A, 9B, 10B, 11A, 12A, 13B. Add up your points, and compare the total to the following scale: 1–3 (very low in sensation seeking), 4–5 (low), 6–9 (average), 10–11 (high), 12–13 (very high).

Adapted from Zuckerman, M. (1994). Behavioral expressions and biosocial bases of sensation seeking. New York: Cambridge University Press.

Chapter 9

Depressants and Inhalants

KEY TERMS

- GHB
- sedatives
- hypnotics
- depressants
- benzodiazepines
- barbiturates
- inhalants
- rohypnol
- GABA
- epilepsies

Online Learning Center Resources

www.mhhe.com/ray

Log on to our Online Learning Center (OLC) for access to the following additional resources.

- Chapter definitions
- Learning objectives
- Student interactive question-and-answer sites
- Self-scoring chapter quiz

The OLC also offers web links for study and exploration of health topics. Here are some examples of what you'll find:

www.iconbazaar.com/molecules/drugs/depressants/

This website provides 3-D animated depictions of depressants. Click a type of depressant drug to see a 3-D molecule animation.

www.geocities.com/SouthBeach/Cove/8430/ddepr.html

The pros, cons, and other facts about drugs are provided here. There is a list of various depressant drugs. Click on the name of a drug to see a biography and points to remember about it.

www.usdoj.gov/dea/concern/inhalants.htm

The U.S. Department of Justice's Drug Enforcement Administration sponsors this web page about inhalants. The information here warns about household products that can be abused as inhalants and explains government regulations pertaining to them.

Drugs in the Media

The Legacy of Samantha Reid

We have previously discussed the importance of emotional "prairie fires" in the passage of many of the drug laws in the United States. From the time of the 1906 Pure Food and Drugs Act to the present, public media have played a

Drugs in the Media Continued...

critical role in spreading the word about the tragic consequences related to the use of one or another type of drug. That publicity often leads to legislation generated in the heat of emotion. A recent example is the passage through Congress of a law requiring that gamma hydroxy butyrate **(GHB)** be listed as a Schedule I controlled substance. President Clinton quickly signed the law, and it went into effect in March 2000. This is an unusual process in that decisions about the scheduling of drugs are supposed to be made in a nonpolitical way on the basis of scientific evidence. Previous reviews of GHB by the federal agency responsible for making these decisions had determined that the substance, although posing risks of abuse and the possibility of overdose deaths, should not be listed on Schedule I. Why did Congress take this decision out of the hands of the Food and Drug Administration and the Drug Enforcement Administration?

The answer to that question is Samantha Reid, a 15-year-old Michigan student who died after some male friends apparently put GHB into her soft drink without her

knowledge. When she and another young woman passed out, the young men waited to see whether they would recover, rather than getting them quickly to the hospital. One eventually recovered from her coma; Samantha did not. This tragic death and the subsequent formation of the Samantha Reid Foundation, dedicated to exposing the dangers of GHB, were widely reported by the *Detroit News* and other U.S. news media. Testimony by Samantha's mother left no doubt about her message that young people needed more protection from this potentially dangerous substance. The result was the toughest thing Congress knew how to do—not only list the drug as a federal controlled substance but also list it on Schedule I, even though it was currently undergoing clinical testing as a treatment for narcolepsy.

Regardless of the merits of this decision, what is important is to realize how much of our current legacy of drug laws evolved through a similar series of emotional responses to tragic events.

Downers, depressants, sedatives, hypnotics, gin-in-a-pill: known by many names, these prescription drugs all have a widespread effect in the brain that can be summed up as decreased neural activity. What are the behavioral effects? As suggested by one of the proposed names, if you know what alcohol does, you know what these drugs do. They come from several different chemical classes but are grouped together because of their common psychological effects. At low doses these drugs might be prescribed for daytime use to reduce anxiety (as **sedatives**). At higher doses many of the same drugs are prescribed as sleeping pills (**hypnotics**).

This group of prescription drugs is often referred to as *sedative-hypnotics*, part of a larger group of substances considered to be CNS **depressants.** The most widely *used* depressant is alcohol, which is discussed in detail in Chapters 11 and 12. The most widely *prescribed* types of sedative-hypnotics fall into the chemical grouping called the **benzodiazepines,** which in the past 40 years have largely replaced the **barbiturates.** A similar depressant effect is produced by most of the **inhalants**—the glues, paints, solvents, and gasoline fumes that some young people (and a few older people) breathe to get "high."

HISTORY AND PHARMACOLOGY

Before Barbiturates

Chloral Hydrate

The "knockout drops" (or "Mickey Finn") they used to slip in the sailor's drink in those old movies were a solution of chloral hydrate. First synthesized in 1832, chloral hydrate was not used clinically until about 1870. It is rapidly metabolized to trichloroethanol, which is the active hypnotic agent. When taken orally, chloral hydrate has a short onset period (30 minutes), and 1 to 2 g will induce sleep in less than an hour. This agent does not cause as much depression of the respiratory and cardiovascular systems as a comparable dose of the barbiturates and has fewer aftereffects.

In 1869, Dr. Benjamine Richardson introduced chloral hydrate to Great Britain. Ten years later he called it "in one sense a beneficent, and in another sense a maleficent substance, I almost feel a regret that I took any part whatever in the introduction of the agent into the practice of healing."[1] He had learned that what humankind can misuse, some will abuse. As early as 1871, he referred to its nontherapeutic use as "toxical luxury" and lamented that chloral hydrate addicts had to be added to "alcohol intemperants and opium-eaters." Chloral hydrate addiction is a tough way to go; it is a gastric irritant, and repeated use causes considerable stomach upset.

Paraldehyde

Paraldehyde was synthesized in 1829 and introduced clinically in 1882. Paraldehyde would probably be in great use today because of its effectiveness as a CNS depressant with little respiratory depression and a wide safety margin, except for one characteristic: it has an extremely noxious taste and an odor that permeates the breath of the user. Its safety margin and its ability to sedate patients led to widespread use of paraldehyde in mental hospitals before the 1950s. Anyone who ever worked in, was a patient in, or even visited one of the large state mental hospitals during that era probably still remembers the odor of paraldehyde, which was often detectable on entering the building.

Bromides.

Bromide salts were used so widely in patent medicines to induce sleep in the nineteenth century that the word *bromide* entered our language as a reference to any person or story that was tiresome and boring. The bromides are little used today, now that they have been removed from OTC sleep preparations. Bromides accumulate in the body, and the depression they cause builds up over several days of regular use. There are serious toxic effects with repeated hypnotic doses of these agents. Dermatitis and constipation are minor accompaniments; with increased intake, motor disturbances, delirium, and psychosis can develop. Very low (ineffective) doses of bromides remained in some OTC medicines until the 1960s.

(GHB): gamma-hydroxybutyrate; chemically related to GABA; used recreationally as a depressant.

sedatives: drugs used to relax, calm, or tranquilize.

hypnotics: drugs used to induce sleep.

depressants: drugs that slow activity in the CNS.

benzodiazepines: (ben zo die *ay* zah peens) a chemical grouping of sedative-hypnotics.

barbiturates: (bar *bitch* er ates) a chemical group of sedative-hypnotics.

inhalants: volatile solvents inhaled for intoxicating purposes.

Barbiturates

More than 2,500 barbiturates have been synthesized. Barbital (Veronal) was the first to be used clinically, in 1903. Its name gave rise to the practice of giving barbiturates names ending in *-al*. The second barbiturate in clinical use, phenobarbital (Luminal), was introduced in 1912. Amobarbital (Amytal) in 1923, as well as pentobarbital (Nembutal) and secobarbital (Seconal), both introduced in 1930, are well-established examples of the barbiturates.

As Table 9.1 indicates, barbiturates are typically grouped on the basis of the duration of their activity. In general, the drugs that are the most lipid-soluble are the ones that have both the shortest time of onset (i.e., they are absorbed and enter the brain rapidly) and the shortest duration of action (i.e., they leave the brain quickly and tend to be more rapidly metabolized). These different time courses are important for our understanding of the different uses of these drugs and their different tendencies to produce dependence.

Suppose you want a drug to keep a person calm and relaxed during the daytime (a sedative). You don't want the person to become drowsy, and you want to produce as stable and smooth a drug effect as possible. Therefore, you would choose a *low* dose of a *long-acting* barbiturate, say 30 to 50 mg of phenobarbital. On the other hand, for a sleeping-pill (hypnotic) effect, you want the person to become drowsy, you want the drug to act fairly quickly after it is taken, and you don't want the person to still be groggy the next morning. Therefore, you would choose a *higher* dose of a *shorter-acting* drug, say 100 to 200 mg of amobarbital or secobarbital. Both of these types of prescription were fairly common 40 years ago, before the introduction of the benzodiazepines.

Although a large fraction of phenobarbital is excreted unchanged in the urine, the majority of this drug and nearly all of the shorter-acting drugs is metabolized in the liver. The barbiturates are one of the classes of drugs that stimulate

TABLE 9-1

Groupings of Available Barbiturates

Type	Time of onset	Duration of action
Short-acting Pentobarbital (Nembutal) Secobarbital (Seconal)	15 minutes	2 to 3 hours
Intermediate-acting Aprobarbital (Alurate) Amobarbital (Amytal) Butabarbital (Butisol)	30 minutes	5 to 6 hours
Long-acting Mephobarbital (Merbaral) Phenobarbital (Luminal)	1 hour	6 to 10 hours

the activity of the microsomal enzymes of the liver. Some of the tolerance that develops to the barbiturates is the result of an increased rate of deactivation caused by this stimulation. The induction of these enzymes by the barbiturates might also cause the more rapid metabolism of other drugs, perhaps requiring an adjustment of the dose.

Tolerance can develop to the barbiturates, as well as both psychological and physical dependence. In addition, they depress respiration and, in large doses or in combination with alcohol, can completely stop one's breathing. For many years barbiturate sleeping pills were chosen above all others by people wishing to commit suicide. Also, accidental overdoses occurred when sleeping pills were taken after an evening of heavy drinking.

Although the majority of individuals who took barbiturates were not harmed by them, there was a great deal of concern about both the addiction liability and the danger of overdose. These concerns led to the ready acceptance of new sedative or hypnotic agents that appeared to be safer.

Meprobamate

The first modern antianxiety agents (*anxiolytics*) developed from a muscle relaxant called mephenesin, which was patented in 1946 and was a commercial success but had a short duration of action. One compound patented in 1952 not only was longer lasting but was believed to be a unique type of CNS depressant. Clinical trials in 1953 supported this belief, and the compound was approved by the FDA and released for prescription use in 1955. Meprobamate, the generic name, became widely known by the brand name Miltown, and it represented the drug revolution of the 1950s to many people.

The boom in meprobamate use was tremendous. In the year it was introduced, sales of Miltown went from $7,500 in May to over $500,000 in December. The happy pills had arrived! A publicity agency and excessive prescribing by physicians combined to make Miltown a public nuisance and the unnamed object of comment concerning overuse by the American Psychiatric Association and the World Health Organization in 1957. *Miltown* became such an overused word that physicians began prescribing meprobamate under its other brand name, Equanil.

It gradually became clear that meprobamate, like the barbiturates, can also produce both psychological and physical dependence. Physical dependence can result from taking a bit more than twice a normal daily dose. In 1970, meprobamate became a Schedule IV controlled substance, and although it is still available for prescription under several brand names, the benzodiazepines have largely replaced it.

Although reports of overdose deaths from meprobamate alone are rare, in retrospect it seems ironic that the medical community so readily accepted meprobamate as being safer than barbiturates. Meprobamate was sold only in anxiolytic doses for daytime sedation. Barbiturates produce physical dependence at doses above 400 mg, or twice a maximum *hypnotic* dose. If barbiturates had been sold only as 30 mg phenobarbital for daytime sedation, many fewer cases of physical dependence or overdose would have been reported. Let this be an object lesson: by deciding that the "barbiturates" were addicting and deadly, the focus was on the chemical class, rather than on the dose and the manner in which the drug was used. Thus, a new, "safer" chemical was accepted without considering that its safety was not being judged under the same conditions. This mistake has occurred frequently with psychoactive drugs. In fact, it occurred again with methaqualone.

Methaqualone

With continued reports of overdoses and physical dependence associated with secobarbital and amobarbital sleeping pills, in the 1960s the market was wide open for a hypnotic that would be less addicting and less dangerous. Maybe it was too wide open.

The methaqualone story is one where everyone was wrong—the pharmaceutical industry, the FDA, the DEA, the press, and the physicians. Methaqualone was originally synthesized in India, tested, and found to be ineffective as an antimalarial drug. But it was a good sedative, so in 1959 it was introduced as a prescription drug in Great Britain. It never sold well, but after the thalidomide disaster, there was increased interest in a "safe" nonbarbiturate sleeping pill. Mandrax (250 mg of methaqualone and 25 mg of an antihistamine) was introduced in 1965 in a massive advertising campaign to physicians. The campaign worked, and 2 million prescriptions were issued for Mandrax in 1971 in Great Britain. The drug had already found its way into the street, where it was widely abused: by heroin users, by high school students, by anyone who wanted a cheap but potent "down." Misuse was so great that Great Britain tightened controls on it in 1970 and then again in 1973.

Germany introduced methaqualone in 1960 as a nonprescription drug, had its first methaqualone suicide in 1962, and discovered that 10 to 22 percent of the drug overdoses treated in this period were a result of this drug. In 1963, Germany reduced the problem by making methaqualone a prescription drug. From 1960 to 1964, Japan experienced a major epidemic of methaqualone abuse, causing over 40 percent of all overdoses admitted to hospitals. Japan tightened controls almost to the maximum possible on methaqualone and stemmed the tide.

Apparently no one in the United States was paying much attention to these problems in other countries, because in 1965, after three years of testing, Quaalude and Sopor, brand names for methaqualone, were introduced in the United States as prescription drugs with a package insert that read "Addiction potential not established." In June 1966, the FDA Committee on the Abuse Potential of Drugs decided that there was no need to monitor methaqualone, since there was no evidence of abuse potential! Thus, from 1967 to 1973 the package insert read "Physical dependence has not clearly been demonstrated."

In the early 1970s in this country, *ludes* and *sopors* were familiar terms in the drug culture and in drug-treatment centers. Physicians were overprescribing a hypnotic drug that they believed to be nonaddicting and safer than the barbiturates. Most of the methaqualone sold on the street was legally manufactured and then either stolen or obtained through prescriptions. At any rate, sales zoomed, and front-page reporting of its effects when misused helped to build its reputation as a drug of abuse. In 1973, 8 years after it was introduced into this country, 4 years after American scientists began saying it was addicting, 11 years after the first suicide, methaqualone was put on Schedule II. By 1985, methaqualone was no longer available as a prescription drug, and it is now listed on Schedule I.

Was methaqualone really very different from the barbiturates? For a while physicians thought it was safer. Street users referred to it as the "love drug" (one of many drugs to have been called this) or "heroin for lovers," implying an *aphrodisiac* effect. In reality the effect is probably not different from the disinhibition produced by alcohol or other depressants. Methaqualone causes the same kind of motor incoordination as alcohol and the barbiturates. Both psychological and physical dependence can develop to methaqualone as easily and rapidly as with the barbiturates, and for a few years methaqualone was also near the top of the charts for drug-related deaths (DAWN coroners' reports, Chapter 2). If it was different, it wasn't much different.

Benzodiazepines — sub. for barbiturates — most widley prescribed drug

The first of the benzodiazepines was chlordiazepoxide, which was marketed under the trade name Librium (possibly because it "liberates" one from anxieties). Chlordiazepoxide was synthesized in 1947, but it was 10 years before its value in reducing anxiety was suggested, and it was not sold commercially until 1960. The discovery of this class of drugs was a triumph for behavioral research; a drug-company pharmacologist found that mice given the right dose of chlordiazepoxide would loosen their grip on an inclined wire screen and fall to the floor of the test cage. When this experiment had been done with barbiturates, the mice promptly fell asleep. With Librium, the relaxed mouse continued to walk around, sniffing the cage in a normal manner.[2] This drug was marketed as a more selective "antianxiety" agent that produced less drowsiness than the barbiturates and had a much larger safety margin before overdose death occurred in animals. Clinical practice bore this out: physical dependence was almost unheard of, and overdose seemed not to occur except in combination with alcohol or other depressant drugs. Even strong psychological dependence seemed rare with this drug. The conclusion was reached that the benzodi-azepines were as effective as the barbiturates and much safer. Librium became not only the leading psychoactive drug in sales but also the leading prescription drug of all. It was sup-planted in the early 1970s by diazepam (Val-ium), a more potent (lower-dose) agent made by the same company. From 1972 until 1978, Val-ium was the leading seller among all prescrip-tion drugs. Since then no single benzodiazepine has so dominated the market, but Xanax (a brand name for alprazolam) is currently the most widely prescribed brand name among this class of drugs.

As these drugs became widely used, reports again appeared of psychological dependence, oc-casional physical dependence, and overdose deaths. Diazepam was one of the most fre-quently mentioned drugs in the DAWN system coroners' reports, although almost always in combination with alcohol or other depressants. What happened to the big difference between the barbiturates and the benzodiazepines? One possibility is that it might not be the chemical class of drugs that makes the big difference but the dose and time course of the individual drugs. It's obvious that *overdose* deaths are more likely when a drug is sold in higher doses, such as those prescribed for hypnotic effects. *Psycho-logical dependence* develops most rapidly when the drug hits the brain quickly, which is why in-travenous use of heroin produces more depen-dence than oral use, and why smoking crack produces more dependence than chewing coca leaves. So a drug that has a rapid onset of action will be more likely to produce psychological de-pendence than a slow-acting drug. *Physical de-pendence* occurs when the drug leaves the system more rapidly than the body can adapt— one way to reduce the severity of withdrawal symptoms is to reduce the dose of a drug slowly over time. Drugs with a shorter duration of ac-tion leave the system quickly and are much more likely to produce withdrawal symptoms than are longer-acting drugs.

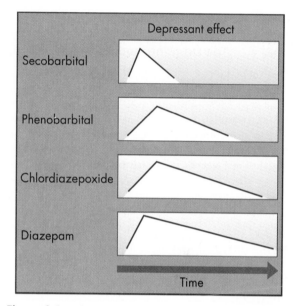

Figure 9.1 Schematic diagram of the relative time courses of two barbiturates and two benzodiazepines af-ter oral administration.

Figure 9.1 gives a schematic picture of the time course of the depressant actions of some of these drugs. Secobarbital, a short-acting barbitu-rate, has a relatively rapid onset, which should make it more likely than other barbiturates to produce psychological dependence. Also, be-cause its depressant action is terminated fairly quickly, withdrawal symptoms would be quite dramatic if the person had been taking large doses. Because this drug was used primarily as a sleeping pill, relatively large doses were pre-scribed. Thus, in the days when barbiturates were widely prescribed, secobarbital was associ-ated with overdoses and both physical and psychological dependence. Phenobarbital, a long-acting barbiturate, has a slower onset of action, which should be less likely to produce psychological dependence. Because the depres-sant action is terminated more slowly, drug clearance occurs slowly and withdrawal symp-toms are minimized. Because phenobarbital was

Targeting Prevention

The Drug-Induced Rape Prevention and Punishment Act

In 1996, the U.S. Congress debated what to do in response to widespread concerns about the use of rohypnol as a "date-rape" drug. One proposal was to make the drug a Schedule I controlled substance—after all, it was not a prescription drug in the United States and therefore could be considered to have "no medical use," one of the defining criteria for inclusion in Schedule I. However, the drug was legally available in more than 60 other countries, and Schedule I status would compel the United States to pressure those countries to outlaw it also. Instead, Congress passed the Drug-Induced Rape Prevention and Punishment Act. This act makes it a federal crime to give someone a controlled substance without the recipient's knowledge, with the intent of committing a violent crime. During the debate it was af-

firmed that rape is considered to be a crime of violence. Under this law, the maximum penalty is 20 years in prison and a $250,000 fine. A urine test is available for rohypnol, so any woman who suspects that she may have been given the drug can request that the test be conducted. It would then be possible, under this act, to charge the person suspected of giving her the drug. Even if no rape took place, it might be difficult for the drug-giver to argue that such was not his intention, given the reputation this drug has.

You might start a discussion among a group of your friends about date rape. What is their perception of this problem? What drugs have they heard about in conjunction with date rape? Are they aware of this federal law and its implications?

---

prescribed mostly in low sedative doses, it was rarely associated with overdose.

The first benzodiazepine was chlordiazepoxide, which was sold in low doses for daytime use and has a slow onset of action and an even longer duration of action than phenobarbital. Chlordiazepoxide produced few problems with either compulsive use or withdrawal symptoms, and overdoses were almost unheard of. Diazepam has a more rapid onset than chlordiazepoxide, but because of slow metabolism and the presence of active metabolites, it also has a long duration of action. We might expect a drug with these characteristics to produce more psychological dependence than chlordiazepoxide but only rarely to produce withdrawal symptoms. This is exactly what happened. To summarize this pharmacology object lesson, there might be greater differences among the barbiturates and among the benzodiazepines than there are between these two classes.

As if to underscore the basic similarity that exists among all the depressant drugs, in the 1990s a new version of the "Mickey Finn" was

HealthQuest Activities

In Module 9, you'll find "Roofies" under *Our Changing World.* This article addresses the use of Rohypnol, also known as the date-rape drug. After reading the article, consider whether you've ever been in a situation in which someone could have given you the drug while you were unaware. What are the risks you take when using Rohypnol? Look through recent newspapers and magazines to see if you can find any reports of crimes committed using Rohypnol. Rohypnol is sometimes taken in an alcoholic beverage or with other drugs. Now look under *Drug Interactions, OTC Drugs.* Read about the possible side effects of mixing sedatives and hypnotics.

In the same module, go to *Drug F/X Exploration.* Assess your dependence on and read about the effects of barbiturates, inhalants, and Valium. If you are interested in reading more about inhalants, see the article under *Specifics On.*

popularized. **Rohypnol** (flunitrazepam), a benzodiazepine sold as a hypnotic in many countries around the world but not in the United States, hit the news when reports surfaced of its being put into the drinks of unsuspecting women by their dates. The combination of rohypnol and alcohol was reputed to produce a profound intoxication, during which the woman would be highly suggestible and unable to remember what had happened to her. Thus, rohypnol became widely known as the "date-rape" drug (see Targeting Prevention box). In 1997, the drug's manufacturer changed the formulation of the pill so that when it dissolves in a drink it produces a characteristic color.[3]

MECHANISM OF ACTION

An important key to understanding the effects of these sedative-hypnotic agents was found in 1977 when it was reported that radioactive diazepam molecules had a high affinity for specific receptor sites in brain tissue. Other benzodiazepine types of sedatives also bound to these receptors, and the binding affinities of these various drugs correlated with their behavioral potencies in humans and other animals. These benzodiazepine receptors did not bind any of the known neurotransmitters, nor did they bind any of the barbiturates. However, it was soon noticed that the benzodiazepine receptors were always near receptors for the amino acid neurotransmitter g-aminobutyric acid **(GABA).** It now appears that when benzodiazepines bind to their receptor site, they enhance the normally inhibitory effects of GABA on its receptors. The barbiturates act at a separate binding site nearby and increase the actions of GABA on its receptors. The picture emerges of a GABA receptor *complex,* which includes the barbiturate binding site and the benzodiazepine receptor.[4] Drug companies quickly began developing new drugs based on their ability to bind to these sites, and several new sedative-hypnotics

have reached the market in recent years. A recent study using genetically altered mice appears to have separated the antianxiety effect from the hypnotic effect, based on isolating different subtypes of the GABA receptor. This could lead in the future to more selective antianxiety drugs.[5]

Although there have been intensive efforts to isolate an endogenous Valium-like substance from brain tissue, so far none has succeeded. Perhaps the brain does not contain a substance that enhances GABA's inhibitory effect. Another possibility is that there are endogenous sedative-hypnotic substances that have yet to be discovered.

BENEFICIAL USES

As Sedatives

Raze out the written troubles of the brain,
and with some sweet oblivious antidote
Cleanse the stuff'd bosom of that perilous stuff
Which weighs upon the heart . . .

As these lines from Shakespeare's *Macbeth* reveal, humans have often sought a "sweet oblivious antidote" to the cares and woes of living. Alcohol has most frequently been used for that purpose, but the sedative drugs also play a major role in modern society. In the United States in recent decades the barbiturates, then meprobamate, and then the benzodiazepines have been among the most widely prescribed medications. Four benzodiazepines are listed among the top 100 most commonly prescribed

---

Rohypnol: a benzodiazepine; the "date-rape drug."

GABA: an inhibitory neurotransmitter.

TABLE 9-2

Some Popular Benzodiazepines

Type	Half-life (hours)
Anxiolytics	
Alprazolam (Xanax)	6 to 20
Chlordiazepoxide (Librium)	5 to 30
Clonazepam (Klonopin)	30 to 40
Clorazepate (Tranxene)	30 to 200
Diazepam (Valium)	20 to 100
Lorazepam (Ativan)	10 to 20
Oxazepam (Serax)	5 to 15
Hypnotics	
Flurazepam (Dalmane)	40 to 250
Temazepam (Restoril)	5 to 25
Triazolam (Halcion)	1.7 to 3
Zolpidem (Ambien)	

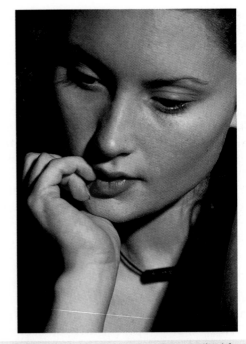

Benzodiazepines are commonly prescribed for anxiety disorders.

medications in the United States: alprazolam (Xanax), clonazepam (Klonopin), diazepam (Valium), and lorazepam (Ativan) (Table 9.2).

The combined sales of the benzodiazepines make them one of the most widely prescribed drug classes. Why? Most psychiatrists refer to the benzodiazepines as antianxiety agents, or anxiolytics. And most psychiatrists seem to accept the widely held view that various types of dysfunctional behavior (e.g., phobias, panic attacks, obsessive-compulsive disorders, psychosomatic problems) might result from various forms of psychological stress that can be lumped under the general classification of "anxieties." So if anxieties produce dysfunctional behavior and these drugs can reduce anxieties, then the drugs will be useful in reducing the dysfunctional behavior. In fact these disorders are now officially referred to as "anxiety disorders" (see Chapter 10). Although this approach seems logical, in reality not all of these conditions respond well to antianxiety drugs. For specific phobias (e.g., fear of spiders), behavior therapy is a more effective treatment. And for obsessive-compulsive disorder, certain antidepressant drugs seem to be most effective. Most of the prescriptions for antianxiety medications are not written by psychiatrists, nor are they written for patients with clearly defined anxiety disorders. In addition, many patients take the drugs daily for long periods of time. What disorder is being treated with such prescriptions? Galen, a second-century Greek physician, estimated that about 60 percent of the patients he saw had emotional and psychological, as opposed to physical, illness. It is currently estimated that for a typical general practitioner, about half of the patients have no treatable physical ailment. Many of these patients who complain of nervousness, distress, or vague aches and pains will be given a prescription for a sedative, such as Xanax. One way to look at this is that the patients may be suffering from a low-level generalized anxiety disorder, and the sedative is reducing the anxiety. A more cynical way of looking at it is that some patients are asking to be protected from the cares and woes of daily living. The physician prescribes something that is relatively safe and can make the patient feel better in a general way. The patient doesn't complain as much and comes back for more pills, so everyone is happy.

Although most physicians would agree that the benzodiazepines are probably overprescribed, in any individual case it may be impossible to know whether the patient just enjoys getting a "feel-good pill" or feels better because of a specific antianxiety effect. Whatever the reason for each individual, based on history there will continue to be a very large and profitable market for prescription sedatives.

As Sleeping Pills

Although one or two beers might relax a person and reduce inhibitions a bit, the effect of larger amounts is more dramatic. If you consume several beers at an active, noisy party, you might become wild and reckless. But if you consume the same number of beers, go to bed, and turn off the lights, you will probably fall asleep fairly quickly. This is essentially the principle on which hypnotic drug therapy is based: a large enough dose is taken to help you get to sleep more quickly.

Insomnia is a fairly common symptom, and in one nationwide household survey about one out of three adults reported some trouble falling asleep, staying asleep, or both.[6] About half of these people felt that their insomnia was serious, but fewer than 10 percent had used a prescription hypnotic drug within the past year. People who complain of insomnia often overestimate how long it takes them to get to sleep and underestimate how much time they actually sleep. Partly because physicians know this and partly because of concern about tolerance, rebound insomnia, dependence, and "hangover" effects, fewer hypnotics are prescribed now than 30 years ago, and they are usually taken for only a few nights at a time rather than continually.

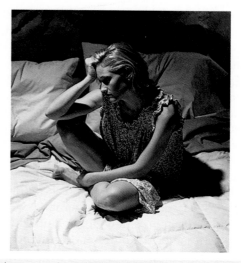

About one-third of adults report trouble sleeping.

Since 1976, when flurazepam (Dalmane) became the leading hypnotic agent, the benzodiazepines have increasingly displaced the barbiturates in the sleeping-pill market. The shorter-acting drug triazolam (Halcion) is now the most commonly prescribed brand of hypnotic. There is an interesting story in this: when barbiturates are used, they produce a fairly rapid tolerance, so that after a few nights of regular use they are no longer effective. To regain the hypnotic effect, it becomes necessary to increase the dose, leading to concerns about addiction. One reason that Dalmane became the hypnotic drug of choice was that research indicated that it still produced hypnotic effects after four weeks of daily use. Dalmane, however, has an active metabolite with a long half-life (well over a day; see Table 9.2). With nightly use there is a buildup of this metabolite in the body. Perhaps the reason Dalmane still works after four weeks is that the total dose of metabolite plus Dalmane is quite large by that time. There is concern that this buildup of Dalmane plus its metabolite might impair the individual's performance during the daytime. Halcion has replaced Dalmane because it has a short half-life, it has no active metabolite, and it should not build up in the body. Most patients are instructed to avoid daily use, but in some cases of severe insomnia chronic use is indicated. Can the short-acting benzodiazepines work under chronic treatment conditions without tolerance or withdrawal symptoms (e.g., rebound insomnia)? There are conflicting reports, but one large study indicated that short-acting benzodiazepines could still be effective after three months of chronic use with no evidence of rebound insomnia on withdrawal.[7]

Although the number of prescriptions for hypnotics has declined considerably over the past 25 years, when a new drug is introduced it displaces some of the older ones and then new concerns are raised about the newer drug and its side effects. By the early 1990s, Halcion sales had reached $100 million per year in the United States and $250 million worldwide. However, concerns were raised about the safety of the drug, and Upjohn, the drug's manufacturer, was sued by a woman who claimed the drug made her so agitated and paranoid that she had killed her own mother. That case was settled out of court, but it brought attention to the drug and to other claims that it produced an unusual number of adverse psychiatric reactions in patients. Halcion has been banned in five countries because of these side effects, but it has survived two FDA reviews in the United States and remains on the market.[8] Although sales have no doubt been harmed by the adverse publicity, Halcion remains the most popular sleeping pill in the United States.

The newest benzodiazapine-like hypnotic on the U.S. market is zolpidem (Ambien). Although it binds only to one subtype of benzodiazepine receptor and has therefore been suggested to be a more specific hypnotic agent,[9] clinically it appears to be similar to Halcion, with rapid onset and short duration of action.

If you or someone you know has trouble sleeping, before resorting to the use of medication it would be wise to follow the suggestions given in the Targeting Prevention box. These tactics will probably help most people deal with their concerns about sleeplessness.

As Anticonvulsants

A thorough description of seizure disorders (the **epilepsies**) is beyond the scope of this book. However, you should know that both the barbiturates and the benzodiazepines are widely used for the control of epileptic seizures. They are effective in reasonably low doses and are often combined with other anticonvulsant drugs for even better effectiveness. There are some practical problems associated with this use, and by now you could guess what some of them are.

Anticonvulsant medications are given chronically, so there is a tendency for tolerance to develop. The dose should be kept high enough to control the seizures without producing undesirable drowsiness. Abrupt withdrawal of these drugs is likely to lead to seizures, so medication changes should be done carefully. In spite of these problems, the sedative drugs are currently a necessary and useful treatment for epilepsy.

CAUSES FOR CONCERN

Dependence Liability

Psychological Dependence

Most people who have used either barbiturates or benzodiazepines have not developed habitual use patterns. However, it was clear with the barbiturates that some individuals do become daily users of intoxicating amounts. Again, the short-acting barbiturates seemed to be the culprits. When Librium, the first benzodiazepine, was in its heyday, relatively little habitual use was reported. As Librium was displaced by the newer, more potent Valium, we saw increasing reports of habitual Valium use, perhaps because its onset, although slower than that of the short-acting barbiturates, is more rapid than that of Librium. Then Xanax, another rapid-acting

Targeting Prevention

Falling Asleep Without Pills

The following procedures are recommended ways of dealing with insomnia. If you occasionally have trouble sleeping, ask yourself which of these rules you typically follow, and which ones you often don't. Are there some of these procedures that you could adopt?

- Establish and maintain a regular bedtime and a regular arising time. Try to wake up and get out of bed at the appointed time, even if you had trouble sleeping the night before. Avoid excessive sleep during holidays and weekends.
- When you get into bed, turn off the lights and relax. Avoid reviewing in your mind the day's stresses and tomorrow's challenges.
- Exercise regularly. Follow an exercise routine, but avoid heavy exercise late in the evening.
- Prepare a comfortable sleep environment. Too warm a room disturbs sleep; too cold a room does not solidify sleep. Occasional loud noises can disturb sleep without fully awakening you. Steady background noise, such as a fan may be useful for masking a noisy environment.

- Watch what you eat and drink before bedtime. Hunger may disturb sleep, as may caffeine and alcohol. A light snack may promote sleep, but avoid heavy or spicy foods at bedtime.
- Avoid the use of tobacco.
- Do not lie awake in bed for long periods of time. If you cannot fall asleep within 30 minutes, get out of bed and do something relaxing before trying to fall asleep again. Repeat this as many times as necessary. The goal is to avoid developing a paired association between being in bed and restlessness.
- Do not nap during the day. A prolonged nap after a night of insomnia may disturb the next night's sleep.
- Avoid the chronic use of sleeping pills. Although sedative-hypnotics can be effective when used as part of a coordinated treatment plan for certain types of insomnia, chronic use is ineffective at best and can be detrimental to sound sleep.

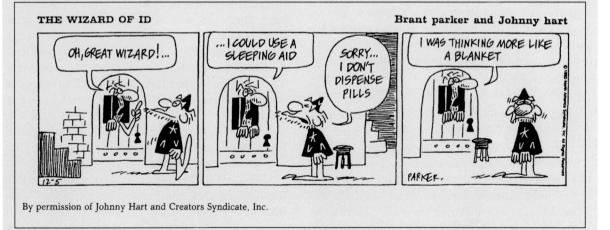

THE WIZARD OF ID — Brant parker and Johnny hart

By permission of Johnny Hart and Creators Syndicate, Inc.

epilepsies: disorders characterized by uncontrolled movements (seizures).

benzodiazepine, became the most widely pre-scribed sedative, and reports of Xanax depen-dence appeared.[10]

Animals given the opportunity to press a lever that delivers intravenous barbiturates will do so, and the short-acting barbiturates work best for this. Animals will also self-inject several of the benzodiazepines, but at lower rates than with the short-acting barbiturates.[11] When hu-man drug abusers were allowed an opportunity to work for oral doses of barbiturates or benzo-diazepines on a hospital ward, they developed regular patterns of working for the drugs. When given a choice between pentobarbital and di-azepam, the subjects generally chose pentobar-bital.[12] These experiments indicate that these sedative drugs can serve as reinforcers of be-havior but that the short-acting barbiturates are probably more likely to lead to dependence than are any of the benzodiazepines currently on the market.

Physical Dependence

A characteristic withdrawal syndrome can occur after chronic use of large enough doses of any of the sedative-hypnotic drugs. This syndrome is different from the narcotic withdrawal syndrome and quite similar to the alcohol withdrawal syn-drome. An early description of the withdrawal from barbiturates is an excellent example:

> Upon abrupt withdrawal of barbiturates from in-dividuals who have been ingesting 0.8 gm. or more daily of one of the shorter-acting barbitu-rates (secobarbital, pentobarbital, amobarbital), signs of barbiturate intoxication disappear in the first 8–12 hours of abstinence, and, clinically, the patient seems to improve. Thereafter, increasing anxiety, insomnia, tremulousness, weakness, dif-ficulty in making cardiovascular adjustments on standing, anorexia, nausea and vomiting appear. One or more convulsions of *grand mal* type usu-ally occur during the second or third day of ab-stinence. Following the seizures a psychosis characterized by confusion, disorientation in time

and place, agitation, tremulousness, insomnia, delusions and visual and auditory hallucinations may supervene. The psychosis clinically resem-bles alcoholic delirium tremens, usually begins and is worse at night, and terminates abruptly with a critical sleep.[13]

This syndrome is different in character from the narcotic withdrawal syndrome, longer last-ing, and probably more unpleasant. In addition, withdrawal from the sedative-hypnotics or alco-hol is potentially life-threatening, with death oc-curring in as many as 5 percent of those who withdraw abruptly after taking large doses.

There has been considerable controversy over the frequency, nature, and severity of withdrawal symptoms after chronic use of the benzodi-azepines. Animal experiments using large intra-venous doses show clearly that a barbiturate-like withdrawal syndrome can be produced with benzodiazepines, with an onset that varies with the half-life of the drug. With Librium and Val-ium, especially when used in low doses, clinical reports of withdrawal are rare. Although the use of short-half-life benzodiazepines began much later than the use of the long-half-life forms, there are a few studies indicating more rapid and more severe withdrawal after the shorter-half-life compounds, as would be expected.[14] The symptoms are rarely as severe as those seen with barbiturates and often consist of increased anxiety, irritability, or insomnia, which can be confused with a return to the predrug condi-tions of anxiety or insomnia for which the drug was initially prescribed.

Because there is a cross-dependence among the barbiturates, the benzodiazepines, and alco-hol, it is theoretically possible to use any of these drugs to halt the withdrawal symptoms from any other depressant. Drug treatment is often used, and a general rule is to use a long-acting drug, given in divided doses until the withdrawal symptoms are controlled. Typically, one of the benzodiazepines is used during detox-ification from any of the CNS depressants.[15]

Toxicity

The major areas of concern with these depressant drugs are the behavioral and physiological problems encountered when high doses of the drug are present in the body (acute toxicity). Behaviorally, all these drugs are capable of producing alcohol-like intoxication with impaired judgment and incoordination. Obviously, such an impaired state vastly multiplies the dangers involved in driving and other activities, and the effects of these drugs combined with alcohol are additive, so that the danger is further increased. On the physiological side, the major concern is the tendency of these drugs to depress the rate of respiration. With large enough doses, as in accidental or intentional overdose, breathing ceases entirely. Again, the combination of these depressants and alcohol is quite dangerous. Although diazepam is usually quite high on the list of drugs associated with deaths in the DAWN coroners' reports, in almost every case the culprit is diazepam in combination with alcohol or another drug, rather than diazepam alone.[16]

Patterns of Abuse

Almost all of the abuse of the sedative-hypnotic agents has historically involved the oral use of legally manufactured products. Two characteristic types of abusers have been associated with barbiturate use, and these two major types probably still characterize a large fraction of sedative abusers. The first type of abuser is an older adult who obtains the drug on a prescription, either for daytime sedative use or as a sleeping pill. Through repeated use, tolerance develops and the dose is increased. Even though some of these individuals visit several physicians to obtain prescriptions for enough pills to maintain this level of use, many would vehemently deny that they are "drug abusers." This type of chronic use can lead to physical dependence. The other major group tends to be younger and consists of people who obtain the drugs simply for the purpose of getting high. Sleeping pills might be taken from the home medicine cabinet, or the drugs might be purchased on the street. These younger abusers tend to take relatively large doses, to mix several drugs, or to drink alcohol with the drug, all for the purpose of becoming intoxicated. With this type of use, the possibility of acute toxicity is particularly high.

INHALANTS

It sometimes seems that some people will do almost anything to escape reality. Gasoline, glue, paint, lighter fluid, spray cans of almost anything, nail polish, and liquid paper all contain volatile solvents that, when inhaled, can have effects that are similar in an overall way to the depressants. High-dose exposure to these fumes makes users intoxicated, often slurring their speech and causing them to have trouble walking a straight line, as if they were drunk on alcohol.

Although most people think first of the abuse of volatile solvents such as glues, paints, and gasoline, other types of substances can be abused through sniffing or inhaling in a similar manner (Table 9.3). Two major groups are the gaseous anesthetics and the nitrites, as well as volatile solvents.

Gaseous Anesthetics

Gaseous anesthetics have been used in medicine and surgery for many years, and abuse of these anesthetics occurs among physicians and others with access to these gases. One of the oldest, nitrous oxide, was first used in the early 1800s and quite early acquired the popular name "laughing gas" because of the hilarity exhibited by some of its users. During the 1800s, there were traveling demonstrations of laughing gas, during which members of the audience would volunteer to become intoxicated for the amusement of others. Nitrous oxide is also one of the

safest anesthetics when used properly, but it is not possible to obtain good surgical anesthesia unless the individual breathes almost pure nitrous oxide, which leads to suffocation through a lack of oxygen. Nitrous oxide is still used for light anesthesia, especially by dentists. It is also often used in combination with one of the more effective inhaled anesthetics, allowing the use of a lower concentration of the primary anesthetic. Nitrous oxide is also found as a propellant in whipping-cream containers and is sold in small bottles ("whippets") for use in home whipping-cream dispensers. Recreational users have obtained nitrous oxide from both sources.

Nitrites

The chemicals amyl nitrite and butyl nitrite cause a rapid dilation of the arteries and reduce blood pressure to the brain, resulting in a brief period of faintness or even unconsciousness. These chemicals have an unpleasant odor and were sold under such suggestive brand names as "Locker Room" and "Aroma of Men." The male-sounding names might also reflect the popularity of these products among some homosexual males who used these "poppers" during sex to enhance the sense of lightheadedness at orgasm. Although many surveys have not separated nitrites from other inhalants, the high school survey began to do so in 1979. It appears that the popularity of the nitrites declined throughout the 1980s and 1990s. Since 1988, the Consumer Product Safety Commission has taken steps to remove these various nitrites from the market.

Volatile Solvents

The modern era of solvent abuse, or at least of widely publicized solvent abuse, can be traced to a 1959 investigative article in the Sunday supplement of a Denver, Colorado, newspaper. This article reported that young people in a nearby city had been caught spreading plastic model

TABLE 9-3

Some Chemicals Abused by Inhalation

Substances	Chemical ingredients
Volatile solvents	
Paint and paint thinners	Petroleum distillates, esters, acetone
Paint removers	Toluene, methylene chloride, methanol, acetone
Nail polish remover	Acetone, ethyl acetate
Correction fluid and thinner	Trichloroethylene, trichloroethane
Glues and cements	Toluene, ethyl acetate, hexane, methyl chloride, acetone, methyl ethyl ketone, methyl butyl ketone, trichloroethylane, tetrachloroethylene
Dry-cleaning agents	Tetrachloroethylene, trichloroethane
Spot removers	Xylene, petroleum distillates, chlorohydrocarbons
Aerosols, propellants, gases	
Spray paint	Butane, propane, toluene, hydrocarbons
Hair spray	Butane, propane
Lighters	Butane, isopropane
Fuel gas	Butane, propane
Whipped cream, "whippets"	Nitrous oxide
Anesthetics	
Current medical use	Nitrous oxide, halothane, enflurane
Former medical use	Ether, chloroform
Nitrites	
Locker room, Rush, poppers	Isoamyl, isobutyl, isopropyl nitrite, butyl nitrite

glue on their palms, cupping their hands over their mouths, and inhaling the vapors to get high. The article contained warning about the dangers of accidental exposure to solvent fumes, and an accompanying photograph showed a young man demonstrating another way to inhale glue vapors—by putting the glue on a handkerchief and holding it over the mouth and nose. The article described the effects as similar to being drunk.

That article both notified the police, who presumably began looking for such behavior, and advertised and described the practice to young people: within the next six months, the city of Denver went from no previously reported cases of "glue-sniffing" to 50 cases. More publicity and warnings followed, and by the end of 1961 the

juvenile authorities in Denver were seeing about "30 boys a month." The problem expanded further in Denver over the next several years, while similar patterns of publicity, increased use, and more publicity followed in other cities. In 1962, the magazines *Time* and *Newsweek* both carried articles describing how to sniff model glue and warning about its dangers, and the Hobby Industry Association of America produced a film for civic groups that warned about glue sniffing and recommended that communities make it illegal to sniff any substance with an intoxicating effect. Sales of model glue continued to rise as the publicity went nationwide.[17]

Since that time, it seems that recreational use of various solvents by young people has occurred mostly as more localized fads. One group of kids in one area might start using cooking sprays, the practice will grow and then decline over a couple of years, and meanwhile in another area the kids might be inhaling a specific brand and even color of spray paint.[18]

Although some "huffers" are adults (e.g., alcoholics without the funds to buy alcohol), most are young. The ready availability and low price of these solvents make them attractive to children. In the high school senior class of 2000, 18 percent of the students reported having used some type of inhalant at some time, whereas 12 percent of the eighth-graders reported using an inhalant within the past year.[19] Inhalant use has traditionally been more common among poor Hispanic youth and on Indian reservations.[20]

Because so many different solvents are involved, it is impossible to characterize the potential harm produced by abuse of glues, paints, correction fluids, and so on, except to say that several of the solvents have been linked to kidney damage, brain damage, and peripheral nerve damage,[21] and many of them produce irritation of the respiratory tract and result in severe headaches. However, several users of various inhalants have simply suffocated. Although most of the children who inhale solvents do so only occasionally and give it up as they grow older and have more access to alcohol, some become dependent and a few will die.

Laws to limit sales of these household solvents to minors or to make it illegal to use them to become intoxicated have been passed in some areas, but typically they have little effect. There are simply too many products too readily available. Look around your own home or on the shelves of a supermarket or discount store—how many products have a warning about using them in an enclosed place? That warning is used by some people to indicate an inhalant to try! This is one type of substance abuse that families and communities should attack with awareness, information, and direct social intervention.

SUMMARY

- The barbiturates, benzodiazepines, inhalants, and other depressant drugs all have many effects in common with each other and with alcohol.
- Depressants may be prescribed in low doses for their sedative effect or in higher doses as sleeping pills (hypnotics).
- Over the past 40 years the barbiturates have been mostly displaced by the benzodiazepines.
- The benzodiazepines are the most widely prescribed type of psychoactive drug.
- The barbiturates and benzodiazepines both increase the inhibitory neural effects of the neurotransmitter GABA.
- Drugs that have a rapid onset are more likely to produce psychological dependence.
- Drugs that have a short duration of action are more likely to produce withdrawal symptoms.
- Overdoses of these depressant drugs can cause death by inhibiting respiration, particularly if the drug is taken in combination with alcohol.
- The abused inhalants include gaseous anesthetics, certain nitrites, and volatile solvents.
- Abuse of inhalants, especially of the volatile solvents, can lead to organ damage, including neurological damage, more readily than with alcohol or other psychoactive substances.

REVIEW QUESTIONS

1. What was the foul-smelling drug that was so widely used in mental hospitals before the 1950s? *proraldahyde*
2. A prescription of 30 mg of phenobarbital would probably have been for which type of use? *seditave*

Web Watch

Activities Related to Depressants and Inhalant Use

Check Out Publications on Depressants
The National Clearinghouse for Drug and Alcohol Information offers a listing of publications about certain types of drugs. Go to the following sites to find and, if you wish, order brochures or other publications about depressants (www.health.org/catalog/catalog.asp?key=5&detail=false) and inhalants (www.health.org/catalog/catalog.asp?key=9&detail=false).

Know the Facts About Barbiturates
What are some examples of barbiturates? What are their common side effects? How can someone safely take a barbiturate for medicinal purposes? Check out the fact sheet at www.noah-health.org/english/illness/mentalhealth/cornell/medications/barbs.html for the answers to these questions and others.

Find Research Results on Inhalant Abuse
Because household products such as glue, lighter fluid, aerosol sprays, and cleaning products are widely available, they are easy to obtain and abuse. Read the research report about inhalant abuse at www.nida.nih.gov/ResearchReports/Inhalants/Inhalants.html. You'll discover basic information about inhalants, patterns of abuse, long-term effects, and special risks.

Learn More About Preventing Inhalant Abuse
At www.inhalants.org you'll find information and answers to frequently asked questions about inhalants. Read about the National Inhalant Prevention Coalition's prevention campaign and its latest survey on the use of inhalants. You'll also find contact information for the coalition and representatives in Washington, DC.

3. What is the relationship between psychological dependence and the time course of a drug's action? *You feel real good real Quick & that's super reinforcing.*

4. What was the first benzodiazepine?

5. What is the current legal and medical status of methaqualone? *Schedule 1   No Medical uses*

6. The barbiturates and benzodiazepines act at which neurotransmitter receptor? *Gappa fight*

7. Why should hypnotic drugs usually be prescribed only for a few nights at a time? *Quickly lose effect without increased dose*

8. What are the characteristics of the sedative-hypnotic withdrawal syndrome? *Jittery, vomit*

9. What happens to a person who takes an overdose of a sedative-hypnotic? *Heart stops, breathing stops & they die*

10. How are the effects of the nitrites different from the effects of inhaled solvent fumes?

REFERENCES

1. Richardson BW: Chloral and other narcotics, I, *Popular Science* 15:492, 1879.
2. Rosenblatt S, Dobson R: *Beyond Valium*. New York: G.P. Putnam's Sons, 1981.
3. Drug linked to assaults is reformulated, *The New York Times* pp Oct 19, 1997.
4. Feldman RS, Meyer JS, Quenzer LF: *Principles of neuropsychopharmacology*. Sunderland, MA: Sinauer, 1997.
5. Low K and others: Molecular and neuronal substrate for the selective attenuation of anxiety, *Science* 290:131–134, 2000.
6. Mellinger GD, Balter MB, Uhlenhuth EH: Insomnia and its treatment: Prevalence and correlates, *Archives of General Psychology* 42:225–232, 1985.
7. Allen RP and others: Efficacy without tolerance or rebound insomnia for midazolam and temazopam after use for one to three months, The *Journal of Clinical Pharmacologies* 27:768–775, 1988.
8. More Halcion headaches, *Newsweek* Mar 7, 1994.
9. Woods JH, Katz JL, Winger G: Abuse and therapeutic use of benzodiazepines and benzodiazepine-like drugs. In Bloom FE and Kupfer DJ, editors: *Psychopharmacology: The fourth generation of progress*. New York: Raven Press, 1995.
10. Longo LP, Johnson B: Addiction: Part I. Benzodiazepines—side effects, abuse risk and alternatives, *American Family Physician* 61:2121–2128, 2000.
11. Griffiths RR and others: Self-injection of barbiturates and benzodiazepines in baboons, *Psychopharmacology* 75:101–109,1981.
12. Griffiths RR, Bigelow G, Liebson I: Human drug self-administration: Double-blind comparison of pentobarbital, diazepam, chlorpromazine and placebo, The *Journal of Pharmacology and Experimental Therapeutics* 210:301–310, 1979.

13. Fraser HF and others: Death due to withdrawal of barbiturates, *American Journal of Internal Medicine* 38: 1319–1325, 1953.

14. Roy-Byrne PP, Hommer D: Benzodiazepine withdrawal: Overview and implications for the treatment of anxiety, *American Journal of Internal Medicine* 84:1041–1052, 1988.

15. Gitlin M: *The psychotherapist's guide psychopharmacology.* New York: Free Press, 1996.

16. *Preliminary estimates from the Drug Abuse Warning Network,* SAMHSA Advance Report Number 17, U.S. Department of Health and Human Services, August 1996.

17. Brecher EM: *Licit and illicit drugs.* Boston: Little, Brown, 1972.

18. Beauvais F: Volatile solvent abuse: Trends and patterns. In Sharp CW and others, editors: *Inhalant abuse: A volatile research agenda,* NIDA Research Monograph 129, NIH Publ No 93–3480, Washington, DC, 1992.

19. *2000 Monitoring the Future survey released.* News release from the National Institute on Drug Abuse, Dec 14, 2000.

20. Crider RA, Rouse BA: *Epidemiology of inhalant abuse: An update,* NIDA Research Monograph 85, DHHS Publ No (ADM) 88–1577, US Public Health Service, 1988.

21. Rosenberg N, Sharp CW: Solvent toxicity: A neurological focus. In Sharp CW and others, editors: *Inhalant abuse: A volatile research agenda,* NIDA Research Monograph 129, NIH Publ No 93–3480, Washington, DC, 1992.

Chapter 10

Psychotherapeutic Drugs

KEY TERMS

- anxiety disorders
- psychosis
- schizophrenia
- bipolar disorder
- depression
- phenothiazines
- neuroleptic
- antipsychotics
- monoamine oxidase (MAO) inhibitor
- tricyclic
- SSRIs
- lithium

Online Learning Center Resources

www.mhhe.com/ray

Log on to our Online Learning Center (OLC) for access to the following additional resources.

- Chapter definitions
- Learning objectives
- Student interactive question-and-answer sites
- Self-scoring chapter quiz

The OLC also offers web links for study and exploration of health topics. Here are some examples of what you'll find:

pharmacology.about.com/health/pharmacology/cs/nervous_system/index.htm

This website, especially designed as a reference guide for pharmacists, offers information about drugs for various psychological disorders. It also includes links and news about treatments.

www.noah-health.org/english/illness/mentalhealth/cornell/medications/betablock.html

This web page contains a fact sheet about beta blockers. It contains information about those commonly used in psychiatry—their uses, side effects, and safe administration.

www.mentalhealth.com/book/p42-sc3.html

Check out this website to find answers about treatment for schizophrenia. The site lists the medications used to treat the disorder, warnings, side effects, and other information. There are also booklets available to order.

Drugs in the Media

Mental Illness at the Movies

Although most of us know at least one person who is being treated with medication for depression or for ADHD (Chapter 8), the fact that these and most other mental disorders can be controlled to some degree with medication means

Drugs in the Media Continued. . .

that we do not experience firsthand many of the most troubling behavior problems that lead to a diagnosis of a serious mental disorder. Films and television programs have attempted to portray characters struggling with mental disorders, and some of these portrayals can be informative. In fact, a 1999 book, *Movies and Mental Illness*,[1] uses the viewing of popular films as an instructional aid to learning about abnormal psychology.

Can these films also teach us about how medications are used in treating those disorders? Yes, to some extent. Two of the best film depictions of mental institutions, for example, are *The Snake Pit* (1948), starring Olivia de Havilland, and *One Flew over the Cuckoo's Nest* (1975), starring Jack Nicholson. Both films are available in video stores and provide an interesting contrast. Although neither portrays the mental institution in a positive light, one is set in the period before antipsychotic and antidepressant medications were available, and the later film is set at a time when some of the early drugs of those types were widely used.

A more recent portrayal of mental illness by actor Jack Nicholson can be found in the 1998 film *As Good as It Gets*. Nicholson's character suffers from obsessive-compulsive disorder, and for most of the film he refuses to treat the problem with medication. Although the medication itself plays a minor role, it is shown to be an important part of his later improvement. In a series of episodes in 2000 on the NBC television program *ER*, Sally Field's character repeatedly fails to take her medication and demonstrates the social destructiveness of the manic episodes of bipolar disorder.

Next time you are discussing movies with your friends, see if you can come up with other examples of films or television programs that depict the use of psychoactive drugs in the treatment of mental disorders. Are the medications generally treated inappropriately as either cures or as a way to force conformity and compliance? Or are they treated more realistically as beneficial in some ways, yet with both limited effectiveness and unwanted side effects?

For most of today's mentally ill the primary mode of therapy is drug therapy. Powerful psychoactive medications help control psychotic behavior, depression, and mania in thousands of patients, reducing human suffering and health-care costs, yet these drugs are far from cures, and many have undesirable side effects. Should mental disorders be approached with chemical treatments? Do these treatments work? How do they work? What can these drugs tell us about the causes of mental illness? Although we don't yet have complete answers for any of these questions, we do have partial answers for all of them.

MENTAL ILLNESS

The Medical Model

The use of a term such as *mental illness* seems to some to imply a particular model for behavioral disorders or dysfunctions. The medical model has been attacked by both psychiatrists (who are medical doctors) and psychologists (who generally hold nonmedical doctorates such as a Ph.D. or Psy.D).

According to this model, the *patient* appears with a set of *symptoms,* and on the basis of these symptoms a *diagnosis* is made as to which *disease* the patient is suffering from. Once the disease is known, its *cause* can be determined and the patient provided with a *cure*. In general terms the arguments for and against a medical model of mental illness are similar to those for and against a medical model of addiction, presented in Chapter 3. For an infectious disease such as tuberculosis or syphilis, a set of symptoms suggests a particular disorder, but a specific diagnostic test for the presence of certain bacteria or antibodies is used to confirm the diagnosis, identify the cause, and clarify the treatment approach. We know in such cases that once the infection is cleared up, the disorder is cured.

For mental disorders a set of behavioral symptoms is about all we have to define and diagnose the disorder. A person might be inactive, not sleep or eat well, and not say much, and what little they do say might be quite negative. This behavior might lead us to call the person depressed. Does that mean that the person has a "disease" called depression, with a physical cause and a potential cure? Or is to call someone depressed really only to give a description of how he or she is acting, in the same way as we might call someone "crabby," "friendly," or "nerdy"? The behaviors that we refer to as indicating depression are varied and probably have many different causes, most of them not known. And we are far from being able to prescribe a cure for depression that will be generally successful in eliminating these symptoms.

In spite of these attacks on the medical model, it still seems to guide much of the current thinking about behavioral disorders. The fact that psychoactive drugs can be effective in controlling symptoms, if not in curing diseases, has lent a great deal of strength to supporters of the medical model. If chemicals can help normalize an individual's behavior, a natural assumption might be that the original problem resulted from a chemical imbalance in the brain—and that measurements of chemicals in urine, blood, or cerebrospinal fluid could provide more specific and accurate diagnoses and give direction to efforts at drug therapy.[2] This kind of thinking gives scientists great hope, and many experiments have attempted to find the searched-for chemical imbalances, so far with very little success.

Classification of Mental Disorders

Because human behavior is so variable and because we do not know the causes of most mental disorders, classification of the mentally ill into diagnostic categories is difficult. Nevertheless, there are some basic divisions that are widely used and important for understanding the uses of psychotherapeutic drugs. In 1994, the American Psychiatric Association published the fourth edition of its *Diagnostic and Statistical Manual of Mental Disorders* (referred to as the *DSM-IV*).[3] This manual provides criteria for classifying mental disorders into hundreds of specific diagnostic categories. Partly because this classification system has been adopted by major health insurance companies, its terms and definitions have become standard for all mental health professionals.

Anxiety is a normal and common human experience: anticipation of potential threats and dangers often helps us avoid them. However, when these worries become unrealistic, resulting in chronic uneasiness, fear of impending doom, or bouts of terror or panic, they can interfere with the individual's daily life. Physical symptoms may also be present, often associated with activation of the autonomic nervous system (e.g., flushed skin, dilated pupils, gastrointestinal problems, increased heart rate, or shortness of breath).

The term *neurosis* was traditionally used as a general term to refer to such problems as psychosomatic complaints, phobias, and obsessive-compulsive disorder. The *DSM-IV* doesn't use the term *neurosis* but refers to these and other problems as **anxiety disorders** (see the DSM-IV box).

DSM-IV — Anxiety Disorders

Panic Disorder (with or Without Agoraphobia)
Panic disorder is defined by recurrent, unexpected panic attacks and by subsequent concern about future attacks or about the meaning of the attacks. Panic attacks may include shortness of breath, dizziness or faintness, palpitations or accelerated heart rate, trembling, sweating, choking, numbness, fear of dying, or fear of going crazy or doing something uncontrolled.

The agoraphobia *(fear of the marketplace)* that often accompanies panic disorders is a fear of being in places or situations from which escape might be difficult or where help might not be available in the event of either a panic attack or some other incapacitating or embarrassing situation (e.g., fainting or losing bladder control). The person with agoraphobia might avoid going outside the home alone or be afraid of being in a public place or standing in a line.

Specific Phobia
Specific phobia is excessive or unreasonable fear of a specific object or situation (e.g., elevators, flying, heights, or some type of animal).

Social Phobia
Social phobia is a marked and persistent fear of social or performance situations (e.g., speaking in public, entering a room full of strangers, or using a public restroom).

Obsessive-Compulsive Disorder
Obsessions are recurrent and persistent thoughts, impulses, or images that are intrusive and inappropriate and that cause marked anxiety or distress. Compulsions are urgent, repetitive behaviors, such as handwashing, counting, or repeatedly "checking" to make sure that some dreaded event will not occur (e.g., checking that all doors and windows are locked, then checking again and again).

Posttraumatic Stress Disorder
The person has been exposed to an event that involved actual or threatened death or serious injury, and the person reacted with intense fear, helplessness, or horror. The traumatic event is persistently reexperienced through recollections, dreams, or a sudden feeling as if the event were occurring.

Generalized Anxiety Disorder
Generalized anxiety disorder is excessive anxiety and worry about a number of events or activities, such as school or work performance or finances, lasting for a period of six months or longer.

Perhaps because these disorders all seem to have some form of anxiety associated with them, and perhaps because psychiatrists often refer to the sedatives as *antianxiety drugs* (see Chapter 9), we all have a tendency to think of anxiety not as a behavioral symptom but rather as an internal state that *causes* the disorders. That view fits well with the medical model, but we should guard against easy acceptance of the view that these disorders are caused by anxiety and that therefore we can treat them using antianxiety drugs. For one thing, most "antianxiety" drugs have not been demonstrated to be very useful in the treatment of specific phobias, panic disorder, and obsessive-compulsive disorder.

Psychosis refers to a major disturbance of normal intellectual and social functioning in which there is loss of contact with reality. Not knowing the current date, hearing voices that aren't there, and believing that you are Napoleon or Christ are only some examples of this withdrawal from reality. Many people refer to psychosis as reflecting a primary disorder of *thinking,* as opposed to mood or emotion.

Psychotic behavior may be viewed as a group of symptoms that can have many possible causes. One important distinction is between the *organic* psychoses and the *functional* psychoses. An organic disorder is one that has a known physical cause, and psychosis can result

DSM-IV
Diagnosis of Schizophrenia

A. Characteristic symptoms: Two or more of the following:
  1. Delusions (irrational beliefs)
  2. Hallucinations (e.g., hearing voices)
  3. Disorganized speech (incoherent, frequent changes of topic)
  4. Grossly disorganized behavior (inappropriate, unpredictable) or catatonic (withdrawn, immobile)
  5. Negative symptoms (lack of emotional response, little or no speech, doesn't initiate activities)
B. Interference with social or occupational function
C. Duration of at least six months

from many such things, including brain tumors or infections, metabolic or endocrine disorders, degenerative neurological diseases, chronic alcohol use, and high doses of stimulant drugs, such as amphetamine or cocaine. Functional disorders are simply those for which there is no known or obvious physical cause. A person suffering from a chronic (long-lasting) psychotic condition for which there is no known cause will probably receive the diagnosis of **schizophrenia.** There is a popular misconception that schizophrenia means "split personality" or refers to individuals exhibiting multiple personalities. Instead, schizophrenia should probably be translated as *shattered mind.* See the DSM-IV box for the diagnostic criteria for schizophrenia.

Mood disorder refers to the appearance of depressed or manic symptoms. Look back at figure 8.3 on page 185 for one schematic representation of mood in which depression is shown as an abnormally low mood and mania as an abnormally high mood. The important distinction in *DSM-IV,* and in the drug treatment of mood disorders, is between **bipolar disorder,** in which both manic and depressive episodes have been observed at some time, and major **depression,** in

which only depressive episodes are reported. See the DSM-IV box "Diagnosis: Mood Disorders" for diagnostic criteria for manic episode and major depressive episode.

Keep in mind that individual human beings often don't fit neatly into one of these diagnostic categories, and in many cases assigning a diagnosis and selecting a treatment are as much a matter of experience and art as they are of applying scientific descriptions. For example, suppose a person displays both abnormal mood states and bizarre thinking. If it is assumed that the disturbance of thinking is the primary problem and that the person is elated or depressed because of a bizarre belief, then the individual may be diagnosed as schizophrenic. Another professional might see the mood disorder as primary, with the crazy talk supporting a negative view of the world, and give the individual a primary diagnosis of depression.

TREATMENT OF MENTAL DISORDERS

Before 1950

Over the centuries, mental patients have been subjected to various kinds of treatment, depending on the views held at the time regarding the causes of mental illness. Because we are

anxiety disorders: mental disorders characterized by excessive worry, fears, or avoidance.

psychosis: (sy co sis) a serious mental disorder involving loss of contact with reality.

schizophrenia: (skitz o *fren* ee yah) a type of chronic psychosis.

bipolar disorder: a type of mood disorder also known as manic-depressive disorder.

depression: a major type of mood disorder.

DSM-IV — Diagnosis of Mood Disorders

I. Manic Episode
   A. Abnormally and persistently elevated, expansive, or irritable mood
   B. At least three of the following:
      1. Inflated self-esteem or grandiosity
      2. Decreased need for sleep
      3. More talkative than usual or pressure to keep talking
      4. Flight of ideas or feeling that thoughts are racing
      5. Distractibility
      6. Increase in activity
      7. Excessive involvement in pleasurable activities that have a high potential for painful consequences (shopping, sex, foolish investments)
   C. Mood disturbance is sufficiently severe to cause marked impairment in functioning
II. Major Depressive Episode
   A. Five or more of the following, including either No. 1 or No. 2:

1. Depressed mood most of the day, nearly every day
2. Diminished interest or pleasure in most activities
3. Significant changes in body weight or appetite (increased or decreased)
4. Insomnia or hypersomnia nearly every day
5. Psychomotor agitation (increased activity) or retardation (decreased activity)
6. Fatigue or loss of energy
7. Feelings of worthlessness or excessive guilt
8. Diminished ability to think or concentrate
9. Recurrent thoughts of death or suicide, or a suicide attempt or plan for committing suicide
   B. The symptoms cause clinically significant distress or impairment.
   C. Not due to a drug or medical condition and not a normal reaction to the loss of a loved one

---

concerned with drug therapy, a good place to begin our history is in 1917, when a physical treatment was first demonstrated to be effective in serious mental disease. In those days a great proportion of the psychotic patients were suffering from *general paresis,* a syphilitic infection of the nervous system. It was noticed that the fever associated with malaria often produced marked improvement, and so in 1917 "malaria therapy" was introduced in the treatment of general paresis. Of course, the later discovery of antibiotics that could cure syphilis virtually eliminated this particular type of organic psychosis.

In the 1920s, some of the wealthier patients could afford to go in for a course of "narcosis therapy," in which barbiturates and other depressants were used to induce sleep for as long as a week or more. Another use for sedative drugs was in conjunction with psychotherapy: an intravenous dose of thiopental sodium, a rapid-acting barbiturate, would relax a person and produce more talking during psychotherapy. The theory was that such a reduction in inhibitions would enable the patient to express repressed thoughts; thus, the term *truth serum* came to be used for thiopental sodium and for scopolamine, an anticholinergic drug used similarly. Anyone who has ever listened to a person talking after drinking a good bit of alcohol will tell you that although the talk might be less inhibited, it isn't always more truthful. So-called truth serum apparently worked about as well.

In 1933, Manfred Sakel of Vienna induced comas in some schizophrenics by administering insulin. The resulting drop in blood glucose level caused the brain's neurons to first increase their activity and produce convulsions and then decrease their activity and leave the patient in a coma. A course of 30 to 50 of these treatments over a two- to three-month period was believed to be highly effective, and discharge rates of 90 percent were reported in the early years of insulin-shock therapy. Later studies demonstrated that the relapse rate was quite high, and this treatment was abandoned.

Ladislas von Meduna believed, incorrectly, that no epileptic was schizophrenic and no schizophrenic ever had epilepsy. Reasoning that epileptic convulsions prevented the development of schizophrenia, he felt that inducing convulsions might have therapeutic value for schizophrenic patients. His first convulsant drug was camphor, but it had the disadvantage of a lag time of several hours between injection and the convulsions. In 1934, he started using pentylenetetrazol (Metrazol), which induced convulsions in less than 30 seconds and reported improvement in 50 to 60 percent of patients.

The use of a drug was not ideal for inducing convulsions, because even a 30-second interval between injection and loss of consciousness (with the convulsion) produced much anguish in the patient. Ugo Cerletti, after experimenting on pigs in a slaughterhouse, developed the technique of using electric shock to induce convulsions. This method has the advantage of inducing loss of consciousness and convulsion at the moment the electric shock is applied. *Electroconvulsive therapy (ECT)* is hardly ever used now with schizophrenia. Although early work in the 1930s and 1940s suggested high improvement rates, later studies found a reduction of schizophrenic symptoms in only about half of the patients, and the relapse rates were quite high. However, ECT is still used with severely depressed patients who do not respond to medication.[4]

By the 1950s, probably the major drug in use for severely disturbed patients in the large mental hospitals was paraldehyde, a sedative, introduced in Chapter 8. Although it produces little respiratory depression and therefore is safer than the barbiturates, the drug has a characteristic odor, which is still well remembered by those who worked in or visited the hospitals of that era. Sedation of severely disturbed patients

by drugs that make them drowsy and slow them down has been referred to as the use of a "chemical straitjacket."

Antipsychotics

A number of people were involved in the discovery that a group of drugs called the **phenothiazines** had special properties when used with mental patients. Credit is usually given to a French surgeon, Henri Laborit, who first tested these compounds in conjunction with surgical anesthesia. He noted that the most effective of the phenothiazines, chlorpromazine, did not by itself induce drowsiness or a loss of consciousness, but it seemed to make the patients unconcerned about their upcoming surgery. He reasoned that this effect might reduce emotionality in psychiatric patients and encouraged his psychiatric colleagues to test the drug. The first report of these French trials of chlorpromazine in mental patients mentioned that not only were the patients calmed, but the drug seemed to act on the psychotic process itself. This new type of drug action attracted a variety of names: in the United States the drugs were generally called tranquilizers, which some now think is an unfortunate term that focuses on the calming action and seems to imply sedation. Another term used was **neuroleptic,** meaning "taking hold of the nervous system," a term implying an increased amount of control. Although both of these terms are still in wide use, most medical texts now refer to this group of drugs as **antipsychotics,**

---

phenothiazines: (feen o *thigh* uh zeens) a group of drugs used to treat psychosis.

neuroleptic: (noor o *lep* tick) a general term for antipsychotic drugs.

antipsychotics: a group of drugs used to treat psychosis; same as neuroleptic.

reflecting their ability to reduce psychotic symptoms without necessarily producing drowsiness and sedation.

One of the early reports (1955) dealing with the side effects of chlorpromazine on a large number of hospitalized psychotic patients stated:

> It produces marked quieting of the motor manifestations. Patients cease to be loud and profane, the tendency to hyperbolic associations diminished, and the patients can sit still long enough to eat and take care of normal physiological needs . . . .
>
> In the more chronic psychotic states, the effect of the drug is much less immediately dramatic, but for those experienced with the relief of psychotic symptoms from other measures, the use of the drug produces results that are equally gratifying when compared with results in the more acute situations.[5]

The tremendous impact of phenothiazine treatment on the management of hospitalized psychotics is clear from a 1955 statement by the director of the Delaware State Hospital:

> We have now achieved . . . the reorganization of the management of disturbed patients. With rare exceptions, all restraints have been discontinued. The hydrotherapy department, formerly active on all admission services and routinely used on wards with disturbed patients, has ceased to be in operation. Maintenance EST (electroshock treatment) for disturbed patients has been discontinued . . . There has been a record increase in participation by these patients in social and occupational activities.
>
> These developments have vast sociological implications. I believe it is fair to state that pharmacology promises to accomplish what other measures have failed to bring about—the social emancipation of the mental hospital.[6]

Treatment Effects and Considerations

Along with an increase in the use of phenothiazines in the treatment of the mentally ill came an increase in the sophistication of experimental programs that evaluate the effectiveness of various drugs. Results of these studies show clearly that phenothiazine-treated patients improve more than patients receiving placebo or no treatments. In an NIMH study, after six weeks 75 percent of acute schizophrenics receiving phenothiazines showed either moderate or marked improvement, whereas of those receiving placebos, only 23 percent improved. Over the years many more studies have demonstrated consistently that, although phenothiazines are far from a complete cure for every patient, they are significantly better than placebo treatments in reducing psychotic behaviors. The issue of what to call this new type of drug arose early on:

> The inappropriateness of the term "tranquilizer" is evident when the pattern of response produced by antipsychotic drugs is examined. They certainly do more than simply calm patients or put them in a "chemical straitjacket." The core symptoms of schizophrenia are consistently improved: emotional withdrawal, hallucinations, delusions and other disturbed thinking, paranoid projection, belligerence, hostility and blunted affect. On the other hand, somatic complaints, anxiety and tension, symptoms which might ordinarily be favorably affected by a "tranquilizer," are not much changed.[7]

Another aspect of evaluating the effectiveness of drug treatment is determining the incidence of relapse, or symptom recurrence, when treatment is discontinued. It is most likely that discontinuation of drug therapy will lead to relapse in 75 to 95 percent of patients within a year and in more than 50 percent of patients in six months. Almost all studies report that when medication is resumed, there is again a reduction in symptoms.[8]

In the years since 1950, many new phenothiazines have been introduced and several completely new types of antipsychotic drugs have been discovered. The ones on the U.S. market are listed in Table 10.1.[9] These drugs vary considerably in how much sedation accompanies

TABLE 10-1

Antipsychotic Drugs

Generic name	Brand name	Usual dose range (mg/day)
Phenothiazines		
Chlorpromazine	Thorazine	100–2,000
Thioridazine	Mellaril	100–600
Mesoridazine	Serentil	100–400
Trifluoperazine	Stelazine	5–60
Fluphenazine	Permitil, Prolixin	5–60
Perphenazine	Trilafon	8–64
Prochlorperazine	Compazine	10–150
Other chemical classes		
Clozapine	Clozaril	100–900
Haloperidol	Haldol	2–100
Loxapine	Loxitane	30–250
Molindone	Moban	10–225
Olanzepine	Zyprex	5–20
Risperidone	Risperdal	4–16
Thiothixene	Navane	5–60

their antipsychotic effect, and physicians tend to select from among the drugs depending partly on how much sedation they feel is called for. For example, two commonly used antipsychotics are thioridazine (Mellaril), one of the most sedating, and haloperidol (Haldol), one of the least sedating. The drug clozapine (Clozaril) deserves special comment, because it is useful in treating patients who do not respond to other antipsychotics, but it carries a big risk of dangerous side effects. In 1994, another type of antipsychotic drug was introduced. Whereas all previous antipsychotics had acted to reduce the so-called *positive symptoms* of schizophrenia (hallucinations, delusions, "crazy" behavior), the drug risperidone (Risperdal) was reported not only to cause fewer side effects but also to improve the *negative symptoms* such as social isolation and lack of emotional responsiveness.[10] Risperidone was joined in 1996 by another "atypical" antipsychotic, olanzepine (Zyprex).

Mechanism of Antipsychotic Action

For several years it was difficult to know which of the many biochemical effects of these drugs was responsible for their antipsychotic action. The phenothiazines tend to block the receptors for norepinephrine, dopamine, acetylcholine, serotonin, and histamine. The antipsychotic drugs vary widely in how much drug it takes to produce a clinical response (clinical potency) and in biochemical affinity for these various receptors, so it was possible to demonstrate a strong correlation between dopamine-receptor binding and clinical potency. It is therefore now accepted that the primary antipsychotic effect is probably a result of the blockade of dopamine receptors. However, atypical antipsychotics risperidone and olanzepine also block a subtype of serotonin receptor (the 5-HT_2 receptor), which might help account for their slightly different profile of effects.[4]

Side Effects of Antipsychotics

Two positive aspects of the antipsychotics are that they are not addictive and it is extremely difficult to use them to commit suicide. Some allergic reactions might be noted, such as jaundice or skin rashes. Some patients exhibit photosensitivity, a tendency for the skin to darken and burn easily in sunlight. These reactions have a low incidence and usually decrease or disappear with a reduction in dosage. *Agranulocytosis,* low white blood cell count of unknown origin, can develop in the early stages of treatment. Because white blood cells are needed to fight infection, this disorder has a high mortality rate if it is not detected before a serious infection sets in. It is extremely rare with most of the antipsychotics other than clozapine.

The most common side effect of antipsychotic medication involves the nigrostrial dopamine pathway (see Chapter 6). The major effects include a wide range of movement disorders from facial tics to symptoms that resemble those of Parkinson's disease (tremors of the hands when they are at rest; muscular rigidity, including a masklike face; and a shuffling walk). You might remember that Parkinson's disease results from damage to the dopamine neurons in the basal ganglia and that it is now treated with a dopamine precursor, L-dopa. The antipsychotic-drug-induced pseudoparkinsonism is a result of the blockade of dopamine receptors in the basal ganglia. L-dopa is not used to treat these symptoms because it has a tendency to worsen psychotic symptoms. However, before the introduction of L-dopa, Parkinson's disease was treated with anticholinergic drugs, which block receptors in the output pathways from the basal ganglia. These anticholinergic anti-Parkinson drugs are used to control the movement disorders produced by the antipsychotic medications.

The antipsychotic medications vary considerably in their tendency to produce movement disorders, but for most of the drugs this is due to the variance in the amount of anticholinergic activity that the drugs themselves possess. For example, thioridazine, which produces very few movement disorders, is about seven times as potent an anticholinergic as chlorpromazine (Thorazine), which is about nine times as anticholinergic as trifluoperazine (Stelazine), which produces many movement disorders. Haloperidol is almost purely a dopamine antagonist with little anticholinergic activity: it, too, produces a high incidence of movement disorders. Although some physicians prefer to use antipsychotic drugs that produce fewer movement disorders, others prefer to treat the psychotic symptoms with a purer dopamine antagonist and to treat the movement disorders separately as necessary with an anticholinergic, such as benztropine (Cogentin).[11] Clozapine and risperidone might diminish movement disorders through a different mechanism, by blocking serotonin receptors.

Tardive dyskinesia is the most serious complication of antipsychotic drug treatment. Although first observed in the late 1950s, it was not viewed as a major problem until the mid-1970s, 20 years after these drugs were introduced. The term *tardive dyskinesia* means "late-appearing abnormal movements" and refers primarily to rhythmic, repetitive sucking and smacking movements of the lips; thrusting of the tongue in and out ("fly-catching"); and movements of the arms, toes, or fingers. The fact that this syndrome usually occurs only after years of antipsychotic drug treatment, and that the symptoms persist and sometimes increase when medication is stopped, raised the possibility of irreversible changes. The current belief is that tardive dyskinesia is the result of supersensitivity of the dopaminergic receptors. Although reversal of the symptoms is possible in most cases, the best treatment is prevention, which can be accomplished through early detection and an immediate lowering of the level of medication.

A meta-analysis of several large trials of long-term antipsychotic drug treatment using more than 1,600 patients found that pseudoparkinsonism was reported as an adverse reaction in about 20 percent of the patients, whereas tardive dyskinesia was reported for only about 2 percent. Echoing a general principle mentioned in Chapter 1, patients maintained on high doses did not show more improvement than patients on lower doses, but the high-dose patients had more adverse side effects.[12]

Antidepressants

Monoamine Oxidase Inhibitors

The story of the antidepressant drugs starts with the fact that tuberculosis was a major chronic illness until about 1955. In 1952, preliminary reports suggested that a new drug, isoniazid, was effective in treating tuberculosis; isoniazid and similar drugs that followed were responsible for the emptying of hospital beds. One of the anti-tuberculosis drugs was iproniazid, which was introduced simultaneously with isoniazid but was withdrawn as too toxic. Clinical reports on its use in tuberculosis hospitals emphasized that there was considerable elevation of mood in the patients receiving iproniazid. These reports

TABLE 10-2		
Antidepressant Drugs		
Generic name	Brand name	Usual dose range (mg/day)
MAO inhibitors		
Phenelzine	Nardil	45–75
Tranylcypromine	Parnate	20–30
Tricyclics		
Amitriptyline	Elavil, Endep	100–200
Amoxapine	Asendin	200–300
Desipramine	Norpramin	75–200
Doxepin	Sinequan, Adapin	100–200
Imipramine	Tofranil	100–200
Nortriptyline	Pamelor	75–150
Protriptyline	Vivactil	15–40
SSRIs		
Fluoxetine	Prozac	20–40
Paroxetine	Paxil	20–50
Sertraline	Zoloft	50–200
Venlafaxine	Effexor	75–375
Others		
Bupropion	Wellbutrin	200–300
Mirtazapine	Remeron	15–45
Nefazodone	Serzone	200–600
Trazodone	Desyrel	150–200

were followed up, and the drug was reintroduced as an antidepressant agent in 1955 on the basis of early promising studies with depressed patients.

Iproniazid is a **monoamine oxidase (MAO) inhibitor,** and its discovery opened up a new class of compounds for investigation. Although several MAO inhibitors have been introduced over the years, toxicity and side effects have limited their use and have reduced their number. Iproniazid itself was removed from sale in 1961 after being implicated in at least 54 fatalities. Currently there are two MAO inhibitors on the U.S. market (Table 10.2). A major limitation of the use of the MAO inhibitors is that they alter the normal metabolism of a dietary amino acid,

tyramine, such that if an individual consumes foods with a high tyramine content while taking MAO inhibitors, a hypertensive (high blood pressure) crisis can result. Because aged cheeses are one source of tyramine, this is often referred to as the "cheese reaction." A severe headache, palpitations, flushing of the skin, nausea, and vomiting are some symptoms of this reaction, which has in some cases ended in death from a stroke (cerebrovascular accident). Besides avoiding foods and beverages that contain tyramine (besides aged cheeses, chianti wine, smoked or pickled fish, and many others), patients taking MAO inhibitors must also avoid sympathomimetic drugs, such as amphetamines, methylphenidate, and phenylpropanolamine (PPA), an ingredient in OTC weight-control products.

MAO is an enzyme involved in the breakdown of serotonin, norepinephrine, and dopamine, and its inhibition results in increased availability of these neurotransmitters at the synapse. This was the first clue to the possible mechanism of antidepressant action.

Tricyclic Antidepressants

Sometimes when you are looking for one thing, you find something entirely different. The MAO inhibitors were found among antituberculosis agents, and the phenothiazine antipsychotics were found while looking for a better antihistamine. The **tricyclic** antidepressants were found in a search for better phenothiazine antipsychotics. The basic phenothiazine structure consists of three rings, with various side chains for the different antipsychotic drugs. Imipramine resulted from a slight change in the middle of the three rings and was tested in 1958 on a

monoamine oxidase (MAO) inhibitor: a type of antidepressant drug.

tricyclic: (try *sike* lick) a type of antidepressant drug.

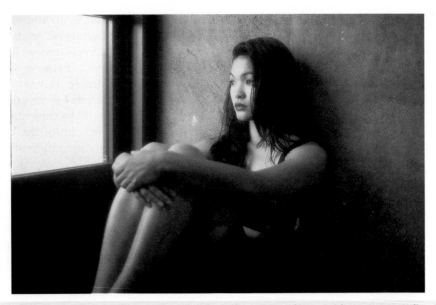

Depression is a serious, debilitating disorder that often responds to antidepressant medication.

group of patients. The drug had little effect on psychotic symptoms but improved the mood of depressed patients. This was the first tricyclic antidepressant, and many more have followed (Table 10.2). Although these drugs are not effective in all patients, most controlled clinical trials do find that depressive episodes are less severe and resolve more quickly if the patients are treated with one of the tricyclic antidepressants than if they are given a placebo.

The first tricyclics were discovered to interfere with the reuptake into the terminal of the neurotransmitters norepinephrine, dopamine, and serotonin. This results in an increased availability of these neurotransmitters at the synapse. Because MAO inhibition also results in increased availability of the same neurotransmitters, there has been considerable speculation that the antidepressant actions of both classes of drugs result from increased synaptic availability of one or more of these neurotransmitters. One of the effective antidepressants, desipramine, was found to have a much greater effect on the

reuptake of norepinephrine than on the reuptake of either dopamine or serotonin, so for a time most theories of antidepressant action focused on norepinephrine.

Selective Serotonin Reuptake Inhibitors

The introduction in 1987 of fluoxetine (Prozac) ushered in the era of the *selective serotonin reuptake inhibitors* (**SSRIs**). Trazodone had already been available and was known to have a greater effect on serotonin than on norepinephrine reuptake, calling the norepinephrine theory into question. Fluoxetine was followed to market by sertraline (Zoloft), paroxetine (Paxil), and venlafaxine (Effexor), and all of these have highly selective effects on serotonin reuptake. These four drugs constitute the category of SSRIs. The most successful of these is Prozac, which rapidly became the most widely prescribed antidepressant drug ever marketed. Prozac is safer than the tricyclic antidepressants in that it is less likely to lead to overdose deaths, so physicians feel more confident about prescribing it. In spite

Taking Sides

Prozac for Everyone?

When Prozac (fluoxetine) was introduced in 1987 as a new, safer antidepressant, no one expected it to become as successful as it did as quickly as it did. People took it, liked it, and told their friends about it, and more people took it. It quickly became the nation's most popular antidepressant drug ever. But few have been as outspoken in favor of the wide-spread use of Prozac as psychologist Jim Goodwin of Wenatchee, Washington. According to a 1994 story by Associated Press writer Aviva Brandt, Goodwin has been called the "Pied Piper of Prozac."

Citing the safety and effectiveness of the drug and its limited side effects, Goodwin, who has taken the drug himself since 1989, has recommended it to virtually all the 700 clients he has seen. Because as a psychologist he couldn't prescribe it himself, he admitted that he was "rather aggressive" in suggesting to people that they obtain a prescription from their family physician. Although Prozac and other antidepressant drugs have been approved for the treatment of major depressive disorder, Goodwin believes that most people suffer from mild depression and can benefit from using the drug. He was quoted as saying, "All of us could probably use a little bit of help with our depressions."

Goodwin's fame and his approach to treating mild depression have generated a storm of criticism from psychiatrists and other psychologists. After all, do most people really need some sort of pill to deal with the trials and tribulations of daily life?

For more on this topic, log on to *www.dushkin.com/online* for current news and links to other popular and informative sites, as well as time-saving web search strategies and study tools.

of reports in the early 1990s of unusual violent or suicidal reactions, which may have reduced sales temporarily, in 2000 Prozac remained the world's leading antidepressant. One factor in its popularity might be that, whereas the tricyclics often lead to weight gain, Prozac use is more often accompanied by weight loss.

Mechanism of Antidepressant Action

It now seems clear that antidepressants work by increasing the availability of either norepinephrine or serotonin at their respective synapses. However, the antidepressant effect of MAO inhibitors, tricyclics, and SSRIs exhibits a "lag period": the patients must be treated for about two weeks before improvement is seen, even though the biochemical effects on MAO or on reuptake occur in a matter of minutes. Although it has been suggested that some patients might benefit more from one type than from another, experiments have so far failed to reveal any rational basis for choosing among the drugs in any individual case, and overall the effectiveness of the drug does not seem to depend on which of the neurotransmitters is more affected.

Current theories of the antidepressant action of these agents focus less on the direct biochemical effects of the drugs than on the reaction of the neurons to those direct effects. For example, after prolonged exposure to all of the antidepressants, there is a decreased number of receptors for both norepinephrine and serotonin, as well as other changes.[13] It might be these long-term adjustments of the brain tissue that result in the antidepressant action.

Well over half of the prescriptions written for antidepressants are written by nonpsychiatrists (family physicians, general practitioners, or internists). In the past, these practitioners frequently prescribed too little for too short a time

---

SSRI: selective serotonin reuptake inhibitors, a type of antidepressant drug.

to decrease the depression. It is understandable, though, because the tricyclics can cause severe side effects: about 1 user in 20 will have disorientation, hallucinations, or other anticholinergic effects. Large doses of the tricyclics can be lethal, so quantities prescribed to suicidal patients need to be restricted. The relative safety of fluoxetine (Prozac) is one major reason for its wide acceptance and prescription, again more often than not written by nonpsychiatrists.

There has been some excitement among those working in laboratories and hospitals about a diagnostic laboratory test for primary unipolar depression: the dexamethasone suppression test (DST). The details need not concern us here, but you should know that the test is only about 40 to 60 percent accurate in identifying patients who are primary unipolar depressives. However, it eliminates about 90 percent of those who are not; that is, it produces few false positive results, but it does produce false negative results. With such a large proportion of depressed people showing a negative (normal) response to this test, one question is whether those who do respond abnormally are either more or less likely to improve when treated with medication. Several studies have found only very slight and inconsistent differences in treatment success between normal and abnormal responders to the dexamethasone test.[14] It appears that this test is of little value in the diagnosis or management of individual patients.

Probably the single most effective treatment for the depressed patient is electroconvulsive shock therapy (ECT). One report summarized the available good studies and showed that in seven of eight studies ECT was more effective in relieving the symptoms of depression than was placebo. Further, in four studies ECT was more effective than the most effective class of antidepressant drugs, and in three other studies the two treatments were equal. One factor that makes ECT sometimes the clear treatment of choice is its more rapid effect than that found with current antidepressant drugs. Reversal of depression might not occur for two or three weeks with drug treatment, but with ECT results sometimes are noticed almost immediately. When there is a possibility of suicide, ECT is thus the obvious choice, and it is possible to use both drug and ECT treatment simultaneously.[4]

Lithium

In the late 1940s, two medical uses were proposed for salts of the element **lithium.** In the United States, lithium chloride, which tastes much like sodium chloride (table salt), was introduced as a salt substitute for heart patients. However, above a certain level lithium is quite toxic, and because there was no control over the dose, many users became ill and several died. This scandal was so great in the minds of American physicians that a proposed beneficial use published in 1949 by an Australian, John Cade, produced little interest in this country.

Cade had been experimenting with guinea pigs, examining the effects of lithium on urinary excretion of salts. Lithium appeared to have sedative properties in some of the animals, so he administered the compound to several disturbed patients. The manic patients all improved, whereas there seemed to be no effect on depressed or schizophrenic patients. This was followed up by several Danish studies in the 1950s and early 1960s, and it became increasingly apparent that the large majority of manic individuals showed dramatic remission of their symptoms after a lag period of a few days when treated with lithium carbonate or other salts.

Three factors slowed the acceptance of lithium in the United States. First, of course, was the salt-substitute poisonings, which gave lithium a bad reputation as a potentially lethal drug. Second, mania was not seen as a major problem in the United States. Remember that manic patients feel energetic and have an unrealistically positive view of their own abilities, and such people are unlikely to seek treatment on their own. Also, patients who became quite

Track Your Daily Mood Changes

Some days are better than others—we all experience that. Try using this psychological "instrument" to measure how your outlook on life changes on a day-to-day basis. Decide on a particular time to mark the scales and try to do them at the same time each day, because your mood also varies with time of day.

Mark a spot on each vertical scale that corresponds to how you're feeling at the moment.

After you've finished the week, look back and see if you can relate the highs and lows to particular events or activities that happened at that time. Do all your scores tend to vary together, or are some areas unrelated to others?

1. How optimistic do you feel about accomplishing something useful or meaningful in the next 24 hours?

	Day 1	Day 2	Day 3	Day 4	Day 5	Day 6	Day 7
Quite certain I will							
Probably will							
Not sure							
Probably won't							
Quite certain I won't							

2. How energetic do you feel at the moment?

	Day 1	Day 2	Day 3	Day 4	Day 5	Day 6	Day 7
Have lots of energy							
Fairly energetic							
About average							
Not much energy							
Almost no energy							

3. How happy or sad are you today?

	Day 1	Day 2	Day 3	Day 4	Day 5	Day 6	Day 7
Very happy							
Happy							
Neither happy nor sad							
Sad							
Very sad							

4. How mentally sharp do you feel today (ability to remember things, ability to think)?

	Day 1	Day 2	Day 3	Day 4	Day 5	Day 6	Day 7
Quite sharp							
Pretty sharp							
Average							
A bit dull							
Very dull and slow							

5. How satisfied are you with yourself today?

	Day 1	Day 2	Day 3	Day 4	Day 5	Day 6	Day 7
Quite satisfied							
Fairly satisfied							
Not sure							
Fairly dissatisfied							
Quite dissatisfied							

Exploring Your Spirituality

Solitude: Therapy for the Soul

Have you taken a moment today to be quiet and just be with yourself? The human mind is such a complex collection of information and feelings that our awareness of what lies within ourselves is often limited, especially during times of great stress or illness. Time alone can help you move away from a busy, fragmented world and draw inward for renewal. It is a time to reflect and to gain new and deeper insights. It can help you break out of negative thought patterns and avoid generalizing difficulties from one area into another. And a strengthened awareness of yourself in both mind and body allows you to experience the fullness of the moment, even feel in sync with the universe.

Solitude can also help you establish your identity, clarify what's important to you, and strengthen your independence. Because most of our hours are spent living with, caring for, or responding to others, it is only when we are alone that we have the opportunity to fully emerge and become ourselves.

Any time you take to pursue this inner awakening will be restorative. You might begin with just five minutes each morning. You will need a place you feel comfortable alone with your thoughts, whether at the kitchen table, in bed, in the shower, at a coffee shop, in the library, or in the garden. Go for a walk, listen to music, weed the garden, write a letter to a friend, paint, read a poem, or just be still and concentrate on your breathing. All of these are solitary actions that, in the end, reconnect you to a life force and to others. Pretty soon you may feel that your time of solitude is more productive than sleep! When you are faced with a difficult project, a household disaster, or something more serious, such as sickness or a loved one's death, these meditative moments will leave you mentally and spiritually equipped to deal with any event.

It's not selfish to carve out whatever time you need alone to refresh yourself. A nourished spirit gives you the grace to be more tolerant of yourself and others. Through your appreciation of a deep, rich inner reality, you will feel rapture in the mystery and gift of just being alive.

---

manic and lost touch with reality would probably have been called schizophrenic in those days, perhaps at least partly because a treatment existed for schizophrenia. In fact, the antipsychotic drugs can control mania in most cases. The third and possibly most important factor is economic and relates to the way new drugs are introduced in the United States: by companies that hope to make a profit on them. Lithium is one of the basic chemical elements (number 3 on the periodic chart) and its simple salts had been available for various purposes for many years, so it would be impossible for a drug company to receive an exclusive patent to sell lithium. A company generally must go to considerable expense to conduct the research necessary to demonstrate safety and effectiveness to the FDA. If one company had done this, as soon as the drug was approved any other company could also have sold lithium, and it would have been impossible for the first company to recoup its research investment. After several years of frustration, the weight of the academically conducted research and the clinical experience in Europe was such that several companies received approval to sell lithium in 1970.

Treatment with lithium requires 10 to 15 days before symptoms begin to change. Lithium is both safe and toxic. It is safe because the blood level can be monitored routinely and the dose adjusted to ensure therapeutic, but not excessive, blood levels. Patients develop tolerances to the minor side effects of gastrointestinal disturbances and tremors. Excessively high blood levels cause confusion and loss of coordination,

lithium: (*lith* ee um) a drug used in treating mania and bipolar disorder.

TABLE 10-3

Drug Treatment Two-Year Outcome in Unipolar and Bipolar Patients

	Percentage of patients with relapses during treatment	
	First 4 months	Next 20 months
Unipolar subjects		
Lithium	30	41
Imipramine	32	29
Placebo	73	85
Bipolar subjects		
Lithium	22	18
Imipramine	46	67
Placebo	54	67

unipolar a relapse means an episode of depression, whereas for bipolar patients relapse can mean either a depressed or a manic period.

The results were relatively clear: lithium was very effective in preventing relapses in bipolar subjects, whereas imipramine treatment showed no clinical improvement compared with a placebo. With unipolar subjects imipramine was superior to lithium, but both drugs were superior to placebo treatment. It is of interest to note one major difference between the unipolar and bipolar patients: 55 percent of the next-of-kin relatives of bipolar patients had some type of psychiatric illness, compared with only 28 percent of the unipolar patients. This suggests a stronger genetic component in bipolar mood disorders than in unipolar disorders.

which can progress to coma, convulsions, and death if lithium is not stopped and appropriate treatment instituted.

The clinical use and effectiveness of lithium have had some interesting effects in several areas. The mechanism of action is still not clear, but one biochemical effect is that lithium increases the synthesis of serotonin in the brain. Of primary importance in the therapeutic use of lithium is the realization that lithium acts as a mood-normalizing agent in individuals with bipolar (manic-depressive) illness. Lithium will prevent both manic and depressed mood swings. It has only moderate effects on unipolar depressions.

These very selective clinical effects of lithium have forced better diagnostic decisions and have given a new basis for belief that unipolar and bipolar mood disorders are not the same illness. This fact is most clearly seen in Table 10.3, which shows the treatment outcome of one study.[15] Lithium, a placebo, or imipramine (a tricyclic) was given to hospitalized patients, who were later discharged and observed for a prolonged period. For patients diagnosed as

CONSEQUENCES OF DRUG TREATMENTS FOR MENTAL ILLNESS

There is no question that the use of modern psychopharmaceuticals, which began in the mid-1950s in the United States, has affected the lives of millions of Americans who have been treated with them. But the availability of these effective medications has also brought about revolutionary changes in our society's treatment of and relationship with our mentally ill citizens. Figure 10.1 depicts what happened to the population of our large mental hospitals from 1946 to 1998.[16] These hospitals had grown larger and larger and held a total of over half a million people in the peak years of the early 1950s. The year in which chlorpromazine was first introduced in the United States, 1955, was the last year in which the population of these hospitals increased. Since then the average population has continued to decline. Remember that the antipsychotics do not cure schizophrenia or other forms of psychosis, but they can control the symptoms to a great degree, allowing the patients to leave the hospital, live at home, and often earn a living.

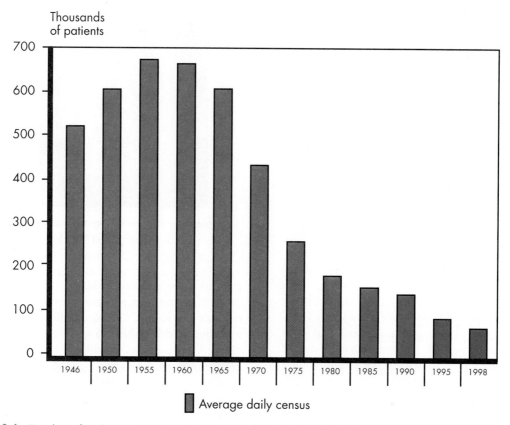

Thousands
of patients

Figure 10-1   Number of patients in nonfederal psychiatric hospitals, 1946–1998.

These drugs began the liberation of mental patients from hospitals, where many of them had previously stayed year after year, committed for an indefinite time.

The movement out of mental hospitals was accelerated in the 1960s with the establishment of federally supported community mental health centers. The idea was to treat mental patients closer to home in a more natural environment, at lesser expense, and on an outpatient basis. Needless to say, the opportunity for such a program to work was greatly enhanced by the availability of potent, effective psychopharmaceuticals, especially the antipsychotics.

The mental health professions have been greatly affected by these drugs. It is probably safe to say that the majority of psychiatrists in practice today spend less time doing psychotherapy than did their colleagues in the 1950s. In fact, for many psychiatrists the first issue is to establish an appropriate drug regimen, and only after the initial symptoms are controlled will they engage in much talk therapy. For some psychiatrists the prescription pad has completely replaced the couch as their primary tool. This may be sensible in terms of overall cost effectiveness, but it has certainly altered the doctor/patient relationship.

HeathQuest Activities

Psychotherapeutic drugs may be provided to patients with a doctor's prescription. In Module 9, look under *Key Articles* and read "Directions for Prescription Drug Use." This article offers information about the FDA's goals for prescription drug instructions. What important issues come to mind when you read this article? When you are taking prescription drugs, are you careful to follow the instructions on the label? Have you ever taken prescription drugs that were not prescribed to you? Did you ever experience any side effects as a result of taking prescription drugs intended for someone else or of not following directions carefully?

In the same module under *Specifics On,* read "Drug Interactions-Polydrug Abuse." Discuss the article with classmates. Do you think the information offered in the article is accurate? What experiences have you had with polydrug abuse? What might be a good way of educating your fellow students about the dangers of polydrug abuse?

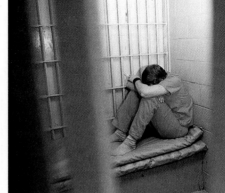

Prisons may hold more mentally ill persons than do state mental hospitals.

Concomitant with the liberation of patients from hospitals and their return to the communities came a concern with their civil rights. Indefinite commitment to a hospital had been declared unconstitutional, and all states have since developed procedures to protect the rights of individual patients. Hearings are required before a person can be committed for treatment against his or her will, and it is usually necessary to demonstrate a clear and present danger to the patient's own person or to others. Periodic reviews of the patient's status are called for, and if at any time the immediate danger is not present, the patient must be released. No one would want to argue that mental patients should not have these rights, but the availability of psychoactive medications helps create difficult situations. A patient who is dangerously psychotic might be admitted for treatment, and after a few weeks on an antipsychotic drug might be sufficiently in

control to be allowed to leave the hospital. However, if the patient remains suspicious or simply doesn't like to take the medication, he or she will eventually stop taking it and again become psychotic. Or patients might be released into the community, perhaps functioning with medication or perhaps not, too sick to really take care of themselves but not sick enough to present an immediate danger. Often, the eventual result is violation of a law, leading to imprisonment. According to an August 31, 2000, ABC news report, more mentally ill persons are jailed each year than are admitted to state mental hospitals. About one-third of all homeless people in the United States have some form of serious mental illness. The plight of our homeless, rootless, mentally ill citizens has been the subject of magazine and television reports, and efforts are being made to change the way these people are treated.

SUMMARY

- The medical model of mental illness has been widely criticized, yet psychotherapeutic drugs are often discussed in the context of this model.

- Diagnosis of mental disorders is difficult and controversial, but the *DSM-IV* provides a standard diagnostic approach for most purposes.
- The introduction of antipsychotics in the mid-1950s started a revolution in mental health care and increased interest in psychopharmacology.
- The antipsychotics are helpful for the majority of schizophrenics, but they often produce movement disorders, some of which resemble Parkinson's disease.
- The major groups of antidepressant drugs are the MAO inhibitors, the tricyclics, and the SSRIs.
- Fluoxetine (Prozac) has quickly become the largest-selling antidepressant drug in history.
- Lithium is useful in treating mania and in preventing mood swings in bipolar disorder.
- The number of people occupying beds in mental hospitals has declined since 1955, largely because psychotherapeutic drugs allow people to be released after shorter stays.

REVIEW QUESTIONS

1. Give two examples of anxiety disorder.
2. Is schizophrenia a functional or an organic psychosis?
3. Besides sadness, what are some other indicators of a major depressive episode?
4. What type of drug is chlorpromazine, and where was it first tested on patients?
5. What is tardive dyskinesia, and how does it respond to a reduction in the dose of an antipsychotic drug?
6. Which type of drug was discovered while testing an antituberculosis agent?
7. How do the SSRIs differ from the older tricyclics in terms of their actions in the brain?
8. What were two of the three reasons it took so long for lithium to be available for use in the United States?

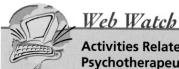

Web Watch

Activities Related to Psychotherapeutic Drugs

What Questions Should You Ask Your Doctor?
Go to www.aacap.org/publications/factsfam/medquest. htm. This site, which was developed by the American Academy of Child and Adolescent Psychiatry, provides a list of questions to ask about psychiatric medication. There is also contact information for other references.

The Side Effects of Psychiatric Medicines
There are many side effects that may afflict those taking psychiatric medications, particularly as they begin treatment. The site www.noah-health.org/english/illness/mentalhealth/cornell/medications/side_effects.html provides a reference guide to consumers who wish to find out more about managing common side effects. The guide lists and identifies temporary and long-term side effects and offers suggestions on how to manage them.

Do You Know the Facts About Antidepressants?
At www.noah-health.org/english/illness/mentalhealth/cornell/medications/antidepres.html, you will find a fact sheet about antidepressant medications. This includes facts about medication names, results, disorders, and symptoms that are treated by certain medicines, common side effects, and other information about safe use.

9. If clozapine is so dangerous, why is it prescribed at all?
10. Why is Prozac the most widely prescribed antidepressant drug ever?

REFERENCES

1. Wedding D, Boyd M: *Movies and mental illness.* New York: McGraw-Hill, 1999.
2. Feldman RS, Meyer JS, Quenzer LF: *Principles of neuropsychopharmacology.* Sunderland, MA: Sinauer, 1997.

3. American Psychiatric Association: *Diagnostic and statistical manual of mental disorders* (4th ed.). Washington, DC: Author.

4. Gitlin M: *The psychotherapist's guide to psychopharmacology.* New York: Free Press, 1996.

5. Goldman D: Treatment of psychotic states with chlorpromazine, *Journal of the American Medical Association* 157:1274–1278, 1955.

6. Freyhan FA: The immediate and long-range effects of chlorpromazine on the mental hospital. In Smith, Kline and French Laboratories: *Chlorpromazine and mental health.* Philadelphia: Lea & Febiger, 1955.

7. Veterans Administration: Drug treatment in psychiatry, Washington, DC: U.S. Government Printing Office, 1970.

8. Kessler KA, Waletzky JP: Clinical use of the antipsychotics, *American Journal of Psychiatry* 138:202, 1981.

9. *Physician's desk reference.* Oradell, NJ: Medical Economics, 1998.

10. Janssen launches new treatment for schizophrenia, *Drug Topics* Apr 11, 1994.

11. Poling A and others: *Drug therapy for behavior disorders.* New York: Pergamon Press, 1991.

12. Bollini P and others: Antipsychotic drugs: Is more worse? A meta-analysis of the published randomized control trials, *Psychological Medicine* 24:307, 1994.

13. Barondes SH: Molecules and mental illness. New York: W.H. Freeman, 1993.

14. Kathol RG, Carter JL: Use of HPA axis tests in patients with major depression. In *Pharmacotherapy of Depression.* Amsterdam JD, editor: New York: Marcel Dekker, 1990.

15. Pokorny AD, Prein RF: Lithium in treatment and prevention of affective disorder, *Diseases of the Nervous System* 35:327, 1974.

16. American Hospital Association: *Hospital statistics, 2000 edition,* Chicago: Author, 2000.

Section IV

Alcohol

Alcohol: social lubricant, adjunct to a fine meal, or demon rum? People today are no different from people throughout the centuries: many use alcohol, and many others condemn its use. This love-hate relationship with alcohol has been going on for a long time. The last two decades have brought a slight swing of the pendulum: health-conscious Americans are opting for low-alcohol or no-alcohol drinks, consumption of hard liquor is down, and we receive frequent reminders to use alcohol responsibly, not to drink and drive, and not to let our friends drive if they've been drinking. Let's take a closer look at the world's number one psychoactive substance.

Chapter 11

Alcohol in the Body

Online Learning Center Resources

www.mhhe.com/ray

Log on to our Online Learning Center (OLC) for access to these additional resources.

- Chapter definitions
- Learning objectives
- Student interactive question-and-answer sites
- Self-scoring chapter quiz

The OLC also offers web links for study and exploration of health topics. Here are some examples of what you'll find:

www.irsc.org/fas.htm

This website is an index of links about fetal alcohol syndrome. It includes news, research, disability links, information about fetal alcohol syndrome, feedback, and an area where visitors can suggest a site.

www.wfu.edu/Student-Services/Student-Health-Service/AUDIT.htm

At this site, you can complete the Alcohol Use Disorders Identification Test (AUDIT). The score will let you know if you have a drinking problem. The test is sponsored by Wake Forest University Student Health Services.

arfnet.arf.org/alcohol.nsf.newform

Use this online assessment to evaluate your drinking behavior. There are 21 questions listed. After answering the questions, submit your answers, and you receive a personalized feedback report.

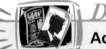

Drugs in the Media

Advertising Alcohol on Television

When it comes to the world portrayed on television, both in programs and in advertising, it seems that beer is OK (there are lots of beer ads and a few more or less

Drugs in the Media Continued...

positive references to beer drinking on some programs), wine is a little less OK, but distilled spirits are apparently not OK. In spite of issues raised by groups concerned about beer ads that seem to be aimed partly at children (e.g., the Budweiser frogs and lizards), advertising of beer on television has not been particularly restricted. In contrast, depending on where you live you might never see television ads for distilled spirits.

After Prohibition, purveyors of distilled spirits did not advertise on radio, and later they did not advertise on television. This was a voluntary ban by the radio, television, and liquor industries, not something mandated by any federal agency. In 1996, Seagram became the first liquor manufacturer to break the voluntary ban, and a few other companies followed suit. The ads are shown on local TV stations in several large cities, usually later at night. According to a December 7, 2000, article in *The New York Times,* in 1999 $18 million was spent to advertise liquor on television and radio combined—not a great deal in relation to beer advertising or in relation to the amount spent to advertise distilled spirits in magazines and newspapers.

The major television networks have not accepted liquor advertising, and it seems unlikely they will do so soon. One might imagine that they would eventually give in to generate more advertising revenue. However, several politicians and political watchdog groups keep a close eye on this and all television advertising of alcoholic beverages. The television networks do not want to do anything to encourage Congress to hold hearings on all forms of advertising for all alcoholic beverages. Imagine yourself as an executive for a television network or for Anheuser-Busch, being questioned by a congressional committee about the meaning and purpose of the "Whasuuuup?" Budweiser ads. Apart from the embarrassment of explaining how these ads target mature adults rather than those under 21, the networks and their current advertisers worry that federal legislation might restrict the advertising of wine and beer along with hard liquor.

ALCOHOLIC BEVERAGES

Fermentation and Fermentation Products

Many thousands of years ago Neolithic humans discovered "booze." Beer and berry wine were known and used about 6400 B.C. and grape wine dates from 300 to 400 B.C. Mead, which is made from honey, might be the oldest alcoholic beverage; some authorities suggest it appeared in the Paleolithic Age, about 8000 B.C. Early use of alcohol seems to have been worldwide: beer was drunk by the Native Americans whom Columbus met.

Fermentation forms the basis for all alcoholic beverages. Certain yeasts act on sugar in the presence of water, and this chemical action is fermentation. Yeast recombines the carbon, hydrogen, and oxygen of sugar into ethyl alcohol and carbon dioxide. Chemically, $C_6H_{12}O_6$ (glucose) is transformed into C_2H_5OH (ethyl alcohol) + CO_2 (carbon dioxide).

fermentation: (fer men *tay* shun) the production of alcohol from sugars through the action of yeasts.

Most fruits, including grapes, contain sugar, and the addition of the appropriate yeast (which is pervasive in the air wherever plants grow) to a mixture of crushed grapes and water will begin the fermentation process. The yeast has only a limited tolerance for alcohol; when the concentration reaches 15 percent, the yeast dies and fermentation ceases.

Cereal grains can also be used to produce alcoholic beverages. However, cereal grains contain starch rather than sugar, and before fermentation can begin the starch must be converted to sugar. This is accomplished by means of enzymes formed during a process called *malting*. In American beer the primary grain is barley, which is malted by steeping it in water and allowing it to sprout. The sprouted grain is then slowly dried to kill the sprout but preserve the enzymes formed during the growth. This dried, sprouted barley is called malt, and when crushed and mixed with water, the enzymes convert the starch to sugar. Only yeast is needed then to start fermentation.

Distilled Products

To obtain alcohol concentrations above those that can be reached by fermentation, distillation must be used. **Distillation** is a process in which the solution containing alcohol is heated, and the vapors are collected and condensed into liquid form again. Alcohol has a lower boiling point than water, so there is a higher percentage of alcohol in the distillate (the condensed liquid) than there was in the original solution.

There is still debate over who discovered the distillation process and when the discovery was made, but many authorities place it in Arabia around A.D. 800. The term *alcohol* comes from an Arabic word meaning "finely divided spirit" and originally referred to that part of the wine collected through distillation—the essence of the wine. In Europe, only fermented beverages were used until the tenth century, when the Italians first distilled wine, thereby introducing

"spirits" to the Western world. These new products were studied and used in the treatment of many illnesses, including senility. The prevalent feeling about their medicinal value is best seen in the name given these condensed vapors by a thirteenth-century professor of medicine at the French University of Montpelier: *aqua vitae,* "the water of life." Around the end of the seventeenth century, the more prosaic Dutch called the liquid *brandy,* meaning "burnt wine."

The name *whiskey* comes from the Irish-Gaelic equivalent of *aqua vitae* and was already commonplace around 1500. The distillation of whiskey in America started on a large scale toward the end of the eighteenth century. The chief product of the area just west of the Appalachian Mountains—western Pennsylvania, western Virginia, and eastern Kentucky—was grain. It was not profitable for the farmers to ship the grain or flour across the mountains to the markets along the eastern seaboard. But 10 bushels of corn could be converted to 1 barrel of whiskey, which could be profitably shipped east, so distillation started on a grand scale.

In the United States the alcoholic content of distilled beverages is indicated by the term **proof.** The percentage of alcohol by volume is one-half of the proof number: for instance, 90-proof whiskey is 45 percent alcohol. The word *proof* developed from a British Army procedure to gauge the alcohol content of distilled spirits before there were modern techniques. The liquid was poured over gunpowder and ignited. If the alcohol content was high enough, the alcohol would burn and ignite the gunpowder, which would go "poof" and explode. That was proof that the beverage had an acceptable alcohol content, about 57 percent.

ALCOHOL AS A CONSUMER ITEM

Alcoholic beverages are of considerable economic importance in the United States, with Americans spending over $100 billion a year on alcoholic beverages.[1] The average American

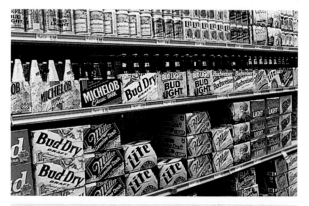

The leading brands of beer actually represent only a few brewers.

household reports spending about $3.00 per week for alcohol consumed at home and just over $2.00 per week for alcohol consumed away from home. Both the apparent frequency of drinking within the general population and the total per capita alcohol consumption reached a peak in about 1980 and have declined gradually since then.

Beer

Beer is made by adding barley malt to other cereal grains, such as ground corn or rice. The enzymes in the malt change the starches in these grains into sugar; then the solids are filtered out before the yeast is added to the mash to start fermentation. Hops (dried blossoms from only the female hop plant) are added with the yeast to give beer its distinctive, pungent flavor. One-fourth pound of hops is enough to flavor a 31-gallon barrel of beer. Most of the beer sold today in America is *lager,* from the German word *lagern,* meaning "to store." To brew lager, a type of yeast is used that settles to the bottom of the mash to ferment. After fermentation and before packaging, the beer is stored for a period to age. In most commercial beers today, alcohol content is a little over 4 percent. Because most American

beer is sold in bottles or cans, the yeast must be removed to prevent it from spoiling after packaging. This is usually accomplished by heating it (pasteurization), but some brewers use microfilters to remove the yeasts while keeping the beer cold. The carbonation is added at the time of packaging.

Ale requires a top-fermentation yeast, warmer temperatures during fermentation, and more malt and hops, which produce a more flavorful beverage. *Malt liquor* is brewed much like lager but is aged longer, and it has less carbonation, more calories, and 1 percent to 3 percent more alcohol. If you were asked to produce a "light" beer, with fewer calories, a lighter taste, and less alcohol, what would you do—add water? That's only part of the answer, because light beers have about 10 percent less alcohol and 25 to 30 percent fewer calories. The mash is fermented at a cooler temperature for a longer time, so that more of the sugars are converted to alcohol. *Then the alcohol content is adjusted by adding water,* resulting in a beverage with considerably less remaining sugar and only a bit less alcohol. Although no-alcohol beer has been around since Prohibition, the introduction of several new brands by the major U.S. brewers resulted in significant sales increases during the 1990s.

The beer-drinking, free-lunch saloon with nickel beer and bucket-of-suds-to-go disappeared forever with Prohibition. And so did a couple of thousand breweries. Two years after Prohibition ended there were 750 brewers, but by 1941 that number had dwindled to 507. From 1960 to the mid-1970s, about 10 beer makers vanished each year, until in 1976 there were fewer than 50.

distillation: (dis ti *lay* shun) the evaporation and condensing of alcohol vapors to produce beverages with higher alcohol content.

proof: a measure of a beverage's alcohol content; twice the alcohol percentage.

This declined to about 40 in the early 1980s and then began to increase again as small, local "boutique" breweries began to sprout up, especially on the West Coast. These were followed by the increasing popularity of *microbreweries,* or *brewpubs,* which make beer for sale only on the premises. These specialty brewers now capture 1 percent of the overall beer market in gallons but presumably a larger share of the beer dollar because of their higher average sale price.

Table 11.1 points to a couple of sales trends. First, you might notice that the top 10 brands are manufactured by only 3 brewers. As a result of mergers and consolidations during the 1980s, 6 major brewing companies now control over 90 percent of the beer market in the United States. The industry leader, Anheuser-Busch, controls over 40 percent of the total market. In fact, its top-selling beer, Budweiser, accounts for over 20 percent of all beer sales. The other trend to notice is that 3 of the top 4 beers are light beers, which have increased in popularity and now constitute 35 percent of the U.S. beer market.[2]

Imported beers have become increasingly popular in the past 20 years. The largest-selling imported beer is Corona, from Mexico. Overall, Mexican and Canadian beers are the biggest imports. In spite of this increased appetite for foreign beers, imports still represent only about 5 percent of total U.S. sales. One way to look at what has happened to the beer market recently is that the craft beers produced by new, small breweries combined with an increased variety of imports and the no-alcohol beers to add many new choices for the beer connoisseur, but Budweiser alone outsells all of these specialty beers combined.

Americans drink almost 25 gallons of beer for every man, woman, and child each year, and that hasn't changed much in the past decade. We're somewhat behind the Irish and Australians, though, at over 30 gallons, and the Germans and Czechs, who drink about 40 gallons per capita. On a per capita basis, Mexicans and Japanese drink less than half of the amount of beer consumed by Americans.

Figure 11.1 shows the trends in consumption by Americans age 14 or older since 1970. The popularity of beer increased during the 1970s, and consumption has declined somewhat since the peak year of 1981. Overall, beer now accounts for 60 percent of the money Americans spend on alcoholic beverages.

Wine

Wine is one of humankind's oldest beverages, a drink that for generations has been praised as a gift from heaven and condemned as a work of the devil. Although a large volume of wine is now produced in mechanized, sterilized wine "factories," there are many small wineries that operate alongside the industry giants, and the tradition continues that careful selection and cultivation of grapevines, good weather, precise timing of the harvest, and careful monitoring of fermentation and aging can result in wines of noticeably higher quality. An interesting ecological story resulted from the fact that most American wine grapes were originally transplanted from France and Spain. After a late-nineteenth-century disease destroyed almost all of the European vineyards, it became necessary to transplant American vines,

TABLE 11-1

Largest-Selling Beer Brands (1998)

Brand	Brewer
Budweiser	Anheuser-Busch
Bud Light	Anheuser-Busch
MillerLite	Miller
Coors Light	Adolph Coors
Busch	Anheuser-Busch
Natural Light	Anheuser-Busch
Genuine Draft	Miller
High Life	Miller
Busch Light Draft	Anheuser-Busch
Milwaukee's Best	Miller

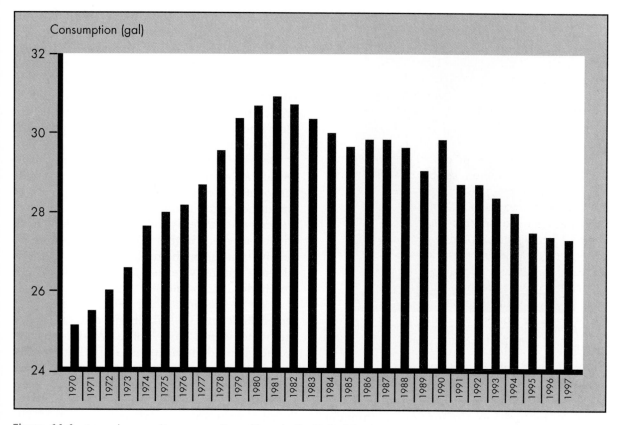

Figure 11-1 Annual per capita consumption of beer in the United States.

which had been protected by isolation, back into Europe. Today most of the French, Italian, and Spanish wine grapes are grown from descendants of those American vines.

There are two basic types of American wines. *Generics* usually have names taken from European land areas where the original wines were produced: Chablis, Champagne, Burgundy, Bordeaux, and Rhine are examples. These are all blended wines, made from whatever grapes are available, and during processing they are made to taste something like the traditional European wines from those regions. However, there is little guarantee of quality in these generic names among American wines. *Varietals* are named after one variety of grape, which by law must

make up at least 51 percent of the grapes used in producing the wine. Chardonnay, pinot noir, and zinfandel are some examples. There are many varietal wines, and traditionally they have been sold in individual bottles and are more expensive than the generics. In some other countries the rules for naming wines are more restrictive. For example, in France the name *Chablis* is carefully protected by law. A French Chablis must come from the Chablis region and be made only from the chardonnay grape. In America many inexpensive dry white wines are labeled Chablis, and they are likely to include a considerable amount of juice from table grapes such as the Thompson seedless. Thus, it is illegal to sell American "Chablis" wines in France

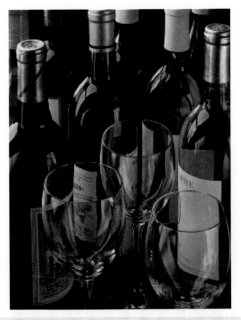

Wine consumption has increased considerably during the past 35 years.

without relabeling them. One varietal that seems to be uniquely Californian is zinfandel. This variety of red grape has been so widely planted that the wine is often packaged in large jugs or boxes and marketed more as a generic. Most white wines are made from white grapes, although it is possible to use red grapes if the skins are removed before fermentation. Red wines are made from red grapes by leaving the skins in the crushed grapes while they ferment. Rose (pronounced *rose-ay*) wines were traditionally made by leaving the skins in for only a day or two, but most inexpensive American rose wine is made by mixing generic red and white wines. During the 1980s, "blush" wines such as white zinfandel became quite popular. With the zinfandel grape, which is red, the skins are left in the crushed grapes for a short while, resulting in a wine that is just slightly pink.

Besides red versus white and generic versus varietal, another general distinction is dry versus sweet. Most table wines are relatively dry, but some are sweeter than others. Also, the sweeter wines are likely to have a "heavier" taste overall, with the sweetness balancing out flavors that might be considered harsh in a dry wine. As a general rule, lighter foods, such as broiled fish, call for a light, dry, white wine, and red wine would be considered an appropriate accompaniment to a steak.

Because carbon dioxide is produced during fermentation, it is possible to produce naturally carbonated sparkling wines by adding a small amount of sugar as the wine is bottled and then keeping the bottle tightly corked. French champagnes are made in this way, as are the more expensive American champagnes, which might be labeled "naturally fermented in the bottle," or "methode Champagnoise." A less expensive way is to do the secondary fermentation in a large sealed tank and then maintain pressure while the wine is put in a bottle. A still cheaper method is used on inexpensive sparkling wines: carbon dioxide is injected into a generic wine during bottling. Champagnes vary in their sweetness, also, with brut being the driest. Sweet champagnes are labeled "extra dry." The *extra* means "not," as in *extraordinary.*

It was discovered many years ago in Spain that, if enough brandy is added to a newly fermented wine, the fermentation will stop and the wine will not spoil (turn to vinegar). Sealing the wine in charred oak casks for aging further refined its taste, and soon *sherry* was in great demand throughout Europe. Other fortified wines, all of which have an alcohol content near 20 percent, include port, Madeira, and Muscatel. Dry sherry is typically consumed before dinner, whereas the sweeter fortified wines may be drunk as a dessert wine.

In the 1960s, Americans consumed less wine than they do now, and most of it consisted of dessert wines. Sales of the sweet wines have decreased, and sales of the drier table wines increased to several times their 1960 level, bringing total wine sales up with them. The

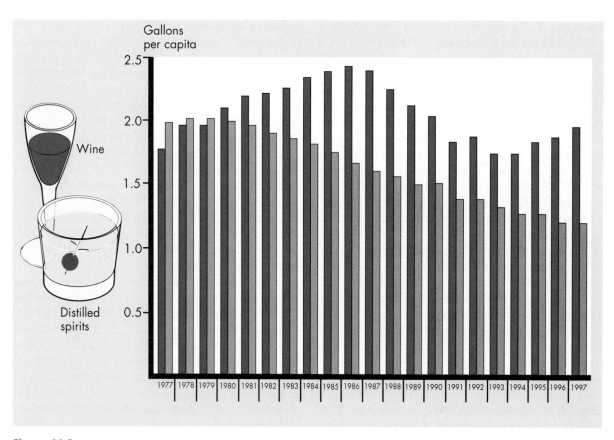

Figure 11-2   Annual per capita consumption of wine and distilled spirits in the United States.

trend toward increased wine drinking continued until 1986, as Figure 11.2 demonstrates.[3] There was a decline in per capita wine consumption during the 1990s.

Part of the increase in per capita wine consumption in the mid-1980s was due to the introduction of the *wine cooler,* a mixture of wine with various carbonated beverages. These sweet, bubbly drinks look and taste a lot like soda pop, a fact that has not been lost on the marketers. They've even been sold in two-liter plastic bottles resembling soft-drink bottles. Wine coolers were first introduced in 1981; by the end of the 1980s wine cooler sales represented 25 percent of the dollar sales for the

American wine industry. The idea of sweet, carbonated, fruit-flavored coolers has now spread, so that both wine-based and malt beverage–based coolers are available in great variety, generally with a final alcohol content similar to that of beer. It appears that these coolers have replaced beer as a common "gateway" alcoholic beverage for many beginning drinkers.

Distilled Spirits

Although brandy, distilled from wine, was probably the first type of spirits known to Europeans, the Celts of Ireland and the Scottish highlands were distilling a crude beverage known as *uisgebaugh*—"water of life"—before 1500. Today's Scotch whisky (without the *e*; it's *whiskey* in the United States and in Ireland, *whisky* in Scotland and Canada) is the distillate of fermented malted barley. The distinctive smoky flavor comes from two sources: the malted barley is dried in kilns in which burning peat provides the heat, so some of the distinctive characteristics of peat are picked up by the malt. With so many casks of sherry wine being sent to the British Isles after the seventeenth century, the Scots began to use the empty casks to age their whisky, and current practice calls for this storage in old sherry casks for at least three years. Pure malt whisky of this type is more popular in the Highlands than elsewhere because of its strong flavors. Most commercial Scotch whisky is blended with lighter-tasting grain spirits to provide a more pleasing drink.

In America the economics of trade resulted in an expanding production of spirits distilled from grain just as our new federal government was forming. In 1789, one of the early distillers who established a good reputation was Elijah Craig, a Baptist minister living in what was then Bourbon County, Kentucky. He began storing his whiskey in charred new oak barrels, originating a manufacturing step still used with most American whiskeys.

By the seventeenth century, improved distillation techniques had made possible the production of relatively pure alcohol. Today's standard product from many large commercial distilleries is 95 percent pure alcohol (190 proof). Into the process goes whatever grain is available at a cheap price and tank loads of corn syrup or other sources of sugars or starches. Out the other end come *grain neutral spirits,* a clear liquid that is essentially tasteless (except for the strong alcohol taste), which might be sold in small quantities as Everclear or for use in medicine or research. More often, it is processed in bulk in various ways. For example, large quantities of grain neutral spirits are now being added to gasoline to produce a less polluting fuel,

which also helps out the American farmer. Besides other industrial uses for ethyl alcohol, such as in cleaners and solvents, bulk grain neutral spirits are also used in making various beverages, including blended Scotch whiskys. One of the first beverages to be made from straight grain neutral spirits was gin. By filtering the distillate through juniper berries and then diluting it with water, a medicinal-tasting drink was produced. First called "jenever" by the Dutch and "genievre" by the French, the British shortened the name first to "geneva" and then to "gin." Gin became a popular beverage in England and now forms the basis for many an American martini.

Another major use for bulk grain neutral spirits is in the production of *vodka.* All American vodkas, and most vodkas from other countries, are simply a mixture of grain neutral spirits and water, adjusted to the desired proof. You may wonder why vodkas of the same proof are priced differently if they are all identical— and they are. The best answer to that question was given by an official of Heublein's, a company that produces both the high-priced Smirnoff vodka and a medium-priced vodka. "That's a very embarrassing question. Shall we say it's a difference in pricing policy?"

The proof at which distillation is carried out influences the taste and other characteristics of the liquor. When alcohol is formed, other related substances, known as **congeners,** are also formed. These may include alcohols other than ethanol, oils, and other organic matter. Luckily they are present only in small amounts, because some of them are quite toxic. Grain neutral spirits contain relatively few congeners and none of the flavor of the grains used in the mash. Whiskey is usually distilled at a lower proof, not more than 160, and thus the distillate contains more congeners and some of the flavor of the grain used. If 51 percent or more of the grain used was rye, then the product is labeled straight *rye whiskey.* When corn constitutes over 51 percent of the grain in the mash, the liquor is called *bourbon.* (To be called *corn whiskey* requires that the mash be 80 percent or more corn.) Both rye and bourbon are then diluted to 120 to 125 proof and aged in new, charred oak barrels for at least two years, and usually longer. Whiskey accumulates congeners during aging, at least for the first five years, and the congeners and the grain used provide the variation in taste among whiskeys.

Until Prohibition almost all whiskey consumed in the United States was straight rye or bourbon manufactured in the United States. Prohibition introduced smuggled Canadian and Scotch whisky to American drinkers, and they liked them. World War II sent American men around the world, further exposing them to this different type of liquor. Scotch and Canadian whiskys are lighter than American whiskey, which means lighter in color and less heavy in taste. They are lighter because Canadian and Scotch whiskys are typically *blended* whiskys, made from about two-thirds straight whisky and one-third grain neutral spirits. After World War II, U.S. manufacturers began selling more blended whiskey. Seagram's 7-Crown has been one of the most popular blended American whiskeys. If you were so inclined, you could make your own blended whiskey by mixing two bottles of straight bourbon with one bottle of vodka, which would soften the whiskey flavor and lighten the color.

Liqueurs, or cordials, are similar in some ways to the fortified wines. Originally the cordials were made from brandy, but rather than mixing the brandy with wine, it was mixed with other flavorings derived from herbs, berries, or nuts. After dilution with sugar and water, the beverages are highly flavored, sweet, and usually about 20 to 25 percent alcohol. Some of the old recipes are still closely guarded secrets of a particular group of European monks. The late twentieth century saw an increase in popularity for these drinks, which are usually consumed in small amounts and have only about half the alcohol content of vodka or whiskey. Many new types were introduced, from Bailey's Irish

Cream to varieties of schnapps. Modern American peppermint, peach, and other types of schnapps are made from grain neutral spirits, which are diluted, sweetened, and flavored with artificial or natural flavorings.

Americans have changed their tastes in distilled spirits. For many years domestic whiskey dominated sales, but the trend toward lighter taste and increased "mixability," which began with imported and domestic blended whiskeys, also led to increased sales of gin, vodka, and rum. In 1983, domestic vodka finally surpassed domestic whiskey to become the leading single type of distilled spirits consumed by Americans. Sales of imported whisky have declined more slowly, and 1983 also marked the first time that sales of domestic whiskey fell behind sales of imports. Sales of vodka, gin, and rum peaked in 1983 and have declined somewhat since then. The resulting trend in overall per capita consumption of distilled spirits was downward during the 1980s and 1990s, as was shown in Figure 11.2.

ALCOHOL PHARMACOLOGY

Absorption

Some alcohol is absorbed from the stomach, but the small intestine is responsible for most absorption. In an empty stomach the overall rate of absorption depends primarily on the concentration of alcohol. Alcohol taken with or after a meal is absorbed more slowly. This is because the food remains in the stomach for digestive action, and the protein in the food retains the alcohol with it in the stomach. Plain water, by decreasing the concentration, slows the absorption of alcohol, but carbonated liquids speed it up. The carbon dioxide acts to move everything quite rapidly through the stomach to the small

---

congeners: (*con* je nurz) other alcohols and oils contained in alcoholic beverages

intestine. It is because of this emptying of the stomach and the more rapid absorption of alcohol in the intestine that champagne has a faster onset of action than noncarbonated wine.

Metabolism

As a "food" item, alcohol has a couple of unusual characteristics. First, it requires no digestion and is absorbed unchanged into the bloodstream. Second, although alcohol does contain usable calories (it produces energy when it is metabolized), alcohol itself cannot be stored or converted into lipids or protein so that this energy can be stored for later use. You might think that this means that alcohol itself cannot contribute to weight gain, but that is not so. With alcohol in the system, other calories that might be burned are not. In fact, one report indicated that alcohol actually decreases the rate at which humans burn fat for energy.[4]

A 1990 study attracted a great deal of attention when it was reported that, compared with men, women absorb a greater proportion of the alcohol they drink. It seems that some metabolism of alcohol actually takes place in the stomach, where the enzyme alcohol dehydrogenase is present. Because this stomach enzyme is more active, on the average, in men than in women, women might be more susceptible to the effects of alcohol.[5]

Once absorbed, alcohol remains in the bloodstream and other body fluids until it is metabolized, and over 90 percent of this metabolism occurs in the liver. A small amount of alcohol, less than 2 percent, is normally excreted unchanged—some in the breath, some through the skin, and some in the urine.

The primary metabolic system is a simple one: the enzyme *alcohol dehydrogenase* converts alcohol to *acetaldehyde*. Acetaldehyde is then converted fairly rapidly by aldehyde dehydrogenase to acetic acid. With most drugs a constant *proportion* of the drug is removed in a given amount of time, so that with a high blood level the amount metabolized is high. With alcohol,

Drugs in Depth

The "Flushing" Reaction and Alcohol Consumption in Asia

About half of all Asians carry a gene that renders their livers' aldehyde dehydrogenase much less effective, and each time they drink there is a buildup of acetaldehyde, a toxic by-product of alcohol metabolism. This leads to a variety of reactions, including a facial flush, sweating, and nausea.

In spite of this common reaction, alcohol use, and especially heavy drinking, is becoming increasingly accepted in Japan, Korea, and China. Mixed drinks are sold in vending machines on the streets in Japan, and Japanese and Korean businesspeople are increasingly likely to pressure each other to go out drinking, often to the point of intoxication. Perhaps this is part of an attempt to adopt what are viewed as American practices, but the rapid increase in heavy drinking promises to lead to severe social problems for these nations. South Korea is now reported to have the highest per capita consumption of distilled spirits in the world.[7]

the *amount* that can be metabolized is constant at about 0.25 to 0.3 ounces per hour, regardless of the blood alcohol concentration (BAC). The major factor determining the rate of alcohol metabolism is the activity of the enzyme alcohol dehydrogenase. Exercise, coffee consumption, and so on have no effect on this enzyme, so the sobering-up process is essentially a matter of waiting for this enzyme to do its job at its own speed.

Acetaldehyde might be more than just an intermediate step in the oxidation of alcohol. Acetaldehyde is quite toxic; though its blood levels are only one-thousandth of those of alcohol, this substance might cause some of the physiological effects now attributed to alcohol. One danger in heavy alcohol use might be in the higher blood levels of acetaldehyde (see the Drugs in Depth box).

The second enzyme system is much more complicated and at this time has many more known ramifications. The liver responds to chronic intake of alcohol by increasing the levels of liver microsomal enzymes (see Chapter 7). This gives rise to some interesting situations. In a person who drinks alcohol heavily over a long period of time, there is an increase in the activity of the microsomal enzymes. As long as there is alcohol in the system, alcohol gets preferential treatment and the metabolism of other drugs is *slower* than normal. When heavy alcohol use stops and the alcohol has disappeared from the body, the high activity level of the enzymes continues for four to eight weeks. During this time other drugs are metabolized more *rapidly*. To obtain therapeutic levels of the drugs metabolized by this enzyme system (e.g., the benzodiazepines), it is necessary to administer less drug to the drinking alcoholic and more drug to the just-nondrinking alcoholic. Thus, alcohol increases the activity of one of the two enzyme systems responsible for its own oxidation. The increased activity of this microsomal pathway might be a partial basis for the tolerance to alcohol that is shown by heavy users of alcohol.[6]

Central Nervous System Effects

Alcohol is like any other general anesthetic: it depresses the CNS. It was used as an anesthetic until the late nineteenth century, when nitrous oxide, ether, and chloroform became more widely used. However, it was not just new compounds that decreased alcohol's use as an anesthetic; alcohol itself has some major disadvantages. In contrast to the gaseous anesthetics, alcohol is almost completely metabolized in the body and the rate of oxidation is slow. This gives alcohol a long duration of action that cannot be controlled. A second disadvantage is that the dose effective in surgical anesthesia is not much lower than the dose that causes respiratory arrest and death. Finally, alcohol makes blood slower to clot.

The exact mechanism for the CNS effect of alcohol is not clear. Until the mid-1980s, the most widely accepted theory was that alcohol

acted on all neural membranes, perhaps altering their electrical excitability. However, with increased understanding of the role of the GABA receptor complex in the actions of other depressant drugs (see Chapter 9), many scientists now believe that the same receptor complex might play a special role in the action of alcohol. The study of GABA receptors led to the discovery of an experimental drug, RO 15-4513, which appeared to be a specific antidote or antagonist for many of the behavioral effects of alcohol. In a dramatic demonstration, intoxicated rats that had been unable to roll over and stand up appeared, within two minutes after an injection of RO 15-4513, to be "sober" and walking normally. This drug antagonizes alcohol's enhancement of GABA action and is able to overcome some (but not all) of the depressant actions of alcohol.[8] It is not likely that a sober-up pill will be on the market at any time soon. Even if such a drug were available, the company selling it would be potentially liable for accidents occurring when a person who was over the legal BAC limit used its product to sober up.

At the lowest effective blood levels, complex, abstract, and poorly learned behaviors are disrupted. As the dose increases, better learned and simpler behaviors are also affected. Inhibitions can be reduced, with the result that the overall amount of behavior increases under certain conditions. Even though alcohol can result in an increase in activity, most scientists would not call alcohol a stimulant. Rather, the increased behavioral output is usually attributed to decreased inhibition of behavior.

If the alcohol intake is "just right," most people experience a high, a happy feeling. Below a certain **blood alcohol concentration** (BAC) there are no mood changes, but at some point

blood alcohol concentration; also called blood alcohol level: a measure of the concentration of alcohol in blood, expressed in grams per 100 ml (percentage).

TABLE 11-2

Blood Alcohol Concentration and Behavioral Effects

Percent BAC	Behavioral effects
0.05	Lowered alertness, usually good feeling, release of inhibitions, impaired judgment
0.10	Slower reaction times and impaired motor function, less caution
0.15	Large, consistent increases in reaction time
0.20	Marked depression in sensory and motor capability, intoxication
0.25	Severe motor disturbance, staggering, sensory perceptions, great impairment
0.30	Stuporous but conscious—no comprehension of what's going on
0.35	Surgical anesthesia; about LD_1, minimal level causing death
0.40	About LD_{50}

we become uninhibited enough to enjoy our own "charming selves" and uncritical enough to accept the "clods" around us. This point seems to be when the alcohol has disrupted social inhibitions and impaired good judgment but has not depressed most behavior. We become witty, clever, and quite sophisticated. Fortunately, those around us at this time might also have slightly impaired judgment, so they can't say any different.

Another factor contributing to the feeling of well-being is the reduction in anxieties as a result of the disruption of normal critical thinking. The reduction in concern and judgment can range from not worrying about who'll pay the bar bill to being sure that you can take that next curve at 60 mph.

These effects depend on the BAC—also called blood alcohol level (BAL). BAC is reported as the number of grams of alcohol in 100 ml of blood and is expressed as a percentage. For example, 100 g in 100 ml is 100 percent, and 100 mg of alcohol in 100 ml of blood is reported as 0.10 percent.

Before suggesting relationships between BAC and behavioral change, two factors must be mentioned. One is that the rate at which the BAC rises is a factor in determining behavioral effects. The more rapid the increase, the greater the behavioral effects. Second, a classic study using a variety of simple visual, motor, and visual-motor tests showed disruption of performance at an average BAC of 0.05 percent in abstainers, 0.07 percent in moderate drinkers, and 0.10 percent in heavy drinkers.[9] These results show clearly that behavioral and CNS tolerance to alcohol does develop. They also indicate that the better performance of the heavy drinker compared with the moderate drinker after equal amounts of alcohol is not caused by the greater rate of alcohol metabolism in heavy drinkers. A higher BAC is necessary to impair the performance of a chronic, heavy drinker than to impair a moderate drinker's performance.

A partial explanation might be that the heavy drinker is better motivated to conceal the alcohol-induced impairment and probably has had more practice. Performance differences might reflect only the extent to which the two groups have learned to overcome the disruption of nervous system functioning. Another explanation might be that the CNS in the heavy drinker develops a tolerance to alcohol, which does not exist in the moderate drinker. It is established that neural tissue becomes tolerant to alcohol, and tolerance can apparently develop even when the alcohol intake is well spaced over time.

Table 11.2 describes some general behavioral effects of increasing doses of alcohol. These relationships are approximately correct for moderate drinkers. There are some reports that changes in nervous system function have been obtained at concentrations as low as 0.03 to 0.04 percent.

The vomiting reflex can be activated by alcohol at a BAC of about 0.12 percent or even lower, but only if that level is approached rapidly. With slow, steady drinking the BAC increases gradually, and at high concentrations the vomiting center is depressed. The individual can then continue drinking up to lethal concentrations if he or she remains conscious.

The surgical anesthesia level and the minimum lethal level are perhaps the two least precise points in the table. In any case, they are quite close, and the safety margin is less than 0.1 percent blood alcohol. Death resulting from acute alcohol intoxication usually is the result of respiratory failure when the medulla is depressed.

The relationship between BAC and behavior is similarly, but more enjoyably, described in the following, which is modified from Bogen:

At less than 0.03%, the individual is dull and dignified.

At 0.05%, he is dashing and debonair.

At 0.1%, he may become dangerous and devilish.

At 0.2%, he is likely to be dizzy and disturbing.

At 0.25%, he may be disgusting and disheveled.

At 0.3%, he is delirious and disoriented and surely drunk.

At 0.35%, he is dead drunk.

At 0.6%, the chances are that he is dead.[10]

The relationship between BAC and alcohol intake is relatively simple and reasonably well understood. Remember, alcohol is not appreciably excreted from, or stored anywhere in, the body before metabolism. When taken into the body, alcohol is distributed throughout the body fluids, including the blood. However, alcohol does not distribute much into fatty tissues, so a 180-pound lean person will have a lower BAC than a 180-pound fat person who drinks the same amount of alcohol.

Table 11.3 demonstrates the relationships among alcohol intake, BAC, and body weight for hypothetical, *average* females and males. The chart distinguishes between the sexes because the average female has a higher proportion of

body fat and therefore, for a given weight, has less volume in which to distribute the alcohol. It's worth spending a bit of time to try to understand this table and to try one of the blood alcohol calculators on the Internet (see the Targeting Prevention box) because you can learn a lot about how much you can probably drink to avoid going above a specified BAC.

First, Table 11.3 makes the simplifying assumption that all of the alcohol is absorbed quickly and "in one hour," so that there is little opportunity for metabolism. If the 150-pound female had a tank of water weighing about 100 pounds (12.5 gallons, or 45 liters) and just dumped 1 ounce (28.3 g) into it and stirred it, the concentration would be about 0.6 g/liter, or 0.06 g/100 ml (0.06%). Figure 11.3 shows a

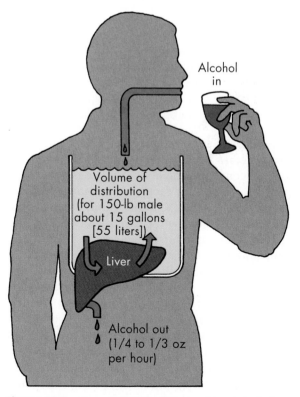

Alcohol in

Volume of distribution (for 150-lb male about 15 gallons [55 liters])

Liver

Alcohol out (1/4 to 1/3 oz per hour)

Figure 11-3 The relationship between blood alcohol concentration and alcohol intake.

TABLE 11-3

Relationships Among Gender, Weight, Alcohol Consumption, and Blood Alcohol Concentration

Absolute alcohol (ounces)	Beverage intake*	Blood alcohol concentrations (g/100 ml)					
		Female (100 lb)	Male (100 lb)	Female (150 lb)	Male (150 lb)	Female (200 lb)	Male (200 lb)
$^1/_2$	1 oz spirits† 1 glass wine 1 can beer	0.045	0.037	0.03	0.025	0.022	0.019
1	2 oz spirits† 2 glasses wine 2 cans beer	0.090	0.075	0.06	0.050	0.045	0.037
2	4 oz spirits† 4 glasses wine 4 cans beer	0.180	0.150	0.12	0.100	0.090	0.070
3	6 oz spirits† 6 glasses wine 6 cans beer	0.270	0.220	0.18	0.150	0.130	0.110
4	8 oz spirits† 8 glasses wine 8 cans beer	0.360	0.300	0.24	0.200	0.180	0.150
5	10 oz spirits† 10 glasses wine 10 cans beer	0.450	0.370	0.30	0.250	0.220	0.180

*In one hour
†100-proof

schematic of such a tank. The 150-pound average male has a tank with more water in it, so his alcohol concentration after 1 ounce is about 0.05 percent. The major factor determining individual differences in BAC is the volume of distribution, so find your own weight on Table 11.3 and estimate how many drinks could be poured into your tank to obtain a BAC of 0.05 percent.

Second, notice that several beverages are equated to 0.5 ounce of absolute alcohol. A 12-ounce can or bottle of beer at about 4.2 percent alcohol contains $12 \times 0.042 = 0.5$ ounce of alcohol. The same amount is found in a glass of wine containing about 4 ounces of 12 percent alcohol, 1 ounce of 100-proof spirits, or 1.25 ounces of 80-proof spirits. Each of these can be equated as a standard "drink."

We have not yet taken metabolism into account, but we can do so with one more simple calculation. As we already know, alcohol is removed by the liver at essentially a constant rate of 0.25 to 0.3 ounce of ethanol per hour. There are some individual differences in this rate, but most people fall within this range no matter what their body size or drinking experience, unless they have consumed so much alcohol that the liver is damaged. To be on the safe side, estimate that you can metabolize about 0.25 ounce per hour, and note that this is one-half of one of our standard drinks (1 beer, 1 shot, or 1 glass of wine). Over the course of an evening, if your rate of intake equals your rate of metabolism, you will maintain a stable BAC. If you drink faster than 1 drink every 2 hours, your BAC will climb.

Targeting Prevention

Estimating Blood Alcohol Calculations

Table 11.3 in the text is one way to estimate blood alcohol level based on gender, weight, and number of drinks. However, there are now available several more dynamic blood alcohol calculators on the Internet. If you do an Internet search on the term "blood alcohol calculator," you will find several of these. Whether or not you consume alcohol yourself, it is instructive to understand how your own body (and brain) will respond to various numbers of alcoholic drinks. Try a few of the Internet calculators to see how their results compare with each other and to Table 11.3. An important thing for you to learn is how many drinks it is likely to take in order to bring your BAC to 0.08, which will soon be the legal limit for driving in all of the United States, as it currently is in some states and several other countries.

The extra drinks, those over the 1 every 2 hours, will be added to your tank. Let's take an example from the chart: a 150-pound male goes to the bar at 8 P.M. and consumes 6 beers before midnight. During that 4 hours his liver metabolizes the alcohol from 2 of the beers, so he still has 4 drinks, or 2 ounces of ethanol, in his system. His BAC at midnight should be about 0.10 percent, making him legally intoxicated and unfit to drive home. If he had had 2 fewer beers (4 over the 4-hour period), his BAC would have been about 0.05 percent. In other words, once the 2 drinks for 4 hours of metabolism are accounted for, you simply add up the extra drinks and look up the estimated BAC on the chart. If you want to do other calculations for yourself, follow these 2 steps: first, calculate the number of "drinks" metabolized at the rate of half a drink per hour. Second, pour the remaining drinks into the tank for a person of that size using Table 11.3. A 100-pound female who had kept up with our 6-pack-consuming friend would have metabolized the same 2 beers, but the 4 remaining ones would have left her in pretty bad shape at 0.18 percent. If

our friend were driving home in a "dangerous and devilish" state, she might be too "dizzy and disturbed" to notice.

Let's take a brief look at some nonstandard drinks. What if our male friend had been drinking "3.2" beer? Each 12-ounce beer at 3.2 percent has almost 0.4 ounce of alcohol instead of 0.5, so 6 of them contain 2.3 ounces. After metabolizing 1 ounce in 4 hours, his tank has 1.3 ounces, or enough to put him at about 0.065 percent. He's better off than when he drank the 6 regular beers, but it's wrong to say that 3.2 beer is not intoxicating. Alcohol is alcohol, no matter what beverage it comes from. As an exercise, figure out how many 3.2 beers it would take to put this guy over the 0.10 percent line. Some wine coolers contain 12 ounces of about 5 percent alcohol, more than 1 of our standard drinks, so you might try some calculations with drinks containing 0.6 ounces.

What's a safe BAC? After we remember that nothing in this world is totally safe, let's say that if you are going to drink and want to remain in reasonable control of your faculties you should probably stay below 0.05 percent. Individuals differ considerably in their sensitivities to alcohol, however, so the best rule is to learn about your own sensitivity and not to feel compelled to keep up with anyone else's drinking. And alcohol-induced impairment is dose-related and depends on what you're trying to do. Carrying on bar conversation places fewer demands on your nervous system than driving on a Los Angeles freeway during rush hour, where any alcohol at all might interfere.

BAC gives a good estimate of the alcohol concentration in the brain, and the concentration of alcohol in the breath gives a good estimate of the alcohol concentration in the blood. The concentration in the blood is almost 2,100 times the concentration in air expired from the lungs, making breath samples accurate indicators of BAC. Such breath samples are easily collected by police and can be the basis for conviction as a drunk driver in most states.

HealthQuest Activities

Complete "Consequences of Alcohol Abuse" in Module 8. The article explains the dangerous results of alcohol abuse. Have you or has someone in your family ever experienced these consequences? Together with your classmates, create an informational pamphlet or display to share with other students on your campus. You may wish to set up an educational booth about the consequences of alcohol abuse during a special event at your school. Ask others for feedback when they visit your booth. Do they or do they not feel these consequences are great enough to deter them from abusing alcohol?

Read "Alcohol, Violence, and Aggression" under *Key Articles* in Module 8. Are you surprised at the links between alcohol and violent or aggressive behavior? List several movies or television shows that link alcohol and violence or aggression. Do you think these are accurate portrayals of behavior as outlined in the article? Also, scan recent magazines and newspapers for violent crimes linked to alcohol abuse. How many can you find?

Blackouts

Alcohol-induced blackouts are periods of time during alcohol use in which the drinking individual appears to function normally but later, when the individual is sober, he or she cannot recall any events that occurred during that period. The drinker might drive home or dance all night, interacting in the usual way with others. When the individual cannot remember the activities, the people, or anything else, that's a blackout. Most authorities include it as one of the danger signs suggesting excessive use of alcohol. The limited amount of recent research on this topic is probably related to ethical concerns about giving such high doses of alcohol to experimental subjects. An article from 1884 titled "Alcoholic Trance" referred to the syndrome:

This trance state is a common condition in inebriety, where . . . a profound suspension of memory and consciousness and literal paralysis of certain brain-functions follow.

This trance state may last from a few moments to several days, during which the person may appear and act rationally, and yet be actually a mere automaton, without consciousness or memory of his actual condition.[11]

Sexual Behavior

Lechery, sir, it provokes, and
unprovokes; it provokes the desire,
but it takes away the performance.[12]

Alcohol, because it is a depressant drug, decreases inhibitions and at least makes the thought of sexual activity more likely. The amount of sexual behavior might increase after moderate alcohol intake, but there is considerable anecdotal evidence that the quality decreases.

Whether alcohol enhances sexual activity through pharmacological mechanisms or through attitudes and beliefs is not clear. Those who believe alcohol to be an aid to sexual pleasure are more likely to drink, and the act of drinking can provide a sort of license to be more relaxed and to behave less responsibly. In fact, one clear finding is that alcohol use by adolescents is associated with increased risky sex (not using a condom, engaging in promiscuity).[8]

A sophisticated and well-designed study[13] using college women as subjects explored the relationships among the dose of alcohol ingested (0.05, 0.25, 0.50, and 0.75 alcohol per kg body weight), self-reports of sexual arousal, and vaginal vasocongestion. There were two experimental conditions—watching an erotic-pornographic film and watching a nonerotic film of a tour of a computer facility—and two sets of instructions, one suggesting that alcohol would increase sexual arousal and the other suggesting that alcohol would decrease sexual arousal. The subjects were tested about 40 minutes after alcohol intake. Each subject was tested under each alcohol dose, and in each session both the erotic and the nonerotic film were viewed.

Several results are worthy of note. The instructional set did not generally alter the expected effect of alcohol: most of the college women expected alcohol to increase sexual arousal. On the self-report measure, (1) sexual arousal increased with alcohol intake and (2) the percentage of subjects reporting arousal to the erotic film increased as the amount of alcohol ingested increased.

The erotic film elicited much greater vaginal vasocongestion than the computer film, providing some validity to vaginal vasocongestion as a measure of sexual arousal. Importantly, the amount of increase in vaginal vasocongestion decreased as the dose of alcohol increased. For women, increased alcohol intake results in self-reports of increased sexual arousal along with a decrease in a physiological measure of arousal.

A similar study[14] was carried out on college men by the same research team. The physiological measure of arousal was also vasocongestion—speed, amount, and duration of penile erection. The doses of alcohol ingested were 0.08, 0.4, 0.8, and 1.2 g/kg. All three measures of penile vasocongestion decreased as the dose of alcohol was increased. Self-reports of degree of arousal were highly correlated with the extent of vasocongestion.

Alcohol Withdrawal—Delirium Tremens

The physical dependence associated with prolonged heavy use of alcohol is revealed when alcohol intake is stopped. *The abstinence syndrome that develops is medically more severe and more likely to cause death than withdrawal from narcotic drugs.* In untreated advanced cases, mortality can be as high as one in seven. For that reason it has long been recommended that the initial period of **detoxification** (allowing the body to rid

itself of the alcohol) be carried out in an inpatient medical setting, especially for alcoholics who have been drinking very heavily or have other medical complications.

The progression of withdrawal, the abstinence syndrome, has been described in the following way:

- Stage 1: tremors, excessively rapid heartbeat, hypertension, heavy sweating, loss of appetite, and insomnia
- Stage 2: hallucinations—auditory, visual, tactile, or a combination of these; and, rarely, olfactory signs
- Stage 3: delusions, disorientation, delirium, sometimes intermittent and usually followed by amnesia
- Stage 4: seizure activity

Medical treatment is usually sought in stage 1 or 2, and rapid intervention with a sedative drug, such as chlordiazepoxide, will prevent stage 3 or 4 from occurring. The old term **delirium tremens** is used to refer to severe cases including at least stage 3.

Tremors are one of the most common physical changes associated with alcohol withdrawal and can persist for a long period after alcohol intake has stopped. The classic drunk, bending over to sip from a cup, attests to the frequency of tremors. Anxiety, insomnia, feelings of unreality, nausea, vomiting, and many other symptoms can also occur.

The withdrawal symptoms do not develop all at the same time or immediately after abstinence begins. The initial signs (tremors, anxiety)

---

detoxification: an early treatment stage, in which the body eliminates the alcohol or other substance.

delirium tremens: (de *leer* ee um *tree* mens) an alcohol withdrawal syndrome that includes hallucinations and tremors.

Exploring Your Spirituality

Overcoming Codependence

A term used to describe the relationship between drug-dependent people and those around them is *codependence*. This term implies a kind of dual addiction: the alcoholic is addicted to the alcohol, and the person close to the alcoholic is addicted to the alcoholic. Family members and friends often are in denial about the addiction and, so, "enable" the alcohol-dependent person; they inadvertently support the drinking behavior by denying that a problem exists.

Unfortunately, this behavior harms both parties. The alcoholic's treatment may be delayed, and codependent people often pay a heavy price. Codependence can be as serious as alcohol, some people say, because many codependents think about killing themselves. They may become drug- or alcohol-dependent themselves, or they may suffer psychological problems related to guilt, depression, anxiety, and loss of self-esteem.

Codependents often retain a high quality of spiritual strengths, despite a disease that may cause them to feel helpless and full of despair. The family and friends of alcoholics often have a deep sense of commitment, compassion, selflessness, determination, and courage, as well as the ability to see goodness in others. A sense of detachment, however, is something they may need to develop in order to loosen the grip of this opportunistic disease.

One of the 12-step programs (based on Alcoholics Anonymous; see Drugs in Depth box in Chapter 12) and the spiritual principles underlying it can foster recovery from codependence, including a sense of detachment. Detachment may seem at first like a concept in conflict with compassionate qualities. It is not, according to Darlene Entenmann. She writes at www.hopeand-healing.com that detachment is realizing you are not the cause of, or the cure for, someone else's addiction. Detachment is being able to care about someone without doing so in inappropriate ways that prevent that person from becoming responsible for himself or herself. It is recognizing what you have, and do not have, the power to change.

Detachment is realizing that you do not know the future but can know the serenity of turning over your future to a higher spiritual power. The only control you have may be control of your attitude.

---

might develop within a few hours, but the individual is relatively rational. Over the next day or two, hallucinations appear and gradually become more terrifying and real to the individual. Huckleberry Finn described these in his father quite vividly:

> Pap took the jug, and said he had enough whisky there for two drunks and one delirium tremens. He drank and drank . . .
>
> I don't know how long I was asleep, but . . . there was an awful scream and I was up. There was pap looking wild, and skipping around every which way and yelling about snakes. He said they was crawling up on his legs; and then he would give a jump and scream, and say one had bit him on the cheek—but I couldn't see no snakes. He started and run round . . . hollering

> "Take him off! he's biting me on the neck!" I never see a man look so wild in the eyes. Pretty soon he was all fagged out, and fell down panting; then he rolled over . . . kicking things every which way, and striking and grabbing at the air with his hands, and screaming . . . there was devils a-hold of him. He wore out by and by. . . . He says . . .
>
> "Tramp-tramp-tramp; that's the dead; tramp-tramp-tramp; they're coming after me; but I won't go. Oh, they're here; don't touch me—don't! hands off—they're cold; let go . . ."
>
> Then he went down on all fours and crawled off, begging them to let him alone . . .
>
> By and by he . . . jumped up on his feet looking wild . . . and went for me. He chased me round and round the place with a claspknife, calling me the Angel of Death, and saying he would

kill me, and then I wouldn't come for him no more. . . . Pretty soon he was all tired out . . . and said he would rest for a minute and then kill me.[15]

The sensation of snakes or bugs crawling on the skin should ring a bell with the abuser—this also occurs after high doses of stimulant drugs. In the context of alcohol withdrawal, it is an indication that the nervous system is rebounding from constant inhibition and is hyperexcitable.

Optimal treatment of patients during the early stages involves the administration of a benzodiazepine, such as chlordiazepoxide or diazepam (see Chapter 9). Because of the high degree of cross-dependence between alcohol and chlordiazepoxide, one drug can be substituted for the other and withdrawal continued at a safer rate.[16]

There is increasing recognition that some withdrawal symptoms can last for up to several weeks. Unstable blood pressure, irregular breathing, anxiety, panic attacks, insomnia, and depression are all reported during this period. These phenomena have been referred to as a protracted withdrawal syndrome, and they can trigger intense cravings for alcohol. Thus, some alcoholics might benefit from residential or inpatient treatment for up to six weeks, simply to prevent relapse during this critical period. To keep the alcoholic from resuming drinking for longer periods is a difficult task that is discussed in Chapter 12.

Physiological Effects

Peripheral Circulation

One effect of alcohol on the CNS is the dilation of the peripheral blood vessels. This increases heat loss from the body but makes the drinker feel warm. The heat loss and cooling of the interior of the body are enough to cause a slowdown in some biochemical processes. This dilation of the peripheral vessels argues against giving alcohol to individuals in shock or extreme cold. Under these conditions blood is needed in the central parts of the body, and heat loss must be diminished if the person is to survive.

Fluid Balance

One of the actions of alcohol on the brain is to decrease the output of the antidiuretic hormone (ADH, also called vasopressin) responsible for retaining fluid in the body. It is this effect, rather than the actual fluid consumption, that increases the urine flow in response to alcohol. This diuretic effect can lower blood pressure in some individuals.

Hormonal Effects

Even single doses of alcohol can produce measurable effects on a variety of hormonal systems: adrenal corticosteroids are released, as are catecholamines from the adrenal medulla, and the production of the male sex hormone testosterone is suppressed. It is not known what significance, if any, these effects have for occasional, moderate drinkers. However, chronic abusers of alcohol can develop a variety of hormone-related disorders, including testicular atrophy and impotence in men and impaired reproductive functioning in women.

ALCOHOL TOXICITY

Hangover

The Germans call it "wailing of cats" *(Katzenjammer)*, the Italians "out of tune" *(stonato)*, the French "woody mouth" *(gueule de boise)*, the Norwegians "workmen in my head" *(jeg har tommeermenn)*, and the Swedes "pain in the roots of the hair" *(hont i haret)*.[17] Hangovers aren't much fun. And they aren't very well understood, either. Even moderate drinkers who only occasionally overindulge are well acquainted with the symptoms: upset stomach, fatigue, headache, thirst, depression, anxiety, and general malaise.

Some authorities believe that the symptoms of a hangover are the symptoms of withdrawal from a short- or long-term dependence to alcohol. The pattern certainly fits. Some alcoholics report continuing to drink just to escape the pain of the hangover. This behavior is not unknown to moderate drinkers, either: many believe that the only cure for a hangover is some of "the hair of the dog that bit you"—alcohol. And it might work to minimize symptoms, because it spreads them out over a longer period of time. There is no evidence that any of the "surefire-this'll-fix-you-up" remedies are effective. The only known cures are an analgesic for the headache, rest, and time. Some of the ways to reduce the probability and the severity of a hangover are evident from the following discussion.

A study titled "Experimental Induction of Hangover"[18] provided support for two factors as contributing to the hangover syndrome: (1) the higher your BAC, the more likely you are to have a hangover, (2) with the *same* BAC, bourbon drinkers were more likely (two out of three) than vodka drinkers (one out of three) to have a hangover. This fits with the belief that some hangover symptoms are reactions to congeners. Congeners are natural products of the fermentation and preparation process, some of which are quite toxic. Congeners make the various alcoholic beverages different in smell, taste, color, and, possibly, hangover potential. Beer, with a 4 percent alcohol content, has only a 0.01 percent congener level, whereas wine has about 0.04 percent and distilled spirits between 0.1 and 0.2 percent congener level. Gin, being a mixture of almost pure alcohol and water, has a congener content about the same as wine, whereas a truly pure mixture of alcohol and water (vodka) has the same congener level as beer. Aging distilled spirits does not decrease the level of congeners—it increases their level about threefold.

Still other factors contribute to the trials and tribulations of the "morning after the night before." Thirst means that the body has excreted more fluid than was taken in with the alcoholic beverages. However, this does not seem to be the only basis for the thirst experienced the next day. Another cause might be that alcohol causes fluid inside cells to move outside the cells. This cellular dehydration, without a decrease in total body fluid, is known to be related to, and might be the basis of, an increase in thirst.

The nausea and upset stomach typically experienced can most likely be attributed to the fact that alcohol is a gastric irritant. Consuming even moderate amounts causes local irritation of the mucosa covering the stomach. It has been suggested that the accumulation of acetaldehyde, which is quite toxic even in small quantities, contributes to the nausea and headache. The headache can also be a reaction to fatigue. Fatigue sometimes results from a higher than normal level of activity while drinking. Increased activity frequently accompanies a decrease in inhibitions, a readily available source of energy, and a high blood sugar level. One of the effects of alcohol intake is to increase the blood sugar level for about an hour after ingestion. This can be followed several hours later by a low blood sugar level and an increased feeling of fatigue. Although hangover cures might be just around the corner, for now the only sure cure is time.

When alcohol intake occurs regularly and in large quantities over a period of years, physical dependence on the drug follows. Abrupt withdrawal from alcohol results in dangerous changes in body physiology. Before the dependence on addiction to alcohol reaches this point, physical symptoms sometimes develop, with facial appearance the first to be affected. The capillaries around the conjunctiva of the eyes become enlarged, and the skin of the face, forehead, and under the eyes becomes puffy and filled with fluid. In an individual with a fair complexion, the skin might appear continually flushed and, after prolonged use, a purple "whiskey nose" might develop. The frequent hoarseness of the alcoholic results from the accumulation of fluid in the mucous membranes of the nose, pharynx, larynx, and vocal cords. Continual ingestion of alcohol leads to an inflamed stomach associated with nausea and loss of appetite.

Chronic Disease States

The relationship of alcohol use to many diseases has been studied extensively and still continues. Let's review some of the major health concerns discussed in the National Institute on Alcohol Abuse and Alcoholism's (NIAAA's) 1993 report to Congress on alcohol and health.[8] As a general rule, heavy alcohol use, either directly or indirectly, affects every organ system in the body. The alcohol or its primary metabolite, acetaldehyde, can irritate and damage tissue directly. Because alcohol provides empty calories, many heavy drinkers do not eat well, and chronic malnutrition leads to tissue damage. Separating the effects of alcohol exposure from those of malnutrition relies to a great extent on experiments with animals, so that some animals can be fed adequate diets and exposed to high concentrations of alcohol, whereas other animals are fed diets deficient in certain vitamins or other nutrients.

Brain Damage

Perhaps the biggest concern is the damage to brain tissue that is seen in chronic alcoholics. It has been reported for years that the brains of deceased alcoholics demonstrate an obvious overall loss of brain tissue: the ventricles (internal spaces) in the brain are enlarged, and the fissures (sulci) in the cortex are widened. Modern imaging techniques, first CT scans and then MRIs, have demonstrated this tissue loss in living alcoholics as well. This generalized loss of brain tissue is probably a result of direct alcohol toxicity rather than malnutrition and is associated with *alcoholic dementia,* a global decline of intellect. Patients with this type of organic brain syndrome might have difficulty swallowing in addition to impaired problem solving, difficulty in manipulating objects, and abnormal electroencephalograms. Another classical alcohol-related organic brain syndrome has two parts, which so often go together that the disorder is referred to as **Wernicke-Korsakoff syndrome.** *Wernicke's disease* is associated with a deficiency of thiamine (vitamin B_1) and can sometimes be corrected nutritionally. The symptoms include confusion, ataxia (impaired coordination while walking), and abnormal eye movements. Most patients with Wernicke's disease also exhibit *Korsakoff's psychosis,* characterized by an inability to remember recent events or to learn new information. Korsakoff's psychosis can appear by itself in patients who maintain adequate nutrition, and it appears to be mostly irreversible. There has been great controversy about the specific brain areas that are damaged in Wernicke-Korsakoff syndrome, as well as about the relationship between the two parts of the disorder.

Important practical questions include the following. Exactly how much alcohol exposure is required before behavioral and/or anatomical evidence can be found indicating brain damage? And how much of the cognitive deficit seen in alcoholic dementia can be reversed when drinking is stopped and adequate nutrition is given? Both have been the subject of several experiments. As for the first question, there is no definitive answer. Some of the studies on moderate drinkers have included individuals who consume up to 10 drinks per day! Most studies with lower cutoffs for moderate drinking have not found consistent evidence for anatomical changes in the brain. As for recovery, several studies have reported both behavioral improvement and apparent regrowth of brain size in alcoholics after some months of abstinence. However, not all such studies find improvement, and some have found improvement in some types of mental tasks but not in others. There is some room for hope, especially in younger alcoholics.

Wernicke-Korsakoff syndrome: (*wer nick ee core sa kof*) chronic mental impairments produced by heavy alcohol use over a long period of time.

Liver Disorders

Fatty acids are the usual fuel for the liver. When present, alcohol has higher priority and is used as fuel instead. As a result, fatty acids (lipids) accumulate in the liver and are stored as small droplets in liver cells. This condition is known as alcohol-related *fatty liver*, which for most drinkers is not a serious problem. If alcohol input ceases, the liver uses the stored fatty acids for energy. Sometimes the droplets increase in size until they rupture the cell membrane, causing death of the liver cells. Before the liver cells die, a fatty liver is completely reversible and usually of minor medical concern.

Sometimes, with prolonged or high-level alcohol intake, another phase of liver damage is observed. This is alcoholic hepatitis, which is a serious disease and includes both inflammation and impairment of liver function. Usually this occurs in areas of the liver where cells are dead and dying, but it is not known if an increasingly fatty liver leads to alcoholic hepatitis. It is known that you can have alcoholic hepatitis in the absence of a fatty liver, so this form of tissue damage might be due to direct toxic effects of alcohol.

Cirrhosis is the liver disease everyone knows is related to high and prolonged levels of alcohol consumption. It's not easy to get cirrhosis from drinking alcohol—you have to work at it. Usually it takes about 10 years of steady drinking of the equivalent of a pint or more of whiskey a day. Not all cirrhosis is alcohol-related, but a high percentage is, and cirrhosis is the seventh leading cause of death in the United States. In large urban areas it is the fourth or fifth leading cause of death in men ages 25 to 65. In cirrhosis, liver cells are replaced by fibrous tissue (collagen), which changes the structure of the liver (Figure 11.4). These changes decrease blood flow and, along with the loss of cells, result in a decreased ability of the liver to function. When the liver does not function properly, fluid accumulates in the body, jaundice develops, and

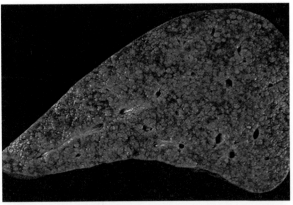

(a)

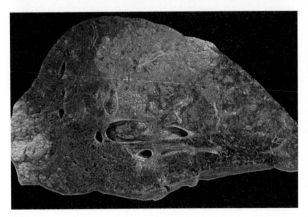

(b)

Figure 11-4   (a) Normal liver (b) cirrhotic liver.

other infections or cancers have a better opportunity to establish themselves in the liver. The yellow color of the jaundiced individual's skin (and in the whites of the eyes) is the result of bile pigment distributed throughout the body, but, most important, it is a sign that the liver is not functioning properly and that toxins are beginning to accumulate in the blood. Cirrhosis is not reversible, but stopping the intake of alcohol will retard its development and decrease the serious medical effects. The liver has a large reserve capacity and is able to function adequately with mild cirrhosis. One of the important unanswered questions is why not all alcoholics develop cirrhosis. Also, when comparing countries, there is an imperfect correlation between alcohol consumption and rates of cirrhosis. France, Portugal, Italy, and Spain, which are among the top per capita consumers of alcohol, also have the highest rates of cirrhosis. But Switzerland, which reports much lower per capita alcohol consumption than the United States, has a higher rate of cirrhosis than the United States. Differences in susceptibility to cirrhosis might reflect different drinking patterns, inherited susceptibilities, nutritional differences, or other factors.

In alcoholics with severely damaged livers, liver transplants have been quite successful—a 64 percent survival rate after two years. The success rate has been helped by the fact that most of these recipients do not resume drinking after the transplant.

Heart Disease

Another area of concern is the effect of alcohol on the heart and circulation. There is no doubt that heavy alcohol use is associated with increased mortality resulting from heart disease. Much of this is due to damage to the heart muscle (cardiomyopathy), but there is also an increased risk of the more typical heart attack resulting from coronary artery disease. Heavy drinkers are also more likely to suffer from high blood pressure and strokes. An interesting twist to this story is that several studies have found a *lower* incidence of heart attacks in moderate drinkers than in abstainers, and for several years there has been discussion about this protective effect of moderate alcohol consumption and the possible mechanism for it. It has been pointed out that the abstainers in such studies might include both abstaining alcoholics who once drank heavily and others who quit on their doctor's advice because of poor health. However, one study separated those who never drank

from the "quitters" and still reported fewer heart attacks and lower overall mortality in moderate drinkers, with increased mortality for both abstainers and heavy drinkers.[19] It has been proposed that alcohol increases high-density lipoproteins (HDL, sometimes called "good cholesterol"), some of which seem to protect against high blood pressure. The reduced blood clotting produced by alcohol could also play a role. There has been some speculation that red wine might have better effects than other forms of alcohol due to the presence of antioxidants in the grapes from which the wine is made. But the scientific evidence supports only a beneficial effect of alcohol on heart attacks, with an optimal effect occurring at about one drink per day.[20]

Cancer

Alcohol use is associated with cancers of the mouth, tongue, pharynx, larynx, esophagus, stomach, liver, lung, pancreas, colon, and rectum. There are many possible mechanisms for this, from direct tissue irritation to nutritional deficiencies to the induction of enzymes that activate other carcinogens. There is a particularly nasty interaction with cigarette smoking that increases the incidence of cancers of the oral cavity, pharynx, and larynx. Also, suppression of the immune system by alcohol, which occurs to some extent every time intoxicating doses are used, probably increases the rate of tumor growth.

The Immune System

The immune deficits seen in chronic alcoholics are associated with at least some increase in the frequency of various infectious diseases,

---

cirrhosis: (sir *oh* sis) an irreversible, frequently deadly liver disorder associated with heavy alcohol use.

including tuberculosis, pneumonia, yellow fever, cholera, and hepatitis B. Alcohol use might be a factor in AIDS, for several reasons: loss of behavioral inhibitions probably increases the likelihood of engaging in unprotected sex; alcohol could increase the risk of HIV infection in exposed individuals; and alcohol could suppress the immune system and therefore increase the chances of developing full-blown AIDS once an HIV infection is established. Although one epidemiological study did not find an acceleration of HIV-related disease in infected individuals who drank, heavy alcohol use is probably not a good idea for anyone who is HIV-positive.

After all is said and done, there is no evidence that the occasional drinking of one or two drinks has overall negative effects on the physical health of most individuals. An important exception to this statement might be drinking during pregnancy.

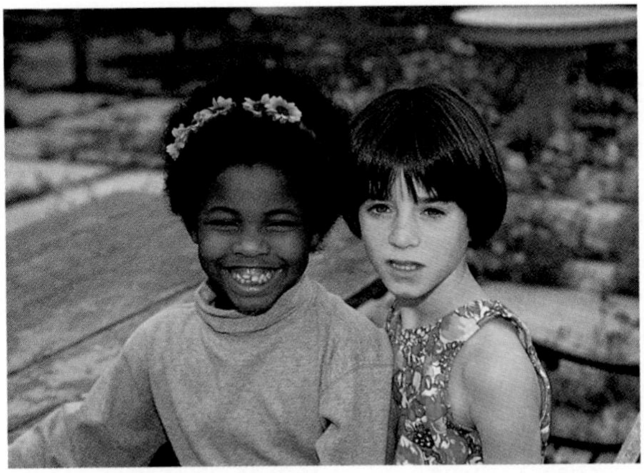

FETAL ALCOHOL SYNDROME

The unfortunate condition of infants born to alcoholic mothers was noted in an 1834 report to the British Parliament: they have a "starved, shriveled, and imperfect look." Until fairly recently most scientists and physicians believed that any effects on the offspring of heavy alcohol users were the result of poor nutrition or poor prenatal care. Those beliefs changed, however, when a 1973 article reported the following:

> Eight unrelated children of three different ethnic groups, all born to mothers who were chronic alcoholics, have a pattern of craniofacial, limb, and cardiovascular defects associated with prenatal-onset growth deficiency and developmental delay. This seems to be the first reported association between maternal alcoholism and aberrant morphogenesis in the offspring.[21]

That publication signaled the recognition of **fetal alcohol syndrome** (FAS), a collection of physical and behavioral abnormalities that seems to be caused by the presence of alcohol

Figure 11-5 Two girls born with fetal alcohol syndrome. Symptoms include small eyes, flattened bridge of the nose, and flattening of the vertical groove between the nose and mouth.

during development of the fetus (Figure 11.5). There are three primary criteria for diagnosing FAS, at least one of which *must* be present:

1. Growth retardation occurring before and/or after birth
2. A pattern of abnormal features of the face and head, including small head circumference, small eyes, or evidence of retarded formation of the midfacial area, including a flattened bridge and short length of the nose and flattening of the vertical groove between the nose and mouth (the philtrum)
3. Evidence of CNS abnormality, including abnormal neonatal behavior, mental retardation, or other evidence of abnormal neurobehavioral development

Each of these features can be seen in the absence of alcohol exposure, and other features might also be present in FAS, such as eye and ear defects, heart murmurs, undescended testicles, birthmarks, and abnormal fingerprints or palmar creases. Research also found a high frequency of various abnormalities of the eyes, often associated with poor vision.[22] Thus, the diagnosis of

FAS is a matter of judgment, based on several symptoms and often on the physician's knowledge of the mother's drinking history.

A large number of animal studies have been done in a variety of species, and they indicate that FAS is related to peak BAC and to duration of alcohol exposure, even when malnutrition is not an issue. In mice and other animal models, with increasing amounts of alcohol there is an increase in mortality, a decrease in infant weight, and increased frequency of soft-tissue malformation. The various components of the complete FAS reflect damage occurring at different developmental stages, so heavy alcohol exposure throughout pregnancy is the most damaging situation, followed by intermittent high-level exposure designed to imitate binge drinking.

By no means do all infants born to drinking mothers show abnormal development. If they did, it would not have taken so long to recognize FAS as a problem. Estimates of the prevalence of FAS in the overall population have ranged from 0.4 per 1,000 births to 2.9 per 1,000. Estimating the prevalence among problem drinkers or alcohol abusers is more of a problem. There is the difficulty not only of diagnosing FAS but also of diagnosing alcohol abuse. If the physician knows that the mother is a heavy drinker, this can increase the probability of noticing or diagnosing FAS, thus inflating the prevalence statistics among drinking mothers. FAS itself seems to occur in 23 to 29 per 1,000 births among women who are problem drinkers. If all alcohol-related birth defects (referred to as **fetal alcohol effect,** or FAE) are counted, the rate among heavy-drinking women is higher, from 80 to a few hundred per 1,000. Maternal alcohol abuse might be the most frequent known environmental cause of mental retardation in the Western world.

In addition to the risk of FAS, the fetus of a mother who drinks heavily has a risk of not being born at all. Spontaneous abortion early in pregnancy is perhaps twice as likely among the 5 percent of women who are the heaviest drinkers. The data on later pregnancy loss (stillbirths) are not as clearly related to alcohol for either animals or humans.

An important question, and one that can never be answered in absolute terms, is whether there is an acceptable level of alcohol consumption for pregnant women (see the Taking Sides box). The data on drinking during pregnancy rely on self-reports by the mothers, who are assumed to be at least as likely as everyone else to underreport their drinking. In addition, almost every study that has been done has used different definitions of heavy drinking, alcohol abuse, and problem drinking. It is clear that the heaviest drinkers in each study are the most at risk for alcohol-related problems with their children, but we don't really know if the large number of light or moderate drinkers are causing significant risks. Based on the dose-related nature of birth problems in animal studies, one might argue that any alcohol use at all produces some risk, but at low levels the increased risk is too small to be revealed except in a large-scale study. In 1981, the U.S. surgeon general recommended that "pregnant women should drink absolutely no alcohol because they may be endangering the health of their unborn children." Maybe that's going a bit too far. The bottom line is this: scientific data do not demonstrate that occasional consumption of one or two drinks definitely causes FAS or other alcohol-related birth defects. On the other hand, neither do the data prove that low-level alcohol use is safe nor do they indicate a safe level of use. Remember

fetal alcohol syndrome: facial and developmental abnormalities associated with the mother's alcohol use during pregnancy.

fetal alcohol effect: individual developmental abnormalities associated with the mother's alcohol use during pregnancy.

Taking Sides

Protecting the Unborn from Alcohol

Increased concern about fetal alcohol syndrome has led to some significant changes in the status of pregnant women, at least in certain instances and certain locations. Waiters have refused to serve wine to pregnant women, women have been arrested and charged with child abuse for being heavily intoxicated while pregnant, and others have been charged with endangerment for breastfeeding while drunk. These social interventions represent concerns for the welfare of the child. However, to women already concerned about their own rights because of the issue of government regulation of abortion, such actions seem to be yet another infringement, yet another signal that the woman's rights are secondary to the child's.

We know that heavy alcohol consumption during pregnancy does increase the risk to the child of permanent disfigurement and mental retardation. We also know that, even among the heaviest drinkers, the odds still favor a normal-appearing baby (less than 10 percent of the babies born to the heaviest-drinking 5 percent of mothers exhibit full-blown FAS).

Do you think that men are more likely than women to support limiting the rights of pregnant women to drink while they are pregnant? You might ask a group of both men and women to give you answers to the following questions.

How strongly do you agree (5 = strong agreement, 1 = strong disagreement) with the following statements?

1. Women who repeatedly get drunk while they are pregnant should be kept in jail if necessary until the baby is born.
2. All bartenders should be trained not to serve any drinks at all to a woman who is obviously pregnant.
3. If a man and a pregnant woman are drinking together and both become intoxicated, both the man and the woman should be arrested for child abuse.

For more on this topic, log on to www.dushkin. com/online for current news and links to other popular and informative sites, as well as time-saving web search strategies and study tools.

from Chapter 7 that it is not within the realm of science to declare something totally safe, so it will be impossible ever to set a safe limit on alcohol use. It is good to know that most women decrease their alcohol use once they have become pregnant, and many decrease it further as pregnancy progresses.

SUMMARY

- Alcohol is made by yeasts in a process called fermentation. Distillation is used to increase the alcohol content of a beverage.
- Beer has the lowest alcohol content of the traditional beverages and is consumed in much greater volumes than wine or liquor. Beer consumption has not changed greatly in the past decade.

- Wine consumption increased until the mid-1980s and has declined somewhat since then.
- Consumption of distilled spirits, especially of the stronger-tasting whiskeys, has declined considerably over the past 15 years.
- Alcohol is metabolized by the liver at a constant rate, which is not much influenced by body size.
- The exact mechanism by which alcohol affects the nervous system is still not known but might involve the neurotransmitter GABA.
- By the use of simple calculations and Table 11.3, it is possible to estimate a person's blood alcohol concentration if you know how many drinks he or she consumed over what period of time.
- Alcohol appears to enhance interest in sex but to impair physiological arousal in both sexes.

- The alcohol withdrawal syndrome is referred to as delirium tremens.
- Chronic heavy drinking can lead to neurological damage, as well as damage to the heart and liver. However, light drinking has been associated with a decrease in heart attacks.
- Recognition of fetal alcohol syndrome and fetal alcohol effect since 1973 has led to educational and other programs aimed at preventing this important cause of mental retardation.

REVIEW QUESTIONS

1. What is fortified wine, and why was it invented?
2. Grain neutral spirits are 95 percent alcohol. What is its proof?
3. The largest-selling brand of beer has about what share of the overall domestic market?
4. The experimental drug RO 15-4513 has what effect on an intoxicated rat? *Makes it sober*
5. What is the typical behavior of a person with a BAC of 0.20 percent?
6. Describe the stages of alcohol withdrawal syndrome in a very heavy drinker.
7. Why does bourbon produce more hangover symptoms than vodka?
8. What are the behavioral characteristics of Korsakoff's psychosis?
9. How might alcohol play a role in contracting AIDS?
10. What are the three defining characteristics of FAS?

REFERENCES

1. Shaken and stirred: The state of the liquor industry, *Washington Post*, Nov 12, 1996.
2. Data courtesy of *Modern Brewery Age.* 1998.

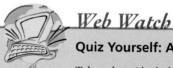

Web Watch

Quiz Yourself: Alcohol Risks

Take the Alcohol Quiz at library. thinkquest.org/29500/addictions/alcohol.quiz.shtml to learn about the effects of alcohol on the body and the risks that come with these effects.

Quiz Yourself: Alcoholism

The website www.mayohealth.org/mayo/9707/htm/ alcohol.htm offers various assessments about alcoholism. Complete the assessments "Assess Yourself" and "Assess Someone Else" to find out whether or not your lifestyle or a friend's lifestyle gives evidence of struggling with alcoholism.

Quiz Yourself: Drinking Behavior

The site www.indiana.edu/~caps/flyers/selfalcohol. html is sponsored by the Indiana University Health Center and offers an assessment of your drinking and related behavior. Explore your own approach to drinking in certain situations. This site also offers advice and resources for help.

3. Williams GD and others: *NIAAA surveillance report #51: Apparent per capita alcohol consumption.* Bethesda, MD: USPHS, 1999.
4. Suter PM and others: The effect of ethanol on fat storage in healthy subjects, *New England Journal of Medicine* 326:983, 1992.
5. Frezza M and others: High blood alcohol levels in women: The role of decreased gastric alcohol dehydrogenase activity and first-pass metabolism, *New England Journal of Medicine* 322:95, 1990.
6. NIAAA: *Alcohol alert,* Bethesda, MD: USPHS, 1997.
7. Gibbons B: Alcohol, the legal drug, *National Geographic,* Feb, 1992.
8. *Eighth special report to the U.S. Congress on alcohol and health.* Bethesda, MD: USPHS, 1993.
9. Goldberg L: Quantitative studies on alcohol tolerance in man, *Acta Physiologica Scandinavica* 5(16): 1–128, 1943.
10. Bogen E: The human toxicology of alcohol. In Emerson H, editor: *Alcohol and man.* New York: Macmillan, 1932.
11. Crothers TD: Alcoholic trance, *Popular Science* 26:189, 191, 1884.
12. Shakespeare W: *Macbeth,* Act II, Scene 1.
13. Wilson GT, Lawson DM: Effects of alcohol on sexual arousal in women, *Journal of Abnormal Psychology* 85(5):489–497, 1976.

14. Briddell DW, Wilson GT: Effects of alcohol and expectancy set on male sexual arousal, *Journal of Abnormal Psychology* 85(2):225–234, 1976.

15. Twain M: *The adventures of Huckleberry Finn,* 1885.

16. Mayo-Smith ME: Pharmacological management of alcohol withdrawal: a meta-analysis and evidence-based practice guideline, *Journal of the American Medical Association* 278:144–151, 1997.

17. Brody J: Personal health, *The New York Times,* p C13, Dec 27, 1976.

18. Chapman LF: Experimental induction of hangover, *Quarterly Studies on Alcohol* (Suppl 5), pp 67–86, 1970.

19. DeLabry LO and others: Alcohol consumption and mortality in an American male population: Recovering the u-shaped curve—findings from the normative aging study, *Journal of Studies on Alcohol* 53:25–32, 1992.

20. Alcohol and the heart: Consensus emerges, *Harvard Health Letter* 6(5): 1996.

21. Jones KL and others: Pattern of malformation in offspring of chronic alcoholic mothers, *Lancet* 1(7815):1267–1271, 1973.

22. Stromland K, Hellstrom A: Fetal alcohol syndrome: An opthalmological and socioeducational prospective study, *Pediatrics* 97:845–850, 1996.

Chapter 12

Alcohol and Society

KEY TERMS

temperance

prohibition

expectancies

alcoholism

balanced placebo

genetic marker

Antabuse

controlled drinking

abstinence

Online Learning Center Resources

www.mhhe.com/ray

Log on to our Online Learning Center (OLC) for access to these additional resources.

- Chapter definitions
- Learning objectives
- Student interactive question-and-answer sites
- Self-scoring chapter quiz

The OLC also offers web links for study and exploration of health topics. Here are some examples of what you'll find:

www.habitsmart.com/chkup.html

This website asks you to view your alcohol risk from a new perspective. It assesses the number of drinks and specific amounts of alcohol you consume over a period of time, your drinking patterns, and various drinking situations. It not only addresses how much you drink but also why.

www.edc.org/hec/pubs/cara

Environmental approaches to substance-abuse prevention are outlined on this website. The articles posted are about assessment, problem-oriented prevention, scanning exercises, analysis exercises, response, and students' voices in prevention. Take the Party Risk Assessment and the On-Sale Alcohol Outlet Risk Assessment and look over selected publications and resources.

www.promprac.gmu.edu/articles/digest1.html

Check out this article "Dealing with Alcohol Abuse on Campus," posted on this website. This article addresses the numbers of college students engaged in alcohol abuse around the country and outlines prevention efforts.

Drugs in the Media

Linking Alcohol with Violence in the News

Among the nation's drinkers, many are underage and more than one-third "binge drink" (defined as the consumption of five or more drinks at a time for men and four or more for women). Since the term *binge drinking* was first used by the Harvard School of Public Health in a study of alcohol use by Massachusetts college students in the 1990s, the news media have focused greater attention on alcohol-related tragedies among college students, including acute alcohol poisoning, falls, drownings, automobile collisions, homicides, and sexual assaults.

Among the general public, however, one of the interesting things about the involvement of alcohol in violence is that it's so common that it often is *not* seen as newsworthy. For example, a few years ago a local newspaper article in a small town reported an incident that occurred in the wee hours of a Saturday morning. Two men got into an argument over a piece of leftover meatloaf, and one stabbed the other with a butcher knife. The article didn't mention alcohol involvement, but it seemed likely. A curious reader happened to be a sheriff's deputy and was able to get a copy of the arrest report. Sure enough, both men had high BACs (one was above 0.20%).

Such incidents are more common than you might think. Another example is that of a man in Los Angeles who was reportedly having trouble parking his car properly in front of a nightclub. Some bystanders were taunting him, and he proceeded to shoot one of the hecklers. Again, the newspaper didn't mention that he had been drinking, but the circumstances indicate a high probability that he was.

Some newspapers have recently begun to make more of an effort to look into the connection between alcohol and violence, or at least to state in the report that "it is not known" whether alcohol was involved, if they are not certain. But often the issue is not addressed at all. Check out the Saturday and Sunday newspapers for two or three weeks, and listen to local television weekend news coverage. One neighbor shooting another on a Sunday afternoon because the victim shoveled snow onto the shooter's driveway? Too much beer during a televised football game, maybe? See how many reports you can find for which it seems likely that alcohol was a contributing factor. Does the news report state or imply that drinking was involved, or does it avoid the issue entirely? In any newspaper reports you find of violence on college campuses, is the issue of alcohol involvement discussed more often than in the reports of violence among the general population?

ALCOHOL USE AND "THE ALCOHOL PROBLEM"

Historians seem to agree that, at the time of America's revolution against the English in the late 1700s, most Americans drank alcoholic beverages and most people valued these beverages compared with drinking water, which was often contaminated. The per capita consumption of alcohol was apparently much greater than current levels, and little public concern was expressed. Even the early Puritan ministers, who were moralistic about all kinds of behavior, referred to alcoholic drink as "the Good Creature of God." They denounced drunkenness as a sinful misuse of the "Good Creature" but clearly placed the blame on the sinner, not on alcohol itself.[1]

Because American colonial history and American law evolved from English law, it is worth noting that England had tried to control drunkenness as early as 1327 by limiting the number of establishments that could sell alcoholic beverages. Drunkenness apparently continued, and this first law was repealed. Other regulations were passed over the years, but none of them attacked alcohol per se; nor did they attempt to prevent "normal," moderate use of alcoholic beverages.

A new view of alcohol as the *cause* of serious problems began to emerge in America soon after the Revolution. That view took root and still exists as a major influence in American culture today. It is so pervasive that some people have a hard time understanding what is meant by the "demonization" of alcohol (viewing alcohol as a demon, or devil). The concept is important, partly because alcohol was the first psychoactive substance to become demonized in American culture, leading the way for similar views of cocaine, heroin, and marijuana in this century. What we are referring to is a tendency to view a substance as an *active* (sometimes almost purposeful) source of *evil,* damaging everything it touches. Whenever harmful consequences result from the use of something (firearms and nuclear energy are other possible examples), there are those who find it easiest to simply view that thing as "bad" and avoid all contact with it. Such a view of alcohol might be personally convenient for an alcoholic if it helps him or her to stay sober, but it is too simple an explanation for the social scientist or policy maker who needs to understand the complex interplay between alcohol and human society. The danger is that alcohol (or marijuana, cocaine, or heroin) can become a scapegoat, thus causing us to ignore all the other factors contributing to whatever problem we might be concerned about. Later in this chapter, we will examine this social interplay in more detail. For now, let's ask how this "new" idea about alcohol as a demon developed about 200 years ago.

The Temperance Movement in America

The first writings indicating a negative view of alcohol itself are attributed to a prominent Philadelphia physician named Benjamin Rush, one of the signers of the Declaration of Independence. Rush's 1784 pamphlet, "An Inquiry into the Effects of Ardent Spirits on the Mind and Body," was aimed particularly at distilled spirits (*ardent* means "burning" "fiery"), not at the weaker beverages, such as beer and wine. As a physician, Rush had noticed a relationship between heavy drinking and jaundice (an indicator of liver disease), "madness" (perhaps the delirium tremens of withdrawal, what we now call Korsakoff's psychosis), and "epilepsy" (probably the seizures seen during withdrawal). All of those are currently accepted and well-documented consequences of heavy alcohol use and were reviewed in Chapter 11. However, Rush also concluded that hard liquor damaged the drinker's morality, leading to a variety of antisocial, immoral, and criminal behaviors. Although the correlation between these types of behavior and alcohol use had been documented many times, Rush believed that this was a direct toxic action of distilled spirits on the part of the brain responsible for morality. Rush then introduced for the first time the concept of *addiction* to a psychoactive substance, describing the uncontrollable and overwhelming desires for alcohol experienced by some of his patients. For the first time this condition was referred to as a *disease* (caused by alcohol), and he recommended total abstinence from alcohol for those who were addicted.[1]

Other physicians readily recognized these symptoms in their own patients, and physicians became the first leaders of the **temperance**

---

temperance: (temp a rance) the idea that people should drink beer or wine in moderation but drink no hard liquor.

movement. What Rush proposed, and most early followers supported, was that everyone should avoid distilled spirits entirely, because they were considered to be toxic, and should consume beer and wine in a *temperate,* or moderate, manner. Temperance societies were formed in many parts of the country, at first among the upper classes of physicians, ministers, and businesspeople. In the early 1800s, it became possible, and fashionable, for the middle classes to join the elite in this movement, and hundreds of thousands of American businesspeople, farmers, lawyers, teachers, and their families "took the pledge" to avoid spirits and to be temperate in their use of beer or wine.

In the second half of the nineteenth century, things changed. Up to this time there had been little consumption of commercial beer in the United States. It was only with the advent of artificial refrigeration and the addition of hops, which helped preserve the beer, that there was an increase in the number of breweries. The waves of immigrants who entered the country in this period provided the necessary beer-drinking consumers. At first, encouraged by temperance groups that preferred beer consumption to the use of liquor, breweries were constructed everywhere. However, alcohol-related problems did not disappear. Instead, disruptive, drunken behavior became increasingly associated in the public's mind with the new wave of immigrants—Irish, Italians, and eastern Europeans, more often Catholic than Protestant—and they drank beer and wine. Temperance workers now advocated total abstinence from all alcoholic beverages, and pressure grew to prohibit the sale of alcohol altogether.

Prohibition

The first state **prohibition** period began in 1851 when Maine passed its prohibition law. Between 1851 and 1855, 13 states passed statewide prohibition laws, but by 1868 nine had repealed them.

The National Prohibition Party, organized in 1874, provided the impetus for the second wave of statewide prohibition, which developed in the 1880s. From 1880 to 1889 seven states adopted prohibition laws, but by 1896 four had repealed them.

In 1899, a group of educators, lawyers, and clergymen described the saloon as the "working-man's club, in which many of his leisure hours are spent, and in which he finds more of the things that approximate luxury than in his home. . . ." They went on to say: "It is a centre of learning, books, papers, and lecture hall to them. It is the clearinghouse for common intelligence, the place where their philosophy of life is worked out, and their political and social beliefs take their beginnings."[2] Truth lay somewhere between those statements and the sentiments expressed in a sermon:

> The liquor traffic is the most fiendish, corrupt and hell-soaked institution that ever crawled out of the slime of the eternal pit. It is the open sore of this land. . . . It takes the kind, loving husband and father, smothers every spark of love in his bosom, and transforms him into a heartless wretch, and makes him steal the shoes from his starving babe's feet to find the price for a glass of liquor. It takes your sweet innocent daughter, robs her of her virtue and transforms her into a brazen, wanton harlot. . . .
>
> The open saloon as an institution has its origin in hell, and it is manufacturing subjects to be sent back to hell.[3]

Prohibition was not just a matter of "wets" versus "drys" or a matter of political conviction or health concerns. Intricately interwoven with these factors was a middle-class, rural, Protestant, evangelical concern that the good and true life was being undermined by ethnic groups with a different religion and a lower standard of living and morality. One way to strike back at these groups was through prohibition.

Between 1907 and 1919, 34 states enacted legislation enforcing statewide prohibition, whereas only two states repealed their prohibition laws. By 1917, 64 percent of the population lived in dry territory, and between 1908 and 1917 over 100,000 licensed bars were closed.

It should also be remembered that the fact that there was a state prohibition law did not mean that the residents did not drink. They did, both legally and illegally. They drank illegally in speakeasies and other private clubs. They drank legally from a variety of the many patent medicines that were freely available. A few of the more interesting ones were Whisko, "a nonintoxicating stimulant" at 55 proof; Golden's Liquid Beef Tonic, "recommended for treatment of alcohol habit" with 53 proof; and Kaufman's Sulfur Bitters, which "contains no alcohol" but was in fact 20 percent alcohol (40 proof) and contained no sulfur.

In August 1917, the U.S. Senate adopted a resolution, authored by Andrew Volstead, that submitted the national prohibition amendment to the states. The U.S. House of Representatives concurred in December, and 21 days later, on January 8, 1918, Mississippi became the first state to ratify the Eighteenth Amendment. A year later, January 16, 1919, Nebraska was the 36th state to ratify the amendment, and the deed was done.

As stated in the amendment, a year after the 36th state ratified it, national prohibition came into effect—on January 16, 1920. The amendment was simple, with only two operational parts:

Section 1. After one year from the ratification of this article the manufacture, sale or transportation of intoxicating liquors within, the importation thereof into, or the exportation thereof from the United States and all territory subject to the jurisdiction thereof for beverage purposes is hereby prohibited.

Section 2. The Congress and the several States shall have concurrent power to enforce this article by appropriate legislation.

The beginning of prohibition was hailed in a radio sermon by popular preacher Billy Sunday:

The reign of tears is over. The slums will soon be a memory. We will turn our prisons into factories and our jails into storehouses and corncribs. Men will walk upright now, women will smile, and the children will laugh. Hell will be forever for rent.[1]

The law did not result in an alcohol-free society, and this came as quite a surprise to many people. Apparently the assumption was that prohibition would be so widely accepted that little enforcement would be necessary. Along with saloons, breweries, and distilleries, hospitals that had specialized in the treatment of alcoholics closed their doors, presumably because there would no longer be a need for them.[4]

It soon became clear that people were buying and selling alcohol illegally and that enforcement of prohibition was not going to be easy. The majority of the population might have supported the idea of prohibition, but such a large minority insisted on continuing to drink that *speakeasies, hip flasks,* and *bathtub gin* became household words. Organized crime became both more organized and vastly more profitable as a result of prohibition.

The popular conception is that prohibition was a total failure, leading to its repeal. That is not the whole picture. Prohibition did have the apparent effect of reducing overall alcohol intake. Hospital admissions for alcoholism and deaths from alcoholism declined sharply at the beginning of prohibition. During the 1920s, it appears that the prohibition laws were increasingly violated, particularly in large eastern cities, such as New York, and the rates of alcoholism and alcohol-related deaths began to

prohibition: laws prohibiting all sales of alcoholic beverages in the United States in the period of 1920–1933.

increase.[5] But even toward the end of the "noble experiment," as Prohibition was called by its detractors, alcoholism and alcohol-related deaths were still lower than before Prohibition.

If Prohibition did reduce alcohol-related problems, why was it repealed? In 1926, the Association Against Prohibition was founded by a small group of America's wealthiest men, including the heads of many of the largest corporations in America. Their primary concern seems to have been the income taxes they were paying. Historically, taxes on alcohol had been one of the primary sources of revenue for the federal government. Indeed, the federal government relied heavily on alcohol taxes before the income tax was initiated in 1913. A major hope of the repeal supporters was that income taxes could be reduced. There was also fear that the widespread and highly publicized disrespect for the Prohibition law encouraged a sense of "lawlessness," not just among the bootleggers and gangsters but in the public at large. The Great Depression, which began in 1929, not only made more people consider the value of tax revenues but also increased fears of a generalized revolt. If Prohibition weakened respect for law and order, it had to go.[1]

The Eighteenth Amendment was repealed by the Twenty-First Amendment, proposed in Congress on February 20, 1933, and ratified by 36 states by December 5 of that year. So ended an era. The Twenty-First Amendment was also short and sweet:

> Section 1. The eighteenth article of amendment of the Constitution of the United States is hereby repealed.
>
> Section 2. The transportation or importation into any State, Territory, or possession of the United States for delivery or use therein of intoxicating liquors, in violation of the laws thereof, is hereby prohibited.

When national Prohibition ended, America did not return overnight to the pre-1920s levels of alcohol consumption. Sales increased until after World War II, at which point per capita consumption was approximately what it had been before Prohibition. Thus, the prohibition of alcohol, much like the current prohibitions of marijuana and heroin, did work in that it reduced alcohol availability, alcohol use, and related problems. On the other hand, even at its best it did not allow us to close all the jails and mental hospitals, and it encouraged organized crime and created expensive enforcement efforts.

Regulation After 1933

After national Prohibition, control over alcohol was returned to the states. Each state has since had its own means of regulating alcohol. Although a few states remained totally dry after national Prohibition, most allowed at least beer sales. Thus, the temperance sentiment that beer was a safer beverage continued to influence policy. In many cases, beer containing no more than 3.2 percent alcohol by weight was allowed as a "nonintoxicating" beverage. Even states that remained dry, such as Kansas and Oklahoma, allowed 3.2 percent beer. As we saw in Chapter 11, alcohol is alcohol, and 3.2 percent beer *is* intoxicating.

Over the years the general trend was for a relaxation of laws: states that did not allow sales of liquor became fewer until in 1966 the last dry state, Mississippi, became wet. The minimum age to purchase alcoholic beverages was set at 21 in all states except New York and Louisiana before 1970, when the national voting age was lowered to 18. During the 1970s, 30 states lowered the drinking age to 18 or 19. Per capita consumption rates, which were relatively stable during the 1950s, increased steadily from 1965 through 1980. However, times have changed; pushed by concerns over young people dying in alcohol-related traffic accidents, in the 1980s Congress authorized the Transportation Department to withhold a portion of the federal highway funds for any state that did not raise its minimum drinking age to 21. In 1988, the final state raised its drinking age, making 21 the uniform drinking age all across the United States.

Taxation

Federal taxes on alcoholic beverages are a significant means of gathering money for the federal government. Although most of the federal revenue comes from individual income taxes, taxes on alcohol produce about 1 percent of the total collections by the Internal Revenue Service ($7.2 billion in 1999). The states also collect almost $4 billion each year in excise taxes and license fees for alcoholic beverages. When all these are added up, over half the consumer's cost for an average bottle of distilled spirits is taxes. In 1991, after hearing arguments that taxes on alcoholic beverages had not kept up with inflation, Congress initiated a significant tax increase: the beer tax doubled to $18 per barrel, the tax on bottled wine increased sixfold to about 22¢ per bottle, and the tax on distilled spirits rose less than 10 percent to $13.50 per gallon of 100-proof liquor.[6] There was some controversy about how much such an increase would affect sales, especially because at the same time most producers increased their own prices by about 5 percent. The total increase in cost to the consumer (averaging about 10 percent more) did result in about a 2 percent decrease in sales of beer and liquor during the first half of the year. Domestic wine sales decreased even more, almost 9 percent. That such large price increases resulted in fairly modest declines in purchases might indicate that very large tax increases would be needed if part of the goal were to reduce alcohol intake significantly.

WHO DRINKS? AND WHY?

Cultural Influences on Drinking

Comparing alcohol use in various cultures around the world gives us a chance to look at ethnic and social factors that lead to differences in patterns of alcohol use. For example, both the Irish and the Russian cultures are associated with heavy drinking, especially of distilled spirits. This has been attributed to several factors, including early invasions by the hard-drinking Vikings at a time when each of these regions was beginning to develop a national identity. Also, both regions experienced frequent famine, and they were not exposed to the notion of individual potential that characterized the Renaissance or to the notions of individual responsibility and sobriety that came with the Protestant Reformation.[7] Americans of Irish descent have been studied and found to have higher rates of alcohol-related problems than other ethnic groups. A comparison of Irish Americans with Italian Americans is of interest: the Irish forbid children and adolescents from learning to drink, but they seem to expect adult men to drink large quantities. They value hard liquor more than beer and promote drinking in pubs, away from family influences. By contrast, Italian families give their children wine from an early age in a family setting but disapprove of intoxication at any age.[8]

The French drink primarily wine and consume it in the family setting and with meals, so it might be expected that they would not have many heavy drinkers or drinking-related problems. Unfortunately, the French consume more alcohol per capita than any other nation and have the highest rates of alcoholism, suicide, and deaths from cirrhosis of the liver.[9] The French associate wine drinking with virility, and French working men have traditionally consumed large amounts of wine during the work day (it was not unusual for a French laborer to consume a liter of wine with lunch). In today's postindustrial society, fewer farm and factory workers translates to a drop in the consumption of lower-quality wines. That, combined with a greater tendency to stay home and watch television instead of going to a bistro in the evenings, has led to a decrease in wine consumption in France, but it is still high relative to other countries.

Regional Differences in the United States

In the United States it has been true for many years that about one-third of the adult population label themselves as abstainers. The two-thirds who use alcohol consume an amount that averages out to about three drinks per day. Most of us don't drink anything near that amount—in fact, another consistent finding is that half the alcohol is consumed by about 10 percent of the drinkers.

Whites are more likely to drink than blacks, northerners more than southerners, younger adults more than older, Catholics and Jews more than Protestants, nonreligious more than religious, urban more than rural, large-city dwellers more than small-city residents, and college-educated people more than those with only a high school or grade school education.

Figure 12.1 shows estimated overall alcohol consumption combining beer, wine, and distilled spirits (about half the total U.S. alcohol consumption comes from beer) for each state, based on sales.[10] Nevada and New Hampshire have the highest per capita sales, followed by the District of Columbia. The District of Columbia is the leader in consumption of wine, whereas Nevada consumes the most beer. Note the generally low consumption in the southern states and the generally higher consumption in the western states, with the notable exception of Utah, which has a large Mormon population. These differences in per capita sales reflect

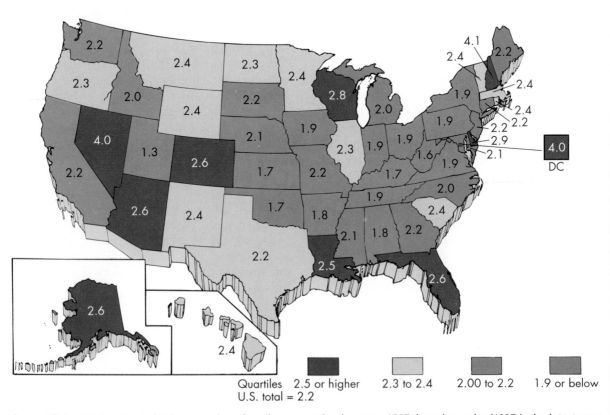

Figure 12-1   Total estimated U.S. per capita ethanol consumption by state, 1997, based on sales (1997 is the latest year for which statistics are available).

differences in the proportion of drinkers in various parts of the country. If the sales figures are divided by the estimated number of drinkers rather than by the total population, it appears that southern drinkers might consume at higher levels than northern drinkers.[11]

One theory about heavy drinking proposes that the populations of people who experience a great deal of social stress and tension (as in cities) and who approve of the use of alcohol to release tension and stress drink more and have more drinking problems. One study compared the various states with regard to such stress indicators as business failures, unemployment, divorces, abortions, disasters, percentage of new residents, and high school dropout rates. On the overall state stress index, Nevada and Alaska scored the highest, Iowa and Nebraska the lowest. Alcohol norms were rated based on the percentage of fundamentalist or Mormon church members, the percentage of dry areas in the state, the number of liquor outlets per capita, and the number of hours per week allowed for drinking in bars. On this scale Mississippi and Utah were the most restricted, Nevada and Wisconsin the least. Overall, both the stress index and the drinking norms were significantly correlated with indicators of heavy drinking and alcohol-related arrests.[12]

Gender Differences

Looking at individual people, efforts to relate personality factors to drinking have not been terribly enlightening. Researchers have been studying the learned **expectancies** each of us has about what alcohol is for and what it does. We learn much of what we expect alcohol to do even before we take our first drink, from books, movies, and other people. One study reported that men who have strong expectations that alcohol will lead to increased social and physical pleasure and to sexual enhancement are most likely to drink heavily, whereas among women the heaviest drinkers are those who believe that alcohol will reduce tension.[13] You can see how these different expectancies might lead to different types of drinking

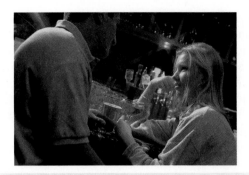

Alcohol abuse by college students usually takes place through binge drinking, five or more drinks in a row.

in different situations, thus complicating attempts to predict simply who drinks and how much. Combining those differences in beliefs about alcohol with a greater pharmacological effect of alcohol on the average woman, as reviewed in Chapter 11, means that men and women differ with respect to predictions of problem drinking and alcoholism.

Drinking Among College Students

The college years have traditionally been associated with alcohol use, and in 1999 the proportion of drinkers was indeed about 10 percent higher among 18- to 22-year-old college students than among others of that age (e.g., about 63 percent of college students reported drinking within the past month, compared with about 52 percent of other 18- to 22-year-olds in the NIDA household survey described in Chapter 1).[14] Colleges and universities have followed the lead established by the federal government's mandating a uniform 21-year-old drinking age, and many campuses have banned the sale or advertising of alcohol. Many fraternities have banned keg parties and the use of alcohol during "rush," partly

---

expectancies: learned beliefs about the effects of alcohol or another drug.

out of concern for legal liability for the consequences if a guest becomes intoxicated and has an accident. In spite of the changes in laws and rules, drinking behavior itself has not changed much in the past few years. In fact, there is some evidence that, among college drinkers, there might be a slightly increased incidence of some alcohol-related problems, such as fighting, vandalism, poor grades, trouble with the police, and missing class because of hangovers.[15] These adverse consequences might result from more students drinking off campus in less controlled and less friendly environments. One ray of hope is that today's college students are less likely than those of the early 1980s to drive after drinking.

Health Quest Activities

Making decisions about alcohol while reading about the risks may differ from making a decision when faced with peer pressure. Complete the "Alcohol Decision Maze" in Module 8. Do you think the decisions you made about alcohol consumption were wise? Do you often feel pressured by others to drink or abuse alcohol when you would rather not? Do you drive after drinking or ride with someone who has been drinking? When you make up your mind ahead of time about how much alcohol you will drink in an evening, do you usually stick with it? What could you do to be more careful when drinking?

In Module 8, under *Our Changing World*, you'll find the article "Responsible Drinking Behavior." After reading the article, take a poll of classmates or other students. Ask the following questions. Do you believe you practice responsible drinking behavior? How many days a week do you drink? How many alcoholic beverages do you consume on the days that you drink? In the past month, how many times have you driven after drinking or ridden with someone who has been drinking? Make a chart reporting your findings and share it in class.

Time-Out and Alcohol Myopia

It has been pointed out that many of the effects experienced by drinkers are based on what they expect to happen, which interacts somewhat with the pharmacological effects of alcohol. One important component of alcohol use is that drinking serves as a social signal, to the drinker and others, indicating a "time-out" from responsibilities, work, and seriousness. Sitting down with a drink indicates "I'm off duty now" and "Don't take anything I say too seriously." Steele and Josephs have proposed[16] that alcohol induces a kind of social and behavioral myopia, or nearsightedness. After drinking, people tend to focus more on the here and now and to pay less attention to long-term consequences. That might be why some people are more violent after drinking, whereas others become more helpful to others even if there is personal risk or cost involved. The idea is that alcohol releases people from their inhibitions, largely because the inhibitions represent concerns about what might happen, whereas the intoxicated individual focuses on the immediate irritant or the person who needs help right now.

SOCIAL PROBLEMS

Driving Under the Influence

Attention was focused in the early 1980s on the large number of traffic fatalities involving alcohol. The total number of traffic fatalities in 1980 was over 50,000, but by 1983 that had dropped to nearer 40,000, where it has remained since.[17] It is difficult to estimate exactly how many of those fatalities are *caused* by alcohol, but we can obtain some relevant information. Many states mandate that the coroner measure blood alcohol in all fatally injured drivers. Based on those measurements, estimates have been made of the number of alcohol-related traffic crash fatalities. From the peak of over 42 percent in 1982, by 1997 the percentage had declined to around 30 percent.[17]

Several studies have demonstrated that the danger of combining alcohol with automobiles is dose-related. At a BAC of 0.08 percent the relative risk of being involved in a fatal crash is about three times as great as for a sober driver. A British study on younger, less experienced drivers (and drinkers) found that the relative risk at 0.08 percent was about five times as great. The risk rises sharply for all drivers above 0.10. Similarly, the risk of involvement in a personal injury crash increases with BAC, as does the risk of involvement in a fatal pedestrian accident. As with other dose-response curves, these data provide strong evidence that the relationship between drinking and accidents is causal and not merely related to the lifestyles of individuals who drink.

Some other interesting facts have emerged from studies of alcohol and accidents. Alcohol-related traffic fatalities are not a random sample of all fatalities. Single-vehicle fatalities are more likely to involve alcohol than are multiple-vehicle fatalities in which the fatally injured person was driving the striking vehicle. The probability of alcohol involvement is lower if the fatally injured individual was driving a vehicle that was struck by another driver. Alcohol-related fatalities are a greater proportion of the fatalities occurring during dark hours than of those occurring in daylight and are a greater proportion of fatalities occurring on the weekend than of those occurring during the week. In fact, if someone is killed in a struck vehicle during daylight hours on Monday through Thursday, the odds are less than 1 in 10 that the victim was impaired by alcohol. The odds are more like 9 in 10 for a single-vehicle accident occurring in the early morning hours on a weekend.[18]

When you hear that about 85 percent of all the fatally injured drivers who had been drinking were male, that sounds like a big difference, and it is. But it is important to remember that 75 percent of all fatally injured drivers are male, whether or not drinking is involved. That men are more likely to be involved in alcohol-related

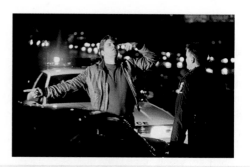

Drinking and driving can have serious—even fatal—consequences.

traffic fatalities reflects three important facts: any given car is more likely to have a male than a female driver, men might take more chances when driving even when they're sober, and male drivers are more likely than female drivers to have been drinking.

Who is responsible for all these alcohol-related traffic accidents? One question is whether there are certain individuals, such as problem drinkers, responsible for much of the drunk driving. In one study of drivers involved in fatal crashes who had BACs of 0.10 percent or more, 11 percent had previous convictions for driving under the influence (DUI).[18] Problem drinkers, although a relatively small fraction of the drinking population, are more likely on a given day to be driving around with a high BAC. On the other hand, almost 90 percent of the intoxicated drivers involved in fatal crashes have never been convicted of DUI in the past. Therefore, whereas individual problem drinkers cause more than their share of traffic accidents, the majority of alcohol-related traffic accidents are caused by individuals who have not been identified as problem drinkers. Anyone who drinks and drives is a potential threat.

Younger drivers have more than their share of alcohol-related accidents. In 1994, persons aged 16 to 24 made up 14 percent of the U.S. population yet were involved in 28 percent of the alcohol-related traffic accidents.[17]

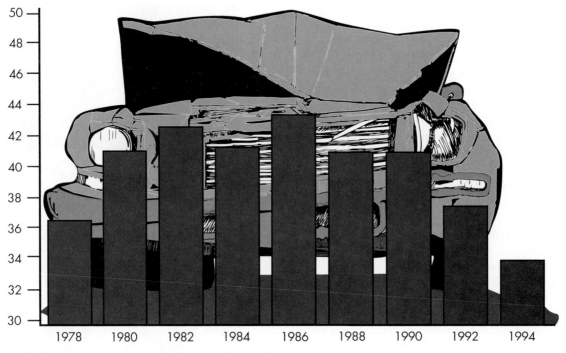

Figure 12-2   Percentage of alcohol-related traffic fatalities.

What can be done about this problem? Current efforts focus mainly on three fronts: identifying repeat offenders and keeping them off the roads, publicizing in the mass media the dangers of drinking and driving, and targeting younger drinkers for special prevention efforts. Although it is impossible to determine the effectiveness of any one of these measures, Figure 12.2 indicates that the total effort has worked to reduce alcohol-related fatalities. In 2000, the U.S. Congress passed legislation requiring states to reduce the BAC for DUI conviction from 0.10 to 0.08.

Crime and Violence

Homicide

The correlation between alcohol use and homicides is well known to police and judicial systems all around the world. Based on several studies of police and court records, the proportion of murderers who had been drinking before the crime ranged from 36 percent in Baltimore to 70 percent in Sweden.[19] It is also interesting that, across all these studies, about 50 percent of the murder victims had been drinking. These data certainly imply that homicide is more likely to occur in situations in which drinking also occurs, but they leave open the question as to whether alcohol plays a causal role in homicides.

Assault and Other Crimes of Violence

As with homicide, studies of assault, spousal abuse, and child abuse reveal correlations with drinking: heavier drinkers are more likely to engage in such behaviors, and self-reports by offenders indicate a high likelihood that they had been consuming alcohol before the violent act.[20]

However, scientists are still cautious in trying to determine how much of a causal role alcohol plays in such activity. For example, if fights are likely to occur when men get together in groups at night and drinking is likely to occur when men get together in groups at night, how much of a role does alcohol itself play in increasing the chances of violence? Similarly, if both heavy drinking and violent arguments are characteristics of dysfunctional family situations, how much of the ensuing family violence can be blamed on the use of alcohol? Unfortunately, it has proven difficult to perform controlled experimental studies on these complex problems, so the answers remain unclear.[21]

Suicide

Most studies show that alcohol is involved in about one-third of all suicides. Suicide *attempts* seem to have a different background than successful suicides, but alcoholism is second only to depression as the diagnosis in suicide attempters. The relationship between alcoholism and depression is a strong one and has been the subject of many studies. One interesting finding is that people who were alcoholics first and probably became depressed as a result of their repeated failures and shortcomings have a better prognosis than those who showed clear signs of clinical depression before they became alcoholics.[20]

WHO IS AN ALCOHOLIC?

Defining **alcoholism** is not an easy thing to do. The term has different meanings to different authorities, so picking any one of them gets you into a discussion right away. How one defines alcoholism has important implications for the approaches that are taken in treatment, the treatment goals, and how one measures success. Our immediate concern is how many and what types of people will be included in the group defined as alcoholics.

When we see a man who drinks to the point of drunkenness every day, who has lost his job

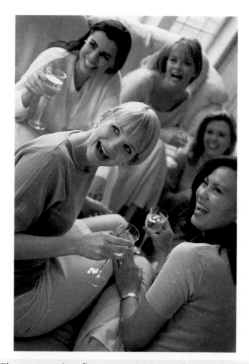

The street wino fits our stereotype of an alcoholic, but most alcoholics are not as easy to spot.

and family, who has a damaged liver, and who will suffer from delirium tremens if he doesn't drink for a day, then everyone can agree that he is an alcoholic. Some definitions have focused on the *physiological* aspects of this model alcoholic and define alcoholism on the basis of obvious liver or brain damage, tolerance, or withdrawal symptoms. Other definitions have focused on the *psychosocial* aspects, using criteria such as daily use or interference with personal, social, or occupational behavior. The problem arises when we leave the stereotypical, model alcoholic and start looking at ourselves and our friends and neighbors. There are lots of people who do not have obvious symptoms of

alcoholism: alcohol dependence or addiction.

liver or brain damage and who don't get the "shakes" if they don't drink on a given day but who drink regularly, depend on drinking at least as an important aspect of their individual and social lives, and who suffer some level of interference with their personal, social, or occupational lives. In fact, it is probably true that almost anyone who drinks at all will occasionally drink too much and have a hangover at work, be embarrassed socially, or fail to accomplish a personal goal on that day. How do we decide when such a person becomes an alcoholic? As far as this text is concerned, it is not possible to develop a universal decision rule. The term has too many meanings to too many people to be specific in our definition and still do justice to this important topic. What we will do is examine several of the ways in which this issue has been addressed.

Probably the most significant influence on American attitudes about alcoholism was a 60-year-old book called *Alcoholics Anonymous.* This book described the experiences of a small group of people who formed a society whose "only requirement for membership is a desire to stop drinking." That society has now grown to include more than 1.5 million members in over a hundred countries. A central part of their belief system is that alcoholism is a progressive disease characterized by a loss of control over drinking and that alcoholism can never be cured. People who do not have the disease might drink and even become intoxicated, but they do not "lose control over alcohol." There is a suspicion that the alcoholic is different even before the first drink is taken. The only treatment is to arrest the disease by abstaining from drinking. This *disease model* of alcoholism has received support from many medical practitioners and has been endorsed by the American Medical Association and other professional groups. In one sense, this description of alcoholism as a disease is a reaction against long-held notions that excessive drinking is only a symptom of some other underlying pathology, such as depression, or some type of personality

defect. Traditional psychoanalysts practicing many years ago might have treated the alcoholic by trying to discover the unconscious conflicts or personality deficiencies that caused the person to drink. One important consequence of defining alcoholism as a *primary* disease is to recognize that the drinking itself might be the problem and that treatment and prevention should be aimed directly at alcoholism.

However, there are many scientific critics of the disease concept. If alcoholism is a disease, what is its cause? How are alcoholics different from nonalcoholics, except that they tend to drink a lot and have many alcohol-related problems? Let's accept for the purpose of discussion that those who go into hospitals or treatment programs with a primary diagnosis of alcoholism are alcoholics. What are their characteristics? Although sequential stages have been described for this "progressive disease," most individual alcoholics don't seem to fit any single set of descriptors. Some don't drink alone, some don't drink in the morning, some don't go on binges, some don't drink every day, and some don't report strong cravings for alcohol. Experiments have shown that alcoholics do retain considerable control over their drinking, even while drinking—it's not that they completely lose control when they start drinking, but they might have either less ability or less desire to limit their drinking because they do drink excessively. Although an "alcoholic personality" has been defined that characterizes many alcoholics who enter treatment, the current belief is that these personality factors (impulsive, anxious, depressed, passive, dependent) reflect the years of intoxication and the critical events that led to the decision to enter treatment rather than preexisting abnormalities that caused the alcoholism.

The American Psychiatric Association's *Diagnostic and Statistical Manual of Mental Disorders,* fourth edition (*DSM-IV,* 1994)[22] is probably the closest thing there is to a single official, widely accepted set of labels for behavioral disorders, including substance abuse and dependence (see Chapter 3). The *DSM-IV* does not separately define these for alcohol but includes alcohol as one of the psychoactive substances. This manual implies, but does not directly state, that the term *alcoholism* may refer to alcohol abuse, which is defined in psychosocial terms (a maladaptive pattern of use indicated by continued use despite knowledge of having persistent problems caused by alcohol) or alcohol dependence, which involves more serious psychosocial characteristics and includes the physiological factors of tolerance and withdrawal among the possible symptoms.

In 1989, it may have appeared that the U.S. Supreme Court had decided the issue of whether alcoholism is or is not a disease. Two veterans of the armed services had filed for educational benefits after the 10-year eligibility period after their service had elapsed. The Veterans Administration denied their benefits, even though extensions of the eligibility period could be granted if the individual was delayed in education by physical or mental disorders "not the result of their own willful misconduct." These individuals argued that they were alcoholics and that, because alcoholism was a disease over which they had no control, they should be allowed the extension. Newspapers, magazines, and television commentators widely touted the case as deciding once and for all whether alcoholism is truly a disease or whether it should be considered more akin to misbehavior (willful misconduct).[23] On one side were legions of treatment professionals and alcoholics (or ex-alcoholics, if there can be such a thing) who believe very strongly in the disease model on which most programs of treatment and recovery are based. On the other side were a smaller number of professionals and academics who argued that we have gone too far in the "medicalization" of alcohol, with every wife-beater and criminal claiming the illness and being sent off for treatment. They argued that people must be held accountable for their behavior and misbehavior regarding alcohol. The Supreme Court ruled in favor of the Veterans

Administration, but we cannot conclude from that that alcoholism is not truly a disease. We should recognize by now that alcoholism is one of those complex concepts that means different things to different people in different contexts, not something that can be defined perfectly and absolutely. "Disease" is the same kind of concept. We could pick an official definition of alcoholism, which we should recognize as being somewhat arbitrary, and an official definition of disease, similarly somewhat arbitrary, and then match them up to see if alcoholism is truly a disease. A more sensible conclusion would be that there are probably contexts in which it makes sense to think of alcoholism as a disease, other contexts in which it probably does not make sense to think that way, and perhaps many contexts in which it is not at all clear.

Why are some people able to drink in moderation all their lives, whereas others repeatedly become intoxicated, suffer from alcohol-related problems, and continue to drink excessively? So far, no single factor and no combination of multiple factors has been presented that allows us to predict which individuals will become alcoholics. Multiple theories exist, including biochemical, psychoanalytic, and cultural approaches. At this period of scientific history, probably the most attention is being focused on understanding two types of factors: cognitive and genetic. The importance of cognitive factors with regard to alcohol's effects is perhaps best demonstrated by a series of experiments conducted by Marlatt and his colleagues on loss of control in alcoholics and social drinkers.[24] The experimental subjects are given drinks that either do or do not contain alcohol, and half of each group are told that the drinks do contain alcohol, whereas the other half of each group are told that the drinks do not have alcohol in them (this is referred to as a **balanced placebo** design). Of course, there's a limit to how much alcohol you can give a person before he or she will be able to detect it with no doubt, but the most interesting results from these studies are when people have not actually had any alcohol but believe that they have. Both alcoholics and social drinkers report more intoxication and consume more drinks when they are told the drinks have alcohol, regardless of the actual alcohol content. It is important that alcoholics actually given small amounts of alcohol (equivalent to one or two drinks) do not report becoming intoxicated and do not increase their drinking if they are led to expect that the drink contains no alcohol. Therefore, it would seem that, if alcoholics do lose control when they begin drinking, it might be because they have come to *believe* that they will lose control if they drink (this is sometimes referred to as the *abstinence violation effect*). These balanced placebo experiments have been replicated several times by others. In such experiments, which contrast the pharmacological effects of alcohol with the cognitive effects of expecting to drink alcohol, typically alcohol itself can be shown to impair information-processing ability and motor performance regardless of expectation. Expectancy of alcohol increases alcohol consumption, sexual arousal, and aggressiveness.[25] The most obvious interpretation of such results is that alcohol use provides a social excuse for behaving in ways that would otherwise be considered inappropriate, and it is enough for one to believe that one has drunk alcohol for such behaviors to be released.

There is considerable evidence in support of the idea that some degree of vulnerability to alcoholism might be inherited. Alcoholism does tend to run in families, but some of that could be due to similar expectancies developed through similar cultural influences and children learning from their parents. Studies on twins provide one way around this problem. Monozygotic (one-egg, or identical) twins share the same genetic material, whereas dizygotic (two-egg, or fraternal) twins are no more genetically related than any two nontwin siblings. Both types of twins are likely to share very similar cultural and family learning experiences. If one adult twin is diagnosed as alcoholic, what is the likelihood that the other twin will also receive that

diagnosis (are the twins concordant for the trait of alcoholism)? Almost all such studies report that the concordance rate for monozygotic twins is higher than that for dizygotic twins, and in some studies it is as high as 50 percent. These results imply that inheritance plays a strong role but is far from a complete determinant of alcoholism. Another important type of study looks at adopted sons whose biological fathers were alcoholics. These reports consistently find that such adoptees have a much greater than average chance of becoming alcoholics, even though they are raised by nonalcoholic parents. Although these studies again provide clear evidence for a genetic influence, it is important to remember that most children of alcoholics do not become alcoholics—they simply have a statistically greater risk of doing so. For example, in one study, 18 percent of the adopted-away sons of alcoholics became alcoholic, compared with 5 percent of the adopted-away sons whose parents had not received the diagnosis of alcoholism.

Further evidence for an inherited risk factor in alcoholism comes from experiments on young men (because alcoholism is more common in men) who are drinking but have not yet demonstrated alcoholism. If these young men had an alcoholic parent, they were less affected by a dose of alcohol than were control subjects with no family history of alcoholism. The argument is that these vulnerable individuals might drink more alcohol because they are less able to detect the initial effects of alcohol. Another type of study examined electrical brain-wave responses recorded from the scalp in response to repeated auditory stimuli. Alcoholic men as a group have a smaller response at a particular time point after the stimulus (the P300 wave). In addition, young men who have never drunk alcohol, but whose fathers are alcoholics, as a group show a similarly reduced P300 wave.[26]

In 1990, national attention was focused on a report that a possible **genetic marker** had been found for alcoholism. Studying brain tissue obtained from 35 people who had died from complications of alcoholism, with 35 nonalcoholic brains as controls, researchers found that an unusual form of one type of dopamine receptor was present in 69 percent of the alcoholics' brains but in only 20 percent of the nonalcoholics' brains. The genetic code for this dopamine receptor is located on chromosome 11 in humans. Could this be the long-sought key to an alcoholism gene?[27] The research that has emerged since then does not give a clear answer—some studies have continued to find a relationship between this dopamine receptor type and alcoholism, whereas others have not.[28] Of course, alcoholism is a complicated feature of human behavior, and even if genetic influences are critical, there could be more than one genetic factor involved. Probably it is too much to hope that a single genetic marker will ever be found to be a reliable indicator of alcoholism in all individuals.

TREATMENT OF ALCOHOLISM

Excessive alcohol consumption is an age-old human problem, and one that exacts enormous costs from contemporary society, both in dollars and in wasted human potential. Where do we place the blame for this difficulty? If we believe that the fault is a moral defect in the alcoholic, then we might treat the problem by using the same sort of approach we use with other social transgressions, such as stealing. Historically, these have consisted of social ostracism, imprisonment, and other forms of punishment. If we believe that the fault lies with alcohol itself ("demon rum"), then our treatment consists of attempts to control the availability of alcohol. If we believe that alcoholism is a disease, then we seek medical treatment.

Historically, all these ideas and all these approaches have coexisted. For example, at the turn of the twentieth century it was common to view drunkards as social outcasts and to throw them in jail. At the same time, the temperance movement was rapidly gaining ground in its rush toward the eventual prohibition of alcohol.

Meanwhile, some physicians were advocating the use of morphine, cocaine, and other drugs as preferable substitutes for alcohol.

Alcoholics Anonymous

The formation of Alcoholics Anonymous (AA) in 1935 can now be seen as an important milestone in treatment. This group, which has total abstinence as a goal, has given support to the disease model of alcoholism. One of the basic tenets of this group is that the alcoholic is biologically different from the nonalcoholic person and therefore can never safely drink any alcohol at all. Central to this disease model is the idea that the disease takes away the person's control of his or her own drinking behavior and therefore removes the blame for the problem. AA members are quick to point out that removing blame for the disease does not remove responsibility for dealing with it. By analogy, we would not blame diabetics for being diabetic, but we do expect diabetics to control their diets, take their medication, and so on. Thus, the alcoholic is seen as having the responsibility for managing the disease on a day-by-day basis but need not feel guilty about being different. The major approach used by AA has been group support and a buddy system. The members of AA help each other through difficult periods and encourage each other in their sobriety.

Although AA has been described as a loose affiliation of local groups, each with its own character, they have in common adherence to a

---

balanced placebo: a research design in which alcohol is compared with a placebo beverage, and subjects either believe they are drinking alcohol or believe they are not.

genetic marker: a chemical or physiological characteristic that is known to be caused by a particular gene and that is highly correlated with a disease state.

Drugs in Depth

The 12 Steps of Alcoholics Anonymous

1. We admitted we were powerless over alcohol—that our lives had become unmanageable.
2. Came to believe that a Power greater than ourselves could restore us to sanity.
3. Made a decision to turn our will and our lives over to the care of God *as we understood Him.*
4. Made a searching and fearless moral inventory of ourselves.
5. Admitted to God, to ourselves, and to another human being the exact nature of our wrongs.
6. Were entirely ready to have God remove all these defects of character.
7. Humbly asked Him to remove our shortcomings.
8. Made a list of all persons we had harmed and became willing to make amends to them all.
9. Made direct amends to such people wherever possible, except when to do so would injure them or others.
10. Continued to take moral inventory and when we were wrong promptly admitted it.
11. Sought through prayer and meditation to improve our conscious contact with God *as we understood Him,* praying only for knowledge of His will for us and the power to carry that out.
12. Having had a spiritual awakening as the result of these steps, we tried to carry this message to alcoholics, and to practice these principles in all our affairs.

The Twelve Steps are reprinted with permission of Alcoholics Anonymous World Services, Inc. Permission to reprint the Twelve Steps does not mean that A.A. has reviewed or approved the contents of this publication, nor that A.A. agrees with the views expressed herein. A.A. is a program of recovery from alcoholism *only*—use of the Twelve Steps in connection with programs and activities which are patterned after A.A., but which address other problems, or in any other non-A.A. context, does not imply otherwise.

12-step program of recovery from alcoholism (see the Drugs in Depth box).

Everyone agrees that AA has been helpful for many people and, because it has reached more individuals than any other approach, has undoubtedly helped more people than any other method. Nevertheless, formal evaluations of the success of AA have been few and have not been very positive. For example, studies of court-ordered referrals to AA or to other types of interventions have not shown AA to be more effective. However, AA was developed by and for people who have made a personal decision to stop drinking and who want to affiliate with others who have made that decision, and it might not be the most appropriate approach for individuals who are coerced into attending meetings as an alternative to jail. More appropriate (and more difficult and expensive) evaluations of AA should be done to determine which types of alcoholics are most likely to benefit from this organization's program.

Medical Approaches

One of the most influential contributors to the disease concept of alcoholism was E. M. Jellinek, who portrayed alcoholism as a progressive disease leading characteristically through several stages.[29] In the final and most severe stage, which he called *gamma alcoholism,* the individual has suffered liver and nervous system damage and has a profound physical dependence, so that dangerous withdrawal symptoms appear when alcohol intake is stopped. More recent studies have discounted the notion that all, or even most, alcoholics go through such a consistent set of stages. However, a large number of alcoholics enter treatment with liver and nervous system damage and will suffer withdrawal symptoms. In fact, thousands of people die each year under these circumstances. In such severe cases, it is clear that medical intervention is called for.

Detoxification

The first problem is to get the individual over the immediate crisis. There is some danger of death from respiratory depression at first, simply from alcohol overdose. Clearing the stomach and supporting respiration can get the individual through this first threat. The next hurdle is to

Exploring Your Spirituality

Online Support for Recovery

All of us have heard the expression "You are what you eat." That is, your *body* is made up of what you put in your mouth.

You, your *mind*—the things you like and fear—and your behavior, on the other hand, are influenced perhaps most strongly by *association*—people you spend time with. One reason is that the people you hang around with often determine what you hear and believe. Maybe you've always heard "You can't," "You'll get hurt," or "You're not smart enough." As irrational as it sounds, your brain hears and restrains all those negative messages, and you start believing that you have limited abilities and potential.

Twelve-step programs, such as Alcoholics Anonymous, have helped many people unlearn the negative thought patterns that contribute to self-destructive behavior. With its strong spiritual orientation emphasizing the acknowledgment of a "higher power," AA and its main text, the AA *Big Book,* can provide comfort and structure to people of all ages and backgrounds and of both genders. In recent years, alternatives to AA have emerged that offer acceptance and peer support for special-interest groups, such as recovering alcoholic women, lesbians, racial and ethnic minorities, and those of non-Christian backgrounds. For those who prefer to pursue their goal in a nonspiritual context, an alternative is Rational Recover (RR), based on the theories of psychologist Albert Ellis's Rational Emotive Theory. RR uses a cognitive approach that fosters cohesiveness and provides the emotional support sought by people trying to gain and maintain sobriety.

The first step to recovery is to admit that you have been adversely affected by your problem and that your life has become unmanageable. The second step—seeking help—can begin by simply getting online and checking out the many resources available for help. A couple of useful websites www.open-mind.org/Self-help.htm for general recovery, self-help, support, and mental health resources, and the 12-Step Cyber Café at www.12steps.org. Both have links to many other addiction and recovery resources.

The next step is to begin thinking about taking care of your spiritual, emotional, and physical needs. Associate with people and events that bring out the positive in you. Focus on the things that are necessary and possible to ensure your success while accepting the things that are unchangeable.

---

allow the alcohol to clear the system (detoxification), while preventing convulsions and delirium tremens because of withdrawal. Intravenous administration of diazepam or another benzodiazepine sedative is an accepted method for controlling these potentially dangerous symptoms.

Treatment

Regardless of which approach is taken to try to alter drinking behavior, the next stage of medical treatment is based on the fact that many alcoholics are malnourished and that at least some of the alcohol-related brain damage could be a result of a vitamin (thiamine) deficiency. Thus, an important part of treating chronic alcoholics is providing a nutritious diet supplemented by extra vitamins. There might be other physical problems associated with liver occlusion and altered blood circulation, and these also require symptomatic medical treatment.

Aftercare

Once an individual has been "dried out" and has received the primary treatment, it can be appropriate to provide some long-term medical support. A common approach, which might be considered part of the treatment itself, is the prescribing of disulfiram (**Antabuse**). Alcohol is normally metabolized in the liver through two enzymatic steps. Disulfiram inhibits the enzyme aldehyde dehydrogenase, the second of these

> **Antabuse: (disulfiram)** a drug that alters alcohol metabolism and is used in treating alcoholism.

steps. Alcohol is then converted into acetalde-hyde, but further conversion is prevented and acetaldehyde builds up in the system. High lev-els of acetaldehyde usually produce a severe re-action: headache, nausea, vomiting, throbbing of the head and neck, breathing difficulties, and a host of other unpleasant symptoms. Therefore, a person taking Antabuse can't take a drink without becoming ill, and this threat can be suf-ficient to help many people avoid the impulse to drink. It takes two or three days after a person stops taking disulfiram before a drink can be taken safely, so a person on this treatment must make a decision to stop taking Antabuse for that length of time if he or she wants to drink.

Antabuse treatment has been used in court-ordered treatment programs, but there is con-siderable doubt as to its long-term usefulness in that way. If Antabuse does help, it is by helping those who want to avoid drinking by making it impossible for them to give in to a momentary impulse or to social pressure.

Naltrexone is a drug that was originally de-veloped as a narcotic antagonist and has been used in the treatment of narcotic addiction (see Chapter 16). Research in the early 1990s found that naltrexone given in conjunction with outpa-tient rehabilitation treatment for alcoholism re-duced reported cravings for alcohol, and in the first three months after treatment only about one-fourth of the naltrexone-treated patients re-lapsed, compared with about 50 percent of the placebo control group.[30] Based on such re-search, the FDA in 1994 approved naltrexone for use in the treatment of alcoholism. Although great fanfare accompanied this approval and no doubt many alcoholics will receive naltrexone, it is too early to tell what the long-term impact of this treatment will be.

Behavioral Approaches

One behavioral approach involves teaching cop-ing skills. Some of the same behaviors that are taught in prevention programs are used, such as recognizing peer pressure and practicing ways

to deal with it. In addition, therapists often get patients to pay special attention to high-risk sit-uations and teach alternative behaviors that can be used to get through those difficult times. For example, if the individual is accustomed to hav-ing a drink or two before dinner, it might be sug-gested that a nonalcoholic drink be substituted, that the person assist with the dinner prepara-tions, or even that the dinner hour be moved up to eliminate the difficult time gap. The idea is to help the client to manage his or her behavior to decrease the probability of drinking. Some stud-ies have reported positive results from such treatment approaches, whereas others have not.

Some behavior-management approaches have accepted **controlled drinking** as a desir-able outcome and have attempted to teach methods that limit alcohol intake. Such strate-gies as switching to drinks with lower alcohol content, keeping track of each drink taken, or even learning to recognize a target BAC have been tried. A number of such experiments have reported success in producing a higher percent-age of improved patients (both abstaining and "controlled") than with traditional abstinence-oriented approaches. However, there is enormous controversy about both the success and the desir-ability of controlled-drinking approaches.

Is Controlled Drinking a Realistic Goal?

The notion that alcoholism is a disease that pro-duces a loss of control over drinking seems to be inconsistent with AA's belief that alcoholics do have the responsibility to decide to remain sober. This apparent dilemma is resolved by the commonly used saying "One drink is too much and a thousand not enough." In other words, the belief is that the alcoholic does have control over that first drink and can choose not to take it, but once alcohol has entered her system she is helpless and her drinking is out of control. This seems to be descriptive of binge drinking, in which a problem drinker might not drink at all for days or weeks and then really "tie one

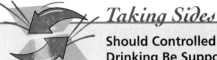

Taking Sides

Should Controlled Drinking Be Supported as a Treatment Goal?

Imagine that you are on the board of directors for your local community mental health center. One of the psychologists there would like to offer an alternative treatment program for alcoholics. In this program the therapist and the client would agree on a goal or set of goals for reducing the client's alcohol intake to a more manageable level, which might be total abstinence or a level of controlled social drinking. Some of your fellow board members are convinced that this is a good option and are willing to approve the program. Others are extremely opposed to the program, based on a strong belief that anyone who is truly an alcoholic can never drink in a controlled way, at least for an extended length of time. How would you vote? What other information would you need to gather to make an informed decision about this issue?

on." But does this notion of loss of control have any further merit? Does it describe the behavior of all alcoholics all of the time? A number of experimental studies have been done with hospitalized alcoholics, and virtually all of them report that alcoholics do not differ fundamentally in the types of events that control drinking, although they do drink more than control subjects. Other descriptive studies of the drinking patterns of large numbers of active alcoholics show a great variety of patterns. Some drink in this binge fashion, whereas others have extended periods of what can be described only as controlled drinking. Also, a surprisingly large number of alcoholics who have been through abstinence-oriented treatment programs are found on later follow-ups to be drinking, but in a controlled manner.[31]

Just about everyone can agree that anyone who has a drinking problem would be best advised to stop drinking and to abstain completely. But there are arguments against having

abstention as the only treatment goal. First, problem drinkers might be reluctant to enter treatment if they are required to accept the label *alcoholic* and the goal of total **abstinence.** Second, about two-thirds of adult Americans are drinkers (and even more among urban, college-educated adults). Thus, assuming that the alcoholic has been part of a social group that accepts or even expects drinking, we are in a sense trying to promote a "deviant" behavior. Third, if abstinence has been tried several times with no success, why not try controlled drinking as a treatment goal? Those opposed to such approaches believe that they are doomed to failure because their definition of alcoholism includes the individual's powerlessness to control drinking. Any apparent successes can be argued away either by agreeing that alcoholics might appear to be under control for a few weeks or months or by saying that the controlled-drinking successes were not really alcoholics when they entered treatment. These experts are concerned that even discussing the possibility might just encourage alcoholics to drink. After all, they've probably been telling themselves and others for years that they could handle it. Do we really need scientists providing support for such self-delusion?

A widely publicized Rand Corporation report added fuel to this controversy. This study, funded by the National Institute on Alcohol Abuse and Alcoholism (NIAAA), examined treatment effectiveness in eight large treatment centers. After establishing clearly that the alcoholics in these programs were seriously impaired (they drank nine times more than the average person), they found that about 70

controlled drinking: the idea that alcohol abusers might be able to drink unlimited amounts of alcohol.

abstinence: no alcohol or drug use at all.

percent of them were improved 18 months after treatment. Their controversial conclusion was this:

> It is important to stress that the improved clients include only a relatively small number who are long-term abstainers. . . . The majority of improved clients are either drinking moderate amounts of alcohol—but at levels far below what could be described as alcoholic drinking—or engaging in alternating periods of drinking and abstinence.[32]

You should be aware that these programs had abstinence as their primary goal, yet controlled drinking seemed to have been the result for a large number of the clients. This report came under immediate and highly emotional attack, as did the Rand Corporation itself and the NIAAA for funding such a study.

The traditional view was vindicated to some extent by the 4-year follow-up of these clients. Of those who had been drinking without symptoms at 18 months, 41 percent had relapsed by the 4-year follow-up, compared with 30 percent of those who had been abstaining at 18 months.[33] This was widely hailed as indicating that abstinence was a more desirable treatment outcome than controlled drinking. However, we should not ignore the fact that the *majority* of those who were drinking in a controlled fashion at 18 months did not relapse and were found to be either controlled drinkers or abstainers at 4 years. At this point it seems reasonable to conclude that abstinence is the preferred goal and the one adopted by the vast majority of programs but that controlled drinking is a realistic option for some alcoholics.

Although research continues on disulfiram, naltrexone, controlled drinking, and other approaches, the mainstay of alcoholism treatment in the United States has been a four- to six-week visit to a residential (inpatient) treatment facility. Most of these programs adopt the AA model of alcoholism as a disease and use individual counseling, group counseling, and family therapy approaches to help the alcoholic "work the steps" (the 12 steps of AA). Because health insurance companies were willing to pay for such treatment, these residential facilities became a growth industry during the 1980s. As health insurance companies began to limit coverage to shorter stays and to fewer clients, most of the treatment facilities that opened during the 1980s were closed during the 1990s.

Is Alcoholism Treatment Effective?

Are the insurance companies getting anything for their money when they pay for someone to go to treatment? The answers to these questions about alcoholism treatment aren't necessarily simple, but we can start by saying a qualified yes. If an individual receives the diagnosis of alcoholism (or alcohol dependence disorder), the prognosis is not good. Most such individuals can be expected to drink again, drink heavily, and have further alcohol-related problems. But it is clear that those who enter treatment do better than those who do not. Thus, statistically, alcoholism treatment is effective. However, the same studies show over and over that most of the people who go through treatment will drink again, with typical first-year relapse rates running about 65 to 75 percent.[21] Therefore, it might seem that treatment is not effective for most of the individuals. A further complication has been hinted at: how do we define relapse? If the goal is 100 percent abstinence, then even one drink at any time after treatment would be considered a relapse and therefore a treatment failure. It is quite possible for people to go through a treatment program, spend a couple of months going to AA meetings and not drinking, think they have the problem licked, try drinking again, drink too much for a month or two, and then go back to AA and quit drinking. Neither recovery nor relapse should be viewed as a permanent condition.

Many studies over the years have examined the characteristics of the treatment programs

Try It!

How Can You Tell Whether You Have a Drinking Problem?

There have been many self-tests published for people to use to determine if they are alcoholics or if they have a drinking problem. None of them should be taken as an absolute test or as a definite answer to that question, because in most cases it is a complex, subjective judgment as to whether someone should seek help. One of the best popularly printed self-tests appeared in a "Dear Abby" column, and it is offered here as a possible guide. If these questions seem to indicate that you or a friend need to seek help, we recommend a visit to a counselor, psychologist, or physician who is experienced in the assessment of chemical dependence. An assessment would probably include the use of a more professional questionnaire, such as the Michigan Alcoholism Screening Test (MAST) or the Alcohol Dependency Scale (ADS).
Check those that apply to you:

___ 1. Have you ever decided to stop drinking for a week or so but lasted for only a couple of days?

___ 2. Do you wish people would stop nagging you about your drinking?

___ 3. Have you ever switched from one kind of drink to another in the hope that this would keep you from getting drunk?

___ 4. Have you had a drink in the morning in the past year?

___ 5. Do you envy people who can drink without getting into trouble?

___ 6. Have you had problems connected with drinking during the past year?

___ 7. Has your drinking caused problems at home?

___ 8. Do you ever try to get "extra" drinks at a party because you did not get enough to drink?

___ 9. Do you tell yourself you can stop drinking anytime you want to, even though you keep getting drunk when you don't mean to?

___ 10. Have you missed days at work (or school) because of drinking?

___ 11. Do you have "blackouts"?

___ 12. Have you ever felt that your life would be better if you did not drink?

If you checked four or more of these, it would be a good idea to seek the guidance of a specialist in chemical dependence or to seek help directly through Alcoholics Anonymous or a similar organization. It's perfectly acceptable to go to an open AA meeting, listen to what is being said, and decide for yourself if the program would be useful to you.

and the characteristics of the clients to determine whether one type of treatment is better than another, which clients do better than others, and whether certain types of clients do better in certain types of programs. Because of the difficulties in measuring relapse and other indicators of success, this type of research is difficult to do, and individual reports can often be criticized on procedural grounds. But several large-scale studies agree that differences among treatment approaches are less important in predicting success than differences among the clients when they enter treatment.

Clients who have jobs, stable family relationships, minimal psychopathology, no history of treatment failures, and minimal involvement with other drugs tend to do better than the clients with no jobs, no meaningful relationships, and so on. What is surprising is that the type of treatment program seems to make little or no difference: residential versus outpatient, shorter versus longer, intensity of therapy, and theoretical approach are all factors that have not consistently influenced outcome. This seems to imply that insurance companies could save money by providing for shorter-term, less intense, outpatient treatment and still have about the same success rate. The companies have paid attention and have placed further restrictions on long-term residential treatment.

One important new approach might have some value in reducing the frequency of severe alcoholism. Medical patients in primary care settings are given a screening survey, and those who are found to be heavy drinkers then are counseled by a physician that their drinking is much higher than average and they should cut down. Surprisingly, several studies have shown this type of intervention to be effective. In one report, two brief counseling sessions with a primary care physician resulted in an average 37 percent reduction in average number of drinks in men and a 47 percent reduction in women, 12 months after the counseling sessions.[34]

SUMMARY

- In colonial America alcohol use was widespread and drunkenness was frowned on, but alcohol itself was not seen as a cause of major social and medical ills.
- Reformers first proposed temperate use of alcoholic beverages, and it was not until the late 1800s that proposals to prohibit alcohol were instituted in several states.
- National prohibition of alcohol did not achieve the results expected by its proponents, but it was successful in reducing total consumption and alcohol-related problems.
- Alcohol use and alcohol-related problems vary widely among different cultural groups and in different regions of the United States.
- Alcohol use is associated with thousands of traffic fatalities and has been correlated with homicide, assault, family violence, and suicide.
- The concept of alcoholism is complex. No single definition or theory is adequate to cover all the people who are called or who call themselves alcoholic.
- One continuing controversy is whether every alcoholic should have abstinence as the only goal or whether controlled drinking is also a worthwhile treatment outcome.
- Although many alcoholics relapse after treatment, not all do, and treatment programs are statistically effective.

REVIEW QUESTIONS

1. What important concepts regarding alcohol's social and medical effects were first introduced by Benjamin Rush in 1784?
2. What were the effects on American society of Prohibition of alcohol during the 1920s?
3. What was the impact on sales of the 1991 increase in U.S. alcohol taxes?

Web Watch

Warning Sighs of Alcohol Abuse
Go to www.wisbar.org/bar/alcohol.html.
This website provides a detailed article on alcoholism
as a disease and its role in society. After you read the
article and the additional information following, scroll
down and take the quiz "Warning Signs for Alcohol
Abuse." Answer the questions as a self-assessment.
You may also refer these questions to a friend to find
out whether he or she is dealing with alcoholism.
When you're finished, read the information on intervention and enabling.

Check Out Publications on Alcohol
Go to www.health.org/catalog/catalog.asp?key=3&
detail=false. Here you'll find a listing of articles about
alcohol as well as informational pamphlets, booklets,
and brochures that you can order.

What Makes a Good Assessment?
Go to silk.nih.gov/silk/niaaa1/publication/assinstr. htm,
read the article "Assessment in Alcoholism Treatment:
An Overview." Find out about the use of assessments
in clinics, client treatment, the setup of a good assessment, and related issues.

4. What are some differences between Irish
American and Italian American cultures relating to alcohol use?
5. Which state has the highest apparent per
capita alcohol consumption and which the
lowest? *New Ham. Most / Lowest Utah*
6. What are some effects of restrictive campus
drinking and alcohol-related problems? *gets moved off campus*
7. What is meant by "alcohol myopia"?
8. What has been the trend since 1980 in alcohol-related traffic fatalities? *decreased*
9. Describe the balanced placebo research design and what types of alcohol effects might
be due to the belief that alcohol has been
consumed, rather than the actual alcohol
itself. *you don't know what your drinking either
alchol or not. some act drunk + nearly aren't.*

10. What is the role of God in the 12 steps of
AA? *The Basis. The Higher power*
11. What three arguments have been given in
favor of controlled drinking as a treatment
outcome?
12. What are some individual client characteristics that predict success in alcoholism
treatment?

REFERENCES

1. The alcohol problem in America: From temperance to
alcoholism, *British Addiction* 79:109–119, 1984.
2. Koren J: *Economic aspects of the liquor problem.* New
York: Houghton Mifflin, 1899.
3. Clark NH: *The dry years: Prohibition and social change in
Washington.* Seattle: University of Washington Press,
1965.
4. Keller M: Alcohol problems and policies in historical
perspective. In Kyvig DE, editor: *Law, alcohol and order.*
Westport, CT: Greenwood Press, 1985.
5. Emerson H: *Alcohol and man.* New York: Macmillan,
1932, reprinted 1981, New York, Arno Press.
6. *U.S. industrial outlook 1992.* Washington, DC: U.S. Department of Commerce, 1992.
7. Segal BM: *The Soviet heavy-drinking culture and the American heavy-drinking subculture.* In Babor TF, editor: *Alcohol and culture: Comparative perspectives from Europe and
America.* New York: New York Academy of Sciences,
1986.
8. Vaillant G: *Cultural factors in the etiology of alcoholism: A
prospective study.* In Babor TF, editor: *Alcohol and culture:
Comparative perspectives from Europe and America.* New
York: New York Academy of Sciences, 1986.
9. Geddes D: France sets records in suicide, alcoholism
and anxiety, *The Times* (London), p 9, June 14, 1986.
10. Williams GD and others: *NIAAA Surveillance Report #51:
Apparent per capita alcohol consumption.* Bethesda, MD:
USPHS, 1999.
11. *Sixth special report on alcohol and health,* DHHS Pub. No.
(ADM) 87-1519, Washington, DC: U.S. Government
Printing Office, 1987.
12. Linsky AS and others: Social stress, normative con-
straints and alcohol problems in American states, *Social
Science and Medicine* 24:875–883, 1987.
13. Mooney DK and others: Correlates of alcohol consumption: Sex, age, and expectancies relate differentially to
quantity and frequency, *Addictive Behavior* 12:235–240,
1987.

14. Office of Applied Studies: *Summary of findings from the 1999 National Household Survey on Drug Abuse, Department of Health and Human Services, Substance Abuse and Mental Health Services Administration,* August 2000.

15. Wet or dry: Schools ponder variety of strategies to curb alcohol problems, *The Bottom Line* 18(3) 18(3):68–72, 1997.

16. Steele CM, Josephs RA: Alcohol myopia, *American Psychologist* 45:921–933, 1990.

17. Yi HY and others: *NIAAA surveillance report #49. Trends in alcohol-related traffic fatalities in the United States, 1975–97.* Bethesda, MD: USPHS, 1999.

18. Insurance Institute for Highway Safety: *Fatality facts 1991,* Washington, DC: Author, 1991.

19. Pernanen K: *Alcohol in human violence,* New York, 1991, Guilford Press.

20. *Eighth special report on alcohol and health,* NIH Pub No 94-3699, Washington, DC: U.S. Public Health Service, 1993.

21. Bushman BJ, Cooper HM: Effects of alcohol on human aggression: An integrative research review, *Personality and Social Psychology Bulletin* 107:341–354, 1990.

22. *Diagnostic and statistical manual of mental disorders* (4th ed.). Washington, DC: American Psychiatric Association, 1994.

23. Alcoholism a disease or foible? *Denver Post,* pp 00, Dec 1988.

24. Wilson GT: Cognitive studies in alcoholism, *Journal of Consulting and Clinical Psychology* 55:325–331, 1987.

25. Hull JG, Bond CF: Social and behavioral consequences of alcohol consumption and expectancy: A meta-analysis, *Personality and Social Psychology Bulletin* 99:347–360, 1986.

26. Schuckit MA: Biological vulnerability to alcoholism, *Journal of Consulting and Clinical Psychology* 55:301–309, 1987.

27. Cowley G: The gene and the bottle, *Newsweek,* Apr 30, 1990.

28. Ackerman SJ: Research on the genetics of alcoholism is still in ferment, *The Journal of NIH Research* 4:61–65, 1992.

29. Jellinek EM: *The disease concept of alcoholism,* New Brunswick, NJ: Hillhouse Press, 1960.

30. Volpicelli JR and others: Naltrexone in the treatment of alcohol dependence, *Archives of General Psychiatry* 49: 876, 1992.

31. Pomerleau O, Pertschuk M, Stinnet J: A critical examination of some current assumptions in the treatment of alcoholism, *Journal of Studies on Alcohol* 37:849–867, 1976.

32. Armor DJ, Polich JM, Stambul HB: *Alcoholism and treatment,* NIAAA Pub No R-1739, Washington, DC: U.S. Government Printing Office, 1976.

33. Polich JM, Armor DJ, Braiker HB: *The course of alcoholism: Four years after treatment.* New York: Wiley, 1981.

34. Fleming MF and others: *Brief physician advice for problem alcohol drinkers: A randomized controlled trial in community-based primary care practices, Journal of the American Medical Association* 277:1039–1045, 1997.

Section V

Familiar Drugs

Some drugs are seen so often that they don't seem to be drugs at all, at least not in the same sense as cocaine or marijuana. However, tobacco and its ingredient nicotine, as well as caffeine in its various forms, are psychoactive drugs meeting any reasonable definition of the term drug. Certainly the drugs sold over-the-counter (OTC) in pharmacies are drugs, and many of them have their primary effects on the brain and behavior. In Section 5, we learn about the psychological effects of all these familiar drugs, partly because they are so commonly used. Also, they provide several interesting points for comparison with the less well known, more frightening drugs.

Chapter 13

Tobacco

Online Learning Center Resources

www.mhhe.com/ray

Log on to our Online Learning Center (OLC) for access to these additional resources.

- Chapter definitions
- Learning objectives
- Student interactive question-and-answer sites
- Self-scoring chapter quiz

The OLC also offers web links for study and exploration of health topics. Here are some examples of what you'll find:

www.nicnet.org

The Nicotine and Tobacco Network is an Arizona program devoted to nicotine and tobacco research. Its site provides the latest news and information on research, prevention, and the dangers of secondhand smoke.

www.tobacco.org

This site provides breaking news and quotes about tobacco. It also posts links, health articles, information on lung cancer awareness and activist groups, and a tobacco time line.

www.dentalcare.com/soap/ journals/dh_news/dhn1001/ aform.htm

This website provides a tobacco use questionnaire.

Drugs in the Media:

Cigarette Smoking in the Movies

In 1989, U.S. tobacco companies voluntarily agreed to halt a long-standing practice, directly paying film producers for what is known as "product placement" in popular films. All sorts of companies do this, and at times, the practice is fairly obvious once you know about it. For example, you might notice that in one movie a particular brand of new automobile appears with unusual frequency.

Drugs in the Media Continued. . .

In another, one type of soft drink can or billboard (and never a competing brand) might be seen in the background of several shots. Despite all the efforts to control more explicit advertising of cigarettes to young people, this practice is especially insidious, because there is research indicating that tobacco use by an adolescent's favorite actor does influence the adolescent's smoking behavior. Thus, this type of product placement is likely to be a very potent form of advertising for cigarette manufacturers. Did the 1989 voluntary ban work?

Apparently not, according to a study reported in the medical journal *The Lancet* in 2001.[1] Researchers from Dartmouth College studied the top 25 U.S. films each year for 10 years (1988–1997, a total of 250 films). The first 3 of those years should have reflected pre-ban film production, compared with the later 7 years. They found that 85 percent of the films portrayed tobacco use (whereas only about one third of adult Americans are smokers). Specific brands were identified in 28 percent of the films. Neither of these statistics was different before versus after the voluntary ban on direct payments for product placement. Films considered suitable for adolescent audiences (those with PG or PG-13 ratings) contained just as many brand appearances as films for adult audiences.

One important difference noted was an increase, rather than a decrease, in the frequency of use of an identified brand by an actor, as opposed to the appearance of a cigarette package or billboard in the background. This suggests that this effective form of hidden advertising in movies is actually increasing rather than decreasing. Although the authors of the study proposed several possible reasons for continued placement of the most widely advertised cigarette brands in movies (such as realism), it is quite possible that cigarette marketers are either ignoring the voluntary ban or are finding less direct ways to pay film producers and actors to display their products.

Long before Columbus stumbled onto the Western Hemisphere, the Indians here were using tobacco. It was one of the many contributions of the New World to Europe: tobacco, corn, sweet potatoes, white potatoes, chocolate, and—so you could lie back and enjoy it all—the hammock. Christopher Columbus recorded that the natives of San Salvador presented him with tobacco leaves on October 12, 1492, a fitting birthday present.

In 1497, a monk who had accompanied Columbus on his second trip wrote a book on native customs that contained the first printed report of tobacco smoking. It wasn't called tobacco, and it wasn't called smoking. Inhaling smoke was called drinking. In that period you either "took" (used snuff) or "drank" (smoked) tobacco.

The word *tobacco* came from one of two sources. *Tobaco* referred to a two-pronged tube used by natives to take snuff. But some early reports confused the issue by applying the name to the plant they incorrectly thought was being used. Another idea is that the word developed its current usage from the province of Tobacos in Mexico, where everyone used the herb. Be that as it may, in 1598, an Italian-English dictionary published in London translated the Italian *Nicosiana* as the herb tobacco, and that spelling and usage gradually became dominant.

One member of Columbus's party, Rodrigo de Jerez, was the poor fellow who introduced tobacco drinking to Europe. He was also the first European to touch Cuba and possibly the first to smoke tobacco. When he continued his habit in Portugal, his friends were convinced the devil had possessed him as they saw the smoke coming out his mouth and nose. The priest agreed, and Rodrigo spent the next several years in jail, only to find on his release that people were doing the same thing for which he had been jailed.

TOBACCO HISTORY

Early Medical Uses

Tobacco was formally introduced to Europe as an herb useful for treating almost everything. A 1529 report[2] indicated that tobacco was used for "persistant headaches," "cold or catarrh," and "abscesses and sores on the head." Between 1537 and 1559, 14 books mentioned the medicinal value of tobacco.

The French physician Jean Nicot went to Lisbon, Portugal, in 1559 to arrange a royal marriage. The marriage never took place, but Nicot became enamored with the medical uses of tobacco. He tried it on enough people to convince himself of its value and sent glowing reports of the herb's effectiveness to the French court. He was successful in "curing" the migraine headaches of Catherine de Medicis, queen of Henry II of France, which made tobacco use very much "in." It was called the *herbe sainte,* "holy plant," and *the herbe à tous les maux,* "the plant against all evils." The French loved it and, although tobacco had been introduced earlier to Paris, Nicot received the credit. By 1565, the plant had been called nicotiane, and Linnaeus sanctified it in 1753 by naming the genus *Nicotiana.* When a pair of French chemists isolated the active ingredient in 1828, they acted like true nationalists and called it nicotine.

In the late sixteenth century,

it was more likely than not that . . . the doctor would prescribe tobacco. . . . Did the patient

suffer from flatulence? The remedy was a tobacco emetic . . . A heavy cough? Smoke of tobacco, deeply inhaled. Pains accompanying gestation or labor? Place a leaf of tobacco, very hot, on the navel. If a form of delirium ensued, blow smoke up the nostrils.[3]

In the 16th century, Sir Anthony Chute[2] summarized much of the earlier material and said, "Anything that harms a man inwardly from his girdle upward might be removed by a moderate use of the herb." Others, however, felt differently: "If taken after meals the herb would infect the brain and liver," and "Tobacco should be avoided by (among others) women with child and husbands who desired to have children."[2]

A few years later in 1617, Dr. William Vaughn phrased the last thought a little more poetically:

> Tobacco that outlandish weede
> It spends the braine and spoiles the seede
> It dulls the spirite, it dims the sight
> It robs a woman of her right.[4]

Dr. Vaughn may have been ahead of his time: a December 1994 report indicated that smokers are 50 percent more likely than nonsmokers to be impotent.[5]

Special note must be made of a series of experiments reported in 1805 by Dr. D. Legare, because his work pushed back the boundaries of ignorance and clearly disproved an old folk remedy. Beyond the shadow of a doubt, Dr. Legare personally proved that, contrary to general opinion, blowing tobacco smoke into the intestinal canal did *not* resuscitate drowned animals or people. The slow advance of medical science through the eighteenth and nineteenth centuries gradually removed tobacco from the doctor's black bag, and nicotine was dropped from *The United States Pharmacopeia* in the 1890s.

The Spread of Tobacco Use

To fully appreciate the history of tobacco, you must know that there are more than 60 species of *Nicotiana,* but only two major ones. ***Nicotiana tobacum,*** the major species grown today in more than a hundred countries, is a large-leaf species. Most important, *tobacum* was indigenous only to South America, so the Spanish had a monopoly on its production for over a hundred years. ***Nicotiana rustica*** is a small-leaf species and was the plant existing in the West Indies and eastern North America when Columbus arrived.

The Spanish monopoly on tobacco sales to Europe was a thorn in the side of the British. When settlers returned to England in 1586 after failing to colonize Virginia, they took with them seeds of the *rustica* species and planted them in England, but this species never grew well. The English crown again attempted to establish a tobacco colony in 1610, when they sent John Rolfe as leader of a group to Virginia. From 1610 to 1612, Rolfe tried to cultivate *rustica,* but the small-leaf plant was weak and poor in flavor, and it had a sharp taste.

In 1612, Rolfe somehow got hold of some seeds of the Spanish *tobacum* species. This species grew beautifully and sold well in 1613. The colony was saved, and every available plot of land was planted with *tobacum.* By 1619, as much Virginia tobacco as Spanish tobacco was sold in London. That was also the year that King James prohibited the cultivation of any tobacco in England and declared the tobacco trade a royal monopoly.

Tobacco became one of the major exports of the American colonies to England. The Thirty Years' War spread smoking throughout central Europe, and nothing stopped its use. Measures such as one in Bavaria in 1652 probably slowed tobacco use, but only momentarily. This law said that "tobacco-drinking was strictly forbidden to the peasants and other common people" and made tobacco available to others only on a doctor's prescription from a druggist.[6]

During the eighteenth century, smoking gradually diminished, but the use of tobacco did not. Snuff replaced the pipe in England. At the beginning of that century, the upper class was already committed to snuff. The middle and lower classes only gradually changed over, but by 1770 very few people were smoking. The reign of King George III (1760–1820) was the time of the big snuff. His wife Charlotte was so addicted to the powder that she was called "Snuffy Charlotte," although for obvious reasons not to her face. On the continent, Napoleon had tried smoking once, gagged horribly, and returned to his 7 pounds of snuff per month.

Tobacco in Early America

Trouble developed in the colonies, which, being democratic, made the richest man in Virginia (perhaps the richest in the colonies) commander in chief of the Revolutionary Army. In 1776, George Washington said in one of his appeals, "If you can't send money, send tobacco."[7] Tobacco played an important role in the Revolutionary War, because it was one of the major products for which France would lend the colonies money. Knowing the importance of tobacco to the colonies, one of Cornwallis's major campaign goals in 1780 and 1781 was the destruction of the Virginia tobacco plantations.

After the war, ordinary Americans rejoiced and rejected snuff as well as tea and all other things British. The aristocrats who organized the republic were not as emotional, though, and installed a communal snuff box for members of Congress. Only in the mid-1930s did this remembrance of things past disappear. However, to emphasize the fact that snuff was a nonessential, the new Congress put a luxury tax on it in 1794.

Nicotiana tobacum: (**ni co she *ann* a toe *back* um**) the species of tobacco widely cultivated for smoking and chewing products.

Nicotiana rustica: (***russ* tick a**) the less desirable species of tobacco, which is not widely grown in the United States.

Chewing Tobacco

If you don't smoke and you don't snuff
How can you possibly get enough?

You can get enough, of course, by chewing, which gradually increased in the United States. Chewing was a suitable activity for a country on the go; it freed the hands, and the wide-open spaces made an adequate spittoon. There were also other considerations: Boston, for example, passed an ordinance in 1798 forbidding anyone from being in possession of a lighted pipe or "segar" in public streets. The original impetus was a concern for the fire hazard involved in smoking, not the individual's health, and the ordinance was finally repealed in 1880. Today it is difficult to appreciate how much of a chewing country we were in the nineteenth century. In 1860, only 7 of 348 tobacco factories in Virginia and North Carolina manufactured smoking tobacco. The amount of tobacco for smoking did not equal the amount for chewing until 1911 and did not surpass it until the 1920s.

The high level of chewing-tobacco production during the Industrial Age led to occasional accidents, as suggested by a quote from a 1918 decision of the Mississippi Supreme Court:

> We can imagine no reason why, with ordinary care, human toes could not be left out of chewing tobacco, and if toes were found in chewing tobacco, it seems to us that somebody has been very careless.[3]

The turn of the twentieth century was the approximate high point for chewing tobacco, the sales of which slowly declined through the early part of that century, as other tobacco products became more popular. In 1945, cuspidors were removed from all federal buildings.

Cigars and Cigarettes

The transition from chewing to cigarettes had a middle point, a combination of both smoking and chewing: cigars. Cigarette smoking was coming, and the cigar manufacturers did their best to keep cigarettes under control. They suggested that cigarettes were drugged with opium, so one could not stop using them and that the paper was bleached with arsenic and, thus, was harmful. They had some help from Thomas Edison in 1914:

> The injurious agent in Cigarettes comes principally from the burning paper wrapper. . . . It has a violent action in the nerve centers, producing degeneration of the cells of the brain, which is quite rapid among boys. Unlike most narcotics, this degeneration is permanent and uncontrollable. I employ no person who smokes cigarettes.[3]

Most cigars had been hand rolled or at least made by hand shaping in a mold, but as sales increased, machines had to be used. Today a good worker hand rolls about 200 cigars in an 8- to 9-hour day. There was an aversion to machine-made cigars, so some advertising was educational. The following is an example of the high level of advertising before television and Madison Avenue:

> Spit is a horrid word, but it's worse on the end of your cigar. Why run the risk of cigars made by dirty yellowed fingers and tipped in spit?[3]

The efforts of the cigar manufacturers worked for a while, and cigar sales reached their highest level in 1920, when 8 billion were sold. As sales increased, though, so did the cost of the product. The whole world knows that "what this country *needs* is a really good five-cent cigar," but how many know that this statement was made by a vice president of the United States as an aside in the Senate, when one of the members was going on at great length about the needs of the country?

Thin reeds filled with tobacco had been seen by the Spanish in Yucatan in 1518. In 1844, the French were using them, and the Crimean War circulated the cigarette habit throughout Europe. The first British cigarette factory was

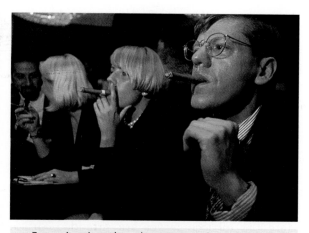

Expensive cigars have become trendy, with "cigar bars," smoke-ins, and magazines devoted to the aficionado.

started in 1856 by a returning veteran of the Crimean War, and in the late 1850s an English tobacco merchant, Phillip Morris, began producing handmade cigarettes. On the continent the use of this new dose form must have developed fairly rapidly. One company in Austria began making double cigarettes in 1865—both ends had a mouthpiece, and the consumer cut them in two—and sold 16 million in 1866.

In the United States, cigarettes were being produced during the same period (14 million in 1870), but it was in the 1880s that their popularity increased rapidly. The date of the first patent on a cigarette-making machine was 1881, and by 1885 over a billion cigarettes a year were being sold. Not even that great he-man, boxer John L. Sullivan, could stem the tide, though in 1905 his opinion of cigarette smokers was pretty clear:

> Smoke cigarettes? Not on your tut-tut. . . . You can't suck coffin-nails and be a ring-champion. . . . You never heard of . . . a bank burglar using a cigarette, did you? They couldn't do it and attend to biz. Why, even drunkards don't use the things. . . . Who smokes 'em? Dudes and college stiffs—fellows who'd be wiped out by a single jab or a quick undercut. It isn't natural to smoke

cigarettes. An American ought to smoke cigars. . . . It's the Dutchmen, Italians, Russians, Turks and Egyptians who smoke cigarettes and they're no good anyhow.[3]

At the turn of the twentieth century, there was a preference for cigarettes with an aromatic component—that is, Turkish tobacco. Camels—a new cigarette in 1913, capitalized on the lure of the Near East while rejecting it in actuality. Camels contained just a hint of Turkish tobacco. Besides, eliminating most of the imported tobacco made the price lower. Low price was combined with a big advertising campaign: "The Camels are coming. Tomorrow there'll be more CAMELS in town than in all of Asia and Africa combined." In 1918, Camels had 40 percent of the market, and they stayed in front until after World War II.

The year 1919 was marked by the first ad showing a woman smoking. To make the ad easier to accept, the woman was pictured as Asian and the ad was for a Turkish type of cigarette. King-size cigarettes appeared in 1939 in the form of Pall Mall, which became the number-one seller. Filter cigarettes as filter cigarettes, not cigarettes that happen to have filters along with a mouthpiece, appeared in 1954 with Winston, which rapidly took over the market and continued to be number one until the mid-1970s. Filter cigarettes captured an increasing share of the market and now constitute over 90 percent of all U.S. cigarette sales.

CURRENT TOBACCO PRODUCTS

Tobacco is grown on about 125,000 American farms, most with only a few acres devoted to tobacco. There's a lot of hand labor involved, requiring about 250 worker-hours for each harvested acre (compared with about 3 worker-hours per acre for wheat). Tobacco seeds are started in seed beds and transplanted, 5,000 to 10,000 plants to an acre, when they are 6 to 8 inches high. In 2 to 3 months, when the tobacco is ready to harvest, the leaves are 1 to $2^1/_2$ feet long, and a typical burley tobacco plant has 10 leaves. The nicotine content of a raw tobacco leaf ranges from 0.3 to 7 percent and varies with the variety, climatic conditions, fertilizer used, and many other factors. Nicotine levels can be manipulated during processing to any desired level.

Burley is one of the major tobaccos used in cigarettes. It is harvested by cutting the stalk close to the ground, then hanging the entire stalk in a curing barn for four to six weeks. The plant uses its stored food, dies, and loses about 80 percent of its weight through moisture loss. This is "air-curing," the method used for most cigarette tobacco grown west of the Appalachians. East of the mountains, "flue-curing" is used to produce *bright* tobacco. Tobacco that is to be flue-cured has the leaves separated from the stalks during harvesting, and heat is added

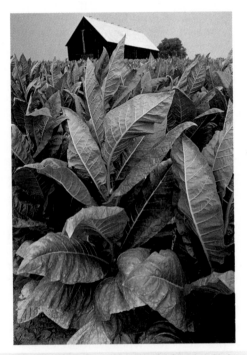

Although labor-intensive, tobacco farming is more profitable per acre than any other legal crop.

to the curing barn, so that the process is complete in less than a week.

After curing, the burley leaves are removed from the stalk and sorted on the basis of color, size, and stalk position. Almost all tobacco is still sold at one of the 136 auction houses in this country. The farmer's hard work is well rewarded, with an average gross income of almost $4,000 per acre (compared with less than $100 per acre for wheat). Overall, tobacco is America's seventh largest legal cash crop.[8]

When the tobacco reaches the buyer's processing plant, modern technology takes over. Here the tobacco leaves are shredded, dried, picked, blown clean of foreign matter and stems, remoisturized to a particular level, and packed in huge wooden barrels called hogsheads. The hogsheads are placed in storehouses, where the tobacco ages for two to three years.

Proper aging is one of the secrets to good tobacco. Aging allows fermentation to occur so that the tobacco gets darker and loses moisture, as well as nicotine (probably about one-third of its original level) and other volatile substances. When the aging is complete, moisture is again added, and various types of tobacco are blended. During the secret blending process, other substances are also added. Glycerine is used to stabilize the moisture content, and a variety of flavorants are included. A 1972 publication by the Reynolds Tobacco Company listed 1,290 flavorants that could be added to tobacco, including such common tastes as chocolate, licorice, and sugar. The blended material is compressed and then cut into hangnail-size strips to prepare it for the cigarette machine.

In the 1870s, James Buchanan Duke thought his cigarette girls were doing very well if they could consistently roll four cigarettes a minute. In 1881, he started the cigarette revolution by using a machine that had just been patented. It produced 200 cigarettes a minute. He would love today's machine. It starts with a roll of cigarette paper $3^1/_2$ miles (5.6 km) long, makes a continuous clotheslinelike tube filled with tobacco, cuts it to length, weighs the cigarettes, (rejecting those over or under the correct weight), and checks them for uniformity. It does all that and still turns out 3,600 cigarettes a minute. Filter cigarettes are made by adding a machine that attaches a double-size filter between two cigarettes and then cuts them apart at the same rapid rate.

Less Hazardous Cigarettes

The cigarettes of the 1950s were quite different from today's cigarettes. For one thing, in the 1950s, it required $2^3/_4$ pounds (1.2 kg) of leaf tobacco to produce 1,000 cigarettes. Now only about $1^3/_4$ pounds (0.8 kg) are required to produce the same number. Besides the addition of filters, two other technological changes have decreased the amount of leaf tobacco per cigarette. One is the use of reconstituted sheets of tobacco. Parts of the tobacco leaf and stems that had been discarded in earlier years are now ground up, combined with various ingredients, and then rolled out as a flat sheet of tobacco. After shredding, this material is combined with normally processed leaf tobacco. Today about 20 percent of all cigarette tobacco is reconstituted sheet.

The second development that reduced the need for tobacco in cigarettes is "fluffing." Tobacco is freeze-dried, and an inert gas is used to expand the tobacco cells, so that they take up more space and absorb more additives. One low-tar cigarette introduced in the early 1970s was able to reduce by 35 percent the tobacco in each cigarette because of its process to fluff the tobacco. Fluffing, of course, reduces the tar, nicotine, and carbon monoxide content of a cigarette, but it also reduces smoking time, perhaps by 15 percent. Carbon monoxide is important because it decreases the oxygen-carrying capacity of the blood, putting more strain on the heart and reducing oxygenation of all the tissues.

For many years the Federal Trade Commission (FTC) measured the tar and nicotine content of cigarettes and published a listing of the results by brand name and type. These were measured by standardized smoking machines. The machine contained a filter, and the word *tar* refers to a complex mixture that remains on the filter after moisture and nicotine have been removed. This tar mixture contains most of the cancer-causing chemicals in tobacco smoke. As you might suspect, cigarettes with less tobacco have less tar and less nicotine, and measurements across brands found very high correlations between the two. Thus, it is possible to speak of the tar and nicotine (T/N) content of a cigarette. Because of the changes in cigarette manufacturing, T/N levels have declined since the 1950s. The average 1950s cigarette delivered about 2.5 mg of nicotine, whereas the average cigarette now delivers about 1 mg of nicotine. Average tar yield has dropped from over 40 mg to under 20 mg per cigarette.

Low T/N cigarettes are associated with a lower health risk, and low T/N is a significant factor in advertising and in brand selection. However, there are a few things you should know about low T/N cigarettes. First is that the measurements are made by a machine that smokes each cigarette in a standard manner (e.g., to within 3 mm of the filter "overwrap"). Manufacturers were able to reduce T/N content by manipulations such as using a longer overwrap or putting airholes around the filter. Smokers could and did smoke differently from the machine (for instance, covering some or all of the air holes while puffing), thus obtaining more tar and nicotine. It seems that smokers aim for a certain nicotine input, and when switched to a low T/N brand they take more puffs and inhale more deeply so as to compensate largely for the change in cigarettes.[9] Obviously, if a smoker compensates in this manner, there might be little value in switching. Also, there is a limit to how low a T/N level the consumer will accept

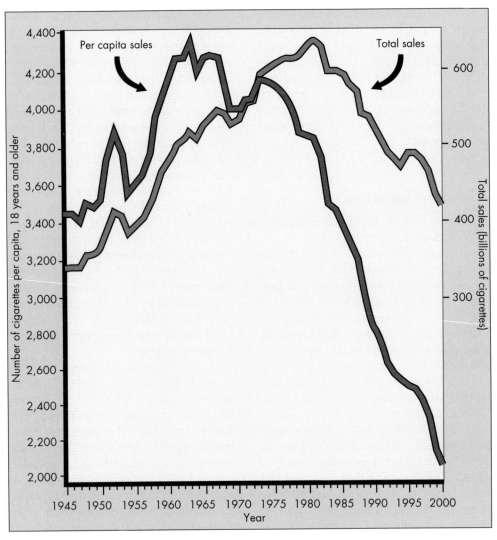

Figure 13-1   Trends in cigarette sales since 1945.

because there is a decrease in satisfaction. At some point (about 8 mg tar and 0.3 mg nicotine), smokers begin to lose interest.

Trends in Smoking Behavior

The health warnings and educational programs certainly had an effect on cigarette consumption (Figure 13.1). After World War II, cigarette sales increased, both on a per capita basis and in total sales. The peak year for per capita sales was 1963. In 1964, the surgeon general's Report on Smoking and Health declared that smoking is a health hazard. For the next several years per capita sales decreased, with a more rapid decrease after 1973. Because of the expanding adult population, total cigarette sales continued to climb slowly, even while per capita sales

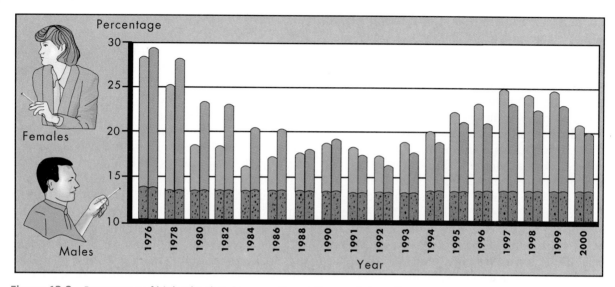

Figure 13-2   Percentage of high school seniors reporting daily use of cigarettes.

dropped. This trend continued until 1981, when the peak was reached with sales of over 640 billion cigarettes. For the past several years both total and per capita sales have declined. Per capita sales are now lower than at any time since World War II.

For many years a much greater percentage of adult men smoked than adult women. The 1970s saw an alarming increase in smoking among young females: for the first time, in 1976, more female than male high school seniors reported smoking (Figure 13.2, data from the annual high school senior survey described in Chapter 1). From then through the mid-1980s, fewer high school seniors of both genders were smoking, but girls retained a higher smoking rate than boys throughout this period of decline. In the mid-1980s, the decline leveled off, and then smoking rates for high school seniors began to increase again. Slightly greater increases among boys have led to essentially no gender difference in the latest reports. Among adult smokers, men still slightly outnumber women; however, the trend is toward equality. Women are also moving toward equality with

men in lung cancer, heart disease, and overall life expectancy.

Smokeless Tobacco

In the early 1970s, many cigarette smokers apparently began to look for alternatives that would reduce the risk of lung cancer. Pipe and cigar smoking enjoyed a brief, small increase, followed by a long period of decline. Sales of **smokeless tobacco** products—specifically, different kinds of chewing tobacco—began to increase. Once limited to western movies and the baseball field as far as public awareness was concerned, smokeless tobacco use grew to become a matter of public concern.

The most common types of oral smokeless tobacco in the United States are loose-leaf (Red Man, Levi Garrett, Beech Nut), which is sold in

---

smokeless tobacco: a term used for chewing tobacco during the 1980s.

a pouch, and **moist snuff** (Copenhagen, Skoal), which is sold in a can. When you see a baseball player on TV with a big wad in his cheek, it is probably composed of loose-leaf tobacco. Sales of loose-leaf tobacco, growing from a traditional base in the Southeast and Midwest, increased by about 50 percent during the 1970s and then declined through the 1980s and 1990s. Moist snuff is not "snuffed" into the nose in the European manner; a small pinch is dipped out of the can and placed beside the gum, often behind the lower lip. One form of moist snuff also comes in a little teabag type of packet, so that loose tobacco fragments don't stray out onto the teeth. Moist snuff, which has its traditional popularity base in the rural West, continued to show sales gains through the 1990s. With all forms of oral smokeless tobacco, nicotine is absorbed through the mucous membranes of the mouth into the bloodstream, and users achieve blood nicotine levels comparable to those of smokers.

Smokeless tobacco enjoys many competitive advantages over smoking. First, it is unlikely to cause lung cancer. Smokeless tobacco is less expensive than cigarettes, with an average user spending only a few dollars a week. In spite of the Marlboro advertisements, a cowboy or anyone else who is working outdoors finds it more convenient to keep some tobacco in the mouth than to try to light cigarettes in the wind and then have ashes blowing in the face. And, believe it or not, chewing might be more socially acceptable than smoking under most circumstances. After all, the user doesn't blow smoke all around, and most people don't even notice when someone is chewing, unless the chewer has a huge wad in the mouth or spits frequently. Many users can control the amount of tobacco they put in their mouths so that they don't have to spit very often. What they do with the leftover **quid** of tobacco is a different story and often not a pretty sight.

The use of chewing tobacco had never completely died out in rural areas, and its resurgence in the past 30 years was strongest there. It is primarily a male phenomenon, and surveys of high school students in Oregon, Colorado, and Louisiana have found 20 to 25 percent of the boys reporting smokeless tobacco use. In one survey of Wyoming junior high school students, about 25 percent of the boys reported being current users of smokeless tobacco, compared with only 1.2 percent of the girls. For the boys, the median reported age of first use was 11 years.[10] Although these studies indicate high rates of regional use, increased sales of smokeless tobacco are not limited to the rural West and South. Promoted by sport celebrities, increased advertising budgets, and sponsorship of auto racing, college rodeo, and skiing, smokeless tobacco use increased among young men in many parts of the country. The high school senior class of 2000 reported that 14.3 percent of the boys and about 1 percent of the girls were using smokeless tobacco in the past month.[11]

Chewing tobacco might not be as unhealthy as smoking it. However, smokeless tobacco is not without its hazards. The one of most concern is the increased risk of cancer of the mouth, pharynx, and esophagus. In spite of the fact that snuff and chewing tobacco are not burned during use, they do contain potent carcinogens, including high levels of tobacco-specific **nitrosamines.** Many users experience tissue changes in the mouth, with **leukoplakia** (a whitening, thickening, and hardening of the tissue) a relatively frequent finding. Leukoplakia is considered to be a precancerous lesion (a tissue change that can develop into cancer). The irritation of the gums can cause them to become inflamed or to recede, exposing the teeth to disease. The enamel of the teeth can also be worn down by the abrasive action of the tobacco. In short, dentists are also becoming more aware of the destructive effects of oral tobacco.

Concerns about these oral diseases led the surgeon general's office to sponsor a conference and produce a 1986 report on that conference, *The Health Consequences of Using Smokeless Tobacco.*[12] This report went into some depth in

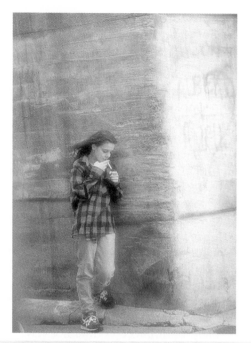

Despite antismoking education, one in five young people still becomes a regular smoker.

reviewing epidemiological, experimental, and clinical data and concluded "the oral use of smokeless tobacco represents a significant health risk. It is not a safe substitute for smoking cigarettes. It can cause cancer and a number of noncancerous oral conditions and can lead to nicotine addiction and dependence." Packages of smokeless tobacco now carry a series of rotating warning labels describing these dangers.

Are Cigars Back?

After many years of declining popularity, cigar smoking reappeared on the cultural scene in the mid-1990s. Yuppies, businesspeople, and celebrities of both sexes began lighting up large, expensive cigars, many of which are made in Florida from tobacco supposedly grown using Cuban seeds. Magazines devoted to cigars, "cigar bars," and radio talk–show discussions of the

merits of various $25 "stogies" all pointed to the trendiness of this phenomenon.[13] Perhaps it was a reaction against the abstinent 1980s, with a slight hope that cigars were safer than cigarettes. All the same, it was another example of the unpredicatable faddishness of people's recreational use of psychoactive substances. At the beginning of the twenty-first century, however, cigar sales showed signs of leveling off.

A SOCIAL AND ECONOMIC DILEMMA

It is now clear that cigarette smoking is deadly. People have been slow to accept this fact, perhaps partly because tobacco, like alcohol and other substances, has long been the subject of emotional diatribes. In 1604, King James of England (the same one who had the Bible translated) wrote and published a strong antitobacco pamphlet stating that tobacco was "harmefull to the braine, dangerous to the lungs." Never one to let morality or health concerns interfere with business, he also supported the growing of tobacco in Virginia in 1610, and when the crop prospered, he declared the tobacco trade a royal monopoly.

New York City made it illegal in 1908 for a woman to use tobacco in public, and in the Roaring Twenties women were expelled from

moist snuff: finely chopped tobacco, held in the mouth rather than snuffed into the nose.

quid: a piece of chewing tobacco.

nitrosamines: (nye *troh* sa meens) a type of chemical that is carcinogenic; several are found in tobacco.

leukoplakia: (luke o *plake* ee ah) a whitening and thickening of the mucous tissue in the mouth, considered to be a precancerous tissue change.

schools and dismissed from jobs for smoking. These concerns were partly for society and partly to "protect women from themselves." Those sensitive to feminist issues will find an analogy to current reactions to drug and alcohol use by pregnant women in this quote from the 1920s:

> Smoking by women and even young girls must be considered from a far different stand point than smoking by men, for not only is the female organism by virtue of its much more frail structure and its more delicate tissues much less able to resist the poisonous action of tobacco than that of men, and thus, like many a delicate flower, apt to fade and wither more quickly in consequence, but the fecundity of woman is greatly impaired by it. Authorities cannot be expected to look on unmoved while a generation of sterile women, rendered incapable of fulfilling their sublime function of motherhood, is being produced on account of the immoderate smoking of foolish young girls.[14]

And those familiar with the 1930s "Reefer Madness" arguments might find it interesting that earlier in the same decade a weed other than marijuana had been blamed for the same ills once laid at alcohol's door:

> Fifty percent of our insanity is inherited from parents who were users of tobacco. . . . Thirty-three percent of insanity cases are caused direct from cigarette smoking and the use of tobacco. . . .
>
> Judge Gimmill, of the court of Domestic Relations of Chicago, declared that, without exception, every boy appearing before him that had lost the faculty of blushing was a cigarette fiend. The poison in cigarettes has the same effect upon girls: it perverts the morals and deadens the sense of shame and refinement. . . .
>
> The bathing beaches have become resorts for women smokers, where they go to show off with a cigarette in their mouths. The bathing apparel in the last ten years has been reduced from knee skirts to a thin tight-fitting veil that scarcely covers two-thirds of their hips. Many of the girl

bathers never put their feet in the water, but sit on the shore, show their legs and smoke cigarettes.[15]

Besides people's tendency to be suspicious of anticigarette claims, there are other potent forces that work to keep billions of cigarettes going up in smoke. Everyone knows that the tobacco industry has a lot of clout. Tobacco founded the English colonies and funded the American Revolution. But more significant is the continued economic importance of these products. Recent downturns in total sales have largely been offset by increased prices and reduced manufacturing costs, so that making and selling tobacco products is still a highly profitable business, with net income representing about 18 percent of sales.[16] It is perhaps not surprising that these companies were involved in some of the largest corporate mergers and leveraged buyouts of the past 20 years. The large profits made by tobacco companies have made them the targets of an increasing number of lawsuits and have allowed them to make multimillion dollar settlements with several states to offset increased medical costs.

A lot of people make their living, either directly or indirectly, from tobacco. Tobacco products are sold in 625,000 retail outlets, and total sales are almost $50 billion. Grocery stores sell more cigarettes than any other outlet, and recently cigarette sales in gasoline stations have been increasing, whereas the number of vending machines has been cut in half in the past 10 years. Cigarette companies were the largest advertisers on television and radio until such ads were banned in 1971. Now they spend their advertising money on magazine and newspaper ads. It has been pointed out that most magazines need those revenues to survive, and they are therefore not likely to print many articles about the dangers of smoking.[17]

Governments, too, derive significant income from tobacco taxes, with almost $6 billion per year going to the federal government and about another $7.5 billion going to the states. Also, at a time in which the trade deficit is of such concern,

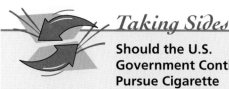

Taking Sides

Should the U.S. Government Continue to Pursue Cigarette Manufacturers?

During the Clinton administration, both the top U.S. tobacco companies and the U.S. Justice Department spent a lot of money on lawyers. The federal government helped arrange the 1998 multistate tobacco settlement, in which the companies agreed to pay $206 billion (over 25 years) to states to recover their increased Medicare costs due to tobacco-related disease; to stop advertisements intended to influence tobacco use by children; and to fund antismoking education program development and implementation. The Justice Department continued action against the tobacco companies, including a lawsuit charging the top five manufacturers with racketeering because they systematically covered up information about the harmful effects of smoking. President Bush seems somewhat less inclined to go after tobacco companies, who continue to protest that they are legitimate businesses making and selling legal products and using standard industry techniques.

The $206 billion settlement already awarded to the states has begun to be passed on to smokers through the greatly increased cost of cigarettes. Do you think the U.S. government should pursue federal legislation to further restrict the activities of the tobacco industry?

For more on this topic, log on to www.dushkin.com/online for current news and links to other popular and informative sites, as well as time-saving web search strategies and study tools.

and more forceful warnings from the surgeon general. The tobacco industry fought back by establishing in 1954 the Council for Tobacco Research to provide funds to independent scientists to study the health effects of tobacco use. A 1993 exposé in the *Wall Street Journal*[18] detailed the manipulation of this "independent" research by tobacco industry lawyers, who arranged direct funding for research casting doubt on smoking-related health problems and who suppressed the publication of findings that threatened the industry. In spite of tobacco industry efforts, by now it is abundantly clear that tobacco is America's true "killer weed" and is a bigger public health threat than all the other drug substances combined, including alcohol. It was not until the late 1990s, however, that a tobacco manufacturer admitted that cigarettes have seriously adverse effects on health. These admissions have come as a part of various settlements in which the companies reimburse states for increased health-care costs associated with smoking.

Adverse Health Effects

There have been so many government and other reports detailing the health hazards of tobacco use that the smoke has now cleared and we can see the overall picture. If we add it all up it comes out like this: although lung cancer is not common, about 85 percent of all lung cancers occur in smokers. Among deaths resulting from all types of cancer, smoking is estimated to be related to 30 percent, or about 150,000 premature deaths per year. However, cancer is only the second leading cause of death in the United States. It now appears that smoking is also related to about 30 percent of deaths from the leading killer, cardiovascular disease, or about 180,000 premature deaths per year. In addition, cigarette smoking is the cause of 80 to 90 percent of deaths resulting from chronic obstructive lung disease—another 80,000 cigarette-related premature deaths per year. The total

it is important to remember that the value of tobacco exports exceeds imports by over $5 billion.[8]

CAUSES FOR CONCERN

Although the first clear scientific evidence linking smoking and lung cancer appeared in the 1950s, acceptance of the evidence was slow to come. Each decade brought clearer evidence

"smoking attributed mortality" is more than 400,000 premature deaths per year in the United States, representing about 20 percent of all U.S. deaths.[19] No wonder these reports keep saying that "cigarette smoking is the chief, single, avoidable cause of death in our society and the most important public health issue of our time."

Think of anything related to good physical health; the research says that cigarette smoking will impair it. The earlier the age at which you start smoking and the more smoking you do, and the longer you do it—the greater the impairment (Figure 13.3). Smoking doesn't do any part of the body any good, at any time, under any conditions (Figure 13.4).

In 1990, the U.S. surgeon general's office released a report on the health benefits of smoking cessation (quitting). This 600-plus-page report not only pointed out once again the increased risk of mortality resulting from smoking but made it clear that quitting smoking has an immediate impact on a person's chances of living to a ripe old age. For example, a 35-year-old man who quits smoking will, on the average, increase his life expectancy by 5.1 years. Even a 65-year-old can add an extra year or more of life by quitting smoking.[20]

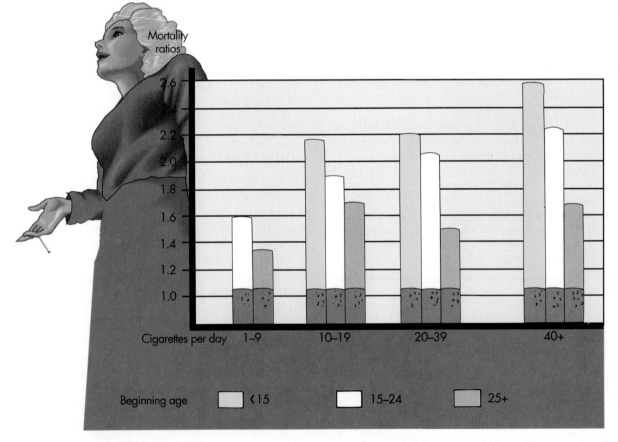

Figure 13-3   Mortality ratios (total deaths, mean ages, 55 to 64) as a function of the age at which smoking started and the number of cigarettes smoked per day.

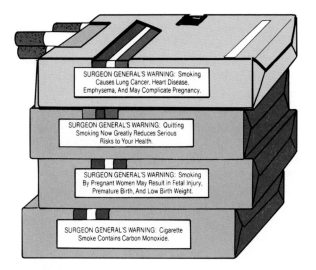

Figure 13-4 Cigarette packages and advertisements are required to "rotate" among different warning labels.

Passive Smoking

There has been a great deal said and written about **passive smoking**—that is, the inhaling of cigarette smoke from the environment by non-smokers. The importance of this issue can best be demonstrated by a couple of court cases. In 1976, the Superior Court of New Jersey ruled in favor of a Mrs. Shimp, a telephone company employee who was allergic to cigarette smoke and who worked in a small office along with some smokers. The judge's opinion established several principles:

> The evidence is clear and overwhelming. Cigarette smoke contaminates and pollutes the air creating a health hazard not merely to the smoker but to all those around her who must rely upon the same air supply. The right of an individual to risk his or her own health does not include the right to jeopardize the health of those who must remain around him or her in order to properly perform the duties of their jobs. The portion of the population which is especially sensitive to cigarette smoke is so significant that it is reasonable to expect an employer to foresee

health consequences and to impose upon him a duty to abate the hazard which causes the discomfort.

In determining the extent to which smoking must be restricted the rights and interests of smoking and nonsmoking employees alike must be considered. The employees' rights to a safe working environment makes it clear that smoking must be forbidden in the work area. The employee who desires to smoke on his own time, during coffee breaks and lunch hours should have a reasonably accessible area in which to smoke.[21]

It is obvious that cigarette smoke can be irritating to others, but is it damaging? Besides the cases of individuals who have lung disorders or are allergic to smoke, is there evidence that cigarette smoke is harmful to exposed nonsmokers? Research is complicated; the smoke rising from the ash of the cigarette (**sidestream smoke**) is higher in many carcinogens than is the mainstream smoke delivered to the smoker's lungs. Of course, it is also more diluted. How many smokers are in the room? How much do they smoke? How good is the ventilation? How much time does the nonsmoker spend in this room? These variables have made definitive research difficult, but enough studies have produced consistent enough findings that the Environmental Protection Agency in 1993 declared secondhand smoke to be a known carcinogen and estimated that passive smoking is responsible for several thousand lung cancer deaths each year. The tobacco companies countered with full-page newspaper ads attacking the methods used by the EPA, but a review of the issue by an independent consumer group found that the EPA

passive smoking: the inhalation of tobacco smoke by individuals other than the smoker.

sidestream smoke: smoke arising from the ash of the cigarette or cigar.

Health Quest Activities

Assess yourself in Module X by completing "Phase 1: Your Risks" of *Tobacco: Are You at Risk?* Make a list of ways you can decrease your exposure to tobacco. If you are strongly at risk, you may also find helpful the suggestions in "Phase 2: Quitting." If you smoke, consider keeping a tally of how many cigarettes you consume each week or month. See if you can decrease this number each week or each month.

The media are filled with messages that influence our decision making, and we are often unaware of the media's power. In the same module, complete the activity *Tobacco Ads and You* to discover how much power advertising has over you. Take note of the tobacco ads you see during the week. If you are a smoker, do these ads make you want to smoke more? If you don't smoke, do the ads glamorize smoking enough to tempt you to take up the practice?

had used accepted techniques and that the tobacco company objections were based on the opinions of a few industry-funded scientists.[22]

Concerns about the effects of secondhand smoke have led to many more restrictions on smoking in the workplace and in public. Most states and municipalities now have laws prohibiting smoking in public conveyances and requiring the establishment of smoking and nonsmoking areas in public buildings and restaurants, and some communities have banned smoking in all restaurants. A few employers have gone so far as to either encourage or attempt to force their employees to quit smoking both on the job and elsewhere, citing health statistics indicating more sick days and greater health insurance costs associated with smoking. This conflict between smoker and nonsmoker seems destined to get worse before it gets better. Although to some this battle might seem silly, it represents a very basic conflict between individual freedom and public health.

Smoking and Health in Other Countries

Cigarette smoking is a social and medical problem worldwide. A 1994 international report estimated that, worldwide, smoking is killing 3 million people a year and that by the year 2020 the rate might be as high as 10 million per year.[23] Throughout the 1970s and 1980s, as sales leveled and declined in developed countries, advertising and promotions in Third World countries (touting cigarettes as delivering "the great taste of America") resulted in large increases in exports of American cigarettes. Asians, in particular, seemed to want American cigarettes, and one of the major efforts was to open Japanese, Taiwanese, and Korean cigarette markets to U.S. imports.[24] There are *no* warnings printed on the packs we sell to them (shades of patent

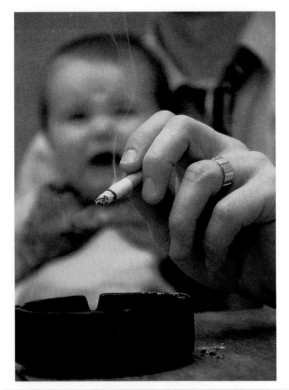

Breathing passive smoke subjects infants and children to dangerous carcinogens.

medicines in the late nineteenth century). Most of the countries U.S. cigarette manufacturers are exporting to are underdeveloped countries with lots of preventable disease and high infant mortality. According to the World Health Organization, "the control of cigarette smoking could do more to improve health and prolong life in these countries than any single action in the whole field of preventive medicine."[25]

Smoking and Pregnancy

The nicotine, hydrogen cyanide, and carbon monoxide in a smoking mother's blood also reach the developing fetus and have significant negative consequences there. On the average, infants born to smokers are about half a pound lighter than infants born to nonsmokers. This basic fact has been known for almost 30 years and has been confirmed in almost 50 studies.[26] There is a dose-response relationship: the more the woman smokes during pregnancy, the greater the reduction in birth weight. Is the reduced birth weight the result of an increased frequency of premature births or of retarded growth of the fetus? Smoking shortens the gestation period by an average of only 2 days, and when gestation length is accounted for, the smokers still have smaller infants. Ultrasonic measurements taken at various intervals during pregnancy show smaller fetuses in smoking women for at least the last 2 months of pregnancy. The infants of smokers are normally proportioned, are shorter and smaller than the infants of nonsmokers, and have smaller head circumference. The reduced birth weight of infants of women smokers is not related to how much weight the mother gains during pregnancy, and the consensus is that a reduced availability of oxygen is responsible for the diminished growth rate. Women who give up smoking early in pregnancy (by the fourth month) have infants with weights similar to those of nonsmokers.

Besides the developmental effects evident at birth, several studies indicate small but consistent differences in body size, neurological problems, reading and mathematical skills, and hyperactivity at various ages. It therefore appears that smoking during pregnancy can have long-lasting effects on both the intellectual and physical development of the child. Several studies have also found an increased risk of sudden infant death syndrome (SIDS) if the mother smokes, but it is not clear if this is related more to the mother's smoking during pregnancy or to passive smoking (the infant's breathing smoke) after birth.

So far we have been talking about normal deliveries of babies. Spontaneous abortion (miscarriage) has also been studied many times in relation to smoking and with consistent results: smokers have more spontaneous abortions than nonsmokers (perhaps 1.5 to 2 times as many). As for congenital malformations, the evidence for a relationship to maternal smoking is not as clear. If there is a small effect here, it could be either related to or obscured by the fact that many smokers also drink alcohol and coffee. One study indicated an increased risk of facial malformations associated with the father's smoking. Neonatal death rates are higher among children of smoking mothers, and this effect is much greater among older women of low socioeconomic status who have had more than three pregnancies.

The overall message is very clear. There are definite, serious risks associated with smoking during pregnancy. In fact, the demonstrated effects of cigarette smoking on the developing child are of the same magnitude and type as those reported for "crack babies," and there are many more pregnant women smoking cigarettes than using cocaine. If a woman smoker discovers herself to be pregnant, that should be a clear signal to her to quit smoking.

PHARMACOLOGY OF NICOTINE

Nicotine is a naturally occurring liquid alkaloid that is colorless and volatile. On oxidation it turns brown and smells much like burning tobacco. Tolerance to its effects develops, along

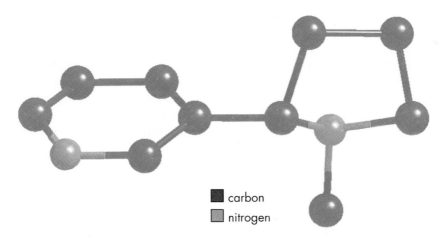

■ carbon
□ nitrogen

Figure 13-5   Nicotine (1-methyl-2 [3-pyridyl] pyrrolidone).

with the dependency that led Mark Twain to re-mark how easy it was to stop smoking—he'd done it several times!

Nicotine was isolated in 1828 and has been studied irregularly since then. It has no thera-peutic actions, so no drug company has exhaus-tively looked at its effects. Because it has proved to be a valuable pharmacological tool for study-ing synaptic functions, as well as being the ac-tive ingredient in tobacco, there is some relevant information. The structure of nicotine is shown in Figure 13.5; it should be noted that there are both *d* and *l* forms, but they are equipotent. It is of some importance that nicotine in smoke has two forms, one with a positive charge and one that is electrically neutral. The neutral form is more easily absorbed through the mucous mem-branes of the mouth, nose, and lungs.

Absorption and Metabolism

Inhalation is a very effective drug-delivery sys-tem; 90 percent of inhaled nicotine is absorbed. The physiological effects of smoking one ciga-rette have been mimicked by injecting about 1 mg of nicotine intravenously.

Acting with almost as much speed as cyanide, nicotine is well established as one of the most toxic drugs known. In humans, 60 mg is a lethal dose, and death follows intake within a few minutes. A cigar contains enough nicotine for two lethal doses (who needs to take a second one?), but not all of the nicotine is delivered to the smoker or absorbed in a short enough period of time to kill a person.

Nicotine is primarily deactivated in the liver, with 80 to 90 percent being modified before ex-cretion through the kidneys. Part of the toler-ance that develops to nicotine might result from the fact that either nicotine or the tars increase the activity of the liver microsomal enzymes that are responsible for the deactivation of drugs. These enzymes increase the rate of deac-tivation and thus decrease the clinical effects of the benzodiazepines and some antidepressants and analgesics. The final step in eliminating de-activated nicotine from the body may be some-what slowed by nicotine itself, since it acts on the hypothalamus to cause a release of the hor-mone that acts to reduce the loss of body fluids.

Physiological Effects

The effect of nicotine on areas outside the cen-tral nervous system has been studied exten-sively. Nicotine mimics acetylcholine by acting

Drugs in Depth

Possible New Painkiller?

One of the early uses of tobacco was as a painkiller. Nicotine itself does have some analgesic properties, but its toxicity limits its usefulness for this. The discovery of a substance in the skin of Ecuadorian "poison-arrow" frogs that binds strongly to nicotinis acetylcholine receptors led in 1997 to the developments of a synthetic analgesic with a novel mechanism. Animal testing with ABT-594 indicates that it may be a potent pain reliever with fewer side effects and less addiction potential than morphine and other opiate analgesics.[37] The drug is now in clinical trials with humans, and soon we will learn whether this potentially revolutionary new type of powerful painkiller will live up to its promise.

at the nicotinic type of cholinergic receptor site and stimulating the dendrite. Nicotine is not rapidly deactivated, and continued occupation of the receptor prevents incoming impulses from having an effect, thereby blocking the transmission of information at the synapse. Thus, nicotine first stimulates and then blocks the synapse. This blockage of cholinergic synapses is responsible for some of nicotine's effects, but others seem to be the result of a second action.

Nicotine also causes a release of adrenaline from the adrenal glands and other sympathetic sites and thus has, in part, a sympathomimetic action. Additionally, it stimulates and then blocks some sensory receptors, including the chemical receptors found in some large arteries and the thermal pain receptors found in the skin and tongue.

The symptoms of low-level nicotine poisoning are well known to beginning smokers and small children behind barns and in alleys: nausea, dizziness, and a general weakness. In acute poisoning, nicotine causes tremors, which develop into convulsions, terminated frequently by death. The cause of death is suffocation resulting from paralysis of the muscles used in respiration. This paralysis stems from the blocking effect of nicotine on the cholinergic system that normally activates the muscles. With lower doses there is actually an increase in respiration rate because the nicotine stimulates oxygen-need receptors in the carotid artery. At these lower doses of 6 to 8 mg there is also a considerable effect on the cardiovascular system as a result of the release of adrenaline. Such release leads to an increase in coronary blood flow, along with vasoconstriction in the skin and increased heart rate and blood pressure. The increased heart rate and blood pressure increase the oxygen need of the heart but not the oxygen supply. Another action of nicotine with negative health effects is that it increases platelet adhesiveness, which increases the tendency to clot. Within the CNS, nicotine seems to act at the level of the cortex to increase somewhat the frequency of the electrical activity, that is, to shift the EEG toward an arousal pattern.

Many effects of nicotine are easily discernible in the smoking individual. The heat releases the nicotine from the tobacco into the smoke. Inhaling while smoking one cigarette has been shown to inhibit hunger contractions of the stomach for up to an hour. That finding, along with a very slight increase in blood sugar level and a deadening of the taste buds, might be the basis for a decrease in hunger after smoking.

In line with the last possibility, it has long been folklore that a person who stops smoking begins to nibble food and thus gains weight. Some studies support such a finding, but one study reported that nicotine might actually increase eating behavior.[27] In addition, there is evidence that smoking increases metabolism rate, so that a weight gain on quitting might be partially due to a decreasing metabolism rate or less energy utilization by the body.

In a regular smoker, smoking results in a constriction of the blood vessels in the skin, along with a decrease in skin temperature and an increase in blood pressure. The blood supply to the skeletal muscles does not change with smoking, but in regular smokers the amount of carboxyhemoglobin in the blood is usually abnormally high (up to 10 percent of all hemoglobin). All smoke contains carbon monoxide; cigarette smoke is about 1 percent carbon monoxide, pipe smoke 2 percent, and cigar smoke 6 percent. The carbon monoxide combines with the hemoglobin in the blood, so that it can no longer carry oxygen. It is this effect of smoking, a decrease in the oxygen-carrying ability of the blood, that probably explains the shortness of breath smokers experience when they exert themselves.

The decrease in oxygen-carrying ability of the blood and the decrease in placental blood flow probably are related to the many results showing that pregnant women who smoke greatly endanger their unborn children.

Behavioral Effects

In spite of all the protests and the cautionary statements you might read or hear, the evidence is overwhelming that nicotine is the primary, if not the only, reinforcing substance in tobacco. Monkeys will work very hard when their only reward consists of regular intravenous injections of nicotine. The more nicotine in a cigarette, the lower the level of smoking. Intravenous injections and oral administration of nicotine will decrease smoking under some conditions—but not all.

An ongoing debate—in smokers as well as researchers—is whether nicotine acts to arouse and activate the smoker or whether it calms and tranquilizes the drug user. One review of the literature pointed to the paradoxical effects of nicotine: "a substantial number of studies have shown that nicotine increases heart rate, blood pressure, and numerous other indices of autonomic arousal; yet rather than producing expected increases of emotional behavior and feelings, it usually decreases emotions."[28]

Most people smoke in a fairly consistent way, averaging one to two puffs per minute, with each puff lasting about two seconds with a volume of 25 ml. This rate delivers to the individual about 1 to 2 μg of nicotine per kg of body weight with each puff. There must be something unique about this dose, because smokers could increase the dose by increasing the volume of smoke with each puff or puffing more often. This dose appears to be optimal for producing stimulation of the cerebral cortex.

Several British studies have shown that smokers are able to sustain their attention to a task requiring rapid processing of information from a computer screen much better if they are allowed to smoke before beginning the task. This could be either because the nicotine produces a beneficial effect on this performance or because when the smokers were not allowed to smoke they were suffering from some sort of withdrawal symptom. Subsequent experiments on both smokers and nonsmokers using an oral nicotine tablet established that nicotine improved performance in both groups, at least for a few minutes.[29]

Addiction to Nicotine

Evidence that nicotine is a reinforcing substance in nonhumans, that most people who smoke want to stop and can't, that when people do stop smoking they gain weight and exhibit other withdrawal signs, and that people who chew tobacco also have trouble stopping led to a need for a thorough look at the addicting properties of nicotine. The 1988 surgeon general's report provided it, in the form of a 600-page tome.[30] This had been a traditionally difficult subject: not that many years ago, psychiatrists were arguing that smoking fulfilled unmet needs for oral gratification and therefore represented a personality defect. It has recently come to light that the cigarette manufacturing company Philip Morris obtained evidence of the addicting nature of nicotine with rats in the early 1980s, but, instead of publishing the results, it fired the researchers and closed the laboratory.[31] Industry executives in 1994 congressional hearings unanimously testified that nicotine was not addicting, still arguing that smoking was simply a matter of personal choice and that many people have been able to quit. As we should know by now, one can theoretically choose to stop using a drug but one has a very difficult time doing so because of the potent reinforcing properties of the substance. That is the case with nicotine. The following conclusions of the 1988 report were pretty strong:

1. Cigarettes and other forms of tobacco are addicting.
2. Nicotine is the drug in tobacco that causes addiction.
3. The pharmacological and behavioral processes that determine tobacco addiction are similar to those that determine addiction to drugs such as heroin and cocaine.

Obviously this statement, although based on an exhaustive review of scientific data, was at one level a political message. It said to Congress and the American people that heroin and cocaine are not in some fundamental way more evil than tobacco. That message met with some predictably negative reactions from the tobacco industry and from some tobacco-state politicians, and the debate continued through the 1994 congressional hearings. Successful lawsuits by former smokers or their survivors finally convinced the tobacco companies that they were going to have to take seriously the issues of toxicity and addictiveness of tobacco products. In 1998, one company even faced criminal charges for growing a high-nicotine strain of tobacco with the presumed intent of manipulating nicotine levels to "hook" more smokers.

For the past several years, research into the mechanism of nicotine dependence has focused on the fact that nicotine produces a release of dopamine in the nucleus accumbens, a major target of the mesolimbic dopamine system,

described in Chapter 5.[32] The brains of chronic nicotine smokers also show a large reduction in one type of monoamine oxidase (MAO), the enzyme that breaks down dopamine and some other neurotransmitters.[33] This slowing of the breakdown of dopamine in chronic smokers might therefore enhance the effect of the dopamine released by each acute dose of nicotine, perhaps contributing to the strength of the dependence on nicotine experienced by most smokers.

HOW TO STOP SMOKING

When you're young and healthy, it's difficult, if not impossible, to imagine dying, being chronically ill, or having such bad **emphysema** that you can't get enough oxygen to walk across the room without having to stop to catch your breath. By the time you're old enough to worry about those things, it's difficult to change your health habits.

Think about this. If you smoke about a pack a day, you increase your probability of dying of lung cancer by about 1100 percent, of any other cancer by about 200 percent, of respiratory disease by about 400 percent, and of other causes by about 200 percent. Looked at another way, smoking two packs of cigarettes a day decreases the remaining years of your life by 20 percent if you're 35, by 24 percent if you're 45, by 29 percent at 55, and by 35 percent at 65.[34]

A lot of people want to stop smoking. A lot of people have already stopped. Are there ways to efficiently and effectively help those individuals who want to stop smoking to stop? With any form of pleasurable drug use, it is easier to keep people from starting to use the drug than it is to get them to stop once they have started. All

---

emphysema: (em fah *see* mah) a chronic lung disease characterized by difficulty breathing and shortness of breath.

Exploring Your Spirituality

The Hidden Costs of Smoking

Have you ever started to hug a smoker and then involuntarily reacted to the strong smell of smoke in his or her hair and clothing? Or have you ever wanted to kiss someone but held back because you had just smoked a cigarette and thought you needed to brush your teeth first? Smoking erects barriers between people. Some nonsmokers are adamant about not wanting people they care about to smoke. They don't want to breathe in smoke themselves, and they want to protect their children from the dangers of passive and side-stream smoke. When the smoker is a relative or friend, it's difficult to feel close to someone who's doing something you strongly disapprove of, such as smoking. And, from the smoker's viewpoint, it's hard to feel comfortable with someone who acts superior and doesn't accept you as you are.

Imagine a family celebration where a smoker would like to have a cigarette after dinner, in the living room, where everyone else is gathered. The nonsmokers, however, tell the smoker to go outside to smoke. What do the children think about all this? Does a "good" relative smoke? If smoking is bad, as a little boy hears often at school, why does his favorite uncle smoke? Is the family celebration marred by the tension?

The physical cost of smoking is obvious when a young smoker has to step out of a basketball game because he's out of breath or coughing. A smoker may find it embarrassing that she can't keep up on an "easy" hike and needs a break after only 10 minutes. No one wants to feel out of shape and limited in ability.

At work, smoking has become politically incorrect. Many companies have a no-smoking policy or allow smoking in designated areas only. Have you ever seen a group of smokers huddled outside a large office building or factory, "dragging" on their cigarettes? Once again, smokers are isolated and feeling the judgment of others about their "weakness."

Smoking takes a physical toll, but it also extracts a spiritual and psychological cost. How does it feel to be unaccepted by much of society? to be the outsider? Why does the smoker have to miss part of a special occasion to go smoke a cigarette? Why must the smoker bow out of a fun outdoor activity—or slow down the rest of the group—because of lack of stamina? Why does the smoker have to feel the resentment of coworkers because he or she takes a smoking break every hour? It's not easy to quit smoking, and many smokers make several attempts before they stick with it. Many who have stopped say they thought about more than their physical health before they tossed that last pack.

---

the educational programs have had an effect on our society and on our behavior. There are now over 40 million former smokers in the United States, and about 90 percent of them report that they quit smoking without formal treatment programs. There is some indication that those who have quit on their own do better than those who have been in a treatment program, but then those who quit on their own also tend not to have been smoking as much or for as long.

One reason it is so hard for people to stop is that a pack-a-day smoker puffs at least 50,000 times a year. That's a lot of individual nicotine "hits" reinforcing the smoking behavior. There are a variety of behavioral treatment approaches to assist smokers who want to quit, and hundreds of research articles have been published on them. Although most of these programs are able to get almost everyone to quit for a few days, by six months 70 to 80 percent of them are smoking again. Some of the programs that combine multiple approaches seem to have better success, with up to 40 percent remaining abstinent for one year.[35]

If nicotine is the critical thing, why not provide nicotine without the tars and carbon monoxide? Prescription nicotine chewing gum became available in 1984, after carefully

Try It!

Test Your Tobacco Awareness

Whether you smoke, chew, or don't use tobacco at all, tobacco is an important economic and political issue in virtually every community and in every country. See how well you do with these questions about tobacco's place in the United States and the world:

1. About what proportion of adults in the United States are smokers?
2. What two countries are the world's largest exporters of tobacco products?
3. About how many Americans die each day from tobacco-related illnesses?
4. What tobacco-related health problem accounts for most deaths among smokers (hint: it's not lung cancer)?
5. Which country produces the most cigarettes?

Answers

1. About one third (most people tend to overestimate the proportion of smokers, which makes smoking seem to be a typical behavior, when in fact, it's not)
2. The United States (#1) and the United Kingdom (Great Britain); Japan is the largest consumer of U.S.-made cigarettes
3. About 1,200 per day, representing about 20 percent of all deaths in the United States.
4. Smoking-related heart disease kills about 180,000 in the United States each year, compared with about 150,000 smoking-related lung cancer deaths.
5. China produces about 30 percent of the world's cigarettes, with the United States a distant second. Most of the cigarettes produced in China are consumed in China.

controlled studies showed it to be a useful adjunct to smoking cessation programs. This gum is now available over-the-counter. In 1991, several companies marketed nicotine skin patches that allow slow release of nicotine to be absorbed through the wearer's skin.[36] Within a few weeks of their introduction, the producers were unable to keep up with the demand and pharmacies had waiting lists of customers. There have been efforts to introduce smokeless cigarettes, as much for the convenience of a smoker who can't light up as an aid to cutting down or quitting. However, various technical problems have led to these smokeless cigarette products being withdrawn.

There is money to be made helping people quit smoking, especially if it can apparently be done painlessly with a substitute. One problem is that the controlled studies done to demonstrate the usefulness of gum or skin patches have been carried out under fairly strict conditions, with a prescribed quitting period, several visits to the clinic to assess progress, and the usual trappings of a clinical research study, often including the collection of saliva or other samples to detect tobacco use. That's a far cry from buying nicotine gum and a patch off the shelf, with no plan for quitting, no follow-up interviews, and no monitoring. No wonder that some people have found themselves, in spite of warnings, wearing a nicotine patch and smoking at the same time.

Is there an effective nondrug program for quitting smoking? Yes and no. A review of programs and techniques, "Behavioral Treatment of Smoking Behavior,"[35] made a point that is relevant here: there is a lot of variability in the effect of any program—some people do very well, some very poorly, and if one program won't work for an individual, maybe another one will. The fact is, we don't know enough yet to know which program will be best for any particular individual. If you want to stop smoking, keep trying programs; odds are you'll find one that works . . . eventually.

SUMMARY

- Tobacco was introduced to Europe and the East after Columbus's voyage to the Americas.
- As with most other "new" drugs, Europeans either loved tobacco and prescribed it for all ailments or hated it and considered it responsible for many ills.
- The predominant style of tobacco use went from pipes to snuff to chewing to cigars to cigarettes.
- The typical modern cigarette is about half as strong in tar and nicotine content as a cigarette of 50 years ago.
- Cigarette smoking declined considerably during the 1960s and 1970s, but about 20 percent of young people still become regular smokers.
- The use of smokeless tobacco increased during the 1980s, causing concerns about increases in oral cancer.
- Although tobacco continues to be an important economic factor in American society, it is also responsible for more annual deaths than all other drugs combined, including alcohol.
- Cigarette smoking is clearly linked to increased risk of heart disease, lung and other cancers, emphysema, and stroke.
- There is increased concern about the health consequences of passive smoking.
- Smoking cessation leads to immediate improvements in mortality statistics, and new products, including nicotine skin patches, are being widely used by those who wish to quit.

REVIEW QUESTIONS

1. Why was nicotine named after Jean Nicot?
2. Which was the desired species of tobacco that saved the English colonies in Virginia?

Web Watch

Learn About Tobacco Addiction

Take the Tobacco Quiz at library.think quest.org/29500/addictions/tobacco.quiz.shtml to find out about the effects of tobacco addiction and ways to quit.

Check Out Publications on Tobacco

The National Clearing House for Drug and Alcohol Information offers a listing of publications about certain types of drugs. Go to www.health.org/catalog/catalog.asp?key=15&detail=false to find and, if you wish, order brochures or other publications about tobacco and nicotine.

Do You Know About Smoking and Pregnancy?

At www.noah-health.org/english/pregnancy/march_of_dimes/substance/nosmoke.html, read the article "Smoking in Pregnancy." Learn about effects such as pregnancy complications, low birth weight, birth defects, and sudden infant death syndrome. You'll also find research sponsored by the March of Dimes. Then go to www.coolware.com/health/medical_reporter/smoking.html and read "If You Smoke and You're Pregnant, Your Baby May Get Burned." This article gives you additional information and survey results on the effects of smoking during pregnancy.

3. What techniques have been used to lower the tar and nicotine content of modern cigarettes?

4. Who smokes more, men or women? What effect does age have on this?

5. What is the significance of tobacco-specific nitrosamines?

6. What are the major causes of death associated with cigarette smoking?

7. What evidence is there that passive smoking can harm nonsmokers?

8. What are the effects of smoking during pregnancy?

9. Nicotine acts through which neurotransmitter in the brain? How does it interact with this neurotransmitter?

10. What is the evidence as to why cigarette smoking is so addictive?

REFERENCES

1. Sargent JD and others: Brand appearances in contemporary cinema films and contribution to global marketing of cigarettes. *The Lancet*, 357:29–32, 2001.
2. Stewart GG: A history of the medicinal use of tobacco, 1492–1860, *Medical History* 11:228–268, 1967.
3. Brooks JE: *The mighty leaf.* Boston: Little, Brown, 1952.
4. Vaughn W, Quoted in Dunphy EB: Alcohol and tobacco amblyopia: A historical survey, *American Journal of Ophthalmology* 68:573, 1969.
5. Mannino DM and others: Cigarette smoking: An independent risk factor for impotence? *American Journal of Epidemiology* 140:1003, 1994.
6. Corti EC: *A history of smoking.* London: George G. Harrap, 1931.
7. Heimann RK: *Tobacco and Americans.* New York: McGraw-Hill, 1960.
8. *Tobacco situation and outlook.* Economic Research Service, U.S. Department of Agriculture, September 2000.
9. Russell MAH: Nicotine intake and its regulation by smokers. In Martin WR and others, editors: *Tobacco smoking and nicotine: A neurobiological approach.* New York: Plenum Press, 1998.
10. Gritz ER, Ksir C, McCarthy WJ: Smokeless tobacco use in the United States: present and future trends, *Annals of Behavioral Medicine* 7:2, 24–27, 1985.
11. Johnston LD and others: *2000 Data from Monitoring the Future Study.* Press release, Dec 14, 2000.
12. *The health consequences of using smokeless tobacco: A report of the advisory committee to the Surgeon General.* NIH Pub. No. 86-2874. Washington, DC: U.S. Government Printing Office, 1986.
13. Hamilton K: Blowing smoke, *Newsweek* July 27, 1997.
14. Lorand A: *Life shortening habits and rejuvenation* Philadelphia: FA Davis, 1927.
15. Eaglin J: The CC cough-fin brand cigarettes. Cincinnati: Raisbeck, 1931.
16. U.S. Public Health Service Office on Smoking and Health: *Smoking, tobacco and health: A fact book.* Washington, DC: US Government Printing Office, 1987.
17. Okie S: The press and cigarette ads: Smoke gets in their eyes. New York: HealthLink, National Center for Health Education, 1987.
18. Smoke and mirrors: How cigarette makers keep health question "open" year after year, *Wall Street Journal* Feb 11, 1993.
19. Bartecchi CE and others: The human costs of tobacco use, *New England Journal of Medicine* 330:907, 1994.
20. *The health benefits of smoking cessation: A report of the surgeon general,* DHHS Pub. No. (CDC) 90-8416. Washington, DC: U.S. Government Printing Office, 1990.

21. *Shimp v. New Jersey Bell Telephone Company,* Superior Court of New Jersey, Chancery Division, Salem County, Docket No C-2904-75, filed Dec 22, 1976.

22. Secondhand smoke: Is it a hazard? *Consumer Reports* Jan 1995.

23. *Mortality from smoking in developed countries.* World Health Organization, Geneva, 1994.

24. Jain M: Foreign tobacco firms puffing way into Asian market, Associated Press newspaper report, Jan 17, 1988.

25. Broady JE: Personal health, *New York Times* July 8, 1981.

26. *The health consequences of smoking for women: A report of the surgeon general.* Washington, DC: U.S. Government Printing Office, 1981.

27. Perkins KA and others: Effects of nicotine on hunger and eating in male and female smokers, *Psychopharmacology* (Berl) 106:53–59, 1992.

28. Gilbert OG: Paradoxical tranquilizing and emotion reducing effects of nicotine, *Psychological Bulletin* 86(4): 643–662.

29. Wesnes K: Nicotine increases mental efficiency: But how? In Martin WR and others, editors: *Tobacco smoking and nicotine: A neurobiological approach.* New York: Plenum Press, 1988.

30. *The health consequences of smoking: Nicotine addiction, a report of the surgeon general,* DHHS Pub. No. (CDC)88-8406. Washington, DC: U.S. Government Printing Office, 1988.

31. Tobacco company suppressed study on nicotine addiction, Associated Press newspaper report, Apr 1, 1994.

32. Ksir C: Behavioral neuropharmacology of nicotine. In Watson RR, editor: *Drugs of abuse and neurobiology.* New York: Raven Press, 1994.

33. Fowler JS and others: Inhibition of monoamine oxidase B in the brains of smokers. *Nature* 379:733, 1996.

34. Rogot E: Smoking and life expectancy among U.S. veterans, Public Health Briefs, *American Journal of Public Health* 68(10):1023–1025, 1978.

35. Glasgow RE, Bernstein DA: Behavioral treatment of smoking behavior. In Prokop CK, Bradley LA, editors: *Medical psychology.* New York: Academic Press, 1981.

36. Transdermal nicotine study group: transdermal nicotine for smoking cessation, *Journal of the American Medical Association* 266:3133–3138, 1991.

37. Strauss E: New nonopioid painkiller shows promise in animal tests, *Science* 279:32, 1998.

Chapter 14

Caffeine

KEY TERMS

- xanthines
- theophylline
- theobromine
- adenosine
- caffeinism

Online Learning Center Resources

www.mhhe.com/ray

Log on to our Online Learning Center (OLC) for access to these additional resources.

- Chapter definitions
- Learning objectives
- Student interactive question-and-answer sites
- Self-scoring chapter quiz

The OLC also offers web links for study and exploration of health topics. Here are some examples of what you'll find:

www.telusplanet.net/public/kwalden/cafequiz.htm

This website hosts a just-for-fun quiz designed for coffee addicts. Answer the questions and find a humorous assessment provided by a fellow caffeine enthusiast.

abcnews.go.com/sections/living/InYourHead/allinyourhead_28.html

The ABC News site includes this article: "Coffee Bean Genes: A yen for Caffeine May Be All in the Family." It discusses the genetic factors that may influence a person's coffee consumption or lead to addiction.

www.cs.unb.ca/~alopez-o/caffaq.html

The New Coffee and Caffeine FAQ is an interactive site at which questions are posted and answers are displayed.

Drugs in the Media

Fancy Coffee Drinks and Humor

During the past 30 years, coffee has experienced a renaissance in the United States. Although overall coffee consumption is flat, specialty coffee is booming, driven by younger drinkers (18- to 24-year-olds). In its 2000 survey of coffee trends, the National Coffee Association found that 45 percent of this market segment had drunk cappuccino in the past year, 24 percent had drunk espresso, 21 percent latte, 29 percent café mocha, and 36 percent iced or ice-blended coffees. Espresso bars and coffee shops continue to proliferate. Starbucks alone had 3,500 outlets at the end of 2000 and expects to have 10,000 stores by 2005. As specialty coffees have enjoyed this phenomenal growth, it is not surprising that their effect on our popular culture has been reflected in the media.

You've probably noticed that coffee bars are settings for social encounters on television and in the movies. Coffee bars are appealing backdrops in the popular TV situation comedies *Friends* and *Frazier*. An interesting phenomenon is how humorous we seem to find all the complicated coffee drinks. Cartoons, jokes, and witty references are common. In these jokes the espresso sophisticate ordering a "half-caf skinny latte, grande" or a "tall cap with three shots" is often contrasted with some plain folks wanting a regular old cup of coffee. The high price of these upscale specialty drinks compared with just plain coffee is another point of some of the humor.

Why do we find this funny? In some ways the humor may be an indirect attempt to poke fun at social-class differences or generational differences using an issue that seems harmless. Another possible way to look at this is to remember from Chapter 1 that an informal method of dealing with social deviance is to make light of it by making it a joke. As a new behavior permeates the social system, its newness and strangeness make it seem somewhat deviant—not yet completely fitting into what we think of as everyday life. These coffee bars and their associated lingo are now becoming so commonplace, however, that they may soon lose their power to provoke a chuckle.

CAFFEINE: THE WORLD'S MOST COMMON PSYCHOSTIMULANT

On a daily basis, more people use caffeine than any other psychoactive drug. Many use it regularly, and there is evidence for dependence and some evidence that regular use can interfere with the very activities people believe that it helps them with. It is now so domesticated that most modern kitchens contain a specialized device for extracting the chemical from plant products (a coffeemaker), but Western societies were not always so accepting of this drug.

How many drugs can lay claim to divine intervention in their introduction to humankind? The **xanthines,** of which caffeine is the best known, have three such legends, and that fact alone tells you that this has been an important class of drugs throughout the ages.

Coffee

The legends surrounding the origin of coffee are at least geographically correct. The best one concerns an Arabian goatherd named Kaldi who couldn't understand why his goats were bounding around the hillside so playfully. One day he followed them up the mountain and ate some of the red berries the goats were munching. "The results were amazing. Kaldi became a happy goatherd. Whenever his goats danced, he danced and whirled and leaped and rolled about on the ground." Kaldi had taken the first human coffee trip! A holy man took in the scene, and

---

xanthines: (*zan* theens) the class of chemicals to which caffeine belongs.

"that night he danced with Kaldi and the goats"—a veritable orgy. The legend continues with Muhammad telling the holy man to boil the berries in water and have the brothers in the monastery drink the liquid so they could keep awake and continue their prayers.[1]

Around A.D. 900, an Arabian medical book suggested that coffee was good for just about everything, including measles and lust reduction. Once something gets into the literature, it's very difficult to change people's minds about it. Women in England argued against the use of coffee over 700 years later, in a 1674 pamphlet titled "The Women's Petition Against Coffee, representing to public consideration the grand inconveniences accruing to their sex from the excessive use of the drying and enfeebling liquor." The women claimed men used too much coffee, and as a result the men were as "unfruitful as those *Desarts* whence that unhappy *Berry* is said to be brought." The women were *really* unhappy, and the pamphlet continued:

> Our Countrymens pallates are become as *Fanatical* as their Brains; how else is't possible they should *Apostatize* from the good old primitive way of Ale-drinking, to run a *Whoreing* after such variety of distructive Foreign Liquors, to trifle away their time, scald their *Chops*, and spend their *Money*, all for a little *base, black, thick, nasty bitter stinking, nauseous* Puddle water.[2]

Some men probably sat long hours in one of the many coffeehouses composing "The Men's Answer to the Women's Petition Against Coffee," which said in part:

> Why must innocent COFFEE be the object of your Spleen? That harmless and healing Liquor, which Indulgent Providence first sent amongst us. . . . Tis not this incomparable fettle Brain that shortens Natures standard, or makes us less Active in the Sports of Venus, and we wonder you should take these Exceptions.[2]

We can all rest easier today and discuss over a cup of coffee the fact that gradually became

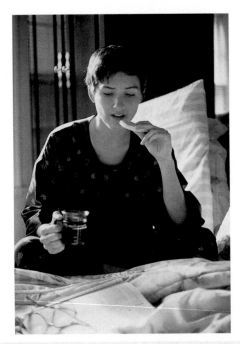

Younger coffee drinkers are a growing customer base for purveyors of gourmet whole-bean coffees.

clear: there is no truth to the idea that coffee diminishes sexual excitability or reduces lust. It is doubtful that the Arabians believed it, either, because the use of coffee spread throughout the Muslim world. In Mecca, people spent so much time in coffeehouses that the use of coffee was outlawed and all supplies of the coffee bean were burned. Prohibition rarely works, and coffee speakeasies began to open. Wiser heads prevailed, and the prohibition was lifted.

The middle of the seventeenth century saw the same play enacted but with a new cast of characters and a different locale. Coffeehouses began appearing in England (1650) and France (1671), and a new era began. Coffeehouses were all things to all people: a place to relax, to learn the news of the day, to seal bargains, and to plot. This last possibility made Charles II of England so nervous that he outlawed coffeehouses, labeling them "hotbeds of seditious talk and slanderous attacks upon persons in high stations." King Charles was no more successful than the Women's Petition had been. In only 11 days the ruling was withdrawn, and the coffeehouses developed into the "penny universities" of the early eighteenth century. For a penny a cup people could listen to and learn from most of the great literary and political figures of the period. Lloyds of London, an insurance house, started in Edward Lloyd's coffeehouse around 1700.

Across the channel, cheap wine made the need for another social drink less essential in France than in England, but French coffeehouses made at least one contribution to Western culture—the cancan. French cabaret owners were not ready to turn the other cheek, and they fought back: one owner was able to persuade his cancan girls to perform without any bloomers. In spite of this, coffeehouses survived, and coffee consumption increased.

Across the Atlantic, coffee drinking increased in the English colonies, although tea was still their preference. Cheaper and more available than coffee, tea had everything, including, beginning in 1765, a 3-pence-a-pound tax on its importation.

The British Act that taxed tea helped fan the fire that lit the musket that fired the shot heard around the world. That story is better told in connection with tea, but the final outcome was that to be a tea drinker was to be a Tory, so coffee became the new country's national drink.

Coffee use expanded as the West was won, and per capita consumption steadily increased in the early 1900s. Some experts became worried about the tendency to "have another cup of coffee," although they believed they could explain it. One wrote:

> The absolute coercion which is imposed on the Americans of the United States by the Prohibition Act with respect to alcohol has necessarily had the result of greatly increasing the use of other excitants and also narcotics. . . . The consumption of coffee has also developed in an

undreamt-of manner. In 1919, 929.2 million pounds were consumed and in 1920 as many as 1,360 million pounds. The consumption therefore increased from 9 to 12.9 pounds per head per year, and is approaching the threshold of abuse.[3]

The funny thing is that Prohibition went away, but coffee consumption continued to rise. We must have been well over the "threshold of abuse" in 1946 when annual per capita coffee consumption reached an all-time high of 20 pounds. The overall trend has been basically downhill since then, in spite of an upsurge of interest in espresso and specialty coffees in the late 1990s.

Some of the decrease in coffee consumption can be attributed to changing lifestyles—sun and fun and convenient canned drinks seem to fit together better, and soft drinks seem to go with fast food. In 1970, Americans still drank more gallons of coffee per capita than of any other nonalcoholic beverage product, but by 1997 Americans were consuming over 50 gallons of soft drinks per person, compared with about 24 gallons of coffee.[4]

If the national drink is not as national as it once was, neither is it as simple. Kaldi and his friends were content to simply munch on the coffee beans or put them in hot water. Somewhere in the dark past, probably when the Meccan warehouses were burned down, the Middle East discovered that roasting the green coffee bean did not ruin it but, in fact, improved the flavor, aroma, and color of the drink made from the bean. For years housewives, storekeepers, and coffeehouse owners bought the green bean, then roasted and ground it just before use. Commercial roasting started in 1790 in New York City, and the process gradually spread through the country. However, one problem is that, although the green bean can be stored indefinitely, the roasted bean deteriorates seriously within a month. Ground coffee can be maintained at its peak level in the home only for a week or two, and then only if it is in a closed container and refrigerated. Vacuum packing of ground coffee was introduced in 1900, a process that maintains the quality until the seal is broken.

Coffee growing spread worldwide when the Dutch began cultivation in the East Indies in 1696. Latin America had an ideal climate for coffee growing, and with the world's greatest coffee-drinking nation just up the road several thousand miles, it became the world's largest producer. Different varieties of the coffee tree and different growing and processing conditions provide many opportunities for varying the characteristics of coffee.

No one really went commercial with a combination of different coffee beans until J. O. Cheek developed a blend in 1892 and introduced it through a famous Nashville hotel: Maxwell House. The coffee was so well received that the hotel owners let the coffee be named after the hotel.

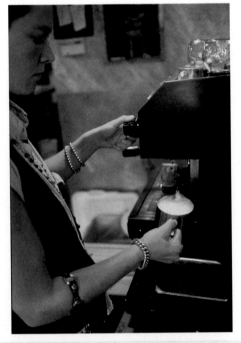

Specialty coffee drinks, such as cappuccino, are expected to continue to gain popularity.

In the early 1950s, about 94 percent of American coffee was from Latin America, but that percentage has steadily declined; today less than half is grown in this hemisphere. Brazil is the principal exporter to the United States, with Colombia second. Both countries grow *arabica*, which has a caffeine content of about 1 percent. *Robusta*, with a caffeine level at 2 percent, is the variety grown in Africa and is usually of a lower grade and price.

The economics of coffee (it is number two in international trade, far behind oil) have as much to do with coffee consumption as does our changing lifestyle. A price increase in the early 1950s—to a dollar a pound—shifted us from being a 40-cups-per-pound nation to being a 60-cups-per-pound nation. This dilution reduced the cost but also the quality of the beverage. Two things happen when prices go up: the quality of the coffee decreases and people drink less coffee.

Instant coffee has been around since before the turn of the twentieth century, but sales began their marked increase in the hustle and bustle after World War II: another decrease in the quality of the beverage but an increase in the convenience. Interestingly, Brazil imports many inexpensive African coffee beans to use in manufacturing instant coffee, because they believe that their coffee is too good to be used in that way.

In the 1980s, health-conscious Americans began to drink more decaffeinated coffee and less regular coffee. There are several ways of removing caffeine from the coffee bean. In the process used by most American companies, the unroasted beans are soaked in an organic solvent, and there have been concerns about residues of the solvent remaining in the coffee. The most widely used solvent has been methylene chloride, and studies have shown that high doses of that solvent can cause cancer in laboratory mice. In 1985, the FDA banned the use of methylene chloride in hair sprays, which can be inhaled during use, but allowed the solvent to be

HealthQuest Activities

Could you be addicted to a drug without realizing it? In Module 9, look under *Unknown Drug Use/Abuse* and read about caffeine. Then go to *Drug Interactions, Food/Beverage* and read about caffeine drinks. Do you believe that a caffeine addiction could be a threat to your health? For the next week, keep a tally of how many caffeinated beverages and foods you consume. List how many times you consume caffeine along with another drug. Compare your findings with those of your classmates. The following week, try to go without eating or drinking anything with caffeine in it. Do you experience side effects, such as headaches, moodiness, drowsiness, or dizziness? Compare these findings with those of your classmates.

used in decaffeination as long as residues did not exceed 10 parts per million. Because the solvent residue evaporates during roasting, decaffeinated coffees contain considerably lower amounts than that, so the assumption is that the risk is minimal. The Swiss water process, which is not used on a large commercial scale in the United States, removes more of the coffee's flavor. The caffeine that is taken out of the coffee is used mostly in soft drinks. One of the largest decaffeinating companies is owned by Coca-Cola.

Today's supermarket shelves are filled with an amazing variety of products derived from this simple bean—pure Colombian, French Roast, decaf, half-caf, flavored coffees, instants, mixes, and even cold coffee beverages. The competition for the consumer's coffee dollar has never been greater, it seems. And Americans are lining up in record numbers at espresso bars to buy cappuccinos, lattes, and other exotic-sounding mixtures of strong coffee, milk, and flavorings. The number of these specialty coffee shops increased from fewer than 200 in 1989 to more than 5,000

in 1994.[5] By 2000, they were found in small towns, shopping malls, and on practically every corner in cities.

Tea

Tea and coffee are not like day and night, but their differences are reflected in the legends surrounding their origins. The bouncing goatherd of Arabia suggests that coffee is a boisterous, blue-collar drink. Tea is a different story: much softer, quieter, more delicate. According to one legend, Daruma, the founder of Zen Buddhism, fell asleep one day while meditating. Resolving that it would never happen again, he cut off both eyelids. From the spot where his eyelids touched the earth grew a new plant. From its leaves a brew could be made that would keep a person awake. Appropriately, the tea tree, *Thea sinensis* (now classed as *Camellia sinensis*), is an evergreen, and *sinensis* is the Latin word for "Chinese."

The first report of tea that seems reliable is in a Chinese manuscript from around A.D. 350, when it was primarily seen as a medicinal plant. The nonmedical use of tea is suggested by an A.D. 780 book on the cultivation of tea, but the real proof that it was in wide use in China is that a tax was levied on it in the same year. Before this time Buddhist monks had carried the cultivation and use of tea to Japan.

Europe had to wait eight centuries to savor the herb that was "good for tumors or abscesses that come from the head, or for ailments of the bladder . . . it quenches thirst. It lessens the desire for sleep. It gladdens and cheers the heart." The first European record of tea, in 1559, says, "One or two cups of this decoction taken on an empty stomach removes fever, headache, stomachache, pain in the side or in the joints. . . ." Fifty years later, in 1610, the Dutch delivered the first tea to the continent of Europe.

An event that occurred 10 years before had tremendous impact on the history of the world and on present patterns of drug use. In 1600, the English East India Company was formed, and

Queen Elizabeth gave the company a monopoly on everything from the east coast of Africa across the Pacific to the west coast of South America. In this period the primary imports from the Far East were spices, and the company prospered. A major conflict developed between Dutch and English trade interests over who belonged where in the East. In 1623, a resolution gave the Dutch East India Company the islands (the Dutch East Indies), and the English East India Company had to be content with India and other countries on the continent.

The English East India Company concentrated on importing spices, so the first tea was taken to England by the Dutch. As the market for tea increased, the English East India Company expanded its imports of tea from China. Coffee had arrived first, so most tea was sold in coffeehouses. Even as tea's use as a popular social drink expanded in Europe, there were some prophets of doom. A 1635 publication by a physician claimed that, at the very least, using tea would speed the death of those over 40 years old. The use of tea was not slowed, however, and by 1657 tea was being sold to the public in England. This was no more than 10 years after the English had developed the present word for it: *tea*. Although spelled *tea*, it was pronounced tay until the nineteenth century. Before this period the Chinese name *ch'a* had been used, anglicized to either *chia* or *chaw*.

With the patrons of taverns off at coffeehouses living it up with tea, coffee, and chocolate, tax revenues from alcoholic beverages declined. To offset this loss, coffeehouses were licensed, and a tax of 8 pence was levied on each gallon of tea and chocolate sold. To keep at home the profits from the expanding tea trade, Britain banned Dutch imports of tea in 1669, which gave the English East India Company a monopoly. Profit from the China tea trade colonized India, brought about the Opium Wars between China and Britain, and induced the English to switch from coffee to tea. In the last half of the eighteenth century the East India

Company carried out a "Drink Tea" campaign unlike anything ever seen before that time. Advertising, patriotism, low cost on tea, and high taxes on alcohol made Britain a nation of tea drinkers.

It was the same profit motive that led to the American Revolution. Because the English East India Company had a monopoly on importing tea to England and thence to the American colonies, the British government imposed high duties on tea when it was taken from warehouses and offered for sale. But, as frequently happens, when taxes went up, smuggling increased. It reached the point in Britain at which more smuggled tea than legal tea was being consumed. The American colonies, ever loyal to the king, had become big tea drinkers, which helped the king and the East India Company stay solvent. The Stamp Act of 1765, which included a tax on tea, changed everything. Even though the Stamp Act was repealed in 1766, it was replaced by the Trade and Revenue Act of 1767, which did the same thing.

These measures made the colonists unhappy over paying taxes they had not helped formulate (taxation without representation), and in 1767 this resulted in a general boycott on the consumption of English tea. Coffee use increased, but the primary increase was in the smuggling of tea. The drop in legal tea sales filled the tea warehouses and put the East India Company in financial trouble. To save the company, in 1773 Parliament gave the East India Company the right to sell tea in the American colonies without paying the tea taxes. The company was also allowed to sell the tea through its own agents, and this would eliminate the profits of the merchants in the colonies.

Several boatloads of this tea, which would be sold cheaper than any before, sailed toward various parts in the colonies. The American merchants would not have made any profit on this tea, and they were the primary ones who rebelled at the cheap tea. Some ships were just turned away from port, but the beginning of the

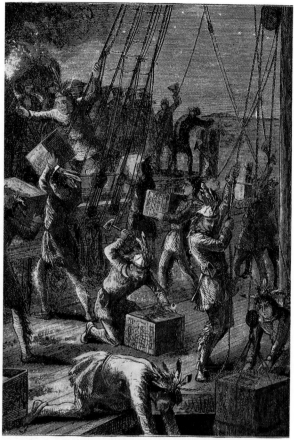

THE DESTRUCTION OF TEA IN BOSTON HARBOR.

The Boston Tea Party contributed to the English preference for tea over coffee.

end came with the 342 chests of tea that turned the Boston harbor into a teapot on the night of December 16, 1773.

The revolution in America and the colonists' rejection of tea helped tea sales in Great Britain—to be a tea drinker was to be loyal to the Crown. Many factors contributed to change the English from coffee drinkers to tea drinkers, and the preference for tea persists today. Although their use of coffee increases yearly and that of tea declines, the English are still tea drinkers. The annual per capita consumption of tea in the United Kingdom is about 8 pounds, second in the world only to Ireland. In comparison, Americans consume less than one pound of tea per person per year.

Most of the tea (about 70 percent) that comes to America starts life on a 4- to 5-foot bush high in the mountains of Sri Lanka (Ceylon), India, or Indonesia. Unpruned, the bush would grow into a 15- to 30-foot tree, which would be difficult to pluck, as picking tea leaves is called. The pluckers select only the bud-leaf and the first two leaves at each new growth. The bud-leaf is called flowering orange pekoe, the second leaf is larger and called orange pekoe, and the third and largest is pekoe (pekoe is pronounced "peck-ho," not "peak-o"). Thus, orange pekoe is not a variety of tea plant but, rather, a size and quality of tea leaf; generally the bud-leaf is of the highest quality and the third leaf is the lowest quality.

In one day a plucker will pluck enough leaves to make 10 pounds of tea as sold in the grocery store. Plucking is done every 6 to 10 days in warm weather as new growth develops on the many branches. The leaves are dried, rolled to crush the cells in the leaf, and placed in a cool, damp place for fermentation (oxidation) to occur. This oxidation turns the green leaves to a bright copper color. Nonoxidized leaves are packaged and sold as green tea, the type used in Chinese restaurants in this country. Oxidized tea is called black tea and accounts for about 98 percent of the tea Americans consume. Oolong tea is greenish-brown, consisting of partially oxidized leaves.

Until 1904, the only choices available were sugar, cream, and lemon with your hot tea. At the Louisiana Purchase Exposition in St. Louis in 1904, iced tea was sold for the first time. It now accounts for 75 percent of all tea consumed in America. Tea lovers found 1904 to be a very good year. Fifteen hundred miles east of the fair, a New York City tea merchant decided to send out his samples in handsewn silk bags rather than tin containers. Back came the orders—send us tea, and send it in the same little bags you used to send the samples. From that inauspicious beginning evolved the modern tea bag machinery, which cuts the filter paper, weighs the tea, and attaches the tag—all this at a rate of 150 to 180 tea bags per minute.

Pound for pound, loose black tea contains a higher concentration of caffeine than coffee beans. However, because about 200 cups of tea can be made from each pound of dry tea leaves, compared with 50 or 60 cups of coffee per pound, a typical cup of tea has less caffeine than a typical cup of coffee. The caffeine content of teas varies widely, depending on brand and the strength of the brew. Most teas have 40 to 60 mg of caffeine per cup.[6]

Most tea is sold in tea bags these days, and the market has been flooded with a variety of tea products. Instant teas, some containing flavorings and sweeteners, are popular for convenience. Flavored teas—which contain mint, spices, or other substances along with tea—offer other options. The biggest boom in recent years has been in so-called herbal teas, which mostly contain no real "tea" at all. These teas are made up of mixtures of other plant leaves and flowers for both flavor and color and have become quite popular among people who avoid caffeine.

It can only gladden and cheer the hearts of tea drinkers to know that the largest seller of tea in America is a company named after a man, born in Scotland of Irish parents, who emigrated to America, became rich and famous in England, and believed in ships with sails right up to the end: Sir Thomas Lipton (1850–1931).

Although tea contains another chemical that derived its name from the tea plant, **theophylline** ("divine leaf") is present only in very small, nonpharmacological amounts in the beverage. Theophylline is very effective at relaxing the bronchial passages and is widely prescribed for use by asthmatics.

Chocolate

Now we come to the third legend, concerning the origin of the third xanthine-containing plant. Long before Columbus landed on San Salvador,

Quetzalcoatl, Aztec god of the air, gave humans a gift from paradise: the chocolate tree. Linnaeus was to remember this legend when he named the cocoa tree *Theobroma*, "food of the gods." The Aztecs treated it as such, and the cacao bean was an important part of their economy, with the cacao bush being cultivated widely. Montezuma, emperor of Mexico in the early sixteenth century, is said to have consumed nothing other than 50 goblets of *chocolatl* every day. The *chocolatl*—from the Mayan words *choco* ("warm") and *latl* ("beverage")—was flavored with vanilla but was far from the chocolate of today. It was a thick liquid, like honey, that was sometimes frothy and had to be eaten with a spoon. The major difference was that it was bitter; the Aztecs didn't know about sugarcane.

Cortez introduced sugarcane plantations to Mexico in the early 1520s and supported the continued cultivation of the *Theobroma cacao* bush. When he returned to Spain in 1528, Cortez carried with him cakes of processed cocoa. The cakes were eaten, as well as being ground up and mixed with water for a drink. Although chocolate was introduced to Europe almost a century before coffee and tea, its use spread very slowly. Primarily this was because the Spanish kept the method of preparing chocolate from the cacao bean a secret until the early seventeenth century. When knowledge of the technique spread, so did the use of chocolate.

During the seventeenth century, chocolate drinking reached all parts of Europe, primarily among the wealthy. Maria Theresa, wife of France's Louis XIV, had a "thing" about chocolate, and this furthered its use among the wealthy and fashionable. Gradually it became more of a social drink, and by the 1650s chocolate houses were open in England, although usually chocolate was sold alongside coffee and tea in the established coffeehouses.

In the early eighteenth century there were health warnings in England against the use of chocolate, but use expanded. Its use and importance are well reflected in a 1783 proposal in the

TABLE 14-1

Caffeine in Beverages and Foods

Item	Caffeine (mg)	
	Average	Range
Coffee (5 oz cup)		
Brewed, drip method	115	60–180
Brewed, percolater	80	40–170
Instant	65	30–120
Decaffeinated, brewed	3	2–5
Decaffeinated, instant	2	1–5
Tea (5 oz cup)		
Brewed, major U.S. brands	40	20–90
Brewed, imported brands	60	25–110
Instant	30	25–50
Iced (12 oz glass)	70	67–76
Cocoa beverage (5 oz cup)	4	2–20
Chocolate milk beverage (8 oz glass)	5	2–7
Milk chocolate (1 oz)	6	1–15
Dark chocolate, semisweet (1 oz)	20	5–35
Baker's chocolate (1 oz)	26	26
Chocolate-flavored syrup (1 oz)	4	4

U.S. Congress that the United States raise revenue by taxing chocolate as well as coffee, tea, liquor, sugar, molasses, and pepper.

Although the cultivation of chocolate never became a matter to fight over, it, too, has spread around the world. The New World plantations were almost destroyed by disease at the beginning of the eighteenth century, but cultivation had already begun in Asia, and today a large part of the crop comes from Africa.

Until 1828, all chocolate sold was a relatively indigestible substance obtained by grinding the cacao kernels after processing. The preparation had become more refined over the years, but it still followed the Aztec procedure of letting the pods dry in the sun, then roasting them before removing the husks to get to the kernel of the plant. The result of grinding the kernels is a thick liquid called chocolate liquor. This is baking chocolate. In 1828, a Dutch patent was issued for the manufacture of "chocolate powder" by removing about two-thirds of the fat from the chocolate liquor. The chocolate powder was the forerunner of today's breakfast cocoa.

The fat that was removed, cocoa butter, became important when someone found that, if it was mixed with sugar and some of the chocolate powder, it could easily be formed into slabs or bars. In 1847, the first chocolate bars appeared, but it was not until 1876 that the Swiss made their contribution to the chocolate industry by inventing milk chocolate, which was first sold under the Nestlé label. By FDA standards, milk chocolate today must contain at least 12 percent milk solids, although better grades contain almost twice that amount.

When chocolate turns white, it might still be all right to eat, but it is probably old, because the white color comes from the separation of the cocoa butter. Someday when you have the time, you can check on whether your piece of chocolate is all chocolate and properly manufactured. Put it on your tongue: it should melt at body temperature. But be careful! One chocolate lover has said, "Each of us has known such moments of orgastic anticipation, our senses focused at their finest, when control is irrevocably abandoned. Then the tongue possesses, is possessed by, what it most desires; the warm, liquid melting of thick, dark chocolate."[7]

The unique xanthine in chocolate is **theobromine**. It has physiological actions that closely parallel those of caffeine but is much less potent in its effects on the central nervous system. The average cup of cocoa contains about 200 mg of theobromine but only 4 mg of caffeine. Table 14.1 compares the caffeine contents of various forms of coffee, tea, and chocolate.

theophylline: (thee *off* a lin) a xanthine found in tea.

theobromine: (thee oh *broh* meen) a xanthine found in chocolate.

OTHER SOURCES OF CAFFEINE

Soft Drinks

The early history of cola drinks is not shrouded in the mists that veil the origins of the other xanthine drinks, so there is no problem in selecting the correct legend. And that's what the story of Coca-Cola is: a true legend in our time. From a green nerve tonic in 1886 in Atlanta, Georgia, that did not sell well at all, Coca-Cola has grown into "the real thing," providing "the pause that refreshes," and selling more than 2 billion cases a year worldwide. And that includes mainland China, where it's called "Ke Koy Ke Le"—which means "tasty happiness."[8]

Dr. J. C. Pemberton's green nerve tonic in the late 1800s contained caramel, fruit flavoring, phosphoric acid, caffeine, and a secret mixture called Merchandise No. 5. A friend of Dr. Pemberton, F. M. Robinson, suggested the name by which it is still known: Coca-Cola. The unique character of Coca-Cola and its later imitators comes from a blend of fruit flavors that makes it impossible to identify any of its parts. An early ad for Coca-Cola suggested its varied uses:

> The "INTELLECTUAL BEVERAGE" and TEMPERANCE DRINK contains the valuable TONIC and NERVE STIMULANT properties of the Coca plant and Cola (or Kola) nuts, and makes not only a delicious, exhilarating, refreshing and invigorating Beverage, (dispensed from the soda water fountain or in other carbonated beverages), but a valuable Brain Tonic, and a cure for all nervous affections—SICK HEADACHE, NEURALGIA, HYSTERIA, MELANCHOLY, &c.[9]

Coca-Cola was touted as "the new and popular fountain drink, containing the tonic properties of the wonderful coca plant and the famous cola nut." This was the period of Sherlock Holmes, Sigmund Freud, and patent medicine—all saying very good things about the product of the coca plant: cocaine. In 1903, the company

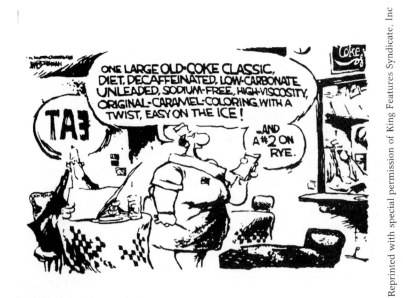

Soft-drink manufacturers offer a wide variety of products to take advantage of every corner of the market.

admitted that there were small amounts of cocaine in its beverage, but soon after that it quietly removed all the cocaine; a government analysis of Coca-Cola in 1906 did not find any.

The name *Coca-Cola* was originally conceived to indicate the nature of its two ingredients with tonic properties. The suggestion of the presence of extracts of coca leaves and cola (kola) nuts in the beverage was supposed to be furthered by the use on each bottle of a pictorial representation of the leaves and nuts. Unfortunately, the artist-glass blower didn't know that the coca and cacao plants were different, so the bottle had kola leaves and cacao pods. In 1909, the FDA seized a supply of Coca-Cola syrup and made two charges against the company. One was that the syrup was misbranded because it contained "no coca and little if any cola" and, second, that it contained an "added poisonous ingredient," caffeine.

Before a 1911 trial in Chattanooga, Tennessee, the company paid for some research into the physiological effects of caffeine, and when all the information was in the company won. The government appealed the decision. In 1916, the U.S. Supreme Court upheld the lower court by rejecting the charge of misbranding, stating that the company had repeatedly said that "certain extracts from the leaves of the coca shrub and the nut kernels of the cola tree were used for the purpose of obtaining a flavor" and that "the ingredients containing these extracts," with the cocaine eliminated, was called Merchandise No. 5. The way this is done today is that coca leaves are imported by a pharmaceutical company in New Jersey. The cocaine is extracted for medical use and the decocainized leaves are shipped to the Coca-Cola plant in Atlanta, where Merchandise No. 5 is produced. A 1931 report indicated that Merchandise No. 5 contained an extract of three parts coca leaves and one part cola nuts, but to this day it remains a secret formula. Then there was the problem of the caffeine:

It is clear that the only question arising under section 7 is whether the caffeine in the Coca Cola

is an "added poisonous or other added deleterious ingredient which may render such article injurious to health."[10]

The question of whether caffeine was an "added poisonous ingredient" was not so readily resolved. Caffeine was added, but it was an essential part of the Coca-Cola formula. In that respect it was not added above and beyond the essential ingredients; it was one of them. The Supreme Court said that the lower courts should decide whether the caffeine made the drink injurious to health. At that time the company substantially reduced the amount of caffeine in its syrup, and the government never felt it had a case worth pursuing beyond that point.

In 1981, the FDA changed its rules, so that a cola no longer has to contain caffeine. If it does contain caffeine, it may not be more than 0.02 percent, which is 0.2 mg/ml, or a little less than 6 mg per ounce. Some consumer and scientist groups believe that all cola manufacturers should indicate on the label the amount of caffeine the beverage contains. This has not happened, even though soft drinks, as with other food products, must now list nutrition information, such as calories, fat, sodium, and protein content.

Table 14.2 lists some popular soft drinks along with their caffeine content in a 12-ounce serving. Diet soft drinks, most now sweetened with aspartame, and caffeine-free colas are commanding a larger share of the market, but regular colas are still the single most popular type of soft drink. As with beers and some other products, the modern marketing strategy seems to be for each company to try to offer products of every type, in order to cover the market. Also as with beers, the large companies are buying up their competitors: in 1990, the Coca-Cola and PepsiCo companies represented more than 70 percent of total shipments. Coca-Cola Classic remains the most popular single brand, with almost 20 percent of the total market. Soft drinks have become increasingly popular. Per capita consumption of soft drinks has continued to edge upward and is now over 50 gallons per year.

TABLE 14-2	
Caffeine in Popular Soft Drinks	
Brand	**Caffeine* (mg)**
Sugar-Free Mr. Pibb	58.8
Mountain Dew	54.0
Mello Yello	52.8
Tab	46.8
Coca-Cola	45.6
Diet Coke	45.6
Shasta Cola	44.4
Mr. Pibb	40.8
Dr Pepper	39.6
Big Red	38.4
Pepsi-Cola	38.4
Diet Pepsi	36.0
Pepsi Light	36.0
RC Cola	36.0
Diet Rite	36.0
Canada Dry Jamaica Cola	30.0
Canada Dry Diet Cola	1.2

*Per 12-oz serving

TABLE 14-3	
Caffeine Content of Nonprescription Drugs	
Drug	**Caffeine (mg)**
Stimulants	
No Doz	100.0
Vivarin	200.0
Analgesics	
Anacin	32.0
Excedrin	65.0
Goody's Headache Powders	32.5
Midol	32.4
Vanquish	33.0
Diuretics	
Aqua-Ban	100.0
Maximum-Strength Aqua-Ban Plus	200.0

Spurred by the huge marketing success of Mountain Dew among young consumers, in the late 1990s several companies introduced high-caffeine drinks with frankly suggestive advertising: "high energy"; "feed the rush"; "blow your mind"; and "raw, primal power."[11] Some of these drinks are no more than caffeine and water; others resemble soft drinks or fruit drinks, adorned with such symbols as lightning bolts. Although the overall market for these products is not yet clear, they have become very popular among young children and teenagers, causing concern about the potential for behavioral disturbance and for dependence.

Over-the-Counter Drugs

Few people realize that many nonprescription drugs also include caffeine, some in quite large amounts. Table 14.3 lists the caffeine content of some of these drugs. Presumably many people who buy "alertness tablets," such as No Doz, are aware that they are buying caffeine. But many buyers of such things as Excedrin might not realize how much caffeine they are getting. Imagine the condition of someone who took a nonprescription water-loss pill, and a headache tablet containing caffeine, who then drank a couple of cups of coffee.

A 1985 report[12] described a study in which 401 men and women were asked to report on their consumption over a 3-day period of all foods, beverages, and medications that might contain caffeine. Only 11 of the 401 did not take in any caffeine at all, and the total intake averaged around 400 mg per day. The sources of this intake in both men and women are reported in Table 14.4.

CAFFEINE PHARMACOLOGY

Xanthines are the oldest stimulants known. *Xanthine* is a Greek word meaning "yellow," the color of the residue that remains after xanthines are heated with nitric acid until dry. The three xanthines of primary importance are caffeine, theophylline, and theobromine. These three chemicals are methylated xanthines and are closely related alkaloids. Most alkaloids are insoluble in water, but these are unique, because they are slightly water soluble.

TABLE 14-4

Caffeine Consumption During a 72-Hour Period Among 173 Men and 228 Women

| Source | (mg) | Men Caffeine consumption | | (mg) | Women Caffeine consumption | |
		% of total caffeine intake	Reported use during study period (%)		% of total caffeine intake	Reported use during study period (%)
Coffee	914.86	79.2	79.29	970.07	76.2	83.8
Tea	111.75	9.7	34.70	125.58	9.9	40.8
Soft drinks	65.79	5.7	28.90	75.82	6.0	28.1
Chocolate beverages	2.43	0.2	10.40	4.32	0.3	18.0
Bar chocolate	7.19	0.6	23.70	5.73	0.5	22.4
OTC drugs	48.32	4.2	21.40	92.17	7.2	26.8
Total	1150.34			1273.69		

These three xanthines have similar effects on the body. Caffeine has the greatest effect. Theobromine has almost no stimulant effect on the central nervous system and the skeletal muscles. Theophylline is the most potent, and caffeine the least potent, agent on the cardiovascular system. Caffeine, so named because it was isolated from coffee in 1820, has been the most extensively studied and, unless otherwise indicated, is the drug under discussion here.

Time Course

In humans, the absorption of caffeine is rapid after oral intake; peak blood levels are reached 30 minutes after ingestion. Although maximal CNS effects are not reached for about two hours, the onset of effects can begin within half an hour after intake. The half-life of caffeine in humans is about three hours, and no more than 10 percent is excreted unchanged.

Cross-tolerance exists among the methylated xanthines; loss of tolerance can take more than two months of abstinence. The tolerance, however, is low grade, and by increasing the dose two to four times an effect can be obtained even in the tolerant individual. There is less tolerance to the CNS stimulation effect of caffeine than to most of its other effects. The direct action on the kidneys, to increase urine output, and the increase of salivary flow do show tolerance.

Dependence on caffeine is real (see the Taking Sides box). People who are not coffee drinkers or who have been drinking only decaffeinated coffee often report unpleasant effects (nervousness, anxiety) after being given caffeinated coffee, but those who regularly consume caffeine report mostly pleasant mood states after drinking coffee. Various experiments have reported on the reinforcing properties of caffeine in regular coffee drinkers; one of the most clear-cut allowed patients on a research ward to choose between two coded instant coffees, identical except that one contained caffeine. Subjects had to choose at the beginning of each day which coffee they would drink for the rest of that day. Subjects who had been drinking caffeine-containing coffee before this experiment almost always chose the caffeine-containing coffee.[13] Thus, the reinforcing effect of caffeine probably contributes to psychological dependence.

There has long been clear evidence of physical dependence on caffeine as well. The most reliable withdrawal sign is a headache, which

Taking Sides

Caffeine-Dependence Syndrome?

As reviewed in Chapter 3, the American Psychiatric Association's *DSM-IV* lists the criteria for substance abuse, substance dependence, substance withdrawal, and substance intoxication. The team that developed the latest revision did not include caffeine among the substances that would be considered to produce substance dependence. However, in 1994 a group of researchers reported the cases of 16 individuals who they considered to meet the general criteria for a *DSM-IV* diagnosis of substance disorder.[33]

Of 99 subjects who responded to newspaper notices asking for volunteers who believed they were psychologically or physically dependent on caffeine, 27 were asked to undergo further testing, which included a psychiatric interview to assess caffeine dependence. Although the *DSM-IV* requires that only 3 of 7 criteria be met for a diagnosis of dependence, this study was more conservative in requiring 3 of the 4 most serious criteria (tolerance, withdrawal, persistent desire or efforts to cut down, and continued use despite knowledge of a persistent or recurrent problem caused by use). Sixteen of the 27 were diagnosed as having caffeine dependence using these criteria. Of those 16, 11 agreed to participate in a double-blind caffeine withdrawal experiment. All were placed on a restricted diet during two 2-day study periods and were given capsules to take at various times of the day to match their normal caffeine intake. During one of the two sessions, each subject was given caffeine, and during the other session the capsules contained a placebo. Neither the subjects nor the interviewers were told on which session they were getting the caffeine. Withdrawal symptoms found during the placebo session included headaches, fatigue, decreased vigor, and increased depression scores. Several of the subjects were unable to go to or stay at work, went to bed several hours early, or needed their spouse to take over child-care responsibilities.

A decision to accept caffeine-dependence syndrome as an official diagnosis would have several implications—some feel that it would trivialize the diagnosis for "serious" drug dependence or complicate questions of insurance payment for treatment of substance dependence. Others feel that this syndrome could be a serious dependence disorder for some coffee drinkers and deserves to be recognized as such.

For more on this topic, log on to www.dushkin. com/online for current news and links to other popular and informative sites, as well as time-saving web search strategies and study tools.

---

occurs an average of 18 to 19 hours after the most recent caffeine intake. Other symptoms include increased fatigue and decreased sense of vigor. These withdrawal symptoms are strongest during the first two days of withdrawal, then decline over the next five or six days.[14]

Mechanism of Action

For years no one really knew the mechanism whereby the methylxanthines had their effects on the CNS. In the early 1980s, evidence was presented that caffeine and the other xanthines block the brain's receptors for a substance known as **adenosine**, which is a neurotransmitter or neuromodulator. Adenosine normally acts in several areas of the brain to produce behavioral sedation by inhibiting the release of other neurotransmitters. Caffeine's stimulant action results from blocking the receptors for this inhibitory effect.[15] Now that this mechanism is understood, it may lead to the development of new chemicals having similar but perhaps more potent effects.

Physiological Effects

The pharmacological effects on the CNS and the skeletal muscles are probably the basis for the wide use of caffeine-containing beverages. With two cups of coffee taken close together (about 200 mg of caffeine), the cortex is activated, the

Exploring Your Spirituality

Get a Mantra, Not a Mocha

With cardiovascular disease the top killer in the United States and stress an ever-present problem in most workplaces, perhaps more of us should trade in our coffee breaks for a meditation break.

A study published in the March 2000 issue of *Stroke: Journal of the American Heart Association* found that meditation may lower heart attack risk by 11 percent and stroke risk by as much as 15 percent. This practice of "restful alertness" may help prevent and treat atherosclerosis, the hardening of the arteries that can lead to a stroke or heart attack. And some doctors have long believed that meditation helps keep blood pressure at low, healthy levels. In addition, during meditation, breathing slows, blood levels of stress hormones drop, brain wave patterns slow down, and muscles relax.

Meditation is one way to take better care of your spiritual well-being, too. Meditation gives people a tool to deal with their stress, and devotees claim it brings an inner peace and appreciation for daily living. It can be an effective way to connect to your deepest desires and to live a more authentic life based on what really matters to you.

Although meditation is not difficult, you will benefit from learning the technique from a teacher. Attend a free introductory class to judge whether an instructor and class will fit your needs. Many people have a tough time sitting still in the beginning. If meditation feels right to you, give yourself a chance to become good at it. It takes practice and patience, especially in our harried, adrenaline-driven society. You might start by listening to a short relaxation tape, which can help guide you to a calm, relaxed state of mind. Some people build up to a 20-minute period of meditation, with their eyes closed and their minds quiet, twice a day. Others find that short meditation breaks throughout the day help keep their stress levels from rising.

Using a specific meditation technique appears to be more beneficial than simply closing your eyes and relaxing. Many people find it difficult to relax and to avoid intrusive thoughts if they have never learned how to do so. Meditation is a more efficient, more effective way to relax deeply, especially when practiced daily. Look into what types of meditation classes are offered in your area. The point is to find a personal practice you're likely to stick with over time.

EEG shows an arousal pattern, and drowsiness and fatigue decrease. This CNS stimulation is also the basis for "coffee nerves," which can occur at low doses in sensitive individuals and in others when they have consumed large amounts of caffeine. In the absence of tolerance, even 200 mg will increase the time it takes to fall asleep and will cause sleep disturbances. There is a strong relationship between the mood-elevating effect of caffeine and the extent to which it will keep the individual awake.

Higher dose levels (about 500 mg) are needed to affect the autonomic centers of the brain, and heart rate and respiration can increase at this dose. The direct effect on the cardiovascular system is in opposition to the effects mediated by the autonomic centers. Caffeine acts directly on the vascular muscles to cause dilation, whereas stimulation of the autonomic centers results in constriction of blood vessels. Usually dilation occurs, but in the brain the blood vessels are constricted, and this constriction might be the basis for caffeine's ability to reduce migraine headaches.

The opposing effects of caffeine, directly on the heart and indirectly through effects on the medulla, make it very difficult to predict the results of normal (that is, less than 500 mg) caffeine intake. At higher levels there is an increase

adenosine: (a *den* o sen) an inhibitory neurotransmitter through which caffeine acts.

in heart rate, and continued use of large amounts of caffeine can produce an irregular heartbeat in some individuals.

The basal metabolic rate might be increased slightly (10 percent) in chronic caffeine users, because 500 mg has frequently been shown to have this effect. This action probably combines with the stimulant effects on skeletal muscles to increase physical work output and decrease fatigue after the use of caffeine.

Behavioral Effects

Stimulation

A hundred years ago, French essayist Balzac spoke with feeling when describing the effects of coffee:

> It causes an admirable fever. It enters the brain like a bacchante. Upon its attack, imagination runs wild, bares itself, twists like a pythoness and in this paroxysm a poet enjoys the supreme possession of his faculties; but this is a drunkenness of thought as wine brings about a drunkenness of the body.[16]

In the original French, the description is even more stimulating and erotic. Unfortunately it does not refer to the effect most people receive from their morning cup of coffee. The hard research data are not so uniformly positive—the effects of caffeine depend on the difficulty of the task, the time of day, and to a great extent on how much caffeine the subject normally consumes. When regular users of high amounts of caffeine (more than 300 mg/day, the equivalent of three cups of brewed coffee) were tested on a variety of study-related mental tasks without caffeine, they performed more poorly than did users of low amounts, perhaps because of withdrawal effects. Although their performance was improved after being given caffeine, they still performed more poorly on several of the tasks than did users of low amounts. It seems as though the beneficial short-term effects can be offset by the effects of tolerance and dependence

> ### Drugs in Depth
>
> #### Caffeine and Panic Attacks
>
> The National Institute of Mental Health (NIMH) has reported that caffeine can precipitate full-blown *panic attacks* in some people.[32] Panic attacks are not common but can be very debilitating for those who suffer them. They consist of sudden, irrational feelings of doom, sometimes accompanied by choking, sweating, heart palpitations, and other symptoms.
>
> In an experiment conducted at NIMH laboratories in Maryland, a group of people who had previously suffered panic attacks were given 480 mg caffeine, equivalent to about 5 cups of brewed coffee. Panic attacks were precipitated in almost half of those people. In a group of 14 people who had never before experienced a panic attack, 2 suffered an attack after receiving 720 mg caffeine.
>
> The results are interesting from a scientific point of view not only because they reveal individual differences in susceptibility to panic but also because of the possible implications for an understanding of the biochemistry of panic disorders. The experiment may also have more immediate and practical implications in that, if a person does experience a panic attack, caffeine consumption should be looked at as a possible cause.

in regular users.[17] There has been a report that high levels of caffeine consumption among college students are associated with lower academic performance.[18]

There is considerable evidence that 200 to 300 mg of caffeine will partially offset fatigue-induced decrement in the performance of motor tasks. Like the amphetamines, but to a much smaller degree, caffeine prolongs the amount of time an individual can perform physically exhausting work.

Headache

Caffeine's vasoconstricitve effects are considered to be responsible for the drug's ability to relieve migraine headaches. However, a study of nonmigraine headache pain found that caffeine reduced headache pain, even in individuals who normally consumed little or no caffeine (in other words, not only headaches resulting from caffeine withdrawal).[19] As for migraine headaches, in 1998, the FDA allowed the relabeling of extra-strength Excedrine, which contains 65 mg caffeine, for over-the-counter use as "Excedrine Migraine."

Hyperactivity

Many studies have looked at the effect of caffeine on the behavior of hyperkinetic children (see Chapter 8), and most have not shown any therapeutic effect. One report[20] of the effects of 3 and 10 mg/kg of caffeine on normal 8- to 13-year-old boys showed decreased reaction times and increased vigilance, along with increased motor activity. That's pretty much what might be expected from a mild stimulant.

Sobering Up

Even the television ads tell you—make coffee that "one last drink for the road." There is not a lot of evidence to support the value of this. Caffeine will not lower blood alcohol concentration, but it might arouse the drinker. As they say—put coffee in a sleepy drunk and you get a wide-awake drunk. You can easily imagine that this might be more dangerous than if the drunk had been left to sleep it off.

CAUSES FOR CONCERN

Caffeine is one of those drugs that seem to always be in trouble. It's always suspected of doing bad things. Because it is probably the most widely used psychoactive drug in the world (it's acceptable to those in most Judeo-Christian as well as Islamic traditions), it is understandable that it would elicit both good and bad reports. Although it is important to point out that there is not yet clear evidence that moderate caffeine consumption is dangerous, the scientific literature has investigated the possible effects of caffeine in cancer, benign breast disease,

reproduction, and heart disease. Part of the problem in knowing for certain about some of these things is that epidemiological research on caffeine consumption is difficult to do well. Coffee drinkers also tend to smoke more, for example, so the statistics have to correct for smoking behavior. Also, some studies have asked only how many cups of coffee people drink per day, without correcting for decaffeinated coffee, tea, colas, or other sources of caffeine or without correcting for differences between weekend and weekday coffee drinking.[21]

Cancer

In the early 1980s, there was a report that coffee drinkers have an increased risk of pancreatic cancers. However, the studies since then have criticized procedural flaws in that report and have found no evidence of such a link. The 1984 American Cancer Society nutritional guidelines indicated that there is no reason to consider caffeine a risk factor in human cancer.

Benign Breast Disease

A relationship has been suggested between use of the methylxanthines and *fibrocystic breast disease*. This is not a form of breast cancer but a condition in which benign lumps form in a woman's breasts, a condition that can be quite painful. The early studies have been criticized for not having proper controls, and in 1984 the AMA's Council on Scientific Affairs concluded that "there is currently no scientific basis for associating methylxanthine consumption with fibrocystic disease of the breast."

A large study[22] of all types of benign breast diseases found no significant relationship to caffeine use. This study, which appeared in 1985, was widely cited as indicating that there might be no such risk associated with caffeine. However, the author who originally reported a positive relationship continued to maintain that patients with fibrocystic disease who stop the use of coffee and other methylxanthines will improve.[23] Conversely, a controlled clinical trial found no such improvement when patients were put on a caffeine-free diet.[24] The bottom line is that there is still no clear evidence that anyone should not drink coffee or colas in moderation. Yet, anyone who has received a diagnosis of sensitive benign breast disease might want to consider stopping consumption of all coffee, tea, colas, and other sources of methylxanthines to see if this will help improve the condition.

Reproductive Effects

Although studies in pregnant mice have indicated that large doses of caffeine can produce skeletal abnormalities in the pups, studies on humans have not found a relationship between caffeine and birth defects.[25] However, studies do strongly suggest that caffeine consumption by a woman can reduce her chances of becoming pregnant,[26] increase the chances of spontaneous abortion (miscarriage), and slow the growth of the fetus so that the baby weighs less than normal at birth.[27] The most controversial of these findings has been the reported increase in spontaneous abortion, which is found in some studies,[28] but not in others.[29] This is an issue of obvious importance, so for now the best advice for a woman who wants to become pregnant, stay pregnant, and produce a strong, healthy baby, is to avoid caffeine, alcohol, tobacco, and any other drug that is not absolutely necessary for her health.

Heart Disease

There are many reasons for believing that caffeine might increase the risk of heart attacks, including the fact that it increases heart rate and blood pressure. Until recently, there were about as many studies that found no relationship between caffeine use and heart attacks as there were studies that found such a relationship. One very interesting report used an unusual

approach. Rather than ask people who had just had heart attacks about their prior caffeine consumption and compare them with people who were hospitalized for another ailment (the typical retrospective study), this study began in 1948 to track male medical students enrolled in the Johns Hopkins Medical School.[30] More than 1,000 of these subjects were followed for 20 years or more after graduation and were periodically asked about various habits, including drinking, smoking, and coffee consumption. Thus, this was a prospective study, to see which of these habits might predict future health problems. Those who drank 5 or more cups per day were about 2.5 times as likely as nondrinkers to suffer from coronary heart disease. This result and recent indications that coffee drinking can increase blood cholesterol levels stimulated more research, including a large-scale retrospective study, which reported that the incidence of nonfatal heart attacks in men under 55 years old was directly related to the amount of coffee consumed, among both smokers and nonsmokers. Those drinking 5 or more cups per day were about twice as likely to suffer a heart attack as those who drank no coffee.[31]

The best research, then, gives a strong suggestion that caffeine can increase the risk of heart attacks. This is of special concern to those with other risk factors (e.g., smoking, family history of heart disease, overweight, high blood pressure, and high cholesterol levels).

Caffeinism

Caffeine is not terribly toxic, and overdose deaths are extremely rare. It is estimated that over 10 g (equivalent to 100 cups of coffee) would be required to cause death from oral caffeine taken by mouth. Death is produced by convulsions, which lead to respiratory arrest.

However, **caffeinism** (excessive use of caffeine) can cause a variety of unpleasant symptoms, and because of caffeine's domesticated social status it might be overlooked as the cause.

For example, nervousness, irritability, tremulousness, muscle twitching, insomnia, flushed appearance, and elevated temperature can all result from excessive caffeine use. There can also be palpitations, heart arrhythmias, and gastrointestinal disturbances. In several cases in which serious disease has been suspected, the symptoms have miraculously improved when coffee was restricted.

SUMMARY

- The ancient plants coffee, tea, and cacao all contain caffeine and two related xanthines.
- Caffeine is also contained in soft drinks and nonprescription medicines.
- Caffeine has a longer-lasting effect than many people realize.
- Caffeine exerts a stimulating action in several brain regions by blocking inhibitory receptors for adenosine.
- In regular caffeine users, headache, fatigue, or depression can develop if caffeine use is stopped.
- Caffeine is capable of reversing the effects of fatigue on both mental and physical tasks, but it might not be able to improve the performance of a well-rested individual, particularly on complex tasks.
- Excessive caffeine consumption, referred to as caffeinism, can produce a panic reaction.
- Daily use of large amounts of caffeine increases the risk of heart attack.
- Caffeine use during pregnancy is not advisable.

REVIEW QUESTIONS

1. What role did the American Revolution and alcohol prohibition play in influencing American coffee consumption?

Web Watch

Finding Alternatives to Caffeine Addiction

According to information presented at www.caffeine blues.com/addiction.htm, almost 80 percent of all Americans are hooked on caffeine. Read about beverages and foods that contain caffeine and the risks and effects of caffeine addiction. Then take the online evaluation to find out whether you're addicted to caffeine, and discover alternatives to caffeine.

Overcoming a Caffeine Habit

At www.wellnessnet.com/testaddict.htm you'll find an addiction quiz, which can be used for caffeine or any other drug. Assess yourself and discover what you can do to avoid or overcome addiction.

Learning About Caffeine and Pregnancy

Read the article "Caffeine in Pregnancy: Is There an Increased Risk for Miscarriage?" at www.mostgene. org/gd/gdvol11d.htm. The article provides statistics and research results on the debated issue of caffeine's effects on pregnancy.

2. What are the differences among black tea, green tea, and oolong?
3. What are the two xanthines contained in tea and chocolate, besides caffeine?
4. Rank the caffeine content of a cup of brewed coffee, a cup of tea, a chocolate bar, and a 12-ounce Coca-Cola.
5. How does caffeine interact with adenosine receptors?
6. What are some of the behavioral and physiological effects of excessive caffeine consumption?
7. Describe the effects of caffeine on migraine headaches, caffeine-withdrawal headaches, and other headaches.

caffeinism: excessive use of caffeine.

8. Give an informed reaction to the statement that caffeine increases the risk of breast cancer.

9. What are three possible ways in which caffeine use by a woman might interfere with reproduction?

10. What is the relationship between caffeine and panic attacks?

REFERENCES

1. Uribe Compuzano A: *Brown gold*. New York: Random House, 1954.
2. Meyer H: *Old English coffee houses*. Emmaus, PA: Rodale Press, 1954.
3. Lewin L: *Phantastica, narcotic, and stimulating drugs*. New York: E.P. Dutton, 1931.
4. U.S. Department of Commerce: *Statistical abstract of the United States*. Washington, DC: U.S. Government Printing Office, 1999.
5. A business built on beans, *Consumer Reports* pp Oct 1994.
6. Groisser DS: A study of caffeine in tea, *American Journal of Clinical Nutrition* 31(10):1727–1731. 1978.
7. Prial FJ: Secrets of a chocoholic, *New York Times* pp May 16, 1979.
8. Sterba JP: Coke brings "tasty happiness" to China, *New York Times* pp Apr 16, 1981.
9. Huisking CL: *Herbs to hormones*. Essex, CT: Pequot Press, 1968.
10. Sixth Circuit Court of Appeals, 1914: 215 *Federal Reporter* 539, June 13, 1914.
11. Barboza D: Caffeine-loaded "extreme beverages" go after the youth market, *New York Times* pp Aug 22, 1997.
12. Weidner G, Istvan J: Dietary sources of caffeine, *New England Journal of Medicine* 313:1421, 1985.
13. Griffiths RR and others: Human coffee drinking: Reinforcing and physical dependence producing effects of caffeine, *J Pharmacol Exp Ther* 239:416–425, 1986.
14. Hughes JR and others: Should caffeine abuse, dependence, or withdrawal be added to DSM-IV and ICD-10? *American Journal of Psychiatry* 149:33, 1992.
15. Feldman RS, Meyer JS, Quenzer LF: *Principles of neuropsychopharmacology*. Sunderland, MA: Sinauer, 1997.
16. Mickel EJ: *The artificial paradises in French literature*. Chapel Hill, NC: University of North Carolina Press, 1969 (Free translation from French) 1969.
17. Mitchell PJ, Redman JR: Effects of caffeine, time of day, and user history on study-related performance. *Psychopharmacology (Berl)* 109:121, 1992.
18. Gilliland K, Andress D: Ad lib caffeine consumption, symptoms of caffeinism, and academic performance, *American Journal of Psychiatry* 138(4):512–514, 1981.
19. Ward N and others: The analgesic effects of caffeine in headache, *Pain* 44:151–155, 1991.
20. Elkins RN and others: Acute effects of caffeine in normal prepubertal boys, *American Journal of Psychiatry* 138(2):178–183, 1981.
21. Schreiber GB and others: Measurement of coffee and caffeine intake: Implications for epidemiological research, *Preventive Medicine* 17:280–294, 1988.
22. Lubin F and others: A case-control study of caffeine and methylxanthines in benign breast disease, *Journal of the American Medical Association* 253:2388–2392, 1985.
23. Minton JP: Caffeine and benign breast disease, *Journal of the American Medical Association* 254:2408, 1985.
24. Allen SS, Froberg DG: The effect of decreased caffeine consumption on benign proliferative breast disease: A randomized clinical trial, *Surgery* 101:720–730, 1987.
25. Dews P and others: Report of Fourth International Caffeine Workshop, *Food Chemistry and Toxicology* 22: 163–169, 1984.
26. Wilcox A and others: Caffeinated beverages and decreased fertility, *Lancet* 1:1453–1455, 1988.
27. Vlajinac HD and others: Effect of caffeine intake during pregnancy on birth weight, *American Journal of Epidemiology* 145:335–338, 1997.
28. Infante-Rivard C and others: Fetal loss associated with caffeine intake before and during pregnancy, *Journal of the American Medical Association* 270:2940, 1993.
29. Mills JL and others: Moderate caffeine use and the risk of spontaneous abortion and intrauterine growth retardation, *Journal of the American Medical Association* 269: 593, 1993.
30. LaCroix AZ and others: Coffee consumption and the incidence of coronary heart disease, *New England Journal of Medicine* 315: 977–982, 1986.
31. Rosenberg L and others: Coffee drinking and nonfatal myocardial infarction in men under 55 years of age, *American Journal of Epidemiology* 128:570–578, 1988.
32. Stewart SA: Caffeine can push the panic button, *USA Today* pp Oct 23, 1985.
33. Strain EC and others: Caffeine dependence syndrome, *Journal of the American Medical Association* 272:1043, 1994.

Try It!

How Much Caffeine Do You Consume?

How many different products do you use that contain caffeine (Review Tables 14.1 to 14.3)? Keep a complete record of your own intake of coffee, tea, soft drinks, and so on for a typical 3-day period (72 hours). From that record, estimate as closely as you can your total caffeine intake in milligrams. If you regularly consume 300 mg or more per day, you might ask yourself if caffeine is interfering with your sleep, work, or studying.

Chapter 15

*O*ver-the-Counter Drugs

Online Learning Center Resources

www.mhhe.com/ray

Log on to our Online Learning Center (OLC) for access to these additional resources.

- Chapter definitions
- Learning objectives
- Student interactive question-and-answer sites
- Self-scoring chapter quiz

The OLC also offers web links for study and exploration of health topics. Here are some examples of what you'll find:

www.ismp.org/Consumer/Read.html

Find out why it's important to read the labels of your medications. The site explains why prescription bottles look alike and are carefully labeled.

www.nacds.org/resources/sound.html

This website offers an extensive list of drug names that look alike or sound alike. The lists include brand and generic drug names and comparisons.

cpmcnet.columbia.edu/texts/guide/hmg34_0008.html

Check out this site for Columbia University's *Complete Home Medical Guide.* It gives instruction on using medications properly and keeping a safe and well-stocked medicine chest. There is also a listing of drugs and uses, helpful tips, and specific writings about medications.

Drugs in the Media

Concern over the Growing Risk of Drug Interaction

As advertising, the Internet, and other media coverage have increased consumers' knowledge of health-care issues, people are taking greater charge of their own health. These more educated consumers are also busier and more impatient for

Drugs in the Media Continued. . .

a quick fix. Patients may put off calling a doctor because it's simply more convenient to pick up an over-the-counter medication at the drugstore than to get the appropriate physician referrals, take time off from work to see the doctor, and go through the hassles of insurance paperwork. Some pharmacists and doctors say, however, that people falsely assume that, if a drug is sold over the counter, it is immune from drug interactions or other complications. With more medications available, and with more people self-medicating, consumers need to be aware of the increasing threat of drug interactions.

In the past 15 years or so, Americans have become less inclined to tough out minor ailments and are quicker to run to the drugstore to seek immediate relief from annoying symptoms. More than half of all Americans take at least two different medications daily, with many taking vitamins and dietary supplements as well, according to an American Society of Health-System Pharmacists (ASHP) survey, reported January 2001, in which 58 percent of the survey respondents said that they had taken an average of two OTC medications or supplements during the week preceding the survey and 40 percent said they use an average of two such products daily.

We're using medicines in ways we've never used them before, and increasingly we're seeing media coverage of the tens of thousands of Americans who are harmed or killed, not by illness but by medication in-

tended to treat it. The federal government recently mandated more consumer-friendly labeling for OTC medications, including a "Warnings" section and a "Do Not Use" section that explains which drugs interact dangerously with other OTC medications. But nearly half of consumers say they do not always read the labels on OTC drugs.

How can we ensure we're taking medications in the safest way possible? The bottom line is to consult your pharmacist, especially as you take more medications and the opportunity for drug interactions grows. You may see multiple physicians; however, if you use the same pharmacist all the time, that pharmacist should develop a complete profile and be able to advise you on all the drugs you're taking. In addition, keep a list of all the drugs you take—including over-the-counter (OTC) medications, supplements, and medicinal foods—for your own awareness and to show to health-care providers. That way you should notice unexpected changes to prescriptions, such as refills that are of the wrong strength, and you'll be able to communicate better with physicians and pharmacists. Finally, if your symptoms persist for more than 10 days despite taking OTC medication, see your doctor. Many viral and bacterial infections clear up after about a week, so chances are there's a more serious problem.

Over-the-counter drugs are those that are self-prescribed and self-administered for the relief of symptoms of self-diagnosed illnesses. The Food and Drug Administration (FDA) estimates that consumers self-treat four times more health problems than doctors treat, often using OTC drugs.

Americans spend over $18 billion a year on OTC products.[1] That's not as much as we spend on prescription drugs, alcohol, cigarettes, or illicit cocaine, but it's enough to keep several OTC drug manufacturers locked in fierce competition for those sales. The two biggest markets are for aspirinlike analgesics and for the collection of cough, cold, and flu products. Do we really need all these nonprescription tablets, capsules, liquids, and creams? How much of what we buy is based on advertising hype, and how much is based on sound decisions about our health? How are we as consumers to know the difference? The FDA is in the process of trying to help us with these decisions.

FDA REGULATION OF OTC PRODUCTS

The 1962 Kefauver-Harris amendment required that all drugs be evaluated for both safety and efficacy. The FDA was not only to set up criteria for new drugs entering the market but also to establish a procedure for reviewing all the OTC drugs already on the market. At first glance this seemed an impossible task, because there were between 250,000 and 300,000 products already being sold (no one knew for sure how many). In addition, each product was likely to change its ingredients without warning, just as the "new" and "improved" soaps and toothpastes do. The FDA made the decision not to study individual products but to review each active ingredient. The reason for this decision is that then, as now, many of the competing brands contain the same ingredients, so there are many fewer ingredients than products. The FDA divided OTC products into 26 classes and appointed an advisory panel for each class. Each panel was to look at the active ingredients contained in the products in its class, to decide for each ingredient whether there was evidence indicating that it was safe and effective for its purpose and to decide what sorts of claims could be made for that ingredient on the label. Several of the 26 classes of OTC drugs to be reviewed by the FDA included psychoactive ingredients: sedatives and sleep aids, analgesics, cold remedies and antitussives, antihistamines and allergy products, and stimulants.

Before the panel could begin work, some rules had to be laid down about what was meant

by such terms as *safe* and *effective*, keeping in mind that no drug is entirely safe and that many might have only limited effectiveness. The FDA uses the acronym **GRAS** ("generally recognized as safe") to mean that, given the currently available information, people who are informed and qualified would agree that the ingredient should be considered safe. "Safe" means "a low incidence of adverse reactions or significant side effects under adequate directions for use and warnings against unsafe use as well as low potential for harm which may result from abuse." Similar acronyms are used for two other important concepts: GRAE ("generally recognized as effective") and GRAHL ("generally recognized as honestly labeled").

> Effectiveness means a reasonable expectation that, in a significant proportion of the target population, the pharmacological effect of the drug, when used under adequate directions for use and warnings against unsafe use, will provide clinically significant relief of the type claimed.

The advisory panel was to rule on each active ingredient and decide whether the evidence indicates that the ingredient is both GRAS and GRAE, or failed on one or both criteria, or if further information was needed.

You'd think that because they simplified the approach and began appointing panels in 1972, this work would be about done. Well, not quite yet. The FDA began to publish "Tentative Final Monographs" on each class in 1985. The idea was to solicit comments from the public and the drug companies before publishing Final Monographs, but the amount of comment was so great that revised Tentative Final Monographs are still appearing. By 1992, 20 years after the process began, only 34 of the proposed 71 monographs had become finalized. Because the process was taking so long, in 1980 the FDA

GRAS: "generally recognized as safe."

commissioner acted to speed up both the reviews and the effects of those reviews. Thus, the FDA began publishing some brief advisory opinions banning certain products or combinations and sent letters to manufacturers and distributors of the products, ordering that the products be removed from the market immediately. In spite of the progress that has been made in reviewing ingredients and removing many products from the market, in 1992 the U.S. General Accounting Office released a critical report, claiming that the FDA still didn't know exactly how many OTC products are being marketed and still couldn't guarantee that everything being sold was both safe and effective.[2] By the late 1990s, the list of therapeutic classes had grown from 26 to over 80. The exact number of OTC products on the market is still not known because they still come and go and change, but we do know that there are more than 100,000, and they contain fewer than 1,000 total active ingredients. Most of those are old ingredients, which were being sold prior to 1972 and survived the review process.[3]

The overall result of this procedure can be seen by taking a trip to your neighborhood drugstore and looking at the lists of ingredients on medications of a given type. You should be struck that all the competing brands contain much the same few ingredients. In some classes, there might be only one approved active ingredient, meaning that all competing brands are essentially identical. The differences among them often are in the long list of other (inactive) ingredients (colorings, flavorings, etc.).

SIMPLIFYING LABELS

Both the safety and effectiveness of OTC drugs depend greatly on their being used according to the directions and warnings on the label. To reduce confusion and make it more likely that consumers will be able to understand the labels, the FDA proposed in 1997 to create uniform standards for labels, with minimum print size,

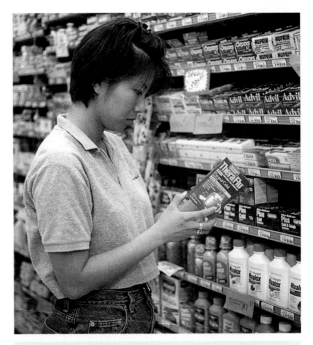

A shopper reading the label on an OTC medication.

topics in a consistent order (active ingredients, directions for use, warnings), and bold, bulleted headings. One important proposal was to make the language clearer and more concise, avoiding medical terminology (e.g., "pulmonary" replaced by "lung").[4] This new, consistent approach to labeling has not been completely adopted, however, and many OTC product labels still appear to be cluttered and confusing.

OVER-THE-COUNTER VERSUS PRESCRIPTION DRUGS

You might remember that it was the 1938 Food, Drug, and Cosmetic Act that established a classification of drugs that would be available only by prescription. The rule is that a drug is supposed to be permitted for OTC sale unless, because of potential toxicity or for other reasons (e.g., if it must be injected), it may be safely sold and used only under a prescription.

Taking Sides

Should There Be a Class of "Pharmacist-Recommended" Drugs?

Professional pharmacists may feel that they "get no respect" from some drug purchasers. Pharmacists are trained to be familiar with not only the prescription orders they fill but also with the ingredients and indications for OTC products. Most feel that consumers should take advantage of their advice on decisions to purchase and use OTC drugs. However, increasing numbers of people are purchasing their OTC medications in grocery and convenience stores, rather than in pharmacies. In addition, there is concern that, as more and more former prescription products are allowed for OTC sale, many people will simply assume that the drugs are safe and will use them carelessly. Pharmacists' organizations have proposed the

establishment of "pharmacist-legend" drugs in the United States, similar to programs that have been used in England and Australia and that are being studied in Canada. Ibuprofen is one drug that Australian pharmacists keep "behind the counter"—no physician's prescription is required, but the pharmacist will dispense it only after giving some advice on its safe use. With such a system, perhaps other drugs (including oral contraceptives?) could become available without a physician's order.

For more on this topic, log on to www.dushkin.com/online for current news and links to other popular and informative sites, as well as time-saving web search strategies and study tools.

Sometimes the only difference between an OTC product and a prescription product is the greater amount of active ingredient in each prescription dose. More often, however, prescription drugs are chemicals that are unavailable OTC. Until the FDA began its OTC Drug Review process, once a new drug was approved for prescription sale it almost never became available OTC. Neither the FDA nor the manufacturers seemed to have much interest in switching drugs to OTC status. However, the FDA advisory panels that reviewed products in a given OTC category sometimes did more than was required of them. In some cases, they recommended that higher doses be allowed in OTC preparations—and as a result we can now buy higher-strength OTC antihistamines. And in several cases the suggestion was that previous prescription-only ingredients, such as ibuprofen, be sold OTC.

Between 1972 and 1992, 20 ingredients were switched to OTC status. Then the FDA established the Nonprescription Drug Advisory Committee, which has an advisory role regarding all the drug categories and has helped move more drugs from prescription to OTC. Drugs recently switched to OTC status include nicotine chewing

gum and patches and the hair-growing drug minoxidil.[3] Several drug manufacturers have now seen the potential for greater markets for some of their products, and it is expected that more and more OTC switches will be based on revised New Drug Applications (NDAs) from the manufacturers.

SOME PSYCHOACTIVE OTC PRODUCTS

Stimulants

Stimulants, one of the original FDA categories, turns out to be one of the simplest categories. The FDA allows stimulants to be sold to "help restore mental alertness or wakefulness when experiencing fatigue or drowsiness." If it sounds like caffeine could do this, you're right! No Doz, a well-known product that has been around for years, has the tried-and-true formula: 100 mg of caffeine (about the equivalent of an average cup of brewed coffee). The recommended dose is two tablets initially, then one every three hours. Another well-known product, Vivarin, contains 200 mg of caffeine, and the initial dose is one tablet.

Thus, although the packages look different and different companies make them, a smart consumer would choose between these two based on the price per milligram of caffeine. Or he or she could choose a less expensive store brand, or buy coffee (usually more expensive), or just get enough rest and save money. The labels warn against using these caffeine tablets with coffee, tea, or cola drinks. The only active ingredient the FDA allows in OTC stimulants is caffeine.[5]

There is a reasonably brisk business in the semilegal field of selling caffeine tablets or capsules resembling prescription stimulants, such as the amphetamines. In fact, many street purchases of speed turn out to contain caffeine as their major ingredient. Some states have tried to ban the sale of these look-alikes, and the FDA has tried to regulate them, but doing so is tough, because caffeine itself is legal. Mail-order advertisements for these products can be found in the backs of various magazines. It is, however, a violation of the controlled substances act to sell something that is represented to be a controlled substance. Although these products no longer use such suggestive names as speed, one does claim the brand name "Amphetrazine." Some companies have manufactured combinations of caffeine with either *ephedrine* or **phenylpropanolamine (PPA)**. You may remember from Chapter 7 that ephedrine is a sympathomimetic derived from a Chinese herbal tea and sold as a bronchodilator. The amphetamine molecule was derived from it. PPA has a structure similar to that of amphetamine and ephedrine and has been sold in weight-control preparations. Each of these has mild stimulant properties of its own. The FDA has ruled that products labeled as stimulants that contain anything other than caffeine as an active ingredient cannot be sold OTC. The FDA also outlawed OTC products labeled for any purpose that contained combinations of caffeine and ephedrine and has taken legal action against several mail-order distributors of such combination products.

OTC products containing only ephedrine have come under recent scrutiny. Although these are allowed for sale as a bronchodilator for asthma, some people are apparently buying them to use as pep or energy, pills. In addition, Oregon has switched ephedrine to prescription-only status over concern that illicit laboratories are using ephedrine as a precursor for making methamphetamine.

Weight-Control Products

The original FDA list of OTC drug categories did not include appetite suppressants or a similar term. Apparently the FDA didn't think it would be dealing with such a product, because, at the time, the use of the prescription amphetamines for this purpose was under widespread attack. However, data were presented indicating that PPA was safe and effective, and by the late 1970s several products were being sold that contained PPA as their only active ingredient. Some studies indicated that caffeine could potentiate the appetite-suppressing effect of PPA, and for a brief period during the early 1980s several of the products included both PPA and caffeine. After the 1983 FDA ruling prohibiting such combinations on the grounds that they might not be safe, all products returned to PPA only. The recommended dose for appetite suppression was 75 mg per day. There was some concern about the safety even of 75 mg doses, with the threat being increased blood pressure resulting from sympathetic stimulation. There was also some controversy about the effectiveness of PPA, given that its effect, as with most appetite suppressant drugs, is small and rather short-lived.

In November 2000, the FDA issued a Public Health Advisory on the safety of PPA, based on a new study showing that women taking PPA had an increased risk of hermorrhagic stroke (bleeding into the brain, usually a result of elevated blood pressure). The FDA requested that all drug companies discontinue marketing products containing PPA and that consumers not use any products containing PPA. Manufacturers and retailers responded quickly, and as of early 2001 no remaining weight-control products contained PPA. Dexatrim, one of the most widely sold products previously based on PPA, was already marketing a "natural" version containing various herbal products, including a small amount of *ma huang* (ephedra).

The FDA has reviewed and ruled against several other products that have been advertised for weight control. Benzocaine-containing candies and gums were supposed to numb the tongue, reducing the sense of taste, but it was never shown that this was an effective way to reduce food intake. Starch blockers, which were supposed to interfere with the absorption of carbohydrates from starchy foods, have never been proved to do so. The FDA asked for all sales to stop until safety and effectiveness could be established, and the government seized the products after promoters failed to comply. Cholecystokinin (CCK) is a hormone that does decrease food intake when injected directly into the brains of experimental animals, but the chemical is quickly destroyed in the digestive tract if taken by mouth. Nevertheless, products claiming to include CCK have been advertised and sold, and the FDA has ordered this practice discontinued. Other unapproved products for weight reduction that have come under FDA scrutiny in recent years include DHEA, arginine and ornithine, spirulina, and glucomannan. None of these products has been demonstrated to be effective in weight loss, despite claims of "burning fat," "natural" weight loss, "Oriental weight-loss secret," and so on.

Sedatives and Sleep Aids

A few years ago the shelves contained a number of OTC sedative, or "calmative," preparations, including Quiet World and Compoz, which contained very small amounts of the acetylcholine receptor blocker *scopolamine* combined with the **antihistamine** methapyrilene. At the same time, sleep aids, such as Sleep-Eze and Sominex, contained just a bit more of the same two ingredients. The rationale for the scopolamine, particularly at these low doses, was under FDA

investigation, but scopolamine had traditionally been included in many such medications in the past. It is quite clear that some antihistamines do produce a kind of sedated state and might produce drowsiness. The FDA advisory panel accepted methapyrilene but eventually rejected scopolamine. For a while all of these medications contained only methapyrilene. Then in 1979, it was reported that methapyrilene caused cancer in laboratory animals, so it was no longer GRAS. Next came pyrilamine maleate, then doxylamine succinate, and then *diphenhydramine*, all antihistamines. The interesting thing about this whole process was that if you bought the same brand from one year to the next, you would get a different formulation each time. But if you bought several different brands at the same time, you stood a good chance of getting the same formulation in all of them.

The sedative category no longer exists for OTC products. One product, Miles Nervine, which went from being a sedative containing bromide salts to a calmative containing whatever they all contained each year, is now Miles Nervine Nighttime Sleep-Aid, containing 25 mg of diphenhydramine. Nytol is also a nighttime sleep aid containing the same ingredient. Sominex and Sleep-Eze are still around, and both contain diphenhydramine.

As we saw in Chapter 9, insomnia is perceived to be a bigger problem than it actually is for most people, and it is rare that medication is really required. Antihistamines can induce drowsiness, but not very quickly. If you do feel the need to use these to get you to sleep more rapidly, take them at least 20 minutes before

---

phenylpropanolamine (PPA): (fen il pro pa *nole* a meen) the active ingredient in OTC weight-control products.

antihistamine: the active ingredient in OTC sleep aids and cough/cold products.

Targeting Prevention

The Medicine Chest

The family medicine chest is often a treasure trove of old tablets, capsules, liquids, and lozenges. Start digging around and see how many different OTC drugs you can find in yours. How old do you think some of them are? If any of them have expiration dates, have the dates passed?

Because formulations change from year to year, there's a good chance the medicines you now have are not the same as the ones being sold in the drugstore. Write down the formulations for a few of your medicine chest drugs. Then go to the drugstore and compare them with the current formulation for the same brand of product. Do you wonder if some of the old ingredients were removed because the FDA no longer considers them safe?

retiring. Their sedative effects are potentiated by alcohol, so it is not a good idea to take them after drinking.

ANALGESICS

People and Pain

Pain is such a little word for such a big experience. Most people have experienced pain of varying intensities, from mild to moderate to severe to excruciating. Two major classes of drugs are used to reduce pain or the awareness of pain, anesthetics and analgesics. Anesthetics (meaning "without sensibility") have this effect by reducing all types of sensation or by blocking consciousness completely. The local anesthetics used in dentistry and the general anesthetics used in major surgery are examples of this class of agent. The other major class, the analgesics (meaning "without pain"), are compounds that reduce pain selectively without causing a loss of other sensations. The analgesics are divided into two groups. Opiates (see Chapter 16) are one group of analgesics, but this chapter primarily

discusses the OTC internal analgesics, such as aspirin, acetaminophen, and ibuprofen.

Although pain itself is a complex psychological phenomenon, there have been attempts to classify different types of pain to develop a rational approach to its treatment. One classification divides pain into two types, depending on its place of origin. Visceral pain, such as intestinal cramps, arises from nonskeletal portions of the body; narcotics are effective in reducing pain of this type. Somatic pain, arising from muscle or bone and typified by sprains, headaches, and arthritis, is reduced by salicylates (aspirin) and related products.

Pain is unlike other sensations in many ways, mostly because of nonspecific factors. The experience of pain varies with personality, gender, and time of day and is increased with fatigue, anxiety, fear, boredom, and anticipation of more pain. Because pain is very susceptible to nonspecific factors, a brief comment is required on the effectiveness of a placebo in reducing pain. Classic studies were done by Beecher, who summarized reports of many investigators on

HealthQuest Activities

In Module 9 you'll find information about OTC drugs under *Drug Interactions*. Read about acetaminophen, antacids, antihistamines, aspirin, cold remedies, and cough medicines. How many of these drugs have you taken before? Have you ever taken one in conjunction with another drug and experienced any of the listed symptoms?

Go to *Drug F/X Exploration* in the same module. Complete the assessment to discover whether or not you have a dependence on antihistamines or aspirin. Have you ever experienced any of the side effects? Collect any OTC medications you have and compare the warnings on the labels with warnings you found in this activity. Are they consistent? Do you think these warnings effectively convey the danger of OTC drug dependence?

the effectiveness of placebos in the reduction of pain.[6] These were real situations with a variety of clinical causes ranging from postoperative pain to the aches associated with the common cold. About 35 percent of the patients in these studies had their pain "satisfactorily relieved" by placebos. That is, when individuals in pain were given an inactive substance along with the suggestion that it would reduce the pain, 35 percent of the patients obtained relief.

This 35 percent proportion is quite high, considering that morphine provides satisfactory relief of pain in only about 75 percent of patients. It was also found that placebos are most effective in reducing pain in stressful situations, whereas morphine has its smallest effect in these stressful situations. As might be expected from the previous statement, placebos are more effective in real-life pain than in experimental pain. The internal analgesics have been repeatedly shown to be more effective at therapeutic doses than placebos for certain kinds of pain.

Aspirin

Salicylates are the most widely used class of internal analgesics. The word itself suggests their long heritage, coming from the Latin *salix,* meaning "willow." Over 2,400 years ago the Greeks used extracts of willow and poplar bark in the treatment of pain, gout, and other illnesses. Aristotle commented on some of the clinical effects of similar preparations, and Galen made good use of these formulations. These remedies fell into disrepute, however, when St. Augustine declared that all diseases of Christians were the work of demons and thus a punishment from God. American Indians, unhampered by this enlightened attitude, used a tea brewed from willow bark to reduce fever. The salicylates were not rediscovered in Europe until about 200 years ago, when an Englishman, the Reverend Edward Stone, combined two bits of the best information then available and put the result to a clinical test. The two pieces of

data he combined were these: (1) listen to old folklore tales and (2) plants acquire the characteristics of the place where they grow. The old folklore kept saying that willow bark was good for pain and whatever else ails you. Stone phrased the second attitude

> As this tree delights in a moist or wet soil where aches chiefly abound, the general maxim that many natural maladies carry their cures along with them, or that their remedies lie not far from their causes, was so very apposite to this particular case that I could not help applying it. That this might be the intention of Providence had some little weight with me.[7]

Stone prepared an extract of the bark and gave the same dose to 50 patients with varying illnesses and found the results to be "uniformly excellent." In the nineteenth century, the active ingredient in these preparations was isolated and identified as salicylic acid. In 1838, salicylic acid was synthesized, and in 1859 procedures were developed that made bulk production feasible. Salicylic acid and sodium salicylate were then used for many ills, especially arthritis.

In the giant Bayer Laboratories in Germany in the 1890s, there worked a chemist named Hoffmann. His father had a severe case of rheumatoid arthritis, and only salicylic acid seemed to help. The major difficulty then, as today, was that the drug caused great gastric discomfort. So great was the stomach upset and nausea that Hoffmann's father frequently preferred the pain of the arthritis. Hoffmann studied the salicylates to see if he could find one with the same therapeutic effect as salicylic acid but without the side effects.

In 1898, he synthesized **acetylsalicylic acid** and tried it on his father, who reported relief from pain without stomach upset. The

acetylsalicylic acid: (a *see* till sal i *sill* ick) the chemical known as aspirin.

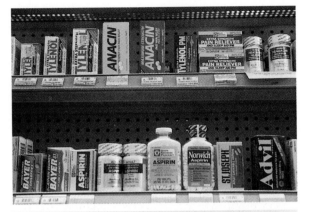

Aspirin works three ways: to block pain, to reduce fever, and to reduce inflammation.

compound was tested, patented, and released for sale in 1899 as *Aspirin*. Aspirin was a trademark name derived from the name *acetyl and spiralic acid* (the old name for salicylic acid).

It is interesting that the two famous compounds that the Bayer Laboratories in Germany were instrumental in introducing to the world are rapidly transformed in the body to their original form after absorption. Both heroin and aspirin were first synthesized in the Bayer Laboratories. Aspirin, either in the gastrointestinal tract or in the bloodstream, is converted to salicylic acid. Taken orally, aspirin is a more potent analgesic than salicylic acid, because aspirin irritates the stomach less and is thus absorbed more rapidly.

Aspirin was marketed for physicians and sold as a white powder in individual dosage packets, available only by prescription. It was immediately popular worldwide, and the U.S. market became large enough that it was very soon manufactured in this country. In 1915, the 5 gram (325 mg) white tablet stamped "Bayer" first appeared, and, for the first time, Aspirin became a nonprescription item. The Bayer Company was on its way. It had an effective drug that could be sold to the public and was known by one name—Aspirin—and the name was trademarked. Before February 1917, when the patent on Aspirin was to expire, Bayer started an advertising campaign to make it clear that there was only one Aspirin, and its first name was Bayer. Several companies started manufacturing and selling Aspirin as aspirin, and Bayer sued. What happened after this is a long story, but you know who lost; aspirin is aspirin—or is it?

Therapeutic Use

Aspirin is truly a magnificent drug. It is also a drug with some serious side effects. Aspirin has three effects that are the primary basis for its clinical use. It is an analgesic that effectively blocks somatic pain in the mild-to-moderate range. Aspirin is also **antipyretic**: it reduces fever. Last but not least, aspirin is an **anti-inflammatory** agent: it reduces the swelling, inflammation, and soreness in an injured area. Its anti-inflammatory action is the basis for its extensive use in arthritis. It is difficult to find another drug that has this span of effects coupled with a relatively low toxicity. It does, however, have side effects that pose problems for some people.

Aspirin is readily absorbed from the stomach but even faster from the intestine. Thus, anything that delays movement of the aspirin from the stomach should affect absorption time. The evidence is mixed on whether taking aspirin with a meal, which delays emptying of the stomach, increases the time before onset of action. It should, however, reduce the stomach irritation that sometimes accompanies aspirin use.

For many years, some aspirin preparations have been *buffered* with additional ingredients meant to neutralize the acidity of aspirin. This is intended to have two effects: first, to reduce stomach irritation and, second, to produce faster relief by moving the aspirin more rapidly into the intestine. There is ample evidence that buffered aspirin does reach the blood somewhat more rapidly, but no one has ever been able to show that this results in faster or stronger pain relief.

The *therapeutic* dose for aspirin is generally considered to be in the range of 600 to 1,000 mg. Most reports suggest that 300 mg is usually more effective than a placebo, whereas 600 mg is clearly even more effective. Many studies indicate that increasing the dose above that level does not increase aspirin's analgesic action, but some research indicates that 1,200 mg of aspirin provides greater relief than 600 mg. In one study,[12] after ingestion of a 650 mg tablet of aspirin, headache and postpartum pain were not reduced significantly from placebo until 45 minutes had elapsed; maximum relief was obtained after 60 minutes. At 4 hours after intake, pain levels were equivalent in the drug and placebo groups; that is, the analgesia was gone. These reports agree with the salicylate blood levels measured in the same patients.

At therapeutic doses, aspirin has analgesic actions that are fairly specific. First, and in marked contrast to narcotic analgesics, aspirin does not affect the impact of the anticipation of pain. It seems probable also that aspirin has its primary effect on the ability to withstand continuing pain. This, no doubt, is the basis for much of the self-medication with aspirin, because moderate, protracted pain is fairly common. The salicylates do not block all types of pain. They are especially effective against headache and musculoskeletal aches and pains, less effective for toothache and sore throat, and almost valueless in visceral pain, as well as in traumatic (acute) pain.

The antipyretic (fever-reducing) action of aspirin does not lower temperature in an individual with normal body temperature. It has this effect only if the person has a fever. The mechanism by which the salicylates decrease body temperature is fairly well understood. They act on the temperature-regulating area of the hypothalamus to increase heat loss through peripheral mechanisms. Heat loss is primarily increased by vasodilation of peripheral blood vessels and by increased perspiration. Heat production is not changed, but heat loss is facilitated so that body temperature can go down.

More aspirin has probably been used for its third major therapeutic use than for either of the other two. The anti-inflammatory action of the salicylates is the major basis for its use after muscle strains and in rheumatoid arthritis.

Most tablets, including aspirin, develop a harder external shell the longer they sit. This hardening effect does not change the amount of the active ingredient, but it does make the active ingredient less effective because disintegration time is increased by the hard exterior coating. Along the same line, moisture and heat speed the decomposition of acetylsalicylic acid into two other compounds: salicylic acid, which causes gastric distress, and acetic acid—vinegar. When the smell of vinegar is strong in your aspirin bottle, discard it.

Effects: Adverse and Otherwise

Aspirin increases bleeding time by inhibiting blood platelet aggregation. This is not an insignificant effect. Two or three aspirins can double bleeding time, the time it takes for blood to clot, and the effect can last 4 to 7 days. There's good and bad in the anticoagulant effect of aspirin. Its use before surgery can help prevent blood clots from appearing in patients at high risk for clot formation. For many surgical patients, however, facilitation of blood clotting is desirable, and the general rule is no aspirin or other salicylates for 7 to 10 days before surgery. The same principle—no aspirin—should hold for women in their last trimester of pregnancy. This might be

---

antipyretic: (an tee pie *reh* tick) fever-reducing.

anti-inflammatory: reducing swelling and inflammation.

particularly important, because aspirin crosses the placental barrier, and neither the short- nor the long-term effects on the fetus are known.

Two possibly big advantages of the anticoagulant effect are of particular interest to men. A *transient ischemic attack (TIA)* results when a tiny clot forms in the brain or the retina, temporarily cutting off the blood supply to a small region. This can be the precursor of a stroke, in which the loss of blood to a brain region results in permanent damage. You won't find this mentioned on aspirin bottles in the store, because the FDA doesn't want people self-diagnosing and self-treating TIAs or strokes, but the professional labeling (for physicians and pharmacists to read), says:

> For reducing the risk of recurrent transient ischemic attacks (TIA's) or stroke in men who have transient ischemia of the brain due to fibrin platelet emboli. There is inadequate evidence that aspirin or buffered aspirin is effective in reducing TIA's in women at the recommended dosage. There is no evidence that aspirin or buffered aspirin is of benefit in the treatment of completed strokes in men or women.[8]

Perhaps even more important, evidence has been building for some time that men who have had one heart attack (myocardial infarction) and who take an aspirin tablet every other day have a reduced risk of a second heart attack. The Canadian government approved aspirin to prevent second heart attacks in 1982, and the FDA tentatively approved this use in 1985. Two large-scale 1988 experiments, one British and one American, make it very clear that this is a real effect. The FDA will include in the professional labeling only, and not to the general public, an indication for aspirin "to reduce the risk of death and/or non-fatal myocardial infarction in patients with a previous myocardial infarction or unstable angina pectoris (chest pain)."[8] Again, the FDA doesn't want people self-diagnosing and self-treating heart attacks. What we don't know, because the study hasn't been done, is whether it would make sense for people who

have not experienced angina or a heart attack but who have other risk factors (e.g., overweight or high incidence of heart disease in the family) to use aspirin to prevent heart attacks. Such studies, as well as studies on women, are currently underway. The aspirin makers would probably like it if everyone over the age of 40 were to start taking an aspirin every other day, and the television ads have become rather suggestive that you should "ask your doctor" about this.

Aspirin will induce gastrointestinal bleeding in about 70 percent of normal subjects. In most cases, this is only about 5 ml per day, but that is five times the normal loss. In some people the blood loss can be great enough to cause anemia. The basis for this effect is not clear but is believed to be a direct eroding by the aspirin tablets of the gastric mucosa. The rule is clear: drink lots of water when you take aspirin or, better yet, crush the tablets and drink them in orange juice or other liquid.

In the early 1980s, there was increasing concern about the relationship of aspirin use to **Reye's syndrome**, a rare disease (fewer than 200 cases per year in the United States). Almost all of the cases occur in people under the age of 20, usually after they have had a viral infection, such as influenza or chicken pox. The children begin vomiting continuously; then they might become disoriented, undergo personality changes, shout, or become lethargic. Some enter comas, and some of those either die or suffer permanent brain damage. The overall mortality rate from Reye's syndrome is about 25 percent.

No one knows what causes Reye's, and it isn't believed to be caused by aspirin. However, there are data that suggest the disease is more likely to occur in children who have been given aspirin during a preceding illness. In late 1984, the results of a Centers for Disease Control and Prevention pilot study were released, indicating that the use of aspirin can increase the risk of Reye's syndrome as much as 25 times. In 1985, makers of all aspirin products were asked to put warning labels on their packages. These labels recommend that you consult a physician before giving aspirin to children or teenagers with chicken pox or flu.

In early 1986, it was reported that fewer parents in Michigan were giving aspirin to children for colds and influenza, and the incidence of Reye's syndrome had also decreased in Michigan.[9] The Michigan study lends further strength to the relationship between aspirin use and Reye's syndrome. No one under the age of 20 should use aspirin in treating chicken pox, influenza, or even what might be suspected to be a common cold.

Aspirin has long been associated with a large number of accidental poisonings of children, as well as with suicide attempts. Although it has now been joined on the DAWN lists (see Chapter 2) by its relatives acetaminophen and ibuprofen, aspirin remains a major cause of emergency room visits and was mentioned in 101 drug-related deaths in the 1998 DAWN data.

Mechanism of Action

Aspirin is now believed to have both a central and a peripheral analgesic effect. The central effect is not clear, but the peripheral effect is well on its way to being understood; it is now known that aspirin modifies the *cause* of pain.

Prostaglandins are local hormones that are manufactured and released when cell membranes are distorted or damaged—that is, injured. The prostaglandins then act on the endings of the neurons that mediate pain in the injured areas. The prostaglandins sensitize the neurons to mechanical stimulation and to stimulation by two other local hormones, histamine and bradykinin, which are more slowly released from the damaged tissue. Aspirin blocks the synthesis of the prostaglandins.

There is now abundant evidence to support this rough outline of the mechanism of the action of aspirin. For one thing, aspirin does not block the pain induced by injections of prostaglandins. Aspirin also has an analgesic effect only in tissues where prostaglandin formation is taking place. A similar explanation

seems most reasonable as the basis for the anti-inflammatory action of aspirin.

The antipyretic action has also been spelled out: a specific prostaglandin acts on the anterior hypothalamus to decrease heat dissipation through the normal procedures of sweating and dilation of peripheral blood vessels. Aspirin blocks the synthesis of this prostaglandin in the anterior hypothalamus, and this is followed by increased heat loss.

Acetaminophen

There are two related analgesic compounds: *phenacetin* and **acetaminophen**. Phenacetin was sold for many years in combination with aspirin and caffeine in the "APC" tablets that fought headache pain "three ways." Phenacetin has been around since 1887 and had long been suspected of causing kidney lesions and dysfunction. In 1964, the FDA required a warning on all products containing phenacetin, which limited their use to 10 days because the phenacetin might damage the kidneys. Phenacetin has now gone to the land of dead drugs: the review panel considered it not to be GRAS.

The only real question is why all these drugs took so long to get off the market. Phenacetin was known to be rapidly converted to acetaminophen, which was the primary active agent. Acetaminophen is equipotent with aspirin in its analgesic and antipyretic effects. The antipyretic mechanism is similar to that of aspirin, but the analgesic effect might be additive to that produced by aspirin. Acetaminophen is not an anti-inflammatory and thus is of minimal value in arthritis, gout, and the like.

Acetaminophen has been marketed as an OTC analgesic since 1955, but it was the big advertising pushes in the 1970s for two brand name products, Tylenol and Datril, that brought

---

acetaminophen: (a seet a *min* o fen) an aspirinlike analgesic and antipyretic.

acetaminophen into the big time. Acetaminophen is usually advertised as having most of the good points of "that other pain reliever" and many fewer disadvantages. To a degree this is probably true: if only analgesia and fever reduction are desired, acetaminophen might be safer than aspirin *as long as dosage limits are carefully observed.* Overuse of acetaminophen can cause serious liver disorders. That statement came true in the 1980s, as more and more reports of acetaminophen-induced liver damage and deaths came in. Acetaminophen has now surpassed aspirin for both drug-related emergency room visits and drug-related deaths, according to the DAWN statistics (see Chapter 2). The FDA doesn't want to advertise on the package that acetaminophen can be lethal, for fear of attracting suicide attempts. So it requires a warning against overdose and includes the statement "Prompt medical attention is critical for adults as well as for children even if you do not notice any signs or symptoms." This statement reflects the fact that damage to the liver might not be noticed until 24 to 48 hours later, when the symptoms of impaired liver function finally emerge. You should remember that acetaminophen is not necessarily safer than aspirin, especially if the recommended dose is exceeded.

Ibuprofen and Other NSAIDs

Since the discovery that aspirin and similar drugs work by inhibiting the synthesis of prostaglandins, the drug companies have been able to use that information to design new and sometimes more potent analgesics, most of which have been available only as prescription products. **Ibuprofen**, which originally was available only by prescription, is now found in several OTC analgesics. In addition to its analgesic potency, ibuprofen is a potent anti-inflammatory and has received wide use in the treatment of arthritis. The most common side effects of ibuprofen are gastrointestinal: nausea, stomach pain, and cramping. There have been reports of

fatal liver damage with overdoses of ibuprofen, so again it is wise not to exceed the recommended dose.

Ibuprofen was the first of several new drugs that are now collectively referred to as "nonsteroidal anti-inflammatory drugs" (**NSAIDs**). Naproxen is also available OTC.

Table 15.1 contains a list of several OTC internal analgesics along with the amounts of each ingredient they contain. The FDA has been discussing whether or not to exclude products that contain both aspirin and acetaminophen. Products containing ibuprofen warn against combining them with aspirin, because that mixture hasn't been thoroughly studied.

COLD AND ALLERGY PRODUCTS

The All-Too-Common Cold

There has to be something good about an illness that Charles Dickens could be lyrical about:

> *I am at this moment*
> *Deaf in the ears,*
> *Hoarse in the throat,*
> *Red in the nose,*
> *Green in the gills,*
> *Damp in the eyes,*
> *Twitchy in the joints,*
> *And fractious in temper*
> *From a most intolerable*
> *And oppressive cold.*[10]

The common cold is caused by viruses: over a hundred have been identified. But in 40 to 60 percent of individuals with colds, researchers cannot connect the infection to a specific virus. That makes it tough to find a cure. Two groups of viruses are known to be associated with colds—the *rhinoviruses* and the more recently identified *coronaviruses.* These viruses are clearly distinct from those that cause influenza, measles, and pneumonia. Success in developing vaccines against other diseases has made some experts optimistic about finding a vaccine for

TABLE 15.1

Ingredients in OTC Analgesics

Brand	Aspirin	Acetaminophen	Ibuprofen	Naproxen	Caffeine	Other
Aleve	—	—	—	200	—	—
Anacin	400	—	—		32	—
Advil	—	—	200		—	—
Bufferin	325	—	—		—	Magnesium carbonate, calcium carbonate, magnesium oxide
Empirin	325	—	—		—	—
Excedrin	250	250	—		65	—
Mediprin	—	—	200		—	—
Nuprin	—	—	200		—	—
Vanquish	227	194	—		33	Magnesium hydroxide, aluminum hydroxide gel

the common cold. Others are pessimistic because of the great variety of viruses and the fact that the rhinoviruses can apparently change their immunologic reactivity very readily.

Viruses damage or kill the cells they attack. The rhinoviruses zero in on the upper respiratory tract, at first causing irritation, which can lead to reflex coughing and sneezing. Increased irritation inflames the tissue and is followed by soreness and swelling of the mucous membranes. As a defense against infection, the mucous membranes release considerable fluid, which causes the runny nose and the postnasal drip that irritates the throat.

Although the incubation period for a cold can be a week in some cases, the more common interval between infection and respiratory tract symptoms is two to four days. Before the onset of respiratory symptoms, the individual might just feel bad and develop joint aches and headaches. When fever does occur, it almost always develops early in the cold.

Most of us grew up believing that colds are passed by airborne particles jet-propelled usually through unobstructed sneezing. ("Cover your mouth! Cover your face!") The old folklore—and the scientists—were wrong. You need to know

four things so you can avoid the cold viruses of others—and avoid reinfecting yourself:

1. Up to 100 times as many viruses are produced and shed from the nasal mucosa as from the throat.
2. There are few viruses in the saliva of a person with a cold, probably no viruses at all in about half of these individuals.
3. Dried viruses survive on dry skin and nonporous surfaces—plastic, wood, and so on—for over three hours.
4. Most cold viruses enter the body through the nostrils and eyes.

Usually colds start by the fingers' picking up viruses and then the individual rubs the eyes or picks the nose. In one study of adults with colds, 40 percent had viruses on their hands but only 8 percent expelled viruses in coughs or sneezes.[11]

ibuprofen: (eye bu *pro* fen) an aspirinlike analgesic and anti-inflammatory.

NSAIDs: nonsteroidal anti-inflammatory drugs, such as ibuprofen.

The moral of the story is clear. To avoid colds, wash your hands frequently, and you may kiss but not hold hands with your cold-infected sweetheart. You don't have to worry about your pets—only humans and some apes are susceptible to colds.

The experimental animal of choice for studying colds has to be the human. In many studies with human volunteers, three types of findings seem to recur. First, not all who are directly exposed to a cold virus develop cold symptoms. In fact, only about 50 percent do. Second, in individuals with already existing antibodies to the virus, there might be only preliminary signs of a developing cold. These signs might last for a brief period (12 to 24 hours) and then disappear. The last finding crosses swords with the folklore, so it is best to quote:

> Chilling experiments with volunteers did not show any particular influence on susceptibility to colds. Some volunteers were given an inoculation followed by a hot bath and made to stand in a draft in wet bathing suits. Some took walks in the rain and sat around in wet clothes. Other subjects were given the same chilling treatments with inoculations which contained no virus. No significant differences were found in these various well-controlled groups.[12]

Theoretically, it is possible to prevent rhinovirus infections by pretreating the individual with interferon or other antiviral drugs. This is of little practical value, however, because most of us don't know when or where we have picked up the virus, or if it's going to infect us at all, until it's too late.

Treatment of Cold Symptoms

There's no practical way to prevent colds and no way to cure the infection once it starts. So why do Americans spend billions each year on cold "remedies"? Apparently, it's in an effort to reduce those miserable symptoms described by Dickens. Cold symptoms are fairly complex, so most cold remedies have traditionally included

Drugs in Depth

Cold Medications and Kids

In a 1991 article in the *Journal of Pediatrics*, Nancy Hutton and her colleagues reported the results of an experiment on 96 children ranging in age from six months to five years. As the children were taken in to be treated for colds, one-third were randomly assigned to receive a placebo, one-third received no drug at all, and one-third received a liquid cold medication containing brompheniramine maleate, phenylephrine, and phenylpropanolamine (one antihistamine and two decongestants). Two days later the parents were asked to rate improvement in the cold symptoms. Two-thirds of those receiving placebo were considered to be improved, as were 57 percent of those receiving no drug. Although 71 percent of the drug-treated group were rated as improved, that was not statistically different from either the placebo or the no-drug group.

An experiment like this can't prove that cold medications don't do any good at all, but several such studies make us question the value of treating children with these drugs, which may make them drowsy and in rare cases can have more serious side effects.

several active ingredients, each aimed at a particular type of symptom. In some ways, the FDA's Cold, Cough, Allergy, Bronchodilator, and Antiasthmatic Advisory Review Panel probably had the most difficult job: multiple symptoms, many ingredients for each symptom, and rapid changes in scientific evidence during the time it studied these products. In the preliminary report, issued in 1976, the panel approved less than half of the 119 ingredients it reviewed. The Tentative Final Monograph was published in 1985,[13] and several ingredients were recommended for approval or for shifting to OTC status that had not been available when the panel started its job. There are three common types of ingredients in modern cold remedies: *antihistamines*, for the temporary relief of runny nose and sneezing; *nasal decongestants*, for the temporary relief of swollen membranes in the nasal passages; and *analgesic-antipyretics*, for the temporary relief of aches and pains and fever reduction. The FDA list in 1985 included 10 approved antihistamines, but by far the most common antihistamine to be found on the shelves is **chlorpheniramine maleate**. The most common nasal decongestant in cold remedies is now pseudoephedrine. The analgesic-antipyretic is usually acetaminophen.

Table 15.2 gives recent formulations for five popular OTC cold remedies. Note that three of them also contain the cough suppressant **dextromethorphan**, which is the most common active ingredient in OTC cough medicines.

It is ironic that the one type of ingredient found in almost every cold remedy since before the FDA began its review continues to be under attack. The FDA advisory panel had serious questions about the data supporting the effectiveness of antihistamines in treating colds. Although some studies have since reported that chlorpheniramine maleate is better than placebo at reducing runny noses, prompting the FDA to approve several antihistamines, more recent controlled experiments have not found any benefit. A 1987 symposium of specialists concluded that ". . . antihistamines do not have a place in the management of upper respiratory infection, though they continue to be useful for allergy." Still more studies have been done that question the effectiveness of antihistamines, and congressional hearings were held in 1992, asking why the FDA still allowed antihistamines in cough and cold remedies.[14]

Allergy and Sinus Medications

There are other related products on your pharmacy shelves. In addition to the cough medicines, there are *allergy* relief pills, which rely mainly on the same antihistamine, chlorpheniramine maleate, to slow down the runny nose. There are sinus medicines that use one of the sympathomimetic nasal decongestants (pseudoephedrine), often combined with an analgesic, to reduce swollen sinus passages and to treat sinus headache.

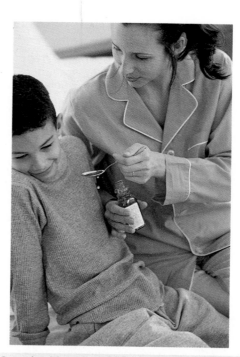

Some health professionals question the value of treating children for colds.

CHOOSING AN OTC PRODUCT

By now you should be getting the idea that, thanks to the FDA's decision to review ingredients rather than individual formulations, you as a consumer can now review and choose from among the great variety of products by knowing just a few ingredients and what they are intended to accomplish. Table 15.3 lists only seven ingredients. Those seven are the major active ingredients to be found in different combinations

---

chlorpheniramine maleate: (clor fen *eer* a meen mal i ate) a common antihistamine in cold products.

dextromethorphan: (dex tro meh *thor* fan) an OTC antitussive (cough control) ingredient.

TABLE 15.2

Ingredients in Selected Brand Name OTC Cold and Allergy Products

Brand	Sympathomimetic	Antihistamine	Analgesic	Cough suppressant	Other
Comtrex*	30 pseudoephedrine HCl	2 chlorpheniramine maleate	325 acetaminophen	10 dextromethorphan	—
Contac*	30 pseudoephedrine HCl	2 chlorpheniramine maleate	500 acetaminophen	15 dextromethorphan	—
Tylenol Cold*	30 pseudoephedrine HCl	2 chlorpheniramine maleate	325 acetaminophen	15 dextromethorphan	—
Dristan	5 phenylephrine HCl	2 chlorpheniramine maleate	325 acetaminophen		—

*mg/tablet
†mg/adult dose (1 oz)

TABLE 15.3

Common OTC Ingredients

Ingredient	Action	Source
Acetylsalicylic acid (ASA; aspirin)	Analgesic-antipyretic	Headache remedies, arthritis formulas, cold and sinus remedies
Acetaminophen	Analgesic-antipyretic	Headache remedies, cold and sinus remedies
Caffeine	Stimulant	"Alertness" medications
Chlorpheniramine maleate	Antihistamine	Cold remedies, allergy products
Dextromethorphan	Antitussive	Cough suppressants, cold remedies
Diphenhydramine	Antihistamine	Sleep aids, some cold remedies
Pseudoephedrine	Sympathomimetic	Cold and sinus remedies

in OTC stimulants, sleep aids, weight-control products, analgesics, cold, cough, allergy, and sinus medications.

Do you want to treat your cold without buying a combination cold remedy? If you have aches and pains, take your favorite analgesic. For the vast majority of colds, the slight elevation in temperature should probably not be treated, because it is not dangerous and can even help fight the infection.[15] Unless body temperature remains at 103°F or above or reaches 105°F, fever is not considered dangerous. If you have a runny nose, you might or might not get relief from an anti-histamine. Generic chlorpheniramine maleate or a store-brand allergy tablet is an inexpensive source. These will probably give you a dry mouth and might produce some sedation or drowsiness (which, of course, is why some of the more sedating antihistamines are used in sleep aids). Do you have a stuffed-up nose? Pseudoephedrine nose drops will shrink swollen membranes for a time. Although oral sympathomimetics will work, nose drops are more effective. You can find these ingredients in sinus preparations (and weight-control products). However, these sympathomimetics should be

Drugs in Depth

Abuse of OTC Dextromethorphan

High school and college students have been "getting high" with large doses of OTC cough suppressants containing dextromethorphan (DM). Possibly, students first came on the effects of DM by drinking large quantities of Robitussin or similar cough syrups containing alcohol. However, the effects reported by those using 4 to 8 oz of Robitussin (up to 720 mg DM) could not be due to the less than one-half ounce of alcohol in them and include visual and auditory hallucinations and in some cases seizures.[16] The altered psychological state may last for several hours. The few cases reported in the literature and individual reports from college students indicate that habitual use (e.g., twice per week or more) is common.

DM has been the standard ingredient in OTC cough suppressants for many years and was originally developed as a nonopiate relative to codeine. DM is not an opiate-like narcotic, produces no pain relief, and does not produce an opiate-like abstinence syndrome. More recent evidence indicates that it may interact with a specific receptor from the opiate family known as the sigma receptor. This apparently safe and simple drug, which is contained in more than 50 OTC products, has more complicated effects when taken in the large doses used by some recreational users.

It's not clear how recent this phenomenon really is. The Swedish government restricted DM to prescription-only use in 1986 as a result of abuse of OTC prepara-

tions, and there were two later reports of DM-caused fatalities in Sweden. In the United States, this has remained a mostly underground activity, apparently spread by word-of-mouth.

One 1995 posting to the alt.psychoactives newsgroup on the Internet described a user's first DM experience, after taking 20 capsules of an OTC cough remedy (600 mg DM):

> . . . 45 minutes worth of itching and for ten seconds it stopped. During one of the most weirdest and stupidest visions, I flew quickly over a mountain. As I did this in that second the itching seemed to go away and it seemed like I wasn't in my body anymore. I flew from one side of a rainbow to another. Then I was flying quickly towards the head of an ostrich and when I got close it only showed the silhouette of the head and I flew into the black nothingness. All that craziness in ten seconds made me laugh out loud as I tried to look at it all soberly. Then the itching came back into my body. No matter how hard I tried the itching never went away.

The itching feeling reported by this user has been reported by others, along with nausea and other unpleasant side effects. In spite of such unpleasantness, some users find it difficult to stop using DM once they have tried it a few times.

used cautiously. There is a rapid tolerance to their effects, and, if they are used repeatedly, a rebound stuffiness can develop when they are stopped. Do you have a cough? Dextromethorphan can be obtained in cough medications.

Why not buy all this in one tablet or capsule? That's a common approach. But why treat symptoms you don't have? During the course of a cold, a runny nose might occur at one time, congestion at another, and coughing not at all. By using just the ingredients you need, when you need them, you might save money, and you would have the satisfaction of being a connoisseur of colds. Then again, given the state of re-

search on the effectiveness of these "remedies," why buy them at all? It's easy for a skeptic to conclude that there's little or no real value in cold remedies. The experts say to rest and drink fluids. But when they actually have a cold, most people are less inclined to be skeptical and more inclined to be hopeful that something will help.

HERBAL PRODUCTS

The 1994 Dietary Supplement Health and Education Act, mentioned in Chapter 5, rescinded the FDA's authority to require premarket safety and effectiveness testing of products that were

Exploring Your Spirituality

Will Aging Baby Boomers Raise Substance-Abuse Rates?

Older adults use prescription drugs three times more frequently than the rest of the population. As baby boomers head into their golden years—the first boomers turn 65 in 2011—the number of people taking medications will skyrocket. If the baby-boom generation used marijuana recreationally in the 1960s, will boomers use marijuana medicinally in their elderly years? If free-spirited baby boomers partied hard as flower children, will they turn to alcohol and drugs to fight the hardships of old age?

Mental health professionals fear that, as baby boomers age, the number of older people abusing drugs and alcohol could jump substantially. First, there will simply be a large number of old people in this generation, about 76 million people born between 1946 and 1964. Second, a large percentage of them will be aging drug users according to Dr. Thomas Patterson, a psychiatrist with the University of California–San Diego. Even if the rate of elderly substance abuse remains steady, at about 17 percent, the number of seniors with drug and alcohol problems will soar.[21]

When you factor in that baby boomer are already using alcohol and drugs at a higher rate than previous generations, the problem looms even larger. Currently about 3.7 million people over 65 are estimated to have substance-abuse problems. About the year 2011, predicts Patterson, that number will jump to about 5 million. And he's not just talking about illegal drugs. Abuse of OTC and prescription drugs could also increase as boomers age. It's become a common notion that, if you have a problem, you take a pill to solve it.[21]

Elderly people's abuse of medications, alcohol, and illicit drugs is worrisome from a physical standpoint because these substances can pose greater health risks in old age, as metabolism changes. Alcohol can do more damage to a 72-year-old liver than it can to a 22-year-old liver. From an emotional and spiritual standpoint, elderly people have weaker support systems to combat feelings of loneliness, isolation, and lack of purpose following retirement and as their contemporaries start to die.

If boomers were more experimental with drugs and alcohol in the past, does that mean that they got it out of their systems, or does it mean that they will continue the pattern into old age? What lifestyle changes might health-care workers encourage to fill emotional voids in older people's lives, which might otherwise be numbed with drugs and alcohol?

---

designated either as food supplements (e.g., vitamins and minerals, amino acids) or herbs and herbal products. This opened the floodgates for the marketing of a wide variety of products that either had not been available before or had been available only in specialty nutrition shops. These products are now widely sold by mail order, on the web, and in drug stores and supermarkets. A few of them have some interesting psychoactive properties or claims associated with them.

St. John's Wort

St. John's Wort (botanical name *Hypericum perforatum*) has been used for centuries and was once known as "the devil's scourge" because it was supposed to prevent possession by demons. In recent years its psychoactive uses have included the treatment of both anxiety and depression. There is limited evidence on the effectiveness of St. John's Wort in the treatment of anxiety, but several studies have indicated some usefulness in treating depression. One summary analysis of 23 clinical trials with daily *Hypericum* doses from 300 to 1,000 mg found it to be superior to a placebo and about as effective as tricyclic antidepressants.[17] However, a careful large-scale study reported in 2001 found no benefit in using St. John's Wort to treat depression.[18]

SAMe

S-adenosyl-L-methionine is a naturally occurring substance found in the body. It is an active form of the amino acid methionine, and it acts as a "methyl donor" in a variety of biochemical pathways. (A methyl group consists of one carbon and three hydrogen atoms.) As long ago as the 1970s, SAMe was tested in Italy for its effectiveness as an antidepressant, and a recent summary analysis found that SAMe was more effective than a placebo, and apparently it is no less effective than tricyclic antidepressants.[19] There is currently less research available on SAMe for this use than for St. John's Wort. Researchers continue to investigate the possibility that, by combining SAMe with approved antidepressants, a more rapid remission of symptoms can be achieved.

Ginkgo Biloba

Extracts from the leaves of the ginkgo biloba tree have a long history of medical use in China. It is not clear which of the identified ingredients in ginkgo are the active agents, and it is not completely clear how effective it is for a variety of uses for which it has been proposed. The substance does reduce blood clotting, so it has been proposed as a blood thinner, which improves circulation. However, combining ginkgo with aspirin, which also reduces clotting, could be dangerous. The most interesting suggestion is that ginkgo biloba extract might improve memory in Alzheimer's patients, due to its presumed ability to increase blood circulation in the brain. A recent study reported minor improvement of functioning in some Alzheimer's patients, which is seen as promising by some researchers but not very interesting by others.[20]

SUMMARY

- A drug can be sold OTC only if it can be used safely when following the label directions.
- The FDA began reviewing OTC ingredients for safety and efficacy in 1972, with the result that most of the various brands of

medicines that are sold for a given use contain the same few ingredients.
- OTC stimulants are based on caffeine.
- OTC sleep aids are based on antihistamines.
- The main ingredient in OTC weight-control products was phenylpropanolamine (PPA), but it was removed from sale in 2000.
- Aspirin has analgesic, antipyretic, and anti-inflammatory actions. Acetaminophen and ibuprofen are related analgesics.
- Cold remedies usually contain an antihistamine, an analgesic, and a decongestant.
- An informed consumer can understand a large fraction of OTC medicines by knowing only seven ingredients.

REVIEW QUESTIONS

1. What do the acronyms GRAS, GRAE, and GRAHL stand for?
2. What is the process that is producing "tentative final monographs" on OTC products?
3. What are the criteria for deciding whether a drug should be sold OTC or by prescription?
4. What is the main ingredient found in look-alike pills for speed?
5. How safe and effective is PPA as a weight-control ingredient?
6. Diphenhydramine is found in what three brand name sleep aids?
7. What effect of aspirin might be involved in its use to prevent TIAs and heart attacks in men?
8. What are the differences in the therapeutic effects of acetaminophen and ibuprofen?
9. What is the most common route for a cold virus to enter a person's system?
10. Which cold symptoms are supposed to be relieved by chlorpheniramine maleate and which by pseudoephedrine?

REFERENCES

1. FDA proposes new, easy to understand labeling for OTC drugs, *Doctor's Guide to Medical and Other News.* Feb 26, 1997.
2. Conlan MF: FDA can't keep track of OTCs, GAO charges in report, *Drug Topics* pp 50–58, Mar 23, 1992.
3. Rheinstein PH: FDA perspective: Prescription to over-the-counter drug switches, *American Family Physician* Sept 15, 1997.
4. Farley D: Label literacy for OTC drugs, *FDA Consumer* May–June, 1997.
5. FDA: OTC stimulant drug products, final monograph, *Federal Register* Feb 29, 1988.
6. Beecher HK: Placebo effects of situations, attitudes and drugs: A quantitative study of suggestibility. In Rickels K, editor: *Non-specific factors in drug therapy.* Springfield, IL: Charles C Thomas, 1968.
7. Smith LH: The clinical pharmacology of salicylates, *California Medicine* 110:411, 413, 1969.
8. FDA: Internal analgesic, antipyretic, and antirheumatic drug products for OTC human use: Tentative final monograph, *Federal Register* Nov 16, 1988.
9. Remington PL and others: Decreasing trends in Reye's syndrome and aspirin use in Michigan—1979 to 1984, Pediatrics 77:93–98, 1986.
10. Dickens C: *The collected letters of Charles Dickens.* Chapman & Hall, 1880.
11. Klumpp TG: The common cold—New concepts of transmission and prevention, *Medical Times* 108(11):98, 1s–3s, 1980.
12. Adams JM: *Viruses and colds, the modern plague.* New York: American Elsevier, 1967.
13. *Federal Register* 50:10, Jan 15, 1985.
14. Conlan MF: House probes antihistamines in OTC cold medications, *Drug Topics* p 59, May 4, 1992.
15. Fever: What to do and what not to do when the heat is on. *FDA Consumer* 19(9):16, Nov 1985.
16. Murray S, Brewerton T: Abuse of over-the-counter dextromethorphan by teenagers, *South Med J* 86:1151, 1993.
17. Linde K and others: St. John's wort for depression: An overview and meta-analysis of randomized clinical trials. *British Medical Journal* 313:253, 1996.
18. Shelton RC: Effectiveness of St. John's Wort in major depression: A randomized controlled trial. *Journal of the American Medical Association* 285:1978–1986, 2001.
19. Bressa, GM. S-adenosyl-l-methionine (SAMe) as antidepressant: Meta-analysis of clinical studies. *Acta Neurol Scand Suppl* 154:7–14, 1994.
20. Le Bars PL and others: A placebo-contolled, double-blind, randomized trial of an extract of ginkgo biloba for dementia. *Jounal of American Medical Association* 278:1327, 1997.
21. Chamberlain C: Baby boom, addiction boom: Will seniors' substance abuse rates rise as boomers age? 2000, www.abcnews.com.

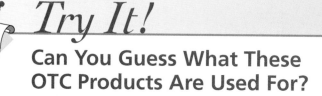

Try It!

Can You Guess What These OTC Products Are Used For?

The following mock product labels include the actual list of ingredients from some OTC products. Your job is to figure out what each product is used for (hint: none of them is a laxative, acne medication, or contraceptive).

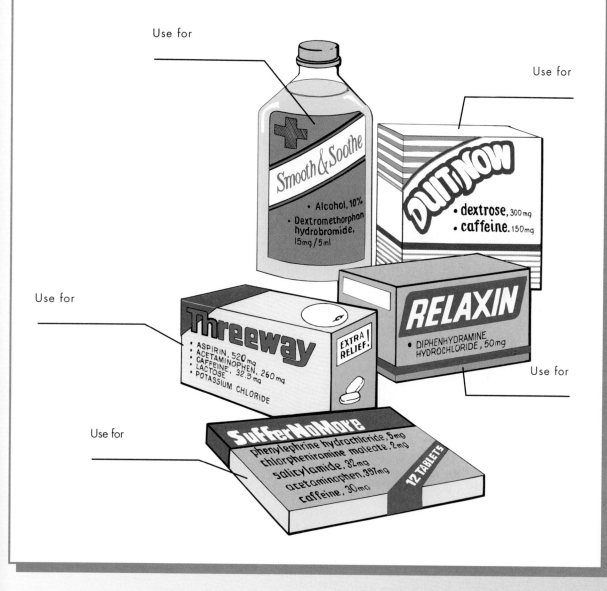

Use for

Use for

Use for

Use for

Use for

Smooth & Soothe
- Alcohol, 10%
- Dextromethorphan hydrobromide, 15mg/5ml

DUITNOW
- dextrose, 300mg
- caffeine, 150mg

Threeway
EXTRA RELIEF!
- ASPIRIN, 520mg
- ACETAMINOPHEN, 260mg
- CAFFEINE, 32.5mg
- LACTOSE
- POTASSIUM CHLORIDE

RELAXIN
- DIPHENHYDRAMINE HYDROCHLORIDE, 50mg

SufferNoMore
- phenylephrine hydrochloride, 5mg
- chlorpheniramine maleate, 2mg
- salicylamide, 32mg
- acetaminophen, 387mg
- caffeine, 30mg

12 TABLETS

Section VI

Restricted Drugs

In contrast to the everyday drugs such as nicotine and caffeine, the drugs discussed in this section include some of the least familiar and most feared substances: heroin, LSD, and marijuana. More recently, the anabolic steroids used by some athletes have also become widely feared by the public, most of whom have no direct contact with the drugs. These substances, along with the stimulants cocaine and amphetamines, are commonly viewed as evil, "devil drugs."

Chapter **16**

*O*piates

KEY TERMS

- opium
- opiate
- morphine
- codeine
- heroin
- black tar
- opioid
- narcotic antagonists
- naloxone
- enkephalins
- endorphins
- methadone
- LAAM

Online Learning Center Resources

www.mhhe.com/ray

Log on to our Online Learning Center (OLC) for access to these additional resources.

- Chapter definitions
- Learning objectives
- Student interactive question-and-answer sites
- Self-scoring chapter quiz

The OLC also offers web links for study and exploration of health topics. Here are some examples of what you'll find:

www.nida.nih.gov/Research Reports/Heroin/Heroin.html

NIDA's report on heroin abuse and addiction is posted at this site. It includes a detailed description of heroin, heroin use in the United States, short- and long-term effects, medical complications, and available treatments.

www.arf.org/isd/pim/list.html

This site offers a pamphlet on opiates, which provides information on abuse, effects, and withdrawal symptoms. All the materials described here are available to order.

www.health.org/pubs/qdocs/ heroin

The National Clearinghouse for Alcohol and Drugs offers many useful brochures and publications. Check out the resources on heroin.

Drugs in the Media

The Rise and Fall of Heroin "Epidemics"

The term *epidemic* refers to a rapidly spreading outbreak of contagious disease or, by extension, to any rapid spread, growth, or development of a problem. Heroin use has always been restricted to a very small proportion of the U.S. population, and it would be an overstatement to say that heroin use has reached or will reach epidemic proportions, if by that we mean that the

Drugs in the Media Continued. . .

problem is widely prevalent. Nevertheless, there are periodic news reports about the most recent "heroin epidemic," amid speculation about its rapid spread.

What usually triggers these reports is the spectacular seizure of a large drug shipment (as was the case in 1988 in England), police reports about new supplies of low-cost heroin (as in a report from San Francisco in 2000), or the arrest of some young heroin users (seen as evidence that a new generation is being affected, as in California in the late 1980s). What is interesting about these scary news accounts, filled with lurid details and predictions of doom, is that the predicted epidemic never really seems to materialize and fades from memory. Once the epidemic has been forgotten, the television and newspaper reporters are primed to warn us about the next epidemic a few years later.

Seizures of drugs, for example, are a notoriously poor way to measure drug use trends. Researchers estimate that authorities capture only about one-tenth of the drugs on the market, but sometimes they get lucky. The amount of drugs seized, however, doesn't answer the question of whether the seizure is a representative portion of a steady market, a growing portion of a shrinking market, or a smaller portion of a growing market.

An October 6, 2000, Maia Szalavitz, at www.NewsWatch.org, criticized the *Los Angeles Times* for a two-part series that called drugs "The Dirty Little Secret of the Dotcom World" (10/01/00 and 10/02/00). The death of Aaron Bunnel of Upside.com from an overdose of heroin, alcohol, and Valium was spotlighted in the first part of the series. Ms. Szalavitz claimed that a biased *Times* struggled to create a drug scare despite lack of evidence that high-tech workers took more drugs than their low-tech peers. In addition to citing more drug seizures (mostly cocaine and the amphetamines) in areas where high-tech companies were located, the *Times'* other line of support for its contention that drug use was growing among dot-commers is that treatment providers said they were seeing more techies among their patients. But with insurance for inpatient substance-abuse care virtually eliminated by HMOs, an overrepresentation of high-tech workers may merely have reflected the fact that these moneyed elite were among the few who could afford to pay for this care—not just that high-tech industries have a growing drug problem.

Keep your eyes and ears open, and it won't be long before you read or hear a news report about an epidemic of heroin use in a part of the United States or in another country (such reports also have appeared in Australia, Burma, and elsewhere). Does the report cite formal studies that help quantify the problem, or does it vaguely point to "ominous signs" of increasing drug use? These reports really attract attention—and increase sales and advertising revenue—so there's always a market for the stories. As we have seen before, most of this kind of illicit drug use is better viewed as occurring in localized areas, taking on more of the character of a fad than of an epidemic.

And soon they found themselves in the midst of a great meadow of poppies. Now it is well known that when there are many of these flowers together their odor is so powerful that anyone who breathes it falls asleep, and if the sleeper is not carried away from the scent of the flowers he sleeps on and on forever. But Dorothy did not know this, nor could she get away from the bright red flowers that were everywhere about; so presently her eyes grew heavy and she felt she must sit down to rest and to sleep. . . . Her eyes closed in spite of herself and she forgot where she was and fell among the poppies, fast asleep. . . . They carried the sleeping girl to a pretty spot beside the river, far enough from the poppy field to prevent her breathing any more of the poison of the flowers, and here they laid her gently on the soft grass and waited for the fresh breeze to waken her.[1]

From the land of Oz to the streets of San Francisco, the poppy has caused much grief—and much joy. **Opium** is a truly unique substance. This juice from the plant *Papaver somniferum* has a history of medical use perhaps 6,000 years long. Except for the past century and a half, opium has stood alone as the one agent from which physicians could obtain sure results. Compounds containing opium solved several of the recurring problems for medical science wherever used. Opium relieved pain and suffering magnificently. Just as important in the years gone by was its ability to reduce the diarrhea and subsequent dehydration caused by dysentery, which is still a leading cause of death in underdeveloped countries.

Parallel with the medical use of opium was its use as a deliverer of pleasure and relief from anxiety. Because of these effects, extensive recreational use of opium has also occurred throughout history. Through all those years, many of its users experienced dependence.

HISTORY OF OPIOIDS

Opium

Early History of Opium

The most likely origin of opium is in a hot, dry, Middle Eastern country several millennia ago, when someone discovered that for 7 to 10 days of its yearlong life *Papaver somniferum* produced a substance that, when eaten, eased pain and suffering. The opium poppy is an annual plant 3 to 4 feet high with large flowers 4 to 5 inches in diameter. The flowers can be white, pink, red, purple, or violet.

Opium is produced and available for collection for only a few days of the plant's life, between the time the petals drop and the seed pod matures. Today, as before, opium harvesters move through the fields in the early evening and use a sharp, clawed tool to make shallow cuts into, but not through, the unripe seed pods. During the night a white substance oozes from the cuts, oxidizes to a red-brown color, and becomes gummy. In the morning the resinous substance is carefully scraped from the pod and collected in small balls. This raw opium forms the basis for the opium medicines that have been used throughout history and is the substance from which morphine is extracted and then heroin is derived.

The importance and extent of use of the opium poppy in the early Egyptian and Greek cultures are still under debate, but in the Ebers papyrus (circa 1500 B.C.) a remedy is mentioned "to prevent the excessive crying of children." Because a later Egyptian remedy for the same purpose clearly contained opium (as well as fly excrement), many writers report the first specific medical use of opium as dating from the Ebers papyrus.

Homer's *Odyssey* (1000 B.C.) contains a passage that some authors believe refers to the use of opium. A party was about to become a real drag because everyone was sad, thinking about Ulysses and the deaths of their friends, when

> Helen, daughter of Zeus, poured into the wine they were drinking a drug, nepenthes, which gave forgetfulness of evil. Those who had drunk of this mixture did not shed a tear the whole day long, even though their mother or father were dead, even though a brother or beloved son had been killed before their eyes.[2]

The drug could only have been opium.

Opium was important in Greek medicine. Galen, the last of the great Greek physicians, emphasized caution in the use of opium but felt that it was almost a cure-all, saying that it

> resists poison and venomous bites, cures chronic headache, vertigo, deafness, epilepsy, apoplexy, dimness of sight, loss of voice, asthma, coughs of all kinds, spitting of blood, tightness of breath, colic, the iliac poison, jaundice, hardness of the spleen, stone, urinary complaints, fevers, dropsies, leprosies, the troubles to which women are subject, melancholy and all pestilences.[2]

Recreational use even then must have been extensive. Galen also commented on the opium cakes and candies that were being sold everywhere in the streets.

Greek and Roman knowledge of opium use in medicine languished during the Dark Ages and thus had little influence on the world's use of opium for the next thousand years. The Arabic world, however, clutched opium to its breast, because the Koran forbade the use of alcohol in any form. Opium and hashish became the primary social drugs wherever the Islamic culture moved, and it did move. The Mohammadans were active fighters, explorers, and traders. While Europe rested through the Dark Ages, the Arabian world reached out and made contact with India and China. Opium was one of the products they traded, but they also sold the seeds of the opium poppy, and cultivation began in these countries. By the tenth century A.D., opium had been referred to in Chinese medical writings.

During this period when the Arabic civilization flourished, two Arabic physicians made substantial contributions to medicine and to the history of opium. Shortly after A.D. 1000, Biruni composed a pharmacology book. His descriptions of opium contained what some believe to be the first written description of **opiate** dependence.[3] In the same period the best-known Arabic physician, Avicenna, was using opium preparations very effectively and extensively in his medical practice. His writings, along with those of Galen, formed the basis of medical education in Europe as the Renaissance dawned, and thus the glories of opium were advanced. (It is strange but true that a physician as knowledgeable as Avicenna, and a believer in the tenets of Islam, should die as a result of drinking too much of a mixture of opium and wine.)

Early in the sixteenth century lived a European medical phenomenon. Paracelsus apparently was a successful clinician and accomplished some wondrous cures for the day. One of his secrets was a potion called laudanum. Paracelsus was one of the early Renaissance supporters of opium as a panacea and referred to it as the "stone of immortality."

Due to Paracelsus and his followers, there was an increasing awareness of the broad effectiveness of opium, and new opium preparations were developed in the sixteenth, seventeenth, and eighteenth centuries. One of these was laudanum as prepared by Dr. Thomas Sydenham, the father of clinical medicine. Sydenham's general contributions to English medicine are so great that he has been called the English Hippocrates. He spoke more highly of opium than did Paracelsus, saying that "without opium the healing art would cease to exist." His laudanum contained 2 ounces of strained opium, 1 ounce of saffron, a dram of cinnamon, and a dram of cloves dissolved in 1 pint of Canary wine, taken in small quantities.

Writers and Opium: The Keys to Paradise

In a momentous year for opium, 1805, Thomas De Quincey, a 20-year-old English youth who had run away from home at 17, purchased some laudanum for a toothache and received change

---

opium: a raw plant substance containing morphine and codeine.

opiate: a drug derived from opium (e.g., morphine and codeine) or a semisynthetic opium-based drug (e.g., heroin).

for his shilling from the apothecary. Here is his description of his response to this dose:

> I took it: and in an hour, O heavens! what a revulsion! what a resurrection, from its lowest depths, of the inner spirit! what an apocalypse of the world within me! That my pains had vanished was now a trifle in my eyes; this negative effect was swallowed up in the immensity of those positive effects which had opened before me, in the abyss of divine enjoyment thus suddenly revealed. Here was a panacea . . . for all human woes; here was the secret of happiness, about which philosophers had disputed for so many ages, at once discovered; happiness might now be bought for a penny, and carried in the waistcoat-pocket; portable ecstasies might be had corked up in a pint-bottle; and peace of mind could be sent down by the mail.[4]

For the rest of his life De Quincey used laudanum. He did not try to conceal the extent of his opium use. Rather, his writings are replete with insight into the opiate-hazed world, particularly his article "The Confessions of an English Opium-Eater," which was published in 1821 (and in book form in 1823). (Throughout this period, *opium eating* was the phrase generally used to refer to laudanum drinking.)

Several other famous English authors also drank laudanum, including Elizabeth Barrett Browning and Samuel Taylor Coleridge. Coleridge's magnificently beautiful "Kubla Khan" was probably conceived and composed in an opium reverie and then written down as best as he could remember it. However, De Quincey is of primary interest here. His emphasis was on understanding the effects that opium has on consciousness, experience, and feeling, and as such he provided some of the most vivid accounts of the power of opium.

Opium does not produce new worlds for the user:

> If a man, "whose talk is of oxen," should become an opium-eater, the probability is, that (if he is not too dull to dream at all)—he will dream about oxen; whereas, in the case before him [De Quincey], the reader will find that the opium-eater boasteth himself to be a philosopher; and accordingly, that the phantasmagoria of his dreams (waking or sleeping, day-dreams or night-dreams) is suitable to one of that character.[5]

Opium does, however, change the way the user perceives the world. For example, "an opium eater is too happy to observe the motion of time."[5]

De Quincey pointed out the sharp contrast between the effects of alcohol and those of opium:

> Crude opium . . . is incapable of producing any state of body at all resembling that which is produced by alcohol. . . . It is not in the quantity of its effects merely, but in the quality, that it differs altogether. The pleasure given by wine is always rapidly mounting, and tending to a crisis, after which as rapidly it declines; that from opium, when once generated, is stationary for eight or ten hours. . . . The one is a flickering flame, the other a steady and equable glow. But the main distinction lies in this—that, whereas wine disorders the mental faculties, opium, on the contrary (if taken in a proper manner), introduces amongst them the most exquisite order, legislation, and harmony. Wine robs a man of his self-possession; opium sustains and reinforces it. Wine unsettles the judgment. . . . Opium, on the contrary, communicates serenity and equipoise to all the faculties.[5]

In spite of all the good things De Quincey said about opium and the effects it had on him, he suffered from its use. For long periods in his life he was unable to write as a result of his opium dependence. As with most things, "Opium gives and takes away. It defeats the steady habit of exertion; but it creates spasms of irregular exertion. It ruins the natural power of life; but it develops preternatural paroxysms of intermitting power."[6]

The publication of De Quincey's book in 1823 and its first translation into French in 1828 spurred the French Romantic writers to explore opium and hashish in the 1840s and later. The only associated American article of note in this period, "An Opium-Eater in America,"[7] appeared in an American magazine in 1842.

The Opium Wars

Although opium and the opium poppy had been introduced to China well before the year A.D. 1000, there was only a moderate level of use there by a select, elite group. Tobacco smoking spread much more rapidly after its introduction. It is not clear when tobacco was introduced to the Chinese, but its use had spread and become so offensive that in 1644 the emperor forbade tobacco smoking in China. The edict did not last long (as is to be expected), but it was in part responsible for the increase in opium smoking.

Up to this period the smoking of tobacco and the eating of opium had existed side by side. The restriction on the use of tobacco and the population's appreciation of the pleasures of smoking led to the combining of opium and tobacco for smoking. Presumably the addition of opium took the edge off the craving for tobacco. The amount of tobacco used was gradually reduced and soon omitted altogether. Although opium eating had never been very attractive to most Chinese, opium smoking spread rapidly, perhaps, at least partly, because smoking results in a rapid effect, compared with the oral use of opium.

In 1729, China's first law against opium smoking mandated that opium shop owners be strangled. Once opium for nonmedical purposes was outlawed, it was necessary for the drug to be smuggled in from India, where poppy plantations were abundant. Smuggling opium was so profitable for everyone—the growers, the shippers, and the customs officers—that unofficial rules were gradually developed for the "game."[2] The background to the Opium Wars is too lengthy and complex to even attempt to sketch it adequately. However, some points must be made to explain why the British went to war so they could continue pouring opium into China against the wishes of the Chinese national government.

Since before 1557, when the Portuguese were allowed to develop the small trading post of Macao, pressure had been increasing on the Chinese emperors to open up the country to trade with the "barbarians from the West." Not only the Portuguese but the Dutch and the English repeatedly knocked on the closed door of China. Near the end of the seventeenth century the port of Canton was opened under very strict rules to foreigners. Tea was the major export, and the British shipped out huge amounts. There was little that the Chinese were interested in importing from the "barbarians," but opium could be smuggled so profitably that it soon became the primary import. The profit the British made from selling opium paid for the tea they shipped back to England.[8] In the early nineteenth century the government of India was actually the British East India Company. As such, it had a monopoly on opium, which was legal in India. However, smuggling it into China was not. The East India Company auctioned chests of opium cakes to private merchants, who gave the chests to selected British firms, which sold it for a commission to Chinese merchants. In this way the British were able to have the Chinese "smuggle" the opium into China. The number of chests of opium, each with about 120 pounds of smokable opium, that were annually imported to China increased from 200 in 1729 to about 5,000 at the century's end to 25,000 chests in 1838.

In the following year, 1839, the emperor of China made a fatal mistake—he sent an honest man to Canton to suppress the opium smuggling. Commissioner Lin demanded that the barbarians deliver all their opium supplies to him and subjected the dealers to confinement in their houses. After some haggling, the representative of the British government ordered the merchants to deliver the opium—20,000 chests worth about $6 million—which was then destroyed and everyone was set free. Pressures mounted, however, and an incident involving drunken American and British sailors killing a Chinese citizen started the Opium Wars in 1839. The British army arrived 10 months later, and in 2 years, largely by avoiding land battles and by using the superior artillery of the royal navy ships, they won a victory over a country of more than 350 million citizens. As victors, the British were given the island of Hong Kong, broad trading rights, and $6 million to reimburse the merchants whose opium had been destroyed.

The Chinese opium trade posed a great moral dilemma for Britain. The East India Company protested until its end that it was not smuggling opium into China, and technically it was not. From 1870 to 1893, motions in Parliament to end the extremely profitable opium commerce failed to pass but did cause a decline in the opium trade. In 1893, a moral protest against the trade was supported, but not until 1906 did the government support and pass a bill that eventually ended the opium trade in 1913.

Morphine

In 1805 in London, 20-year-old De Quincey eased a toothache and fell into the abyss of divine enjoyment. In Hanover, Germany, another 20-year-old worked on experiments that were to have great impact on science, medicine, and the pleasure seekers. In 1806, this German youth, Frederich Sertürner, published his report of more than 50 experiments, which clearly showed that he had isolated the primary active ingredient in opium. The active agent was ten times as potent as opium. Sertürner named it *morphium* after Morpheus, the god of dreams. Use of the new agent developed slowly, but by 1831 the implications of his chemical work and the medical value of **morphine** had become so overwhelming that this pharmacist's assistant was given the French equivalent of the Nobel Prize. Later work into the mysteries of opium found more than 30 different alkaloids, with the second most important one being isolated in 1832 and named **codeine,** the Greek word for "poppy head."

The availability of a clinically useful, pure chemical of known potency is always capitalized on in medicine. The major increase in the use of morphine came as a result of two nondrug developments, one technological and one political. The technological development was the perfection of the hypodermic syringe in 1853 by Dr. Alexander Wood. This made it possible to deliver morphine directly into the blood or tissue rather than by the much slower process of eating opium or morphine and waiting for absorption to occur from the gastrointestinal tract. A further advantage of injecting morphine was thought to exist. Originally it was felt that morphine by injection would not be as dependence-producing as the oral use of the drug. This belief was later found to be false.

The political events that sped the drug of sleep and dreams into the veins of people worldwide were the American Civil War (1861–1865), the Prussian-Austrian War (1866), and the Franco-Prussian War (1870). Military medicine was, and to some extent still is, characterized by the dictum "first provide relief." Morphine given by injection worked rapidly and well, and it was administered regularly in large doses to many soldiers for the reduction of pain and relief from dysentery. The percentage of veterans returning from these wars who were dependent on morphine was high enough that the illness was later called "soldier's disease" or the "army disease."

Heroin

Toward the end of the nineteenth century, a small but important chemical transformation was made to the morphine molecule. In 1874, two acetyl groups were attached to morphine, yielding diacetylmorphine, which was given the brand name Heroin and placed on the market in 1898 by Bayer Laboratories. The chemical change was important because **heroin** is about three times as potent as morphine. The pharmacology of heroin and morphine is identical, except that the two acetyl groups increase the lipid solubility of the heroin molecule, and thus the molecule enters the brain more rapidly. The additional groups are then detached, yielding morphine. Therefore, the effects of morphine and heroin are identical, except that heroin is more potent and acts faster.

Heroin was originally marketed as a nonaddicting substitute for codeine.[9] It seemed to be the perfect drug, more potent yet less harmful. Although not introduced commercially until 1898, heroin had been studied, and many of its pharmacological actions had been reported in 1890.[10] In January 1900, a comprehensive review article, concluded that tolerance and dependence on (habituation) heroin were only minor problems.

> Habituation has been noted in a small percentage . . . of the cases. . . . All observers are agreed, however, that none of the patients suffer in any way from this habituation, and that none of the symptoms which are so characteristic of chronic morphinism have ever been observed. On the other hand, a large number of the reports refer to the fact that the same dose may be used for a long time without any habituation.[11]

The basis for the failure to find dependence probably was the fact that heroin was initially used as a substitute for codeine, which meant oral doses of 3 to 5 mg used for brief periods of time. Slowly the situation changed, and a 1905 text, *Pharmacology and Therapeutics,* took a middle ground on heroin by saying that it "is stated not to give rise to habituation. A more extended knowledge of the drug, however, would seem to indicate that the latter assertion is not entirely correct."[12] In a few more years everyone knew that heroin could produce a powerful dependence when injected in higher doses.

Opiate Abuse Before the Harrison Act

In the second half of the nineteenth century, three forms of opiate dependence were developing in the United States. The long-useful oral intake of opium, and then morphine, increased greatly as patent medicines became a standard form of self-medication. After 1850, Chinese laborers were imported in large numbers to the West Coast, and they introduced opium smoking to this country. The last form, medically the most dangerous and ultimately the most disruptive socially, was the injection of morphine.

Around the turn of the twentieth century the percentage (and perhaps the absolute number) of Americans dependent on one of the opiates was probably greater than at any other time before or since. Several authorities, both then and more recently, agree that no less than 1 percent of the population was dependent on opium, although accurate statistics are not available. In spite of the high level of dependence, it was not a major social problem. In this period,

> The public then had an altogether different conception of drug addiction from that which prevails today. The habit was not approved, but neither was it regarded as criminal or monstrous. It was usually looked upon as a vice or personal misfortune, or much as alcoholism is viewed today. Narcotics users were pitied rather than loathed as criminals or degenerates.[13]

The opium smoking the Chinese brought to this country never became widely popular, although around the turn of the twentieth century about one-fourth of the opium imported was smoking opium. Perhaps it was because the smoking itself occupies only about a minute and is then followed by a state of reverie that can last two or three hours—hardly conducive to a continuation of daily activities or consonant with the outward,

---

morphine: the primary active narcotic agent in opium.

codeine: the secondary active narcotic agent in opium.

heroin: diacetylmorphine, a potent derivative of morphine.

active orientation of most Americans in that period. Another reason that opium smoking did not spread was that it originated with Asians, who were scorned by whites. Similarly, the opium smoking that did occur among whites was found within the asocial and antisocial elements of the culture. Amusingly, even the underworld had its standards of morality, and opium smokers looked down on those who used their drugs by injection. In a New York opium-smoking den early in the twentieth century, "one of the smokers discovered a hypodermic user in the bathroom giving himself an injection. He immediately reported to the proprietor that there was a 'God-damned dope fiend in the can.' The offender was promptly ejected."[13]

The growth of the patent medicine industry after the Civil War has been well documented. Everything seemed to be favorable for the industry, and it took advantage of each opportunity. There were few government regulations on the industry, and as a result drugs with a high abuse potential were an important part of many tonics and remedies, although this fact did not have to be indicated on the label. Because labeling of ingredients was not required, a user who had become aware that he or she was dependent and who wanted to purchase a cure could be sold a remedy labeled as a cure that contained almost as much of the same drug as he had been receiving in the original tonic.

The generally poor level of health care in the country and a large number of maimed and diseased veterans created a need for considerable medical treatment. Patent medicines promised, and in part delivered, the perfect self-medication. They were easily available, not too expensive, and socially acceptable, and they worked. The amount of alcohol and/or opiates in many of the nostrums was certain to relieve the user's aches, pains, and anxieties.

Gradually some medical concern developed over the number of people who were dependent on opiates, and this concern was a part of the motivation that led to the passage of the 1906 Pure Food and Drugs Act. In 1910, a government expert in this area made clear that this law was only a beginning:

> The thoughtful and foremost medical men have been and are cautioning against the free use of morphine and opium, particularly in recurring pain. The amount they are using is decreasing yearly. Notwithstanding this fact, and the fact that legislation, federal, state and territorial, adverse to the indiscriminate use and sale of opium and morphine, their derivatives and preparations, has been enacted during the past few decades, the amount of opium per capita imported and consumed in the United States has doubled during the last forty years. . . . It is well known that there are many factors at work tending to drug enslavement, among them being the host of soothing syrups, medicated soft drinks containing cocaine, asthma remedies, catarrh remedies, consumption remedies, cough and cold remedies, and the more notorious so-called "drug addiction cures." It is often stated that medical men are frequently the chief factors in causing drug addiction.[14]

Data were presented in this paper that tended to support the belief that medical use of opiates initiated by a physician was one, if not the, major cause of dependence in this country at that time. A 1918 government report clearly indicted the physician as the major cause of dependence in individuals of "good social standing."

That physicians widely used opiate medications is understandable in light of articles that had been published, such as one in 1889 titled "Advantages of Substituting the Morphia Habit for the Incurably Alcoholic." The author stated:

> In this way I have been able to bring peacefulness and quiet to many disturbed and distracted homes, to keep the head of a family out of the gutter and out of the lock-up, to keep him from scandalous misbehavior and neglect of his affairs, to keep him from the verges and actualities of delirium tremens horrors, and above all, to save him from committing, as I veritably believe, some terrible crime.[15]

Besides all those good things, a morphine habit was cheap: by one estimate it was 10 times as expensive to be an alcoholic—costing 25 cents a day. The article concluded:

> I might, had I time and space, enlarge by statistics to prove the law-abiding qualities of opium-eating peoples, but of this any one can perceive somewhat for himself, if he carefully watches and reflects on the quiet, introspective gaze of the morphine habitue, and compares it to the riotous, devil-may-care leer of the drunkard.[15]

This middle history period, 1806 to 1914, is rich in material on the use of opiates that gives background to the thesis that, if drugs are widely used, it is because they meet the needs of a culture. An 1880 report called opiate dependence a "vice of middle life." The typical opiate user of this period was a 30- to 50-year-old white woman who functioned well and was adjusted to her life as a wife and mother. She bought opium or morphine legally at the local store, used it orally, and caused few, if any, social problems. She might have ordered her "family remedy" through the mail from Sears, Roebuck—two ounces of laudanum for 18 cents or $1\frac{1}{2}$ pints for $2. Of course, there were problems associated with dependence during this period. There are always individuals who are unable to control their drug intake, whether the drug is used for self-medication or recreation. Because of the high opiate content of patent medicines and the ready availability of dependence-producing drugs for drinking and/or injecting, very high levels of drug were frequently used. As a result, the symptoms of withdrawal were very severe—much worse than today—and the only relief to be found was by taking more of the drug.

Abuse After the Harrison Act

The complex reasons for the passage of the 1914 Harrison Act were discussed in detail in Chapter 4. Remember that this was a fairly simple revenue measure. However, as is true of most laws,

it is not the law itself that becomes important in the ensuing years, but the court decisions and enforcement practices that evolve as the law interacts with the people it affects.

> The passing of the Harrison Act in 1914 left the status of the addict almost completely indeterminate. The act did not make addiction illegal and it neither authorized nor forbade doctors to prescribe drugs regularly for addicts. All that it clearly and unequivocally did require was that whatever drugs addicts obtained were to be secured from physicians registered under the act and that the fact of securing drugs be made a matter of record. While some drug users had obtained supplies from physicians before 1914, it was not necessary for them to do so since drugs were available for purchase in pharmacies and even from mail-order houses.[16]

In 1915, the United States Supreme Court decided that possession of smuggled opiates was a crime, and thus users not obtaining the drug from a physician became criminals with the stroke of a pen. Dependent users could still obtain their supply of drugs on a prescription from a physician, until this avenue was removed by Supreme Court decisions in 1920 and 1922 (see Chapter 4). Even though the *Lindner* case in 1925 reversed these earlier decisions and stated that a physician could prescribe drugs to non-hospitalized users just to maintain their dependence, the doctors had been harassed and arrested enough. Even though it was legal again to prescribe drugs to a dependent user, few physicians would do so. Clinics for the treatment of opiate dependence were closed during the 1920s under pressure from federal officials.

The number of oral opiate users began to decline in response to these pressures, and the primary remaining group were those who injected morphine or heroin. By 1922, about the only source of opiates for a nonhospitalized abuser was an illegal dealer. Because heroin was the most potent opiate available, it was the easiest to conceal and therefore became the illegal dealer's choice. The cost through this source was 30 to 50 times the price of the same drug through legitimate sources, which no longer were available to drug-dependent users. Because of this cost, users wanted to be certain to get the most "bang for their buck," so intravenous injection became more and more common. To maintain a supply of the drug in this way was expensive. Many users resorted to criminal activity, primarily burglary and other crimes against property, to finance their dependence.

During this period, law enforcement agencies and the popular press brought about a change in the attitudes of society toward the drug abusers. Thus sometime during the 1920s,

> the addict was no longer seen as a victim of drugs, an unfortunate with no place to turn and deserving of society's sympathy and help. He became instead a base, vile, degenerate who was weak and self-indulgent, who contaminated all he came in contact with and who deserved nothing short of condemnation and society's moral outrage and legal sanction. The law enforcement approach was accepted as the only workable solution to the problem of addiction.[17]

The Changing Population of Opioid Users

After the Harrison Act there almost certainly was a decline in the number of individuals using opiates orally and thus a drop in white middle-aged users. One paper commented that between World War I and World War II heroin received little publicity and was primarily used by "people in *the life*—show people, entertainers and musicians; racketeers and gangsters; thieves and pickpockets; prostitutes and pimps."[18] The transition from the 1930s to the 1950s in the United States has been best described by an internationally recognized expert who worked in the area of substance abuse through this period:

> If you go back to 1935 the other problems, apart from alcohol, were primarily the opiates and cocaine, usually taken together in the form of the so-called "speed-ball" and then as now . . . drug use was multiple. These individuals that I know

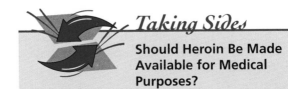

Taking Sides

Should Heroin Be Made Available for Medical Purposes?

Since the 1920s, heroin has been unavailable to physicians for any purpose. It was the first such drug to be so restricted, and its status has now been codified, along with that of LSD and marijuana, under the status of Schedule I controlled substances—those with "no medical use."

However, heroin has been available all along in most countries as a potent pain reliever. It has repeatedly been proposed over the years that heroin should be moved to Schedule II and thus become available for medical use by prescription. Whether heroin is actually a better pain reliever than morphine has been argued for many years—it is more potent, in that less is required for the same effect, but since heroin is converted to morphine in the brain, morphine should be just as effective if given in a higher dose. Regardless of the limited amount of evidence on either side, some physicians believe that heroin should be available in the United States for pain relief. Under some of the proposals, heroin would be available only under restricted circumstances, such as the failure of other potent narcotics to control pain.

As the situation now stands, according to one prominent proponent[47] of medical heroin, the drug is more readily available to a 16-year-old kid on the street than it is to a terminally ill cancer patient in constant pain.

For more on this topic, log on to www.dushkin. com/online for current news and links to other popular and informative sites, as well as time-saving web search strategies and study tools.

used morphine, cocaine, heroin, bromides, phenobarbital or whatever happened to come along but they preferred the opiates and cocaine. The people of those days were really predominately white individuals, they were on the whole members of various criminal trades, pickpockets and so on, and in fact most of them had been involved in these criminal trades either before or after their onset of their career of using drugs. These people more or less disappeared during the Second World War which practically made these drugs unavailable . . . the old fashioned addict, the expert pickpocket, the short change artist couldn't get drugs. This group was succeeded, after the war was over, by a new kind of opiate taker. These were primarily individuals from the minority groups in the big city slums and in contrast to the older addicts who got good drugs, who knew good stuff when they got it, this new group were getting drugs extremely diluted, full of all kinds of other poisons and were a very different kind of people. They were not expert thieves, in fact very inexpert.[19]

In the early years after World War II, heroin use slowly increased in the lower-class, slum areas of the large cities. Heroin was inexpensive in this period; a dollar would buy enough for a good high for three to six people; $2-a-day habits were not uncommon. As the 1950s passed, heroin use spread rapidly. As demand increased, so did both the price and the amount of adulteration.

The 1960s

A brief summary of heroin use from 1940 to 1970 suggests that all the rules changed in late 1961.[18] A critical shortage of heroin developed, prices tripled, and adulteration was carried to new heights. Because this increased profits, the price and adulteration level stayed the same when heroin was again in good supply. It appears that it might have been the large increase in price that disrupted the previous social cohesiveness among abusers, increased the amount of crime, and contributed to the general social disorganization of the ghettos, where most heroin users lived.

In the 1960s, the use of heroin and other drugs skyrocketed. Flower children, hippies, Tim Leary, and LSD received most of the media attention, but within the central core of the large American cities the number of regular and irregular heroin users increased daily. As you might expect, mainstream USA gradually

became concerned with the heroin problem of the large cities. The increase in crime was the key, and because the most visible abusers were African American or Latino, the white majority expressed little patience or tolerance toward people who were dependent on heroin.

Vietnam

The attitude of people in the street toward the relevance of heroin use to their personal lives changed rapidly with the reports that began to filter out of Southeast Asia toward the end of the 1960s. Public anxiety increased dramatically with the possibility that the Vietnam conflict might produce thousands of drug users among the military personnel stationed there.

The Department of Defense established a Task Force on Drug Abuse in 1967; its initial reports emphasized concern over the widespread use of marijuana by troops in combat zones, as well as in rest and rehabilitation areas. In 1970, public and federal concern began to focus on the problem of heroin dependence among service personnel stationed in Southeast Asia.[20]

Heroin was about 95 percent pure and almost openly sold in South Vietnam, whereas purity in the United States was about 5 percent in 1969. Not only was the Southeast Asia heroin undiluted, but it was inexpensive. Ten dollars would buy about 250 mg, an amount that would cost over $500 in the United States. The high purity of the heroin made it possible to obtain psychological effects by smoking or sniffing the drug. This fact, coupled with the completely fallacious belief that dependence occurs only when the drug is used intravenously, resulted in about 40 percent of the users sniffing, about half smoking, and only 10 percent mainlining their heroin.[21]

Some early 1971 reports estimated that 10 to 15 percent of the American troops in Vietnam were dependent on heroin. As a result of the increased magnitude and visibility of the heroin problem, the U.S. government took several rapid steps in mid-1971. One step was to initiate Operation Golden Flow, a urine-testing program for opiates in service personnel ready to leave Vietnam. The testing program, which tested *only* for opiates, was later expanded to include non-military personnel.

In October 1971, the Pentagon released figures for the first three months of testing, which showed that 5.1 percent of the 100,000 personnel tested showed traces of opiates in their urine. Most of the opiate users were in the lower ranks.

In retrospect the Vietnam drug-use situation was "making a mountain out of a molehill," but much was learned. An excellent follow-up study[22] of veterans who returned from Vietnam in September 1971 showed that most of the Vietnam heroin users did not continue heroin use in this country. Only 1 to 2 percent were using narcotics 8 to 12 months after returning from Vietnam and being released from the service, approximately the same percentage of individuals found to be using narcotics when examined for induction into the service.

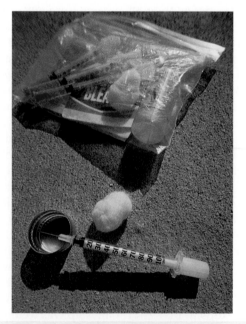

Shooting up heroin.

One of the important things learned from this experience is that narcotic dependence and compulsive use are not inevitable among occasional users. The pattern of drug use in Vietnam also supports the belief that under certain conditions—availability and low cost of the drug, boredom, or unhappiness—a relatively high percentage of individuals will use narcotic drugs recreationally.

The 1970s and 1980s

Beginning in the late 1960s, the federal government made several efforts to estimate the number of heroin users in the United States. This is an impossible task to perform with much accuracy, given that heroin use is conducted in great secrecy and is not uniformly distributed across the country. Nevertheless, several sophisticated statistical techniques were brought to bear, combining various sources of information. Different groups of researchers estimated the number of heroin-dependent individuals from 1970 to the mid-1980s, and the estimates ranged between 400,000 and 500,000.[23] Perhaps because of considerable variability in the estimates, no particular trends or patterns can be seen in these data, and one might argue that heroin dependence didn't really change much over that period.

In 1972, the major source of U.S. heroin was opium grown in Turkey and converted into heroin in southern French port cities, such as Marseilles. This "French connection" accounted for as much as 80 percent of U.S. heroin before 1973. In 1972, Turkey banned all opium cultivation and production in return for $35 million the United States provided to make up for the financial losses to farmers and to help them develop new cash crops. This action, combined with a cooperative effort with the French (also partially funded by the United States), did lead to a reduction in the supply of heroin on the streets of New York in 1973.

This relative shortage did not last for long. In Mexico, opium is processed into morphine by a different process, and the resulting pure heroin has a brown or black color. In 1975, the Drug Enforcement Administration (DEA) estimated that 80 percent or more of all U.S. heroin was from Mexico (depending on its appearance, either called *Mexican brown* or **black tar**). The supply was plentiful, the price low, and the purity high. In 1974, the United States began to finance opium eradication programs in Mexico. Although it is a hopeless task to try to eliminate all such production, these monumental and expensive efforts did slow the importation from Mexico to some extent, and the "epidemic" of the 1970s began to decline.

In the mid-1980s, about half of the U.S. heroin supply apparently originated in Southwest Asia (Afghanistan, Pakistan, Iran). Mexico was the next biggest contributor, with the Golden Triangle area of Southeast Asia (Burma, Laos, and Thailand) producing about 15 to 20 percent of the total. Production of opium and availability of refined heroin from all three of these regions increased during the second half of the 1980s, but the biggest increase came from Southeast Asia, which by 1990 was estimated to be producing 56 percent of the U.S. supply (Figure 16.1).[24]

Current Use of Heroin

It seems as though every few years the media rediscover a new heroin epidemic among young, upper-class or middle-class Americans. And every generation does have its few who dare. Also in every generation a few well-known musicians or entertainers either die from heroin overdoses or make a public announcement of their kicking the habit. One new twist in the 1990s was the popularity of models who were very thin, with sunken eyes and the overall appearance of heroin abusers—"heroin chic" as it was known in the fashion industry.[25] Many expressed fear that glamorizing heroin in this way would attract new users, and self-reported experimental heroin use did increase in the 1990s among high school seniors.

For many years the DEA has used informants to purchase heroin in various regions of the country and has estimated average street price and purity. From the mid-1970s through the mid-1980s the average purity varied from 4 to 6 percent heroin (over 90 percent was something else that the dealers had used to cut the heroin). However, in the late 1980s, increased shipments of increasingly pure heroin began to arrive, and in 1989 the average street purity was estimated to be 25.2 percent, at least four times as strong as in years past. In 1999, the estimated average purity had increased to nearly 40 percent nationwide and over 60 percent in several northeastern cities, including Philadelphia, New York, and Boston. The price of a "bag" has not changed much, so the price per milligram of actual heroin was down considerably.

One big change in the 1990s was that smoking opiates was back, although in a slightly different form than the old opium den. Piggybacking on the smoking of crack cocaine, inner-city users were either mixing the new high-potency heroin with crack or simply heating the heroin and inhaling the vapors from a crack pipe. The increased purity of available heroin has allowed smoking, as well as snorting, to produce the effects users want, while they avoid the use of needles that might spread AIDs or other diseases. However, a couple of mysterious cases of brain damage appeared in New York in 1996, and these were tentatively attributed to smoking heroin by heating it in aluminum foil.[26]

PHARMACOLOGY OF THE OPIOIDS

Chemical Characteristics

Raw opium contains about 10 percent morphine by weight and a smaller amount of codeine. The addition of two acetyl groups to the morphine

---

black tar: a type of illicit heroin usually imported from Mexico.

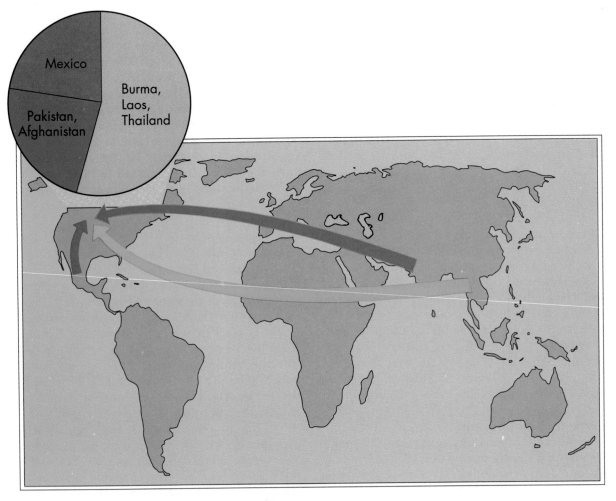

Figure 16.1   Sources of illicit heroin for the United States.

molecule results in diacetylmorphine, or heroin (Figure 16.2). The acetyl groups allow heroin to penetrate the blood-brain barrier more readily, and heroin is therefore two to three times more potent than morphine.

Medicinal chemists have worked hard over the decades to produce compounds that would be effective painkillers, trying to separate the analgesic effect of the opiates from their dependence-producing effects. Although the two effects could not be separated, the research has resulted in a variety of **opioids** that are sold as

pain relievers (Table 16.1). Especially interesting among these is fentanyl, which is approximately a hundred times as potent as morphine. Fentanyl is used primarily in conjunction with surgical anesthesia, although both fentanyl and some of its derivatives have also been manufactured illegally and sold on the streets. In 1994, Abbott Laboratories began to market a prescription fentanyl "lollipop" for children who are facing surgery or other painful procedures. This drug is so potent that, if a child sucks on the lozenge, which is supplied on a plastic stick,

Exploring Your Spirituality

Imitating Fashion Trends Versus Developing a Personal Style

Remember all those haunting images in the mid-1990s of emaciated, hollow-cheeked fashion models, the look known as heroin chic? Even if we did not share a fascination with the drug, it was hard not to be fascinated by the lifestyle and the wasted look of the models. The smug attitude of a model making thousands of dollars a day by sitting in front of a camera, looking stoned, created a curiosity about their lives, a mystery and glamour, that the fashion photos tried to evoke. Do they feel better than we do, know something we don't know, have more fun than we do? The pictures were provocative and visually striking, shot by photographers seeking new ways to influence our perceptions of taste. The models were thin, so thin was chic.

Later came the androgenous "waif" look, epitomized by Kate Moss, and we were again shown an ideal body image that most of us couldn't attain. Finally, at the spring 2001 collections in New York, there was a renewed preference for women who do not look exaggerately thin, but who have ripe curves. The look was clean, fresh, healthy, natural, and more diverse—welcome news for those not inclined to starvation, silicon, or a scalpel.

As with other aspects of fashion, the preferred look for models fluctuates often. People in the modeling business sometimes refer to models as having expiration, or "use by," dates, in an industry always looking for a change. And despite the fickleness of the fashion industry, the "in" look saturating the fashion magazines has a powerful influence on our self-worth and self-esteem. Not surprisingly, studies report that women and girls who read such magazines regularly are more dissatisfied with their bodies than are those who do not. And if you ask a young man to describe his ideal date, his answer may sound a lot like the current model type.

The disparity between ideal body image and reality can affect an individual's spiritual well-being, especially among vulnerable adolescents and young adults. Advertising, the media, and the desire for the respect of others combine to encourage us to look and act a certain way. For those who believe that each person's traits are uniquely valuable, the conflict between a style ideal and the reality of not measuring up presents a spiritual dilemma.

One choice is to try to conform to an ideal, perhaps through dieting, exercise, or surgery to attain a model-type body or perhaps through working extra-long hours to be able to afford a particular lifestyle. But what sacrifices are you willing to make? What if you continue to fail to achieve the goal? How would you feel about yourself then?

An alternative response is to search within yourself for other kinds of self-validation, such as untapped talents and strengths. Or you might look outward, to the real world, where you can see that you're making a positive difference by contributing your capabilities, time, support, and faith to others. If you choose one of these latter approaches, you can put the ideal you see in all the style magazines into perspective and strengthen your feelings of self-worth and self-confidence to be the best, most well-balanced person you can be.

---

within 15 minutes significant sedation and analgesia are obtained. Apparently, Abbott is betting that such a device will find use when children are frightened and in pain and the threat of receiving an anesthetic injection would only increase the child's distress.

In addition to the opioid analgesics, this search for new compounds led to the discovery of **narcotic antagonists,** drugs that block the action of morphine, heroin, or other opioid agonists. The administration of a drug such as **naloxone** or *nalorphine,* can save a person's life by reversing the depressed respiration resulting from a narcotic overdose. If given to an individual who has been taking narcotics and who has become physically dependent, these antagonists

opioids: all naturally occurring and synthetic drugs that stimulate or block morphinelike receptors.

narcotic antagonists: drugs that can block the actions of narcotics.

naloxone: (nal ox own) a narcotic antagonist.

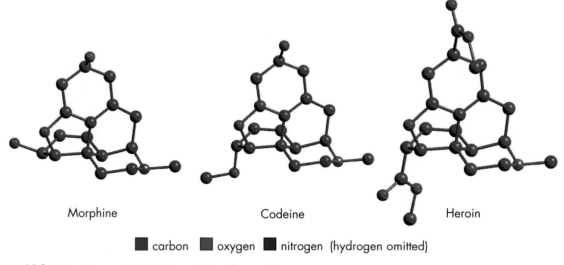

Morphine   Codeine   Heroin

■ carbon ■ oxygen ■ nitrogen (hydrogen omitted)

Figure 16.2   Narcotic agents isolated or derived from opium.

can precipitate an immediate withdrawal syndrome. Both naloxone and the longer-lasting *naltrexone* have been given to dependent individuals to prevent them from experiencing a high if they then use heroin.

Mechanism of Action

In the early 1970s, techniques were developed that led to the discovery of selective opioid receptors in rat brain tissue. For decades before this, theories of opioid drug action had relied on the concept of an opioid receptor, but the finding that such structures actually exist in the membranes of neurons led to the next question: What are opioid receptors doing in the synapses of the brain—waiting for someone to extract the juice from a poppy? The distribution of these receptors didn't agree with the distribution of any known neurotransmitter substance, so scientists all over the world went to work, looking for a substance in the brain that could serve as the natural activator of these opioid receptors. Groups in England and in Sweden succeeded in 1974: a pair of molecules, leu-enkephalin and met-enkephalin, were isolated from brain extracts. These **enkephalins** acted like morphine and were many times more potent. Next came the discovery of a group of **endorphins** (endogenous morphinelike substances) that are also found in brain tissue and have potent opioid effects.

These discoveries opened a number of doors for scientists, some of which have helped answer questions and others of which have led only to more questions. It is now clear that endorphins and enkephalins are contained within neurons and released from terminals to act as neurotransmitters or as modulators of neural activity.[27] Beta-endorphin is contained in a relatively small number of long-axon neurons that interconnect the hypothalamus, the forebrain limbic structures, the medial thalamus, and the locus ceruleus. Enkephalins are found in a larger number of short-axon neurons within the basal ganglia, hypothalamus, amygdala, substantia nigra, and other areas. In addition to these two major types of endogenous opioids, there are dynorphins and other substances that have some actions similar to those of morphine.

TABLE 16.1

Some Prescription Narcotic Analgesics

Generic name	Trade name	Recommended dose (mg)
Natural Products		
Morphine		10–30
Codeine		30–60
Semisynthetics		
Heroin, diamorph	(Not available in the United States)	5–10
Synthetics		
Methadone	Dolophine	2.5–10
Meperidine	Demerol	50–150
Oxycodone	Percodan	2.25–4.5
Oxymorphone	Numorphan	1–1.5
Hydrocodone		5–10
Hydromorphone	Dilaudid	1–4
Dihydrocodeine		32
Propoxyphene	Darvon	32–65
Pentazocine	Talwin	30
Fentanyl	Sublimaze	0.05–0.10

The search for a single endogenous opioid led to the discovery of a wide variety, and another new agonist was reported in 1997.[28] These substances, as well as the natural and synthetic opioid drugs, have actions on at least three types of opioid receptors, the structures of which were discovered in the early 1990s. One of the most important sites of action may be the midbrain central gray, a region known to be involved in pain perception. However, there are many other sites of interaction between these systems and areas that relate to pain, and pain itself is a complex psychological and neurological phenomenon, so we cannot say that we understand completely how opioids act to reduce pain.

In addition to the presence of these endogenous opioids in the brain, large amounts of endorphins are released from the pituitary gland in response to stress. Also, enkephalins are released from the adrenal gland. The functions of these peptides circulating through the blood as hormones are not understood at this point. They could perhaps reduce pain by acting in the spinal cord, but they are unlikely to produce direct effects in the brain because they probably do not cross the blood-brain barrier. In the late 1970s, it was speculated that long-distance runners experience a release of endorphins that might be responsible for the so-called runner's high. Unfortunately, the only evidence in support of this notion was measurements of blood levels of endorphins that seemed to be elevated in some, but not all, runners. These endorphins are presumably from the pituitary and might not be capable of producing a high. It is not known whether exercise alters *brain* levels of these substances.

enkephalins: (en *kef* a lins) morphinelike neurotransmitters found in the brain and adrenals.

endorphins: (en *dor* fins) morphinelike neurotransmitters found in the brain and pituitary gland.

BENEFICIAL USES

Pain Relief

The major therapeutic indication for morphine and the other narcotics is the reduction of pain. After the administration of an analgesic dose of morphine, some patients report that they are still aware of pain but that the pain is no longer aversive. The narcotic agents seem to have their effect in part by diminishing the patient's awareness of and response to the aversive stimulus. Morphine primarily reduces the emotional response to pain (the suffering) and to some extent the knowledge of the pain stimulus.

The effect of narcotics is relatively specific to pain. Fewer effects on mental and motor ability accompany analgesic doses of these agents than accompany equipotent doses of other analgesic and depressant drugs. Although one of the characteristics of these drugs is their ability to reduce pain without inducing sleep, drowsiness is not uncommon after a therapeutic dose. (In the user's vernacular, the patient is "on the nod.") The patient is readily awakened if sleeping, and dreams during the sleep period are frequent.

Intestinal Disorders

Narcotics have long been valued for their effects on the gastrointestinal system. They quiet colic and save lives by counteracting diarrhea. In years past and today in many underdeveloped countries, contaminated food and water have resulted in severe intestinal infections (dysentery). Particularly in the young and the elderly, diarrhea and resulting dehydration can be a major cause of death.

Narcotic drugs decrease the number of peristaltic contractions, which is the type of contraction responsible for moving food through the intestines. Considerable water is absorbed from the intestinal material; this fact, plus the decrease in peristaltic contractions, often results in constipation in patients taking the drugs for pain relief. This side effect is what has saved many lives of dysentery victims. Although modern synthetic narcotic derivatives are now sold for this purpose, old-fashioned paregoric, an opium solution, is still available for the symptomatic relief of diarrhea.

Cough Suppressants

The narcotics also have the effect of decreasing activity in what the advertisers refer to as the cough control center in the medulla. Although coughing is often a useful way of clearing unwanted material from the respiratory passages, at times nonproductive coughing can itself become a problem. Since it was first purified from opium, codeine has been widely used for its *antitussive* properties and is still available in a number of prescription cough remedies. Nonprescription cough remedies contain dextromethorphan, a narcotic analogue that is somewhat more selective in its antitussive effects.

CAUSES FOR CONCERN

Dependence Potential

Tolerance
Tolerance develops to most of the effects of the narcotic drugs, although with different effects tolerance can occur at different rates. If the drug is used chronically for pain relief, for example, it will probably be necessary to increase the dose to maintain a constant effect. The same is true for the euphoria sought by recreational users: repeated use results in a decreased effect, which can be overcome by increasing the dose. Cross-tolerance exists among all the narcotics: tolerance to one reduces the effectiveness of each of the others. Siegel[29] and others have shown that psychological processes can play an important role in the tolerance to narcotics. When a user repeatedly injects an opioid agonist, various physiological effects occur (changes in body temperature, intestinal motility, respiration rate, and so on). With repeated experience the dependent

TABLE 16.2		

Sequence of Appearance of Some of the Abstinence Syndrome Symptoms

	Approximate Hours After Previous Dose	
Signs	Heroin and/or morphine	Methadone
Craving for drugs, anxiety	6	24
Yawning, perspiration, running nose, teary eyes	14	34–48
Increase in above signs plus pupil dilation, goose bumps (pilorection), tremors (muscle twitches), hot and cold flashes, aching bones and muscles, loss of appetite	16	48–72
Increased intensity of above, plus insomnia; raised blood pressure; increased temperature, pulse rate, respiratory rate and depth; restlessness; nausea	24–36	
Increased intensity of above, plus curled-up position, vomiting, diarrhea, weight loss, spontaneous ejaculation or orgasm, hemoconcentration, increased blood sugar	36–48	

person might unconsciously learn to anticipate those effects and to counteract them. Animal experiments have shown that, after repeated morphine injections, a placebo injection produces changes in body temperature opposite to those originally produced by morphine. Thus, some of the body's tolerance to narcotics results from conditioned reflex responses to the stimuli associated with taking the drugs. To demonstrate how important these conditioned protective reflexes can become, Siegel and his colleagues injected rats with heroin every other day in a particular environment. After 15 such injections, the rats were given a much larger dose of heroin, half in the environment previously associated with heroin and half in a different environment. Of the group given the heroin injection in the different environment, most of the rats died. However, of the group given heroin in the environment that had previously predicted heroin, most of the rats lived.[30] Those rats had presumably learned to associate that environment with heroin injections, and conditioned reflexes occurred that counteracted some of the physiological effects of the drug. This is one example of behavioral tolerance.

Physical Dependence

Concomitant with the development of tolerance is the establishment of physical dependence: in a person who has used the drug chronically and at high doses, as each dose begins to wear off, certain withdrawal symptoms begin to appear. These symptoms and their approximate timing after heroin or methadone use are listed in Table 16.2. This list of symptoms might have more personal meaning for you if you compare it to a case of the 24-hour, or intestinal, flu: combine nausea and vomiting with diarrhea, aches, pains, and a general sense of misery, and you have a pretty good idea of what a moderate case of narcotic withdrawal is like: rarely life-threatening but most unpleasant. If an individual has been taking a large amount of the narcotic, then these symptoms can be much worse than those caused by 24-hour flu and can last at least twice as long. Note that **methadone,** a long-lasting synthetic

---

methadone: (*meth a doan*) a long-lasting synthetic opiate.

narcotic, produces withdrawal symptoms that are usually less severe and that always appear later than with heroin. Cross-dependence is seen among the narcotics: no matter which of them was responsible for producing the initial dependence, withdrawal symptoms can be prevented by an appropriate dose of any narcotic agonist. This is the basis for the use of methadone in treating heroin dependence, because substituting legal methadone prevents withdrawal symptoms for as much as a day.

An interesting clue to the biochemical mechanism of withdrawal symptoms has been the finding that *clonidine,* an alpha-adrenergic agonist that is used to treat high blood pressure, can diminish the severity of narcotic withdrawal symptoms. Studies on brain tissue reveal that opioid receptors and alpha-adrenergic receptors are found together in some brain areas, including the norepinephrine-containing cells of the locus ceruleus. Clonidine and morphine produce identical effects on the enzyme activity and neurophysiology of these cells. In other brain areas, opioid receptors are found that are not associated with alpha-adrenergic receptors, which is why clonidine does not produce narcotic-like euphoria and is not a good analgesic.[27]

Psychological Dependence

That opioids produce psychological dependence is quite clear; in fact, experiments with opioids were what led to our current understanding of the importance of the reinforcing properties of drugs (see Chapter 3). Animals allowed to self-administer low doses of morphine or heroin intravenously will learn the required behaviors quickly and will perform them for prolonged periods, even if they have never experienced withdrawal symptoms. This is an example of what psychologists refer to as *positive reinforcement:* a behavior is reliably followed by the presentation of a stimulus, leading to an increase in the probability of the behavior and its eventual maintenance at a higher rate than before. Remember that the rapidity with which the reinforcing stimulus follows the behavior is an important

factor, which is why fewer experiences are needed with a narcotic injected intravenously (fast acting) than with the same drug taken orally (delayed action).

Once physical dependence has developed and withdrawal symptoms are experienced, the conditions are set up for another behavioral mechanism, *negative reinforcement.* In this situation an act (drug taking) is followed by the *removal* of withdrawal symptoms, leading to further strengthening of the habit. In heroin dependence, the rapid and potent euphoric effect resulting from intravenous injection, combined with the appearance of early withdrawal symptoms after only a few hours and their rapid alleviation by another injection, typically leads to the development of a more robust dependence in many users. Remember, however, that heroin was prescribed in low doses and taken orally by many patients for several years during which it was believed to be nonaddictive. Although heroin is more potent than morphine and may have a higher abuse potential because of its more rapid access to the brain, morphine taken intravenously is more likely to produce dependence than heroin taken orally.

The Needle Habit

Each heroin administration is followed by a decrease in discomfort, an increase in pleasure, or both. As a result, the behavior itself of preparing and injecting the drug and the setting in which it occurs acquire pleasurable, positive associations through learning mechanisms. Because of this conditioning, the process of using heroin also becomes rewarding. One occasional user commented on the ritual of heroin use:

> Once you decide to get off it's very exciting. It really is. Getting some friends together and some money, copping, deciding where you're going to do it, getting the needles out and sterilizing them, cooking up the stuff, tying off, then the whole thing with the needle, booting, and the rush, that's all part of it. . . . Sometimes I think that if I just shot water I'd enjoy it as much.[31]

Though it might seem strange, that last statement is true for some individuals who label themselves addicts. These individuals have been called "needle freaks"—at least part of the relief and pleasure they obtain from injecting is a conditioned response to the stimuli (such as needles) associated with heroin use.

A research team headed by a psychiatrist, Charles O'Brien, studied the process of eliminating (extinguishing) the needle habit. A long-acting, experimental narcotic antagonist was administered, and the research volunteers were allowed to shoot up using their own equipment and rituals. Most heroin users shoot up in a bathroom, so the researchers provided a bathroom in which the volunteers could inject their drugs. Under double-blind conditions the users injected either saline or a high or low dose of a narcotic. No matter which the volunteers injected, there was no pharmacological effect from the injected narcotic because of the administration of the antagonist. Both objective and subjective measures were used. Immediately after self-injecting, the research participants reported pleasurable drug effects.[32] Only after three to five injections were the subjective reports neutral. Continued self-injections under these conditions resulted in the participants' reporting that they hated the whole process. Remember that there is variability in any biological system: one participant continued to report euphoria after each injection for 26 trials, and he regularly showed the pupillary constriction that accompanies the injection of a narcotic. That participant was one of those receiving saline, so it was not a question of the narcotic dose being high or the antagonist dose being low.

Toxicity Potential

Acute Toxicity

One specific effect of the narcotics is to depress the respiratory centers in the brain, so that respiration slows and becomes shallow. This is perhaps the major side effect of the narcotic agents and one of the most dangerous, because death resulting from respiratory depression can easily follow an excessive dose of these drugs. The basis for this effect is that the respiratory centers become less responsive to carbon dioxide levels in the blood. It is this effect that keeps heroin/morphine and methadone near the top of the list of mentioned drugs in DAWN coroners' reports. Remember that this respiratory depression is additive with the effects of alcohol or other sedative-hypnotics, and there is evidence that a large fraction of those who die from heroin overdose have elevated blood alcohol concentrations and might better be described as dying from a combination of heroin and alcohol. Narcotic overdose can be diagnosed on the basis of the *narcotic triad:* coma, depressed respiration, and pinpoint pupils. Emergency medical treatment calls for the use of naloxone (Narcan), which antagonizes the narcotic effects within a few minutes.

The behavioral consequences of having morphinelike drugs in the brain are probably less dangerous. Those who inject heroin might nod off into a dream-filled sleep for a few minutes, and opium smokers are famous for their "pipe dreams." It is perhaps not surprising that individuals under the influence of narcotics are likely to be less active and less alert than they otherwise would be. There is a clouding of consciousness which makes mental work more difficult. And opioid users not only are less likely to be interested in sex, but men can even suffer primary impotence as a direct effect of the drug.

Opioid agonists also stimulate the brain area controlling nausea and vomiting, which are other frequent side effects. Nausea occurs in about half of ambulatory patients given a 15 mg dose of morphine. Also, nausea and vomiting are a common reaction to heroin injection among street users.

Chronic Toxicity

Although early in the twentieth century many medical authorities believed that chronic narcotic use weakened the user both mentally and physically, there is no scientific evidence that

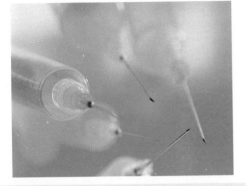

Some communities have needle-exchange programs designed to reduce the spread of HIV and hepatitis B, caused by sharing needles to inject street drugs.

exposure to opioid drugs per se causes long-term damage to any tissue or organ system. Many street users of narcotics do suffer from sores and abscesses at injection sites, but these can be attributed to the lack of sterile technique. Also, the practice of sharing needles can result in the spread of such blood-borne diseases as serum hepatitis and HIV. Again, this is a result not of the drug but of the technique used to inject it.

Patterns of Abuse

The Life of a Heroin User
Only a glimpse of some of the mechanics of a heroin user's life can be presented here. Withdrawal signs might begin about 4 hours after the previous use of the drug, but many addicts report that they begin to feel ill only 6 to 8 hours after the previous dose. That puts most heroin abusers on a schedule of 3 or 4 injections every day. Today's heroin user is not spending a lot of time nodding off in opium dens, as in the good old days. When you have a very important appointment to keep every 6 to 8 hours, every day of the week, every day of the year, you've got to hustle not to miss one of them. Remember, there are no vacations, no weekends off for the regular user, just 1,200 to 1,400 appointments per year to keep.

And each one costs money. Heroin is frequently sold on the street in "dime" bags: $10 for a small plastic bag containing . . . good question—what's in the bag? The material in a $10 bag might have 3 mg or 30 mg. Of course, you might not get *any* heroin, and you can't complain to the Better Business Bureau. At any rate, your habit can cost you $30 to $100 a day.

The variability in amount of heroin is a problem because of the possibility of an overdose (OD). Heroin users should worry about an OD with each new batch of drug used. A sophisticated user buying from a new or questionable source will initially try a much smaller than normal amount of the powder to evaluate its potency.

Once the user has acquired the drug, he or she prepares it for injection. Usually, the user

> mixes the powder with unsterile water, heats the mixture briefly in a spoon or bottle cap with a match or lighter, then draws the heroin into a syringe or eyedropper through cotton, thus filtering out the larger impurities. The heroin is then injected intravenously without any attempt at skin cleansing.[33]

Under these conditions it is not surprising that infections occur. Some users prefer to use an eyedropper with a hypodermic needle attached, because the rubber bulb of the dropper is easier to operate than the plunger of a syringe.

The most common form of heroin use by male users is to inject the drug intravenously—that is, to mainline the drug. A convenient site is the left forearm (for right-handed users), and the frequent use of dirty needles leaves the arm marked with scar tissue. If the larger veins of the arm collapse, then other body areas are used. Many beginning users start by "skinpopping"—subcutaneous injections. Skinpopping increases the danger of tetanus but decreases the risk of hepatitis compared with mainlining. Because of the lack of sterility or even cleanliness, hepatitis, tetanus, and abscesses at the site of injection are not uncommon in street users who inject drugs.

If the user survives the perils of an overdose, escapes the dangers of contaminated equipment, and avoids being caught, there are still other dangers. Heroin is a potent analgesic, and its regular use can conceal the early symptoms of an illness, such as pneumonia. The user's lack of money for, or interest in, food frequently results in malnutrition. With low resistance from malnutrition and the symptoms of illness going unnoticed as a result of heroin use, the user becomes susceptible to serious disease.

If all these dangers are overcome, the user might continue to use opioids to an advanced age. Sometimes, however, the user who avoids illness, death, or arrest and who does not enter and stay in a rehabilitation program or withdraw him- or herself from the drug might no longer feel the need for the drug and gradually stop using it. The data are still very much debated, but this "maturing out" is probably what happens to a large number of heroin abusers. One authority reports that the user who survives remains dependent for only about 8 or 9 years. This is an average, however, and according to this report, the earlier users start, the longer they remain dependent, with maturing out generally occurring around 35 to 45 years of age.[34] Even if the user lives, the street life of a heroin dependent individual isn't a rose garden.

Misconceptions and Preconceptions

Although heroin users haven't received as much press as crack users in recent years, most people have some pretty strongly held beliefs about heroin, derived from television, magazines, movies, and conversations. This section deals with some of the major misconceptions that most people, including many professionals, have about nonmedical use and misuse of narcotics.

One of the most common misconceptions is that mainlining heroin or morphine induces in everyone an intense pleasure unequaled by any other experience. Often it is described as similar to a whole-body orgasm that persists up to five or more minutes. Some users report that they try with every injection to reexperience the extreme

HealthQuest Activities

In Module 9, go to *Drug F/X Exploration* and complete the assessment for heroin. Look under *Drug Interactions, Illicit Drugs* in Module 8. Read about heroin-drug interactions. You'll find information about the dangers of heroin addiction. Do you think heroin addiction is a serious problem in today's society? Do you think heroin is a drug that's easy to obtain? Do you think there are any heroin users on your campus? Discuss your opinions with your classmates.

euphoria of the first injection, but always have a lesser effect. There are studies, however, as well as clinical and street reports, that some people experience only nausea and discomfort after the initial intravenous administration of morphine or heroin. For whatever reasons, some of these users persist and the discomfort decreases—that is, it shows tolerance more rapidly than the euphoric effects. Under these conditions the injections soon result primarily in pleasant effects. To maintain these pleasurable feelings, though, the dose level must gradually be increased. It is true, however, that even with the narcotics some users must partially learn which experiences are defined as pleasurable. One author has referred to the two "powerfully pleasurable effects"—the initial brief rush and then the longer tranquility—and then commented,

> This sequence of events occurs with virtually every nontolerant person, although the first few experiences may be accompanied by vomiting. Even so, the sensations are often pleasurable ("You don't mind vomiting behind smack").[35]

Another misconception has to do with the development of withdrawal symptoms. The heroin user undergoing withdrawal without medication is always portrayed as being in excruciating pain, truly suffering. It depends. With a large habit, withdrawal without medication is truly hell. The opioid abuse scene is changing too rapidly to be definite about today's user, but many street users are described as having "ice cream habits"—they use a low daily drug dose. In one study of individuals who applied for treatment, after being given an injection of the narcotic antagonist naloxone, about one-fifth of the clients showed no withdrawal at all, and about another fifth showed only very mild reactions.[31]

Perhaps the most common misconception about heroin is that, after one shot, you are hooked for life. None of the narcotics, or any other drug, fits into that fantasized category. Becoming dependent takes some time, perhaps a week or more, and persistence on the part of the beginner. Regular use of the drug seems to be more important in establishing physical dependence than the size of the dose used. Becoming physically dependent is possible on a weekend, but it frequently requires a longer period, with three or four injections a day.

There are probably about 500,000 narcotic-dependent individuals in the United States. There may be two to three times as many heroin *chippers*—occasional users. Several reports and studies have appeared on the characteristics of these occasional users, but no consistent differences, compared with heroin-dependent persons, have yet been found other than the pattern of use.

New Users, New Drugs

Heroin dependence will continue to appear in various groups in each new generation. In each generation, low-class junkies are joined by a small group of young, wealthy, "respectable" heroin users, both in the United States and Europe. Black tar first appeared on the streets in 1986. As if the variable nature of street heroin coming from different sources around the world weren't confusing enough, the street scene became further complicated by the presence of various synthetic drugs. Street users learned about fentanyl, a potent prescription narcotic available in sterile solution for injection. Illicit chemists developed derivatives of fentanyl and sold them on the streets as "China White" or

"synthetic heroin." The interesting thing about these designer drugs is that the chemists were able to vary the molecule to produce drugs that had not yet been listed as controlled substances. Since 1988, it has been illegal to make or sell such designer drugs, if they have a chemical structure or a pharmacological effect similar to an already controlled substance.

Another synthetic heroin, MPPP, which is a derivative of meperidine (Demerol), was produced by a few illicit laboratories. However, there is substantial danger of trace amounts of the impurity MPTP being included, and this incredibly toxic substance was responsible for the occurrence of permanent brain damage in several users in the 1980s. MPTP results in the destruction of dopamine neurons, leading to a form of Parkinson's disease.

By the 1990s, heroin was being brought into the United States in larger quantities through a variety of routes. The increased purity of most of the samples increased the danger of overdoses, and the DAWN emergency room and coroners' reports reflected that increased danger. Anyone buying heroin on the street these days faces multiple risks, and the only regulation seems to be that famous old free-market concept *caveat emptor* ("let the buyer beware").

TREATMENT OF NARCOTIC DEPENDENCE

History

Dependence on opium, and later on morphine and heroin, is a very old problem with a long history of varied treatments. A 1902 medical book on the subject of morphinism described a variety of approaches to treatment, concerned mainly with reducing the morphine intake either slowly or more rapidly (over a few days' time) and dealing with the withdrawal symptoms.[36] The danger of relapse was recognized, with the author recommending cold showers, travel abroad, or a temporary change of lifestyle, such as going west to work on a cattle ranch or in a mine. A few years later, the accepted medical "cure" involved the use of high doses of belladonna or some other anticholinergic to maintain a state of delirium for several days, after which the patient was felt to be cured of the narcotic habit.[37]

After the Harrison Act was passed in 1914, narcotics became less freely available and somewhat more expensive, even through legal sources. Not all those already dependent could afford frequent visits to a private physician. So cities around the country established public narcotic clinics to help these people. Most of the clinics gradually detoxified their clients, but some clients (such as those with chronic pain conditions) were considered incurable and were offered "social adjustment" treatment, which meant continued maintenance on a narcotic. After the passage of alcohol prohibition and the establishment of a Bureau of Narcotics, all these clinics were closed down under pressure from federal agents, and by 1925 there was no longer a legal source of treatment that included providing narcotics for maintenance.

Federal prisons had become choked with narcotic abusers by 1930. That and the repeal of Prohibition led to the reorganization of the Bureau of Narcotics under Harry Anslinger and the establishment of two federal treatment facilities, one in Lexington, Kentucky, and the other in Fort Worth, Texas. The center at Lexington was the first and the more important and served as a combination prison farm, treatment center, and research center where the medical and psychological staff searched for a cure for narcotic dependence. The treatment consisted of gradual withdrawal using morphine, followed by a stay of up to a year, during which the clients worked on the farm and took advantage of the recreational facilities, all the while undergoing psychotherapy and participating in various tests and experiments. The relapse rate after this type of treatment appeared to be above 80 percent and never got much better than that.[37] This was

the major approach to treating narcotic dependence into the 1960s, at least partly because Anslinger remained adamantly opposed throughout his career, which ended in 1962, to any outpatient treatment program that included giving narcotics to clients.

Current Medical Approaches

Narcotic Antagonists

Research at Lexington revealed some interesting properties of drugs such as nalorphine, naloxone, and cyclazocine. When given to dependent persons who had been taking morphine, these drugs precipitated a withdrawal syndrome immediately. And these drugs blocked the effects of morphine, heroin, and other narcotics. Could these narcotic antagonists be a cure for heroin abuse? If a dependent individual were first withdrawn from the narcotic and then given the antagonist on a chronic basis, relapse should not be a problem. If a person were to try taking heroin, it would have no effect. Although there would be no negative consequence, other than the waste of money, eventually the individual would learn to stop taking heroin, thus curing the dependence. The problem is, of course, that the individual must be highly motivated to take the antagonist. Some of the antagonists, particularly cyclazocine, produce unpleasant side effects. Naloxone, which produces fairly pure antagonism with few side effects, is a short-acting drug that must be taken several times a day to maintain constant antagonism.

With all these difficulties, reports on the effectiveness of narcotic antagonist treatment have not been very promising. More recent experiments have used naltrexone, a long-acting antagonist that was released for marketing as a prescription drug under the brand name Trexan in 1985. A 50 mg tablet can antagonize the effects of a large dose of heroin for 24 hours and a smaller dose for 2 days or more, and it can therefore be given as infrequently as three times a week. Although naltrexone therapy has been shown to be effective in the treatment of opioid abuse, this therapy appears to be appropriate for only highly motivated individuals because most opioid abusers enrolled in naltrexone therapy programs prematurely discontinue treatment. To circumvent naltrexone compliance problems, a new depot formulation of naltrexone, which requires one administration per month, is currently being studied as a potential treatment medication for opioid abuse. In a recent investigation of depot naltrexone, psychologist Sandra Comer and her colleagues[38] injected recently detoxified heroin-dependent individuals with either 1 or 2 naltrexone injections and evaluated the effects of intravenous heroin over a 6-week period. The single naltrexone injection blocked heroin-related euphoria for 4 weeks, and the double naltrexone injection blocked subjective effects for as long as 6 weeks. We can expect to see depot naltrexone receive continued research attention. An interesting problem arises if a patient on naltrexone is involved in an accident and requires some pain relief. Current practice is to give high doses of hydromorphone (Dilaudid) to overcome the antagonism. This should, of course, be done only in a hospital and with extreme caution.

Methadone Maintenance

Methadone (Dolophine) is a synthetic narcotic analgesic developed in Germany during World War II, and it was found to be a substitute for the then-unavailable opium-based agents. It is quite effective when taken orally, and it has a long duration of action. The long duration means not only that it needs to be taken less frequently to prevent withdrawal symptoms but also that, because the drug leaves the body slowly, the withdrawal symptoms are less severe. Although long approved as a narcotic analgesic, methadone gained fame as a drug useful in treatment programs for heroin dependence.

The initial study in this area was started in 1964 by Dole and Nyswander, a husband-wife

team in New York City. In their initial work, heroin users were given 20 to 30 mg of methadone orally every day; this was gradually increased over four to six weeks to 80 to 120 mg given orally once a day. The theory behind the use of methadone to help rehabilitate heroin users is that the long-lasting effects of methadone prevent withdrawal symptoms and block the pleasurable effects of opiates. It disrupts the

> pattern of swinging between the states of heroin intoxication and the withdrawal syndrome. "There are three states in the heroin addict's life," says Dr. Dole. "He's either 'straight' (feeling normal), 'high,' or 'sick.' He wakes up sick, takes a shot, and gets high. That lasts a couple of hours, maybe, until he begins coming off the high, and then he'll take another shot if he can get it. He spends very little time being straight, so he usually is not able to hold a job or live normally; he's pretty much a lost soul."[39]

The initial report of the effectiveness of this treatment program on 750 criminal heroin abusers was spectacular:

> A four year trial of methadone blockade treatment has shown 94% success in ending the criminal activity of former heroin addicts. The majority of these patients are now productively employed, living as responsible citizens, and supporting families. The results show unequivocally that criminal addicts can be rehabilitated by a well-supervised maintenance program.[40]

Methadone programs expanded rapidly after these reports. Why did we so readily accept the switching of heroin users from one narcotic to another? Could we really condone having government-supported narcotic users walking around the streets? Perhaps programs of this type would not have been possible if Harry Anslinger had not retired in 1962, but one of his major concerns could be avoided. Because methadone can be effective if taken only once or twice a day, the user could be required to go to the clinic and take the drug under supervision. Thus, heroin users were not being supplied with drugs that they could take out on the streets and sell or give to others. Also, there was some confusion over whether methadone was acting purely as a narcotic or whether it had some antagonist properties as well. Note that it was indicated that methadone treatment tended to block the pleasurable effects of heroin and that the program was referred to as methadone "blockade" treatment by its proponents. This apparent blockade was probably a result of the buildup to high doses of methadone used in the initial studies. The heroin users became tolerant to greater levels of narcotic, and the rather small amount of heroin available in most street bags at that time had little effect in a person with such a tolerance. It could be seen as ironic that narcotic dependence was being treated by creating an even greater level of tolerance. Current programs use lower doses, usually under 100 mg per day.

The ethics and morality of the methadone approach were raised early:

> Although there is no question that methadone maintenance treatment is an effective way of reducing the criminalistic activities of drug addicts, it is a question who is being treated: society or the drug takers. . . . Each physician who prescribes methadone to a narcotic addict has this moral question to answer: Is he maintaining the patient on drugs for the good of society or for the good of his individual patient? Is he encouraging a kind of "cop out" by reinforcing the hopeless feeling of drug addicts when he wonders whether he can renounce drug use?[41]

Remember, too, that the 1960s were a time when the majority of problem heroin users were African American and there was simultaneously a focus on racial awareness. The idea that large numbers of people might be expected to spend the rest of their lives, dependent on a substance, becoming passive suppliants who report to a clinic twice daily for counseling, appeared to

some minority leaders to be a frightening experiment in social control.

Despite these concerns, methadone maintenance continues to be accepted as the most effective approach to heroin dependence. Available methadone programs take on a wide variety of forms, ranging from simple storefront drug handouts to more elaborate evaluation, treatment, and job counseling programs. The effectiveness of methadone treatment can be measured in several ways: heroin use declines dramatically, drug-related problems drop, measures of psychological depression decline, commission of nondrug-defined crimes is reduced significantly, and permanent employment is increased. There is some division over the primary reason for the effectiveness of methadone. Early workers emphasized the chemical aspects of the program: preventing withdrawal symptoms and craving and blocking the pleasurable effects of heroin. Others see the need for daily appearances at the clinic and the opportunities for frequent counseling as the major reasons for success, with the methadone merely providing a reason for such tight control. One recent report indicated that some supplementary counseling is beneficial but that high levels of additional support are not cost-effective.[42]

LAAM

In 1993, the FDA approved another synthetic opiate, L-alpha-acetyl-methadol (**LAAM**), for use in treating narcotic-dependent persons. Because LAAM is metabolized in the liver to an active metabolite, it has much longer-lasting effects than methadone. Instead of daily visits, treatment clients are able to take the drug only three times a week, which is the major advantage of LAAM. In addition, however, clients report

LAAM: L-alpha-acetyl-methadol; a very long-lasting synthetic opiate approved for maintenance treatment of narcotic-dependent persons.

feeling less of a narcotic effect from LAAM, which, it is hoped, will ease the transition to a drug-free state.[43]

Both methadone and LAAM maintenance are tightly controlled by the DEA and FDA. Methadone is a regular prescription drug available in both injectable and oral forms for pain relief. But maintenance of opioid-dependent individuals has now been formally defined in federal law, and only oral methadone and LAAM are considered safe and effective for this use by the FDA. And this use is not available to every physician, because the FDA still classifies even methadone maintenance as investigational, allowing its use only under approved protocols and by approved clinics. The average American physician is still prohibited from providing any narcotic to a dependent person for the purpose of maintaining the dependence.

Why don't all heroin users simply sign up for free methadone instead of taking heroin? If their drug-taking behavior were motivated only by the "need" for a narcotic, this would make sense. But let's not forget why most of these people use heroin in the first place: to be part of a subculture, to make a statement about their relationship to the dominant society, or for the experience. And let's not forget that the major reason for continuing to use heroin is probably the positive reinforcement produced by the rapid rise in blood levels of heroin immediately after an intravenous injection (the rush). Slow-acting oral methadone or LAAM won't produce any of these effects.

Buprenorphine

Because a large number of opioid-dependent individuals do not respond to currently available treatment medications, the search for more effective pharmacotherapies continues. One such drug that has received much research attention in this regard is the semisynthetic opioid analgesic buprenorphine. Although not yet FDA-approved for the treatment of opioid dependence, buprenorphine is currently available as an analgesic and is expected to receive FDA

approval for opioid dependence in the near future. Buprenorphine is a partial opioid agonist. This means that it has a relatively large margin of safety and a low overdose potential. Additionally, because buprenorphine has a long duration of action and detaches very slowly from opioid receptors, its occupancy of these receptors blocks the effects of heroin and other opioid agonists. Consistent with this notion, a growing number of scientists have reported that intravenous heroin self-administration is significantly reduced when heroin-dependent research participants are maintained on buprenorphine.[44, 45] These features, along with the fact that buprenorphine requires only once-a-day dosing, should make it a viable future option in the treatment of opioid dependence.

Heroin/Morphine Maintenance

If we are now willing to supply dependent individuals with narcotics, and if they want heroin, why don't we just supply them with heroin and clean syringes and let them inject it intravenously? There are some obvious inconveniences compared with methadone, including the need to administer the drug several times a day and the use of the needles for intravenous injection. Also, there's the aspect of heroin use mentioned by Dole and Nyswander—the intravenous heroin user spends a lot of time reacting to the previous shot or worrying about the next one, with relatively brief periods (only a few hours at a time) of feeling straight. Oral methadone produces less "up and down" in the blood level of the narcotic and can be more conducive to participating in work, school, or other productive activities. But the major impediment to such an approach is probably the long history Americans have of viewing heroin as an evil substance rather than as just another narcotic.

Actually, the public clinics that existed in several cities until around 1920 can give us some idea of the utility of providing the abuser's drug of choice, which was usually morphine but was in some cases heroin or codeine. Although Harry Anslinger said many times in later years

Taking Sides

Tough Moral Stances Versus Harm Reduction

Several authors over the years have pointed out that legal restrictions on the availability of a drug often lead to the use of a more potent (more easily smuggled) and therefore likely more dangerous form of drug use. Examples abound in the history of the opiates: the Chinese tobacco smokers who switched to opium smoking and the opiate abusers in this country who switched to intravenous heroin when narcotics became so expensive.

A more contemporary issue has to do with the availability of sterile needles for intravenous drug users. In several cities, needle exchange programs have been developed whereby dependent individuals are able to obtain clean needles. In other cities, these programs have been met with scorn.

The needle exchange program in Liverpool, England, was one of the first successful demonstrations that the spread of HIV could be slowed if clean needles were readily available, and its designers based their approach on what they call a "harm reduction" model of drug control. At issue is the ultimate goal of our drug-control policies. If it is to reduce the amount of danger and harm to the population in general, then perhaps needle exchange programs and other changes in enforcement practices are in order.

How do you feel? Is it more important to reduce the amount of harm done by drug use, or is it more important for our society to take a firm moral stand in hopes of preventing the further spread of drug use?

For more on this topic, log on to www.dushkin.com/online for current news and links to other popular and informative sites, as well as time-saving web search strategies and study tools.

---

that these clinics did not work and were hotbeds of criminal activity, a 1974 in-depth review of the clinic in Shreveport, Louisiana, gave a more positive assessment.[46] Most of the clients of that program were employed, most were middle-aged, and most had become dependent as a result of medical treatment. The clinic apparently provided an important service for those individuals and has been viewed as a model of what might have been. Of course, that clinic refused admission to people suspected of being criminals and encouraged "bums" or "loafers" to leave town instead of offering them treatment. The individuals it did serve could in no way be seen as representative of today's heroin-abusing population.

A great deal has been said about the British system, in which heroin users can register and receive heroin for purposes of treating their dependence. Actually, for years there really wasn't a system at all. Britain simply never took the step of outlawing the medical use of heroin or the prescribing of narcotics to abusers by physicians. Thus, until 1968, there was no program: British heroin abusers simply obtained a prescription from their physicians just as they would for any other drug. Some Americans, noting that there were few narcotic-dependent individuals in Britain before the 1960s, suggested that the major cause of our much greater narcotic dependence problem lay in our attempts to control it.[16] We'll never know the answer to that one: even though America and England seem quite similar in many ways, they are far from the same society, either now or in the 1920s.

The British were not immune to the social change of the 1960s, and one reflection of that change was that some British youth began to experiment with drugs. Individuals who went to their physicians for heroin and who had developed the dependence recreationally were reported to the Home Office as nontherapeutic heroin users. The number of such individuals increased from 47 in 1959 to 222 in 1963. That might not seem like many, compared with half a million in the United States, but the increase gave support to those who wanted tighter controls. Noting that a few physicians were writing prescriptions for large amounts of heroin, it was concluded that not every physician should be trusted completely where narcotics abusers were concerned. By 1968, the new system had been put in place: British physicians could still prescribe any medication, including heroin, to nondependent persons. But heroin-dependent individuals had to register as such and could receive heroin or cocaine only from specially licensed physicians in drug-dependence clinics, which were established in several areas. During the 1970s, these clinics dispensed less and less heroin and more and more counseling and oral methadone. By 1978, only 9 percent of the clinic clients were receiving heroin, either alone or in combination with other drugs.[47]

In Britain, narcotic dependence has continued to increase, an illicit market for heroin has developed, and crime rates have increased. However, the British still have a much smaller heroin problem than the United States: with a total population about one-fourth that of the United States, Britain probably has less than one-thirtieth the number of heroin abusers.[23] It is certainly ironic that the United States, viewed as the world leader in the control of opioids and in narcotic treatment, continues to be the leader in numbers of heroin users.

Several other countries have explored the idea of providing heroin to users. Switzerland began a program of heroin prescription in 1993 and by 1995 had reported a drop in the proportion of burglaries, robberies, and auto thefts committed by drug users.[48] The Australian parliament voted in 1997 to try such an experiment, but it was vetoed by the prime minister.

Rapid Opioid Detoxification

Around the beginning of the twentieth century, long before treatment of opiate dependence was guided by sound scientific evidence, some physicians treated opiate abusers by administering drugs that produced a state of delirium for several days, after which the opiate abuser would emerge, detoxified and supposedly cured from the opiate habit without remembering the experience of the withdrawal process. This view of equating opiate treatment with withdrawal from opiates came back in a big way in the 1990s, with a new twist.

Opioid-dependent individuals are anesthetized and, while unconscious, are given naltrexone, so that they will experience immediate withdrawal. After 24 hours the patients are released and enter a period of counseling, combined with continued naltrexone treatment. The treatment costs about $7,500 in New York and could obviously generate quite a profit for the providers, who are typically organized as businesses. Although the proponents have made claims of very high success rates with this treatment, traditional treatment specialists are skeptical that this rapid technique will produce long-term abstinence because aftercare (psychosocial intervention) is often deemphasized when rapid opioid detoxification procedures are used.[49] Moreover, few patients continue naltrexone therapy for extended periods. Perhaps depot naltrexone will prove beneficial in this regard.

SUMMARY

- Opium was used in its raw form for centuries, both medicinally and for pleasure.
- Opium had significant influences on medicine, literature, and world politics through the 1800s.
- Dependence on opiates has been recognized for a long time, but no concerted effort to control dependence was tried until the patent medicine era of the late 1800s, combined with opium smoking by Chinese Americans, led to federal regulations in the early 1900s.
- The typical opiate abuser changed from being a middle-aged, middle-class woman using narcotics by mouth to being a young, lower-class man using heroin by intravenous injection.

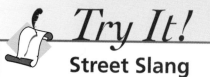

Try It!

Street Slang

Draw lines to match these street terms for drugs and related terms (left-hand column) with the appropriate term or definition in the right-hand column:

Black tar

Chipper

Smack

Dime bag

China white

Works

Jones

Heroin

Fentanyl or a derivative

Withdrawal symptoms

Occasional heroin user

Injecting equipment (syringe or dropper)

$10 worth of heroin

A type of illicit heroin

- Various synthetic narcotics are now available along with the natural products of the opium poppy. These drugs all act at opioid receptors in the brain.
- Opioid receptors are normally acted on by the naturally occurring opioid-like products of the nervous system and endocrine glands, endorphins and enkephalins.
- The narcotic overdose triad consists of coma, depressed respiration, and pinpoint pupils. Death occurs because breathing ceases.
- Illicit heroin comes primarily from Southeast Asia, Southwest Asia, and Mexico.
- Opioid dependents have been offered a wide variety of treatments, but the most effective in reducing crime and relapse has been methadone maintenance.
- A longer-acting synthetic opiate, LAAM, is now available for maintenance treatment.
- Although the British continue to make heroin available for pain relief and treatment of dependent individuals, most British dependent individuals in treatment are now maintained on methadone.

Web Watch

Check Out Publications on Narcotics
The National Clearing House for Drug and Alcohol Information offers a listing of publications about certain types of drugs. Go to the following sites to find and, if you wish, order brochures or other publications about heroin and morphine, www.health.org/catalog/catalog.asp?key=8&detail5false and opiates and narcotics, www.health.org/catalog/catalog.asp?key=11&detail=false.

Read a Heroin Overview
At www.cocaineaddiction.com/other_heroin.html, read an overview of heroin. You will find information on addiction, the history of heroin, its effects, its treatment, study results, and related statistics.

Learn About Heroin Addiction and Treatment
To find information about heroin addiction, go to www.heroinaddiction.com. You'll find updated facts news articles, photos, stories, and links related to heroin addiction. You'll also discover information about the Narcon rehabilitation program.

REVIEW QUESTIONS

1. What two chemicals are extracted from the opium poppy? *morphine/codine*
2. What was the significance of De Quincey's writing about opium eating?
3. What were the approximate dates and who were the combatants in the Opium Wars?
4. How is it possible that heroin was at first sold as a nonaddicting pain reliever?
5. How did the typical opiate abuser change from the early 1900s to the 1920s?
6. Why and when did private physicians and public clinics stop maintaining dependent individuals with morphine and other opiates?
7. What were some of the lessons learned about heroin dependence as a result of the Vietnam experience?
8. What two factors were probably responsible for the increase in the smoking of heroin in 1989 and 1990?
9. What is the effect of a narcotic antagonist on someone who has developed a physical dependence on opioids?
10. What are the enkephalins and endorphins, and how do they relate to plant-derived opiates such as morphine?
11. What are the relative advantages and disadvantages of methadone, LAAM, and heroin maintenance?

REFERENCES

1. Baum LF: *The new wizard of Oz.* New York: Grosset & Dunlap, 1944.
2. Scott JM: *The white poppy: A history of opium.* New York: Funk & Wagnalls, 1969.

3. Hamarneh S: Sources and development of Arabic medical therapy and pharmacology, *Sudhoffs Archiv fur Geschichte der Medizin und der Naturwissenschaften* 54:34, 1970.

4. De Quincey T: *Confessions of an English opium-eater.* New York: EP Dutton, 1907.

5. Turk MH: *Selections from De Quincey.* Boston: Ginn & Co, 1902.

6. De Quincey works, vol 206. Quoted in Lowes JL: *The road to Xanadu.* Boston: Houghton Mifflin, 1927.

7. Blair W: An opium-eater in America. *The Knickerbocker* 20:47–57, 1842.

8. Kramer JC: Opium rampant: Medical use, misuse and abuse in Britain and the West in the 17th and 18th centuries, *British Journal of Addiction*: 377, 1979.

9. Kramer JC: Heroin in the treatment of morphine addiction, *Journal of Psychedelic Drugs* 9(3):193–197, 1977.

10. Dott DB, Stockman R: *Proceedings of the Royal Society of Edinburgh,* p 321, 1890.

11. Manges M: A second report on the therapeutics of heroine, *New York Medical Journal* 71:51, 82–83, 1900.

12. Wilcox RW: *Pharmacology and therapeutics* (6th ed.). Philadelphia: P. Blakiston's Son, 1905.

13. Lindesmith AR: *Addiction and opiates.* Chicago: Aldine, 1968.

14. Kebler LF: The present status of drug addiction in the United States. In *Transactions of the American Therapeutic Society.* Philadelphia: FA Davis, 1910.

15. Black JR: Advantages of substituting the morphia habit for the incurably alcoholic, *The Cincinnati Lancet—Clinic* 22:538–541, 1889.

16. Lindesmith AR: *The addict and the law.* Bloomington: Indiana University Press, 1965.

17. Smith R: Status politics and the image of the addict, *Issues in Criminology* 2(2):157–175, 1966.

18. Preble E, Casey JJ Jr: Taking care of business—the heroin user's life on the street, The *International Journal of the Addictions* 4(1):1–24, 1969.

19. Isbell H: Discussion, Symposium on Problems of Drug Dependence, Fourteenth Annual Conference Veterans Administration Cooperative Studies in Psychiatry, Houston, Texas, Apr. 1, 1969, Highlights of the Conference, Veterans Administration, Washington, DC: U.S. Government Printing Office, 1969.

20. *Inquiry into alleged drug abuse in the armed services.* Report of a special subcommittee of the Committee on Armed Services, House of Representatives, Ninety-second Congress, First Session, Apr 23, 1971. Washington, DC: U.S. Government Printing Office, 1971.

21. *The world heroin problem.* Committee Print, House of Representatives, Committee on Foreign Affairs, Ninety-second Congress, First Session, May 27, 1971. Washington, DC: U.S. Government Printing Office, 1971.

22. Robins LN: *The Vietnam drug user returns,* Special Action Office for Drug Abuse Prevention Monograph, Series A, No. 2, May 1974, Contract No. HSM-42-72-75.

23. Brodsky MD: History of heroin prevalence estimation techniques. In *Self-report methods of estimating drug use,* NIDA Research Monograph No. 57. Washington, DC: U.S. Government Printing Office, 1985.

24. National Narcotics Intelligence Consumers Committee: *The supply of illicit drugs to the United States.* Washington, DC: 1996.

25. Schoemer, K: Rockers, models, and the new allure of heroin, *Newsweek* Aug 26, 1996.

26. Wren CS: View that smoking heroin is safer than injecting is questioned, *New York Times* Dec 1, 1996.

27. Feldman RS, Meyer JS, Quenzer LF: *Principles of neuropsychopharmacology.* Sunderland, MA: Sinauer, 1997.

28. Zadina JE and others: A potent and selective endogenous agonist for the μ-opiate receptor. *Nature* 386:499, 1997.

29. Siegel S: Morphine analgesic tolerance: Its situation specificity supports a pavlovian conditioning model, *Science* 193:323–325, 1976.

30. Siegel S and others: Heroin "overdose" death: Contribution of drug-associated environmental cues, *Science* 216:436–437, 1982.

31. Powell DH: A pilot study of occasional heroin users, *Arch Gen Psychiatry* 28:586–594, 1973.

32. O'Brien CP: "Needle freaks": Psychological dependence on shooting up. In *Medical World News,* Psychiatry Annual. New York: McGraw-Hill, 1974.

33. Louria DB, Hensle T, Rose J: The major medical complications of heroin addiction, *Annals of Internal Medicine* 67:1–22, 1967.

34. Winick C: Maturing out of narcotic addiction, *Bulletin on Narcotics* 14(1):1–8, 1962.

35. Goldstein A: Heroin addiction and the role of methadone in its treatment, *Archives of General Psychiatry* 26:291–297, 1972.

36. Crothers TD: *Morphinism and narcomanias from other drugs,* (reprint ed.). New York: Arno Press, 1981.

37. Latimer D, Goldberg J: *Flowers in the blood: The story of opium.* New York: Arno Press, 1981.

38. Comer SD and others: Time course and effectiveness of a depot formulation of naltrexone in antagonizing IV heroin in humans, *Psychopharmacology,* 2001.

39. Methadone maintenance: How much, for whom, for how long? *Medical World News* pp 53–63, Mar 17, 1972.

40. Dole VP, Nyswander ME, Warner A: Successful treatment of 750 criminal addicts, *JAMA* 206:2708–2714, 1968.

41. Myerson DJ: Methadone treatment of addicts, *New England Journal of Medicine* 281:390–391, 1969.

42. Kraft MK and others: Are supplementary services provided during methadone maintenance really cost-effective? *American Journal of Psychiatry* 154:1214–1219, 1997.

43. Swan N: Treatment practitioners learn about LAAM, *NIDA Notes* 9(1):5, 1994.

44. Mello NK, Mendelson JH, Kuehnle JC: Buprenorphine effects on human heroin self-administration: An operant analysis. *Journal of Pharmacology and Experimental Therapeutics* 223:30–39, 1982.

45. Comer SD, Collins ED, Fischman MW: Buprenorphine sublingual tablets: Effects on IV heroin self-administration by humans. *Psychopharmacology,* 2001.

46. Waldorf D, Orlich M, Reinerman C: *Morphine maintenance: the Shreveport clinic 1919–1923.* Washington, DC: The Drug Abuse Council, 1974.

47. Trebach AS: *The heroin solution.* New Haven, CT: Yale University Press, 1982.

48. Killias M, Uchtenhagen A: On the evaluation of the Swiss heroin prescription projects and its methodology. In *Studies on crime and crime prevention* (Vol. 5). National Council for Crime Prevention, 1996.

49. Mathews J: A solution of substance for substance abuse? *The Washington Post* Dec 3, 1996.

Chapter 17

Hallucinogens

KEY TERMS

animism

phantastica

psychedelic

psychotomimetic

indole

synesthesia

psilocybin

peyote

mescaline

PCP

angel dust

Online Learning Center Resources

www.mhhe.com/ray

Log on to our Online Learning Center (OLC) for access to these additional resources.

- Chapter definitions
- Learning objectives
- Student interactive question-and-answer sites
- Self-scoring chapter quiz

The OLC also offers web links for study and exploration of health topics. Here are some examples of what you'll find:

www.schoolwork.org/drugs.html

This site offers a variety of links to articles and to the web pages of drug-abuse prevention organizations. Scroll down to check out the links to sites on ecstasy, LSD, and PCP.

www.drugwarfacts.org

This site offers up-to-date bar graphs and statistics that tell the story of the war on drugs.

www.drug-abuse.com/information

This site provides information on various kinds of drugs, including PCP, designer drugs, LSD, methamphetamine, and ecstasy.

Drugs in the Media

The Psychedelic Sixties—Reflections in Film, Music, and Literature

In a peculiar interaction between a new drug phenomenon (experimenting with perception-altering drugs, such as LSD) and a time of many radical changes in American society (the civil rights move-ment, the war in Vietnam, the British invasion of popular music led by the Beatles), a cultural mixture was formed that we now call "the psychedelic sixties" (which for most people probably coincided with the

Drugs in the Media Continued. . .

decade 1965 to 1975). All you need to do is to look at popular films from that time or at photographs of relatives to see the influence on hairstyles and clothing. But what was psychedelic about this period, and was it in fact important or interesting from a cultural or an artistic perspective?

One can see the transition in the music of the Beatles. Their early work sounded a lot like mainstream rock and roll, but a visit to India and experimentation with various drugs changed the way they sounded, dressed, and talked. And they in turn influenced many others.

What other writers, artists, and musicians are associated with this phenomenon? The Grateful Dead and Jefferson Airplane may have started it all in music, and Ken Kesey may have started it all in literature, but no

popular figure could ignore the influence. Perhaps its most obvious presentation can be seen by looking at album covers, the cardboard jackets that contained the long-playing record albums of the era. To say that the art form of these music-album covers flowered during that period would be both a pun and an understatement.

The University of Virginia library supports a virtual exhibition on a website, www.lib.virginia.edu/exhibits/sixties/, called The Psychedelic Sixties: Literary Tradition and Social Change. There you can read about the music, the social protests, the literature, and the big events that shaped the period, and you can view enough psychedelic art to satisfy anyone's curiosity.

From the soft, quiet beauty of the sacred *Psilocybe* mushroom to the angry, mottled appearance of the toxic *Amanita,* from the mountains of Mexico to the streets of Anytown, USA, from before history to the end of the twentieth century, humans have searched for the perfect aphrodisiac, spiritual experiences, and other worlds. The plants have been there to help; it's worth repeating that plants have evolved to produce chemicals that alter the biochemistry of animals. If they make us feel sick, we are unlikely to eat them again, and if they kill us, we are certain not to eat them again. But humans long ago learned to "tame" some of these plants, to use them in just the right ways and in just the right amounts to alter perceptions and emotions without too many unpleasant consequences.

ANIMISM AND RELIGION

Animism, the belief that animals, plants, rocks, streams, and so on derive their special characteristics from a spirit contained within the object, is

a common theme in most of the world's religions. Plants that are able to alter our perception of the world and of ourselves fit right into such a view. If the plant contains a spirit, then eating the plant transfers that spirit to the person who eats it, and the spirit of the plant can speak to the consumer, make her feel the plant's joy or provide her with special powers or insights.

In early hunter-gatherer societies, certain individuals became specialists in the ways of these plants, learning when to harvest them and how much to use under what circumstances. These traditions were passed down from one generation to another, and colorful stories were used to teach the principles to apprentices. Our modern term for these individuals is *shaman* or *medicine man/woman* because of their knowledge of drug-containing plants. But because they also were the experts on obtaining power from the spirit world, their function in hunter-gatherer societies had as much to do with the origins of religion as with the origins of modern medicine. These plants and their psychoactive effects were probably important reasons for the development of spiritual and religious traditions and folklore in many societies all over the world.[1]

TERMINOLOGY AND TYPES

The issue of what to call this group of drugs is an old one. In 1931, Lewin referred to a class of **phantastica,** drugs that can create in our minds a world of fantasy. Peyote, psilocybin, and LSD all produce this type of effect. In the 1960s, these drugs were described by enthusiastic users as allowing them to see into their own minds, and the term **psychedelic** ("mind-viewing") was widely used. The term itself implies a beneficial, visionary type of effect, and there is considerable disagreement over whether such effects are really beneficial. Because the drugs are capable of producing hallucinations and some altered sense of reality, a state that could be called psychotic, they have also been referred to as **psychotomimetic** drugs. This term implies that the drugs produce dangerous effects and produce a form of mental disorder, which is also a controversial conclusion.

More recently, proponents have popularized newer terms, such as *entheogen* and *entactogen,* to describe these substances. For example, *entheogen* is used to describe substances (e.g., sacred mushrooms) that are thought to create spiritual or religious experiences, whereas *entactogen,* meaning "to produce a touching within," is used to describe substances, such as MDMA, that are said to enhance feeling of empathy.

Is there a descriptive and unbiased term that will allow us to categorize the drugs and then to examine their effects without prejudice? One thing common to these drugs is some tendency to produce hallucinations, so we will refer to them by the name *hallucinogens.*

PHANTASTICA

Although we will call all of these drugs hallucinogens, there are important differences among them. They can be classified according to their chemical structures, their known pharmacological properties, how much loss of awareness occurs under their influence, and how dangerous they are. The first types we will review are the classical phantastica: they are capable of altering perceptions while allowing the person to remain in communication with the present world. The individual under the influence of these drugs will often be aware of both the fantasy world and the real world at the same time, might talk avidly about what is being experienced, and will be able to remember much of it later. These drugs can be seen as having more purely hallucinogenic effects in that they do not produce much acute physiological toxicity—that is, there is relatively little danger of dying from an overdose of LSD, psilocybin, or mescaline. The two major classes of phantastica, the indole and catechol hallucinogens, are grouped according to their chemical structures.

Indole Hallucinogens

The basic structure of the neurotransmitter serotonin is referred to as an **indole** nucleus. Figure 17.1 illustrates that the hallucinogens LSD and psilocybin also contain this structure. For that reason and the fact that some other chemicals with this structure have similar hallucinogenic effects, we refer to one group of the phantastica as the indoles.

d-Lysergic Acid Diethylamide (LSD)

The most potent and notorious of the hallucinogens, and the one that brought these drugs into the public eye in the 1960s, is not found in nature at all. Although there are naturally occurring compounds that resemble the indole *d*-lysergic acid diethylamide (LSD), their identity as hallucinogens was not known until after the discovery of LSD. LSD was originally synthesized from ergot alkaloids extracted from the ergot fungus *Claviceps purpurea.* This mold occasionally grows on grain, especially rye, and eating infected grain results in an illness called *ergotism.*

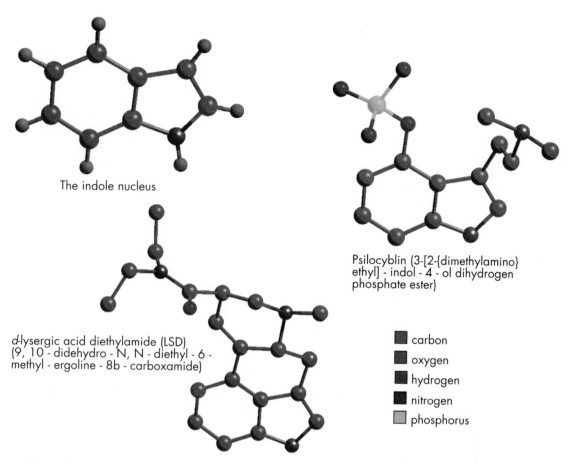

The indole nucleus

Psilocyblin (3-[2-{dimethylamino} ethyl] - indol - 4 - ol dihydrogen phosphate ester)

d-lysergic acid diethylamide (LSD) (9, 10 - didehydro - N, N - diethyl - 6 - methyl - ergoline - 8b - carboxamide)

■ carbon
■ oxygen
■ hydrogen
■ nitrogen
■ phosphorus

Figure 7.1   Indole hallucinogens.

Saint Anthony's Fire.   Grain that has been infected with the ergot fungus is readily identified and is usually destroyed. During periods of famine, however, the grain might be used in making bread. In France between A.D. 945 and 1600, there were at least 20 outbreaks of ergotism, the illness that results from eating infected bread. Although the cause of the illness was established before 1700, only symptomatic treatment exists even today. There are two forms of the disease. In one, there are tingling sensations in the skin and muscle spasms that develop into convulsions, insomnia, and various disturbances of consciousness and thinking. In the other

animism: the belief that objects attain certain characteristics because of spirits.

phantastica: (fan *tass* tick a) drugs that create a world of fantasy.

psychedelic: (sy ka *dell* ick) "mind-viewing." *See into your own mind*

psychotomimetic: (sy cot o mim *et* ick) mimicking psychosis.

indole: (*in* dole) a particular chemical structure found in serotonin and LSD.

form, gangrenous ergotism, the limbs become swollen and inflamed, with the individual experiencing "violent burning pains" before the affected part becomes numb. Sometimes the disease moves rapidly, with less than 24 hours between the first sign and the development of gangrene. Gangrene develops because the ergot causes a contraction of the blood vessels, cutting off blood flow to the extremities.

During the twelfth century, ergotism became associated with Saint Anthony, although the reason for this is not completely clear. It might be that the hospital for the treatment of ergotism was built near the shrine of Saint Anthony because he had suffered from a minor attack of ergotism. Some suggest that the demons he reported battling were the result of the disease.[2] Others believe the illness was called Saint Anthony's fire because those who made the pilgrimage to Egypt, where Saint Anthony had lived, were cured. No matter, those who journeyed to Egypt and those who entered the hospital did lose their symptoms, probably as a result of a diet that did not include ergot-infected rye.

Two interesting articles discussed a possible link between convulsive ergotism and the Salem witch trials of 1692, in which 20 people were executed. The first article[3] built a very strong case that (1) the original symptoms exhibited by the "possessed" 8 girls were similar to those seen in convulsive ergotism and (2) the conditions were right for the growth of the ergot fungus on the rye that was the staple cereal. The second article[4] constructed an equally convincing case that ergotism could not have been involved and that the "possession" was psychological. In fact, we will never know for sure; there are, however, enough similarities and lingering doubts that ergotism seems to remain a possible basis for the Salem incident.

LSD Discovery and Early Research.
In the Sandoz Laboratories in Basel, Switzerland, in 1938, Dr. Albert Hofmann synthesized *lysergsaurediethylamid*, the German word from which *LSD* comes and that names the substance known in English as d-lysergic acid diethylamide. Hofmann was working on a series of compounds derived from ergot alkaloids that had as their basic structure lysergic acid. LSD was synthesized because of its chemical similarity to a known stimulant, nikethamide. It was not until 1943, however, that LSD entered the world of biochemical psychiatry, when Hofmann recorded the following in his laboratory notebook:

> Last Friday, April 16, 1943, I was forced to stop my work in the laboratory in the middle of the afternoon and to go home, as I was seized by a peculiar restlessness associated with a sensation of mild dizziness. Having reached home, I lay down and sank in a kind of drunkenness which was not unpleasant and which was characterized by extreme activity of imagination. As I lay in a dazed condition with my eyes closed (I experienced daylight as disagreeably bright) there surged upon me an uninterrupted stream of fantastic images of extraordinary plasticity and vividness and accompanied by an intense, kaleidoscope-like play of colors. This condition gradually passed off after about two hours.[5]

Hofmann later said, "The first experience was a very weak one, consisting of rather small changes. It had a pleasant, fairy tale–magic theater quality."[6] He was sure that the experience resulted from the accidental absorption, through the skin of his fingers, of the compound with which he was working. The next Monday morning Hofmann prepared what he thought was a very small amount of LSD, 0.25 mg, and made the following record in his notebook:

> April 19, 1943: Preparation of an 0.5% aqueous solution of *∂*-lysergic acid diethylamide tartrate.
>
> 4:20 P.M.: 0.5 cc (0.25 mg LSD) ingested orally. The solution is tasteless.
>
> 4:50 P.M.: no trace of any effect.
>
> 5:00 P.M.: slight dizziness, unrest, difficulty in concentration, visual disturbances, marked desire to laugh.

At this point the laboratory notes are discontinued:

> The last words could only be written with great difficulty. I asked my laboratory assistant to accompany me home as I believed that my condition would be a repetition of the disturbance of the previous Friday. While we were still cycling home, however, it became clear that the symptoms were much stronger than the first time. I had great difficulty in speaking coherently, my field of vision swayed before me, and objects appeared distorted like images in curved mirrors. I had the impression of being unable to move from the spot, although my assistant told me afterwards that we had cycled at a good pace.
>
> Six hours after ingestion of the LSD-25 my condition had already improved considerably. Only the visual disturbances were still pronounced. Everything seemed to sway and the proportions were distorted like the reflections in the surface of moving water. Moreover, all objects appeared in unpleasant, constantly changing colors, the predominant shades being sickly green and blue. When I closed my eyes, an unending series of colorful, very realistic and fantastic images surged in upon me. A remarkable feature was the manner in which all acoustic perceptions (e.g., the noise of a passing car) were transformed into optical effects, every sound causing a corresponding colored hallucination constantly changing in shape and color like pictures in a kaleidoscope. At about 1 o'clock I fell asleep and awakened the next morning somewhat tired but otherwise feeling perfectly well.[5]

The amount Albert Hofmann took orally is 5 to 8 times the normal effective dose, and it was the potency of the drug that attracted attention to it. Mescaline had long been known to cause strange experiences, alter consciousness, and lead to a particularly vivid kaleidoscope of colors, but it takes 4,000 times as much mescaline as LSD. LSD is usually active when only 0.05 mg (50 µg) is taken, and in some people a dose of 0.03 mg is effective.

The first report on LSD in the scientific literature came from Zurich in 1947, but it was 1949 before the first North American study on its use in humans appeared. In 1953, Sandoz applied to the Food and Drug Administration to study LSD as an investigational new drug. Between 1953 and 1966, Sandoz distributed large quantities of LSD to qualified scientists throughout the world. Most of this legal LSD was used in biochemical and animal behavior research.

Besides an interest in trying to develop "model psychoses" in animals and humans so that treatments could be developed, the major thrust of LSD research had to do with its alleged ability to access the "subconscious mind." This notion probably derived from the dreamlike quality of the reports of LSD experiences and the long-held psychoanalytic view that dreams represent subconscious thoughts trying to express themselves. Thus, LSD was widely used as an adjunct to psychotherapy. When a psychiatrist felt that a patient had reached a roadblock and was unable to dredge up repressed memories and motives, LSD might be used for its psychedelic (mind-viewing) properties. Thus, LSD took over as a modern truth serum, replacing sodium pentothal and scopolamine. Whether LSD actually helped these patients in the long run or only seemed helpful to the psychiatrists who believed in it is still being debated.

Two other potentially therapeutic uses were studied: for various theoretical reasons it was believed that LSD might be a good treatment for alcoholics, and initial reports of its effectiveness were quite positive. Later, it was hoped that LSD would allow terminal cancer patients to achieve a greater understanding of their own mortality. Thus, many such patients were allowed to explore their feelings while under the influence of this fantasy-producing agent.

In April 1966, the Sandoz Pharmaceutical Company recalled the LSD it had distributed and withdrew its sponsorship for work with LSD. Large quantities of illegally manufactured LSD of uncertain purity were being used in the street, and Sandoz decided to give the responsibility for the legal distribution of LSD to the federal government.

Scientific study of the hallucinogens declined in the 1970s. The Reverend Walter Clark, a theologian and well-known advocate of controlled research on psychedelic drugs, provided data to support what he wrote in 1975:

> Because of bureaucratic restrictions and public fear of the highly publicized dangers of the drugs both real and supposed, responsible investigators have too often retired from the field, despite their interest in the drugs and the conviction of many that these drugs are exceedingly promising tools in mental health and for the study of the human mind and development.[7]

Dr. Clark was partially whistling in the dark, because marijuana and its active ingredients had the same bureaucratic restrictions and they had been legally studied by thousands of scientists. More probably, hallucinogenic research had reached a dead end, where new ideas were needed and not forthcoming. A 1974 report by a National Institute of Mental Health (NIMH) research task force on hallucinogenic research stated:

> Virtually every psychological test has been used to study persons under the influence of LSD or other such hallucinogens, but the research has contributed little to our understanding of the bizarre and potent effects of this drug.[8]

Partly as a reality-oriented response to this type of evaluation and partly because of the dead ends, the NIMH stopped its in-house LSD research on humans in 1968 and stopped funding university human research on LSD in 1974. The National Cancer Institute and the National Institute on Alcohol Abuse and Alcoholism stopped supporting psychedelic research in 1975 because it was nonproductive. Most of the LSD research since that time has been conducted on animals in an effort to better understand the mechanism of action at a neural level.

Although interest in the therapeutic properties of LSD has faded, there has been a renewed interest in the therapeutic properties of several other types of hallucinogens. This research is usually not funded from U.S. government sources, but much of it is supported by interested private donors through organizations such as the Multidisciplinary Association for Psychedelic Studies.

Secret Army/CIA Research with LSD.

The unveiling of CIA/army human research programs using hallucinogens began with a June 1975 report by the Rockefeller Commission on the CIA. A 43-year-old biochemist, Frank Olson, had committed suicide on November 28, 1953, less than 2 weeks after CIA agents had secretly slipped LSD into his after-dinner drink. This drug had caused a panic reaction in Dr. Olson, and he was taken to New York City for psychiatric treatment. After his suicide, his family was told only that he had jumped or fallen from his 10th-story hotel room in Manhattan. In 1975, when this was uncovered, President Ford quickly apologized to the Olson family at the White House and said the incident was "inexcusable and unforgivable . . . a horrible episode in American history."[9] It was not until October 1976 that enough government red tape was cut through to make it possible to award $750,000 to the Olson family.

Awareness of the Olson death started Congress and journalists digging for more, this time into the military as well. The army's interest in, and human experiments on, the use of psychedelics for warfare and for interrogation of prisoners and spies was not hidden. It was open knowledge in the scientific and military communities that such research was conducted at Edgewood Arsenal in Maryland, where Dr. Olson was poisoned, and at several major universities in the United States.

It was easy to see how the military and intelligence agencies got involved in this work. "American military and intelligence officials watched men with glazed eyes pouring out rambling confessions at the Communist purge trials in Eastern Europe after World War II, and for the first time they began to worry about the threat of mind-bending drugs as weapons."[10] They worried enough to repeatedly contact Dr. Hofmann about the feasibility of large-scale production of LSD,[11] and the CIA considered buying 10 kg in 1953 for $240,000. We can all be pleased that they decided against the purchase, which would have provided 100 million doses.

As the information kept pouring out of government files in the 1975 to 1976 period, it became clear that the army-sponsored research on 585 soldiers and 900 civilians between 1956 and 1967 had been very poorly done. The army and some of the university scientists had violated many of the ethical codes established as a result of the Nuremberg war crimes trials after World War II. Three failures were especially blatant: many of the volunteers were not really volunteers, many of the participants could not quit an experiment if they wanted to, and the participants were not told the nature of the experiment.

This horror story could go on almost without end; mention could be made of CIA agents picking up patrons in bars and secretly putting LSD in their drinks or of the administration of LSD to unsuspecting civilians around the world. The inspector general of the army issued a long report that criticized almost every aspect of the army's involvement with human LSD research: its conception, its execution, and its productivity.[12] This story should all too strikingly bring home the dangers of giving drugs to persons without their knowledge. These drugs can literally be mind-breaking when used incautiously.

Recreational Use of LSD. The illegal LSD story starts with legal psilocybin, or perhaps at West Point, where Timothy Leary discovered Asian mysticism.

The story proper starts in the summer of 1960 in Mexico, where for the first time Leary used the magic mushrooms containing psilocybin. As he later said, he realized then that the old Timothy Leary was dead; the "Timothy Leary game" was over. Working at Harvard University, Leary collaborated with Dr. Richard Alpert and discussed the meaning and implication of this new world with Aldous Huxley.

During the 1960–1961 school year, Leary and Alpert began a series of experiments on Harvard graduate students using pure psilocybin, which they had obtained through a physician. Leary's original work was apparently done under proper scientific controls and with a physician in attendance because drugs were used. The use of a physician was later eliminated, and then other controls were dropped. In fact, Leary believed strongly that the experimenter should use the drug along with the subject, in order to be able to communicate with the subject. This practice removes the experimenter from the role of objective observer and can hardly be classified as seriously scientific.

Leary's drug taking in the role of experimenter and the apparent abandonment of any semblance of a scientific approach were questioned by Harvard authorities and other scientists. Some of the major issues were that no physician was present when drugs were administered, undergraduates were used in drug experiments, and drug sessions were conducted outside the laboratory in Leary's home and at other places off campus. As a result of many factors, Alpert and Leary were dismissed from their academic positions in the spring of 1963.[13]

All was reasonably quiet in 1964 and 1965. Alpert, now known as Baba Ram Dass, separated from Leary and lectured on the West Coast, whereas Leary settled at an estate in Millbrook, New York, which was owned by a wealthy supporter of Leary's beliefs. In 1964, Leary announced that drugs were not necessary to rise above and go beyond one's ego. He reiterated this again in 1966 after he was arrested for possession of marijuana at the Millbrook estate.

Also in 1966, Leary started his religion, the League of Spiritual Discovery, with LSD as the sacrament. The league got off to a slow start, and Leary's home base at Millbrook was under attack around the same time. The concern was that Leary would attract "drug addicts" to Millbrook. When their money runs out, they will murder, rob and steal, to secure funds with which to satisfy their craving."[14]

Leary was the guru of the age, but his sacrament was already being secularized. Increasing numbers of young people were responding to the motto of the League for Spiritual Discovery: "Turn on, tune in, and drop out." Leary phrased it meaningfully:

> Turning on correctly means to understand the many levels that are brought into focus; it takes years of discipline, training, and discipleship. To turn on on a street corner is a waste. To tune in means you must harness rigorously what you are learning. . . .
>
> To drop out is the oldest message that spiritual teachers have passed on. You can get only by giving up.[15]

These were noble words, perhaps, but street-corner turn-ons were becoming more frequent. A combination of many things increased the use of hallucinogens, and especially LSD, during the early and mid-1960s. LSD's promise of new sensations (which were delivered), of potent aphrodisiac effects (which were not forthcoming),[16] of feelings of kinship with a friendly peer group (which occurred) spread the drug rapidly.

In the summer of 1966, delegates to the annual convention of the American Medical Association passed a resolution urging greater controls on hallucinogens. They were a little uptight, as was the nation; in part, the resolution stated that

> these drugs can produce uncontrollable violence, overwhelming panic . . . or attempted suicide or homicide, and can result, among the unstable or those with preexisting neurosis or psychosis, in severe illness demanding protracted stays in mental hospitals.[17]

LSD use appears to have peaked in 1967 and 1968, after which it tapered off. Several factors probably contributed to this decline, including widely publicized "bad trips," prolonged psychotic reactions, worries about possible chromosome damage, self-injurious behavior, and "flashbacks." Concerned, many people began to avoid hallucinogens, whereas others shunned the synthetic LSD for the natural experiences produced by psilocybin or mescaline (actually, into the mid-1970s these natural substances, although in demand, were in short supply, and most street samples of either psilocybin or mescaline contained primarily LSD or PCP).

After a series of arrests on drug charges, Timothy Leary was sent to a minimum security prison in 1969, from which he escaped in 1970. After wandering around the world for a couple of years, he surrendered and was sent back to prison. Before his release in 1976, he stated that he was "totally rehabilitated" and would "never, under any circumstances, advocate the use of LSD or any drug."[18] Touring college campuses on the lecture circuit in the early 1980s, Leary talked about "how to use drugs without abusing them."[19]

LSD Pharmacology. LSD is odorless, colorless, tasteless, and one of the most potent psychochemicals known. Let's remind ourselves about the pharmacological meaning of *potent*: it takes little LSD to produce effects. A drug can be highly potent and yet not produce much in the way of effects. For example, LSD has never been definitely linked to even one human overdose death. In rats, reliable behavioral effects can be produced by 0.04 mg/kg, whereas the LD_{50} is about 16 mg/kg, 400 times the behaviorally effective dose.

Absorption from the gastrointestinal tract is rapid, and most humans take LSD through the mouth. At all postingestion times, the brain contains less LSD than any of the other organs in the body, so it is not selectively taken up by the brain. Half of the LSD in the blood is metabolized every three hours, so blood levels decrease fairly rapidly. LSD is metabolized in the liver and excreted as 2-oxy-lysergic acid diethylamide, which is inactive.

Tolerance develops rapidly, repeated daily doses becoming completely ineffective in three to four days. Recovery is equally rapid, so weekly use of the same dose of LSD is possible. Cross-tolerance has been shown between LSD, mescaline, and psilocybin, and the effects of each can be blocked or reversed with chlorpromazine. Physical dependence or addiction to LSD or to any of the hallucinogens has not been shown.

LSD is a sympathomimetic agent, and the autonomic signs are some of the first to appear after LSD is taken. Typical symptoms are dilated pupils, elevated temperature and blood pressure, and an increase in salivation.

The fact that the indole structure of LSD resembles that of serotonin led first to the idea that LSD works by acting at serotonin receptors. Injections of radioactive LSD into animals demonstrate that serotonin receptors are the primary, but not the only, binding sites for LSD.[20] Electrophysiological recordings from serotonin-containing neurons in the raphe nuclei of rats reveal that LSD injections cause a complete cessation of spontaneous electrical activity at doses comparable to those producing behavioral effects.[21] Thus, there is fairly general agreement that many of the primary CNS effects of LSD are by actions on the serotonin systems.

However, there are several problems with this explanation of LSD effects. A basic problem relates to the fact that mescaline and other catechol hallucinogens have chemical structures more similar to the neurotransmitters dopamine and norepinephrine than to serotonin. However, they have psychological effects that are very similar to those of LSD. Rats trained to press one lever after an injection of LSD and another lever after a saline (placebo) injection will respond on the LSD lever if given other indole or catechol hallucinogens, but not if given PCP,

anticholinergics, stimulants, sedatives, or opiates.[22] Thus, the highly specific "LSD stimulus" in a rat appears to be similar to the stimuli produced by other indole and catechol hallucinogens. It has been suggested that the catechol hallucinogens are flexible enough to assume a shape that would allow them to fit the "LSD receptor," which could be a serotonin receptor.[23]

Whereas most of the behavioral effects of LSD and the catechol hallucinogens can be blocked by drugs that act as serotonin-receptor antagonists, others cannot. Add to this that there are several subtypes of serotonin receptors, some of which are excitatory and others inhibitory, and that LSD can act as either an agonist or an antagonist at different serotonin receptors and you can begin to see how complicated this issue becomes. At the present time, the best evidence seems to indicate that LSD and

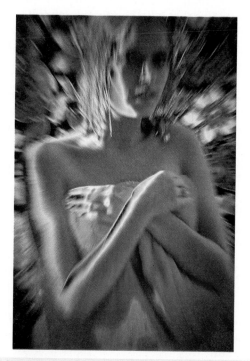

LSD users experience changes in visual perception, such as illusions or hallucinations.

other hallucinogens, including mescaline and psilocybin, act by stimulating the "serotonin-2A" subtype of receptors. Among a large group of hallucinogenic chemicals, there is a high correlation between their potency in binding to this type of receptor from rat brains and their potency in producing hallucinogenic effects in humans. Recent studies from Switzerland provide strong evidence that the hallucinogenic effects of psilocybin in humans are caused by serotonin-2A receptor activation.[24]

The LSD Experience.

Regardless of the chemical mechanism, most scientists feel that the most important effect is the modification of perception, particularly of visual images. Some of the experiences reported, especially after low doses, might best be described as illusions, or perceptual distortions, in which an object that is, in fact, present is seen in a distorted form (brighter than normal, moving, in multiple images). Siegel,[25] who conducted laboratory research on the visual images reported after the ingestion of various drugs, reported that some images can be seen with eyes open or closed and thus are hallucinations rather than illusions. One stage of such hallucinogen-induced imagery consists of form-constants: lattices, honeycomb or chessboard designs, cobwebs, tunnels, alley or cone shapes, and spiral figures. These shapes are generally combined with intense colors and brightness. At another stage, complex images, such as landscapes, remembered faces, or objects, might be combined with the form-constants (e.g., a face might be seen "through" a honeycomb lattice, or multiple images of the face might appear in a honeycomb configuration). Siegel suggested that the perceptual processing mechanisms might be activated at the same time as the sensory inputs are either reduced or impaired, thus allowing vivid perception of images that come from inside, rather than outside, the brain.

Besides changes in visual perception, users also report an altered sense of time, changes in the perception of one's own body (perhaps indicating a reduction in somatic sensory input), and some alterations of auditory input. A particularly interesting phenomenon is that of **synesthesia**, a "mixing of senses," in which sounds might appear as visual images (as reported by Dr. Hofmann on the first-ever LSD trip), or the visual picture might alter in rhythm with music.

Altered perception is combined with enhanced emotionality, perhaps related to the arousal of the sympathetic branch of the autonomic nervous system. Thus, one might interpret the images as exceptionally beautiful or awe-inspiring because of an enhanced tendency to react with intense emotion. Alternatively, an object appearing to break apart or move away from or toward the perceiver might be reacted to with intense sadness or fear. This fear can result in a pounding heart and rapid, shallow breathing, which further frightens the tripper and can lead to a full-blown panic reaction.

Part of the wonder of these agents is that they do not give repeat performances. However, even though each trip differs, the general type of experience and the sequence of experiences are reasonably well delineated. When an effective dose (30 to 100 µg) is taken orally, the trip will last six to nine hours. It can be greatly attenuated at any time through the administration of chlorpromazine intramuscularly.

The initial effects noticed are autonomic responses, which develop gradually over the first 20 minutes. The individual might feel dizzy or hot and cold; the mouth might be dry. These effects diminish and, in addition, are less and less the focus of attention as alteration in sensations, perceptions, and mood begin to develop over the following 30 to 40 minutes. In one study, after the initial autonomic effects, the sequence of events over the next 20 to 50 minutes consisted of mood changes, abnormal body sensation, decrease in sensory impression, abnormal color perception, space and time disorders, and visual hallucinations. One visual effect was described beautifully:

The guide asked me how I felt, and I responded, "Good." As I muttered the word "Good," I could see it form visually in the air. It was pink and fluffy like a cloud. The word looked "Good" in its appearance and so it had to be "Good." The word and the thing I was trying to express were one, and "Good" was floating around in the air.[26]

About one hour after taking LSD, the intoxication is in full bloom, but it is not until near the end of the second hour that changes occur in the perception of the self. Usually these changes center around a depersonalization. The individual might feel that the sensations he or she experiences are not from the body or that he or she has no body. Body distortions are common, the sort of thing suggested by the comment of one user: "I felt as if my left big toe were going to vomit!" Not unusual is a loss of self-awareness and loss of control of behavior.

Two frequent types of overall reactions in this stage have been characterized as "expansive" and "constricted." In the expansive reaction (a good trip) the individual can become excited and grandiose and feel that he or she is uncovering secrets of the universe or profundities previously locked within him- or herself. Feelings of creativity are not uncommon: "If I only had the time, I could write the truly great American novel." The other end of the continuum is the constricted reaction, in which the user shows little movement and frequently becomes paranoid and exhibits feelings of persecution. The prototype individual in this situation is huddled in a corner, fearful that some harm will come to him or her or that the person is being threatened by some aspect of the hallucinations. As the drug effect diminishes, normal psychological controls of sensations, perceptions, and mood return.

Adverse Reactions.   The adverse reactions to LSD ingestion have been repeatedly emphasized in the popular and scientific literature. Because there is no way of knowing how much illegal LSD is being used or how pure the LSD is that people are taking, there is no possibility of determining the true incidence of adverse reactions to LSD. Adverse reactions to the street use of what is thought to be LSD can result from many factors. It is important always to remember that drugs obtained on the street frequently are not what they are claimed to be—in purity, chemical composition, or quantity.

A 1960 study surveyed most of the legal U.S. investigators studying LSD and mescaline effects in humans. Data were collected on 25,000 administrations of the drug to about 5,000 individuals. Doses ranged from 25 to 1,500 µg of LSD and 200 to 1,200 mg of mescaline. In some cases the drug was used in patients undergoing therapy; in other cases the drug was taken in an experimental situation to study the effects of the drug. Only LSD and mescaline used under professional supervision were surveyed.

A 1964 article, "The LSD Controversy," stated:

> It would seem that the incidence statistics better support a statement that the drug is exceptionally safe rather than dangerous. Although no statistics have been compiled for the dangers of psychological therapies, we would not be surprised if the incidence of adverse reactions, such as psychotic or depressive episodes and suicide attempts, were at least as high or higher in any comparable group of psychiatric patients exposed to any active form of therapy.[27]

But it then went on to say:

> It is also important to distinguish between the proper use of this drug in therapeutic or experimental settings and its indiscriminate use and abuse by thrill seekers, "lunatic fringe," and drug addicts. More dangers seem likely for the unstable

synesthesia: (sin ess *thees* ya) the blending of different senses, such as "seeing" sounds.

character who takes the drug for "kicks," curiosity, or to escape reality and responsibility than someone taking the drug for therapeutic reasons under strict medical aegis and supervision.

Panic reactions.   One type of adverse reaction that can develop during the drug-induced experience is the panic reaction, which is typified in the following case history:

A 21-year-old woman was admitted to the hospital along with her lover. He had had a number of LSD experiences and had convinced her to take it to make her less constrained sexually. About half an hour after ingestion of approximately 200 microgm., she noticed that the bricks in the wall began to go in and out and that light affected her strangely. She became frightened when she realized that she was unable to distinguish her body from the chair she was sitting on or from her lover's body. Her fear became more marked after she thought that she would not get back into herself. At the time of admission she was hyperactive and laughed inappropriately. Stream of talk was illogical and affect labile. Two days later, this reaction had ceased. However, she was still afraid of the drug and convinced that she would not take it again because of her frightening experience.[28]

Prolonged psychotic reaction.   When an overt psychosis develops, remedial treatment is not usually so rapid, and the next individual to be described was hospitalized for prolonged treatment. Usually such psychosis occurs in individuals with a precarious hold on reality in the nondrug condition. The flood of new experiences and feelings is too much for this type of person to integrate.

A 23-year-old man was admitted to the hospital after he stood uncertain whether to plunge an upraised knife into his friend's back. His wife . . . reported that he had been acting strangely since taking LSD approximately 3 weeks before admission. He was indecisive and often mute, and shunned physical contact with her. On admission

he was catatonic, mute and echopractic. He appeared to be preoccupied with auditory hallucinations of God's voice and thought he had achieved a condition of "all mind." On transfer to another hospital 1 month after admission, there was minimal improvement.

During his adolescence the patient had alternated between acceptance of and rebellion against his mother's religiosity and warnings of the perils of sex and immorality. He had left college during his 1st year after excessive use of amphetamines. He attended, but did not complete, art school. His marriage of 3 years had been marked by conflict and concern about his masculinity. Increasing puzzlement about the meaning of life, his role in the universe and other cosmic problems led to his ingestion of LSD. Shortly after ingestion he was ecstatic and wrote to a friend, "We have found the peace, which is life's river which flows into the sea of Eternity." Soon afterward, in a brief essay, he showed some awareness of his developing psychosis, writing, "I am misunderstood, I cried, and was handed a complete list of my personality traits, habits, goals, and ideals, etc. I know myself now, I said in relief, and spent the rest of my life in happy cares asylum. AMEN."[28]

It would be easy to blame this young man's psychosis on LSD, but it is also easy to find evidence in his case history of a possible developing schizophrenia, which might have been partly responsible for his wanting to try LSD. Statistically, there is no evidence that LSD use results in increased likelihood of prolonged psychosis (see Table 17.1).

Flashbacks.   One of the frightening and interesting adverse reactions to LSD is the flashback. More than any other reaction, the recurrence of symptoms weeks or months after an individual has taken LSD brings up thoughts of brain damage and permanent biochemical changes. Flashbacks consist of the recurrence of certain aspects of the drug experience after a period of normalcy and in the absence of any drug use.

TABLE 17.1

Estimated Rates of Major Complications Associated with LSD

Groups studied	Number per 1,000 Persons		
	Attempted suicide	Completed suicide	Psychotic reaction over 48 hours
Subjects in experiments	0.0	0.0	0.8
Patients undergoing psychotherapy	1.2	0.4	1.8

The frequency and duration of these flashbacks are quite variable and seem to be unpredictable. They are most frequent just before going to sleep, while driving, and in periods of psychological stress. They seem to diminish in frequency and intensity with time if the individual stops using psychoactive drugs.

Although some of the reactions reported as flashbacks might be nothing more than intense memories or experiences that non-LSD users can also have, such as déjà vu, there remain many reports of "reexperiencing" LSD-like reactions in a frightening way. One group continued to study this phenomenon and reported that psychophysical tests of visual function showed measurable impairments several years after the last use of LSD.[29] A group of 24 ex-LSD users was compared with 20 control subjects. Although there were no differences between the groups in visual acuity, color vision, or several other measures, a significant difference was found in the rate at which a flickering light appeared to "fuse" into a continuous light, especially when the light was presented to the peripheral parts of the visual field. The LSD group also did not adapt to darkness as well as the control group. The authors concluded that their results were consistent with long-term changes in the central nervous system of LSD users.

Beliefs About LSD.   LSD is truly a legend in its own time—actually, there are many legends. People probably have more ideas about what LSD does and does not do than they have about any other drug.

- *Creativity.* One of the most widely occurring beliefs is that these hallucinogenic agents increase creativity or release creativity that our inhibitions keep bottled inside us. There have been several experiments that have attempted to study the effects of LSD on creativity, but there is no good evidence that the drug increases it. In one laboratory study using LSD at doses of 0.0025 or 0.01 mg/kg body weight, "the authors concluded that the administration of LSD-25 to a relatively unselected group of people for the purpose of enhancing their creative ability is not likely to be successful."[30] A recent double-blind, placebo-controlled study found that psilocybin made remote mental associations more available, which might enhance creativity. On the other hand, the research volunteers were less able to focus on their tasks under the influence of psilocybin.[31]

- *Therapy.* Another common belief is that LSD has therapeutic usefulness, particularly in the treatment of alcoholics, even though reports of results with LSD in alcoholism gradually changed from glowing and enthusiastic to cautious and disappointing. One well-controlled study compared the effectiveness of one dose of 0.6 mg of LSD with 60 mg of dextroamphetamine in reducing drinking by alcoholics. No additional therapy, physical or psychological, was used. The authors found that "LSD produced slightly better results early, but after six months the results were alike for both treatment groups."[32] Some investigators reported considerable success with LSD in reducing the pain and depression of patients with terminal cancer. The LSD experiences were part of a several-day program involving extensive verbal interaction between the therapist and patient. Although not successful in every case, the LSD therapy was followed by a reduction in the use of narcotics, "less worry about the future," and "the appearance of a positive mood state." The authors concluded that they had a treatment "which may be highly promising for patients facing fatal illness if implemented in the context of brief, intensive, and highly specialized psychotherapy catalyzed by a psychedelic drug such as LSD." However, federally funded research of this typed ended in the 1970s, when a scientific peer review by NIMH concluded, "Research on the therapeutic use of LSD has shown that it is not a generally useful therapeutic drug as an adjunct to a routine psychotherapeutic approach or as a treatment in and of itself."[33]

- *Chromosome damage.* A credibility gap in the world of drugs developed in 1967 between the press and the public with the publication of a scientific report that LSD caused damage to chromosomes of white blood cells (leukocytes) in vitro. This report was quickly followed by a study showing a higher than normal incidence of chromosomal damage in the white blood cells of LSD users. These data received much attention in the mass media and are thought to be one of the reasons for the decrease in LSD use that has occurred since 1967. Not so widely publicized

were the many follow-up reports that did not show any relationship in vitro or in vivo between white blood cell chromosome damage and LSD use. The popular reports also had a way of neglecting to emphasize (or mention) that the effects were on white blood cells and not on the germ cells, which are the important cells for reproduction. The weight of evidence gathered over the years does *not* support the claim that LSD can cause birth defects or cancer in its human users.

Psilocybin

The magic mushrooms of Mexico have a long history of religious and ceremonial use. These plants, as well as peyote, dropped from Western sight (but not from native use) for 300 years after the Spanish conquered the Aztecs and systematically destroyed their writings and teachings. The mushrooms were particularly suppressed. The name *teonanacatl* can be translated as "God's flesh" or as "sacred mushroom," and either name was very offensive to the Spanish priests.

It was not until the late 1930s that it was clearly shown that these mushrooms were still being used by natives in southern Mexico and the first of many species was identified. The real breakthrough came in 1955. During that year a New York banker turned ethnobotanist and his wife established rapport with a native group still using mushrooms in religious ceremonies. Gordon Wasson became the first outsider to participate in the ceremony and to eat of the magic mushroom. In language quite unlike that of a banker, you can almost hear Wasson's soul cry out as he tries to describe the experience:

> It permits you to travel backwards and forward in time, to enter other planes of existence, even (as the Indians say), to know God.[34]

The most well-known psychoactive mushroom is *Psilocybe mexicana*. The primary active agent in this mushroom is **psilocybin,** an indole that

HealthQuest Activities

Assess your exposure to LSD by completing *Drug F/X Exploration* in Module 9. If you have never used LSD, are you surprised to learn of its effects? If you have used or are currently using LSD, are your own reactions similar to the ones listed here?

In the same module, look under *Specifics On.* Read "Unknown Drug Use/Abuse" and identify the herbal hallucinogens. Do you think these substances are more dangerous or less dangerous than LSD?

the discoverer of LSD, Albert Hofmann, isolated in 1958 and later synthesized.

Another psilocybin-containing mushroom, *Psilocybe cubensis,* grows on cow dung along the U.S. Gulf Coast. Aside from the obvious questions about eating something found on manure, identifying the correct psilocybin-containing mushrooms in the field can be tricky. Most *Psilocybe* species are described as "little brown mushrooms," and there are several toxic look-alikes.

The dried mushrooms are 0.2 to 0.5 percent psilocybin. The hallucinogenic effects of psilocybin are quite similar to those of LSD and the catechol hallucinogen mescaline, and cross-tolerance exists among these three agents.[35]

The psychoactive effects are clearly related to the amount used, with up to 4 mg yielding a pleasant experience, relaxation, and some body sensations. Higher doses cause considerable perceptual and body-image changes, with hallucinations in some individuals. Accompanying these psychic changes are dose-related sympathetic arousal symptoms. There is some evidence that psilocybin has its central nervous system effects only after it has been changed in the body to psilocin. Psilocin is present in the mushroom only in trace amounts but is about 1.5 times as potent as psilocybin. Perhaps the greater CNS effect of psilocin is the result of its higher lipid solubility.

One of Timothy Leary's followers used psilocybin in the now-classic Good Friday study. The Good Friday study was designed to investigate the ability of psilocybin to induce meaningful religious experiences in individuals when the drug is used in a religious setting. Twenty seminarians participated in a double-blind study, with half receiving 30 mg of psilocybin and half placebos, 90 minutes before attending a religious service. Tape recordings of the subjects' experiences were made immediately after the $2\frac{1}{2}$-hour service, which was held in a chapel. Within a week a questionnaire was completed, followed by a similar one 6 months later. The

first was directed at determining the magnitude and type of change that occurred during the experiment; the later one at assessing the durability of the change. Leary later summarized the outcome of the Good Friday study by saying,

> The results clearly support the hypothesis that, with adequate preparation and in an environment which is supportive and religiously meaningful, subjects report mystical experiences significantly more than placebo controls.[36]

The search for beneficial psychological effects of hallucinogens continues to a limited extent, with psilocybin replacing LSD. In addition to the study on creativity, one report suggests that psilocybin is useful in the treatment of obsessive-compulsive disorder.[37]

With access to some spores of the mushroom and proper growing conditions, one can cultivate *Psilocybe* in a closet. As a consequence of illegal production in the United States, the use of this mushroom has continued, with sporadic outbursts of availability. Although occasionally a major mushroom producer is discovered, most of the production seems to be on a local, amateur basis. Young people might obtain a few "shrooms" to consume at a party, usually in small quantities and in combination with alcoholic beverages. Under such circumstances it is difficult to tell how much of an effect is produced by the mushrooms and how much by the social situation and the alcohol.

Morning Glories and Hawaiian Baby Woodroses

Of the psychoactive agents used freely in Mexico in the sixteenth century, *ololiuqui,* seeds of the morning glory plant *Rivea corymbosa,* perhaps had the greatest religious significance. These seeds tie America to Europe even today.

---

psilocybin: (sill o *sy* bin) the active chemical in *Psilocybe* mushrooms.

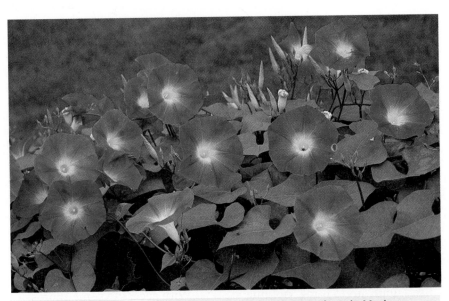

Although morning glory seeds were used as religious plants in Mexico before Columbus, the seeds of most types of morning glories available in the United States have little or no hallucinogenic action.

When Albert Hofmann analyzed the seeds of the morning glory, he found several active alkaloids as well as *d*-lysergic acid amide, which is about one-tenth as active as LSD. The presence of *d*-lysergic acid amide is really quite amazing (to botany majors), because before this discovery in 1960, lysergic acid had been found only in much more primitive groups of plants, such as the ergot fungus.[38]

A different species of morning glory, *Ipomoea violacea*, seems to be the primary source in the United States of most commercial morning glory seeds containing effective amounts of these alkaloids. Considering the psychoactivity of these seeds, the commercial names seem quite appropriate: Pearly Gates, Flying Saucers, Heavenly Blue.

The recreational use of seeds from *Argyreia nervosa*, commonly known as Hawaiian baby woodrose has also been reported.[39] These seeds contain higher levels of *d*-lysergic acid amide than morning glories. However, recreational use of these seeds often has adverse effects, probably because the fuzzy outer coating contains toxic cyanogenic glycosides (which can really make one sick).

DMT

Dimethyltryptamine (DMT) has never been widely used in the United States, although it has a long, if not noble, history. In fact, on a worldwide basis, DMT is one of the most important naturally occurring hallucinogenic compounds, and it occurs in many plants. DMT is the active agent in Cohoba snuff, which is used by some South American and Caribbean Indians in hunting rituals. Although DMT was synthesized in the 1930s, its discovery as the active ingredient in cohoba first led to human examination of its psychoactive properties in 1956.

DMT is ineffective when taken orally and must be snuffed, smoked, or taken by injection. The effective intramuscular dose is about 1 mg/kg body weight. Intravenously, hallucinogenic effects are seen within 2 minutes after doses of 0.2 mg/kg or more and last for less than

30 minutes. The freebase form of DMT can be smoked by adding the crystals to some type of plant, and 20 to 40 mg is the usual dose. The effect is brief, no matter how it is used. Recent, well-controlled human studies have demonstrated that DMT is unique among classic hallucinogens in that tolerance does not develop to its psychological effects.[40]

Ayahuasca

The word *ayahuasca* is from the Quechuan language of the Amazon region, and it means "vine of the soul." The term is used both for the vine *Banisteriopsis caapi* and for the medicinal/divinatory brew made from it. The brew is a traditional South American preparation most commonly combining the *Banisteriopsis* vine, which contains harmaline, with leaves of *Psychotria viridis,* which contains DMT. DMT is normally broken down quickly in the body by the enzyme monoamine oxidase (MAO). This means that, when DMT is taken orally, it is not usually effective. However, harmaline inhibits MAO (see Chapter 10 for a description of MAO inhibitors as antidepressants). Thus, neither plant alone has psychoactive properties, but together they are used by South American tribes as a psychoactive religious sacrament.[41] Doesn't it make you wonder how this combination was discovered before knowledge existed about these chemicals and how they work? Curiosity seekers from North America and Europe have been traveling to the Amazon to experience the effects of ayahuasca, often describing dramatic psychological effects.

Catechol Hallucinogens

The second group of phantastica, although having psychological effects quite similar to those of the indole types, is based on a different structure, that of the catechol nucleus. That nucleus forms the basic structure of the catecholamine neurotransmitters, norepinephrine and dopamine. Figure 17.2 shows the catechol structure and the structures of some catechol hallucinogens. Look for the catechol nucleus in each of the hallucinogens, and then compare these structures with the structure of the amphetamines and other stimulants shown in Chapter 8.

Mescaline

Peyote (from the Aztec *peyotl*) is a small, spineless, carrot-shaped cactus, *Lophophora williamsii* Lemaire, which grows wild in the Rio Grande Valley and southward. It is mostly subterranean, and only the grayish-green pincushion-like top appears above ground.

> In pre-Columbian times the Aztec, Huichol, and other Mexican Indians ate the plant ceremonially either in the dried or green state. This produces profound sensory and psychic derangements lasting twenty-four hours, a property which led the natives to value and use it religiously.[42]

Only the part of the cactus that is above ground is easily edible, but the entire plant is psychoactive. This upper portion, or crown, is sliced into disks, which dry and are known as "mescal buttons." These slices of the peyote cactus remain psychoactive indefinitely and are the source of the drug between the yearly harvests. The Indians' journey in November and December to harvest the peyote is an elaborate ceremony, sometimes taking almost a month and a half. When the mescal buttons are to be used, they are soaked in the mouth until soft, then formed by hand into a bolus and swallowed.

Mescal buttons should not be confused with mescal beans—or with mescal liquor, which is distilled from the fermentation of the agave cactus. Mescal buttons are slices of the peyote cactus and contain **mescaline** as the primary active agent. Mescal beans, however, are dark red

---

peyote: (pay *oh* tee) a type of hallucinogenic cactus.

mescaline: (*mess* ka lin) the active chemical in the peyote cactus.

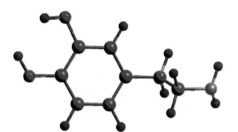

The basic catecholamine structure (dopamine)

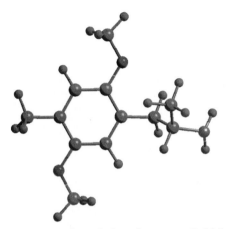

2', 5' dimethoxy -4'- methylamphetamine (DOM)

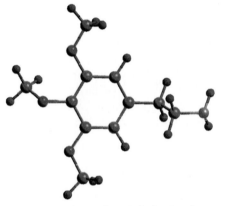

3,4,5 trimethoxyphenylethylamine (mescaline)

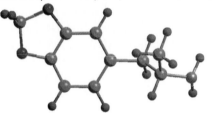

3, 4 methylenedioxy amphetamine (MDA)

■ carbon

■ oxygen

■ hydrogen

■ nitrogen

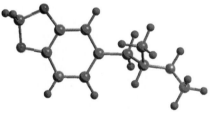

3,4 methylenedioxy methamphetamine (MDMA)

Figure 17.2   Cathechol hallucinogens.

seeds from the shrub *Sophora secundiflora*. These seeds, formerly the basis of a vision-seeking cult, contain a highly toxic alkaloid, cytisine, the effects of which resemble those of nicotine, causing nausea, convulsions, hallucinations, and occasionally death from respiratory failure. The mescal bean has a long history, and there is some evidence that use of the bean diminished and ceased when the safer peyote became available

in the southwestern United States. In the transition from a mescal bean to a mescal button cult there appeared, in some tribes, a period in which a mixture of peyote and mescal seeds was concocted and drunk. These factors contributed to considerable confusion in the early (and some recent) literature.[38]

Although there was evidence that the use of peyote had moved north into the United States

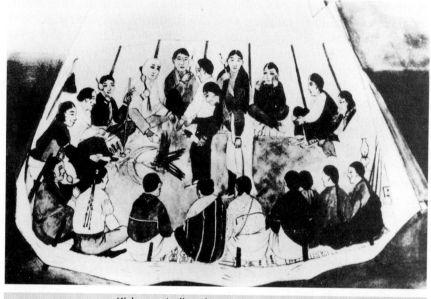

Kickapoo Indians in a peyote ceremony.

as early as 1760, it was not until the late nineteenth century that a peyote cult was widely established among the Indians of the plains. From
that time to the present, Indian missionaries
have spread the peyote religion to almost a quarter of a million Indians, some as far north as
Canada. The development of the present form
of this sect has been summarized:

> The independent groups of the Peyote Religion
> have federated into the Native American Church
> during the 20th century, like the independent
> congregations of the Jesus Cult federated into
> the Catholic Church during the 4th century.
> However, just as not all congregations accepting
> the basic doctrines of Christianity belonged to
> the Catholic Church, so not all groups accepting
> the basic doctrines of Peyotism belong to the Na-
> tive American Church.[43]

The *Native American Church* of the United States
was first chartered in Oklahoma in 1918 and is
an amalgamation of Christianity and traditional
beliefs and practices of the Native Americans.

Peyotism continues to be an important religious practice among the Indians of the United
States between the Rocky Mountains and the
Mississippi. As in all religions, a variety of rituals has developed surrounding the use of peyote
in religious ceremonies. Peyote is also used in
other ways because the Indians attribute spiritual power to the peyote plant. As such, peyote
is believed to be helpful, along with prayers and
modern medicines, in curing illnesses. It is also
worn as an amulet, much as some Christians
wear a Saint Christopher's medal, to protect the
wearer from harm.

In 1971, a psychiatrist working a mental
health program serving the Navajo became concerned about news reports of serious psychiatric
problems resulting from recreational use of hallucinogens. Since his client population included
a high proportion of Native American Church
members, he studied the program's records for
an association. Based on four years' data, he
concluded that peyote use was not associated
with a higher rate of psychopathology but that

peyote users apparently had a lower risk of alcoholism.[44] Of course, the highly ritualistic nature of the peyote ceremony provides safeguards against negative reactions. The informal, recreational use of peyote is more likely to result in undesirable psychological effects.

For many years the use of peyote as a sacrament by the Native American Church was protected by the constitutional guarantee of freedom of religion. In fact, it was that protection that had inspired Timothy Leary to attempt a similar exclusion for LSD in his newly founded 1960s League of Spiritual Discovery. However, in 1990 the Supreme Court ruled that the State of Oregon could prosecute its citizens for using peyote, and the freedom of religion argument was not allowed.[45] A large group of religious and civil liberties organizations asked the Court to reconsider its decision, but it declined to do so. The two defendants in the case were American Indians and members of the Native American Church. Federal law and many state laws specifically exclude sacramental peyote use, and the Court pointed out that Oregon could exclude such use, too. It is not clear what the long-term implications of this ruling might be. That will depend to some extent on whether other states decide to outlaw all use of peyote.

San Pedro Cactus. Another mescaline-containing cactus, *Trichocereus pachanoi,* whose common name is the San Pedro cactus, is native to the Andes Mountains of Peru and Ecuador and has been used for thousands of years as a religious sacrament.[46] The San Pedro is a large, multi-branched cactus, often growing to heights of 10 to 15 feet. Its mescaline content is less than that of peyote, and its recreational use more often results in adverse side effects than in the desired hallucinogenic experience.

Discovery and Early Research on Mescaline. Near the end of the nineteenth century, Arthur Heffter isolated several alkaloids from peyote and showed that mescaline was the primary agent for the visual effect induced by peyote. Mescaline was synthesized in 1918, and most experiments on the psychoactive and/or behavioral effects since then have used synthesized mescaline. More than 30 psychoactive alkaloids have now been identified in peyote, but mescaline does seem to be the agent responsible for the vivid colors and other visual effects. The fact that mescaline is not equivalent to peyote is not always made clear in the literature.

One of the early investigators of the effects of peyote was Dr. Weir Mitchell, who used an extract of peyote and who reported, in part:

> The display which for an enchanted two hours followed was such as I find it hopeless to describe in language which shall convey to others the beauty and splendor of what I saw. Stars, delicate floating films of color, then an abrupt rush of countless points of white light swept across the field of view, as if the unseen millions of the Milky Way were to flow in a sparkling river before my eyes . . . zigzag lines of very bright colors . . . the wonderful loveliness of swelling clouds of more vivid colors gone before I could name them.[47]

Another early experimenter was Havelock Ellis. Interestingly, he took his peyote on Good Friday in 1897, 65 years before the Good Friday experiment with psilocybin. His experience is described in detail in a 1902 article titled "Mescal: A Study of a Divine Plant" in *Popular Science Monthly*, but a brief quotation gives the essence of the experience:

> On the whole, if I had to describe the visions in one word, I should say that they were living arabesques. There was generally a certain incomplete tendency to symmetry, the effect being somewhat as if the underlying mechanism consisted of a large number of polished facets acting as mirrors. It constantly happened that the same image was repeated over a large part of the field, though this holds good mainly of the forms, for in the colors there would still remain all sorts of delicious varieties. Thus at a moment when

uniformly jewelled flowers seemed to be spring-
ing up and extending all over the field of vision,
the flowers still showed every variety of delicate
tone and tint.[48]

Not every individual wants every educational
opportunity. William James, surprisingly, was
one who did not. He wrote to his brother
Henry: "I ate one but three days ago, was violently sick for twenty-four hours, and had no
other symptoms whatever except that and the
Katzenjammer the following day. I will take the
visions on trust." Even Dr. Weir Mitchell, who
had the effect previously recorded, said, "These
shows are expensive. . . . The experience, however, was worth one such headache and indigestion but was not worth a second."

Even if you get by without too much nausea
and physical discomfort, which the Indians also
report, all might not go well. Huxley, whose
1954 *The Doors of Perception*[49] made him a guru
in this area, admitted, "Along with the happily
transfigured majority of mescaline takers there
is a minority that finds in the drug only hell and
purgatory." It is reported that natives sometimes
wished for bad trips when taking this or other
plants. By meeting their personal demons, they
hoped to conquer them and remove problems
from their lives.

Pharmacology of Mescaline.   Mescaline is readily
absorbed if taken orally, but it only very poorly
passes the blood-brain barrier (which explains
the high doses required). There is a maximal concentration of the drug in the brain after 30 to 120
minutes. About half of it is removed from the
body in 6 hours, and there is evidence that some
mescaline persists in the brain for up to 10 hours.
Similar to the indole hallucinogens, the effects
obtained with low doses, about 3 mg/kg body
weight, are primarily euphoric, whereas doses in
the range of 5 mg/kg give rise to a full set of hallucinations. Most of the mescaline is excreted unchanged in the urine, and the metabolites
identified thus far are not psychoactive.

A dose that is psychoeffective in humans
causes pupil dilation, pulse rate and blood pressure increases, and an elevation in body temperature. All of these effects are similar to those
induced by LSD, psilocybin, and most other alkaloid hallucinogens. There are other signs of
central stimulation, such as EEG arousal, after
mescaline intake. In rats the LD_{50} is about 370
mg/kg body weight, 10 to 30 times the dose that
causes behavioral effects. Death results from
convulsions and respiratory arrest. Tolerance
develops more slowly to mescaline than to LSD,
and there is cross-tolerance between them. As
with LSD, mescaline intoxication can be blocked
with chlorpromazine.

Although mescaline and the other catechol
hallucinogens have a structure that resembles
the catecholamine neurotransmitters, it has
been proposed that they might operate via the
same mechanism as LSD, perhaps mainly via
serotonin actions. The fact that the psychological effects of these two chemical classes of
phantastica are so similar in humans, and that
the behavioral effects of either drug in rats are
blocked by serotonin antagonists, suggest a common mechanism, and studies of the structures
of catechol hallucinogens indicate certain similarities to the overall LSD structure.[23]

Amphetamine Derivatives

There is a large group of synthetic hallucinogens
that are chemically related to the amphetamines. However, most of these drugs have little
amphetamine-like stimulant activity. Thanks to
certain chemical substitutions on the ring part
of the catechol nucleus, these drugs are more
mescaline-like (review Figure 17.2).

DOM (STP).   DOM is 2,5-dimethoxy-4-methy-
lamphetamine. In the 1960s and 1970s, DOM
was called STP, and street talk was that the ini-
tials stood for serenity, tranquility, and peace. Its
actions and effects are highly similar to those of
mescaline and LSD, with a total dose of 1 to 3
mg yielding euphoria and 3 to 5 mg a six- to

eight-hour hallucinogenic period. This makes DOM about a hundred times as potent as mescaline but only one-thirtieth as potent as LSD.

DOM has a reputation for inducing an extraordinarily long experience, but this seems to be caused by the very large amounts being used. Some pills of DOM bought on the street contained about 10 mg—a very big dose. Reports by users had suggested that DOM was unlike other hallucinogens and that its effects were enhanced rather than blocked by chlorpromazine. Controlled laboratory work with normal volunteers, however, has clearly shown that the effects of DOM are similar to those of other hallucinogens and that chlorpromazine does attenuate the DOM experience.

An excellent review from the Haight-Ashbury Clinic contains most of the essential information about the rise and fall of DOM use:

> It appears then that DOM produces a higher incidence of acute and chronic toxic reactions than any of the other commonly used hallucinogens. . . . It appears that the effects of DOM are like a combination of amphetamine and LSD with the hallucinogenic effects of the drug very often putting the peripheral amphetamine-like physiological effects out of perspective.[50]

MDA and Others. In addition to DOM, many other amphetamine derivatives have been synthesized and shown to have hallucinogenic properties. Most of these have effects very similar to those of DOM and mescaline, as well as LSD and the indole types. There is some indication that one type of derivative, MDA (review Figure 17.2), has effects that are subjectively somewhat different.[23] MDA, which is somewhat more potent than mescaline, has seen some recreational use through illicit manufacture. Because of the variety of possible hallucinogenic amphetamine derivatives and because most of these chemicals are not specifically listed as controlled substances, illicit drug makers were drawn to this group of chemicals in the production of various designer drugs to be sold on the street as hallucinogens.

MDMA. One of the amphetamine derivatives received special attention in July 1984 when the DEA proposed scheduling it. MDMA is similar in structure to MDA but is apparently quite different from the other hallucinogens. Rats trained to discriminate DOM from saline did show some generalization from the DOM stimulus to MDA but not to MDMA. Furthermore, there is no cross-tolerance between MDA and MDMA.[23] Although there was some use of MDMA on the streets (it is called "Ecstasy" or "XTC"), what was surprising was that a number of psychiatrists came forth who had been quietly using MDMA, a drug that, although not approved by the FDA, was not illegal. These psychiatrists testified against the scheduling of MDMA, insisting that it was not a true hallucinogen and that it had a special ability to promote empathy, thus aiding the psychoanalytic process.[51]

There is some evidence supporting this claim of increased empathy: in a 1987 study, 100 people completed detailed questionnaires describing the effects of their previous use of MDMA.[52] Although such retrospective reports are less reliable than reports obtained during or immediately after the experience, a remarkably common report (90 percent of the individuals) was that they experienced a heightened sense of "closeness" with other people. Other common effects were an increased heart rate, dry mouth, grinding of the teeth, profuse sweating, and other autonomic effects. Although several people reported that objects seemed more "luminescent," very few reported actual visual hallucinations.

The bad news is that this otherwise fairly benign drug might cause brain damage. Several laboratories have reported that rats given MDMA injections show a selective destruction of serotonin neurons in their brains. Then a similar effect was reported in monkeys at only two to three times the normal human dose, and this led many observers to conclude that similar brain damage could occur in human MDMA users. It should be stressed that this effect is not caused by LSD, mescaline, psilocybin, or most other

Exploring Your Spirituality

Living in the Flow

During the 1960s, the spirit of kinship with a peer group helped fuel the spread of LSD. More recently, the feeling of making intense emotional connections seems to have helped spread a "rave" subculture in the United States and elsewhere. This scene, known for its all-night dance parties featuring techno tunes and the drug Ecstacy, has had a dedicated following since the early 1990s. It's not, however, just about the music or the drugs, according to those in the rave community. It's about being in the moment, having a brief conversation with a stranger who affects you, having an emotional internal experience.

What really makes people glad to be alive? What are the inner experiences that make life worthwhile? It's easier to talk about dancing than it is to describe a moment of mystical union with the universe. Joy can find us and lift us in moments of ordinary connection, though, and the opening we feel to life is not unlike that experienced through a spiritual quest or mystical practice. The elation comes when we know we belong—to another, to ourselves, to the mystery that is larger than ourselves.

In our society, celebrations and relaxation often involve moving away from the emotion, numbing ourselves with alcohol or drugs. Dance and music are exceptions to this, but too often we are simply spectators in our lives. Sometimes we discount the small joys in daily living. Sometimes we spoil the good by focusing on the less than perfect or seemingly incompatible. Perhaps we don't want to be let down, so we anticipate disappointment rather than expect success and happiness.

Can you think of a time when joy came unexpectedly and caught you off guard? Maybe it was a sudden realization that made you smile. Perhaps it was something you didn't even know you were looking for. Chances are it was a moment when you felt so alive that, ironically, you forgot yourself. Mihaly Csikszentmihalyi, a University of Chicago psychology professor who has devoted his life's work to studying what makes people happy, satisfied, and fulfilled, describes "flow" as a state of consciousness so focused that you are totally absorbed in an activity and lose track of time. It is a state of complete engagement with life in which you feel strong, alert, in effortless control, unself-conscious, and at the peak of your abilities. Examples of when you might experience flow include after completing a hard task, when feeling the wind in your hair during a walk on the beach, during yoga or sex, and when seeing your child respond to your smile for the first time.

What activities usually make you feel happy and completely engaged? During the next week, be aware of and record what activities give you this feeling of deep enjoyment. Then try to build some of these activities into your daily routine to improve the spiritual and emotional quality of your life.

---

drugs. Although the evidence from the animal studies on MDMA is strong enough to be taken seriously, the evidence of long-term neurotoxic effects of MDMA use in humans is inconclusive.[53] The serotonin reuptake inhibitor fluoxetine (Prozac) (see Chapter 10) blocks the neurotoxicity in rats but does not appear to block the psychoactive effect in humans, and some human users have used fluoxetine with MDMA to reduce the chances of brain damage.[54] Although MDMA has been listed as a Schedule I controlled substance since 1988, it continues to be studied as a potential psycho-therapeutic agent.[55] It is once again ironic but by now no longer surprising—following the listing of MDMA (Ecstacy) as a Schedule I controlled substance, and the attendant publicity about its dangers, it appears to have become more popular than even among young users at "raves."

PCP

In the 1950s, Parke, Davis & Company investigated a series of drugs in the search for an efficient intravenous anesthetic. On the basis of animal studies, the company selected 1-(1-phenylcyclohexyl) piperidine hydrochloride

(PCP, generic name *phencyclidine*) for testing in humans. The studies on monkeys had indicated that **PCP** was a good analgesic but did not produce good muscle relaxation or sleep. Instead, the animals showed a sort of "dissociation" from what was happening: "During the operation the animal had its eyes open and looked about unconcernedly." In 1958, the first report was published on the use of PCP (Sernyl) for surgical anesthesia in humans. Sernyl produced good analgesia without depressing blood circulation or respiration and did not produce irregularities in heartbeat. Loss of sensation occurred within two or three minutes of beginning the intravenous infusion, after about 10 mg of the drug had been delivered. The patients later had no memory of the procedure, did not remember being spoken to, and remembered no pain. Compared with existing anesthetics, which tend to depress both respiration and circulation through general depression of the CNS, this type of "dissociative" anesthetic seemed to be quite safe. However, the psychological reactions to the drug were unpredictable. During administration of the drug a few patients became very excited, and a different anesthetic had to be used. Several patients were "unmanageable" as they emerged from the anesthetic, exhibiting severely manic behavior. This and later reports indicated that many people given anesthetic doses of Sernyl reported changes in body perception and hallucinations, and about 15 percent of the patients experienced a "prolonged confusional psychosis," lasting up to four days after the drug was given. This period of confusion was characterized by feelings of unreality, depersonalization, persecution, depression, and intense anxiety.

News of this new hallucinogen soon reached Dr. Luby, a psychiatrist, who began testing it in both normal and schizophrenic subjects.[56] All the subjects reported changes in perception of their own bodies, with one normal subject saying, "my arm feels like a 20-mile pole with a pin at the end." Another said, "I am a small . . . not human . . . just a block of something in a great big laboratory." There were a number of reports of floating, flying, dizziness, and alternate contraction and expansion of body size. All subjects also showed a thought disorder. Some made up new words, uttered strings of unrelated words, or repeated words or simple phrases. Also, all became increasingly drowsy and apathetic. At times a subject would appear to be asleep but when asked a direct question would respond. When asked, "Can you hear me?" subjects often responded, "No." The majority became either angry or uncooperative. Many of the normal subjects said they felt as if they were drunk from alcohol. All subjects displayed diminished pain, touch, and position sense, and all showed nystagmus (rapid oscillations of the eyes) and a slapping, ataxic walk. Luby and his colleagues felt that PCP was different from LSD or mescaline in that there were few reports of intense visual experiences and many more reports of body image changes. The disorganized thinking, suspiciousness, and lack of cooperation made the PCP state resemble schizophrenia much more than the LSD state.

Thus, by 1960, PCP had been characterized as an excellent anesthetic for monkeys, a medically safe but psychologically troublesome anesthetic for humans, and a hallucinogen different from LSD and mescaline, with profound effects on body perception. Parke, Davis withdrew Sernyl as an investigational drug for humans in 1965 and in 1967 licensed another company to sell Sernylan as an animal anesthetic. It was particularly used with primates, in both research laboratories and zoos. Also, because of its rapid action and wide safety margin, Sernylan was used in syringe bullets to immobilize stray, wild, or dangerous zoo animals. Because of the popular term *tranquilizer gun* for this use, PCP became popularly, and inaccurately, known as an animal "tranquilizer."

Other PCP-like Drugs: Ketamine, Dextromethorphan, and Nitrous Oxide. Even though Sernyl was never marketed for human use, a related chemical from the same series was marketed as a dissociative anesthetic. Ketamine

hydrochloride (Ketalar) has been in continued human use for more than 30 years. A related veterinary product is also available. Although ketamine has more depressant effects than PCP and fewer prolonged reactions, clinical reports indicate that emergence reactions occur in about 12 percent of patients. These reactions include hallucinations and delirium, sometimes accompanied by confusion and irrational behavior. In 1999, widespread reports of ketamine abuse and its notoriety as a party drug (called Special K, or K) caused the Department of Health and Human Service to recommend adding ketamine to the list of Schedule III controlled substances.

Like PCP and ketamine, two more common substances are also capable of causing dissociative effects, perhaps by blocking NMDA-type glutamate receptors in the brain. Nitrous oxide (laughing gas, Chapter 9) and dextromethorphan, an over-the-counter cough suppressant (Chapter 15) can, at very high doses, produce dissociative-type hallucinations similar to those produced by PCP. Unfortunately, at these doses there is also evidence of pathological changes to neurons in the cerebral cortex of animals. Recently, it was reported that the combination of nitrous oxide and ketamine, sometimes used for general anesthesia, produces synergistic neurotoxic effects in animals.[57]

Recreational Use of PCP.   In late 1967, workers at the Haight-Ashbury Medical Clinic obtained samples of a substance being distributed as the "Peace Pill." The drug was analyzed and determined to be PCP, and its identity and dangers were publicized in the community in December 1967. By the next year, it was reported that this drug had enjoyed only brief popularity and then disappeared. It appeared briefly in New York in 1968 as "hog" and at other times as "trank." Into the early 1970s, PCP was apparently regarded as pretty much a "garbage" drug by street people. In the early 1970s, PCP crystals were sometimes sprinkled onto oregano, parsley, or alfalfa and sold to unsuspecting youngsters as marijuana. In this form, it became known as **angel dust**.

Because PCP can be made inexpensively and relatively easily by amateur chemists, when it is available it usually doesn't cost much. Eventually, the rapid and potent effects of angel dust made it a desired substance in its own right. Joints made with PCP sometimes contained marijuana, sometimes another plant substance, and were known as "killer joints" or "sherms" (because they hit the user like a Sherman tank). In the late 1970s, PCP use was the most common cause of drug-induced visits to hospital emergency rooms in many communities, and in some neighborhoods young users could be seen "moonwalking" down the street (taking very high, careful, and slow steps) on any Saturday night.

Some users develop a profound psychological dependence on PCP, in spite of its unpredictability and the behavioral impairment it produces. One user reported:

> Immediately after smoking the Dust I started experiencing the effects. All my troubles seemed to go away. I felt a little drunk and had some trouble walking around the apartment. Objects appeared either very far away or very close and I couldn't really judge distance at all. . . . I liked being apart from things, and felt outside my body for most of the trip. That was fun. Before I smoked I had been troubled about some exams coming up and felt I wasn't really prepared. . . . All that anxiety vanished with the Dust. . . . I felt at peace. It was a good feeling. . . . I want to be there always.[58]

That individual was unusually descriptive about the experience. Most often, a PCP user doesn't say much that makes sense while the drug is having its effects, and later the user doesn't remember much of what happened.

PCP: phencyclidine; originally developed as an anesthetic; has hallucinogenic properties.

angel dust: the street name for PCP sprinkled on plant material.

Taking Sides

Can Ibogaine Cure Drug Dependence?

Ibogaine is a less well-known indole drug that comes from the African shrub *Tabernanthe iboga*. The drug has been used by the local natives as a stimulant at lower doses and a hallucinogen at higher doses.[73] Animal experiments have demonstrated a short-term effect of reducing the self-administration of opioids or of cocaine, although the finding is not consistent. Also, there have been claims that humans who use ibogaine lose their craving for whatever drug they have been addicted to. This has led to proposals to carry out full-scale testing of ibogaine as a possible treatment for addiction. However, these suggestions have been met by a great deal of skepticism from people with long experience in treating addiction, who are used to periodic claims of a miracle cure. Also, there has been considerable reluctance on the part of the federal drug-abuse research agency, NIDA, to promote a large-scale human study of ibogaine. This might be due partly to the drug's reputation as a hallucinogen and due partly to reports of neurotoxicity when high doses were given to animals. Researchers continue to be interested in the possible antidependence properties of both ibogaine and some less toxic chemical relatives.[63]

For more on this topic, log on to www.dushkin.com/online for current news and links to other popular and informative sites, as well as time-saving web search strategies and study tools.

The dependence-producing properties of PCP have also been studied in monkeys, which learn to respond to produce intravenous injections of the drug.[59] This is in contrast to LSD and other hallucinogens, which do not support animal self-administration and do not produce psychological dependence in most users.

Because some PCP users have been reported to behave violently, there is a question as to whether PCP tends to promote violence directly or whether violence is a side effect of the suspicion and anesthesia produced by the drug. Most users do not report feeling violent and feel so uncoordinated that they can't imagine starting a fight. However, police who have tried to arrest PCP users have had trouble subduing them because many of the commonly used arrest techniques rely on restraining holds that result in pain if the arrestee resists. Because the PCP user is anesthetized, these restraint techniques are less effective.[60] Manual restraint by more than one officer might be required to arrest some PCP users, although one might question how different this is from the problem of arresting a violent drunk who is "feeling no pain."

That PCP users might not feel pain has resulted in some gruesome legends about users biting or cutting off their own fingers and so forth. Like earlier stories about LSD users blinding themselves by staring at the sun, these legends cannot be substantiated and most likely have not really occurred. One oft-repeated story probably falls into the category of police folklore. Every cop knows for a fact the story about the PCP user who was so violent, had such superhuman strength, and was so insensitive to pain that he was shot 28 times (or a similar large number of times) before he fell. Although everyone "knows" that this happened, no one can tell you exactly when or where. One might dismiss such folklore as harmless, unless it contributes to events such as the shooting, 6 times at close range, of an unarmed, naked, 35-year-old biochemist who was trying to climb the street sign outside his laboratory. This story really did happen, on August 4, 1977, during the height of the PCP epidemic. The lethal shots were fired by a Los Angeles police officer. The coroner's office reported that the victim's blood did contain traces of a drug similar to PCP.[61] Several years later, Los Angeles police officers involved in the widely publicized videotaped beating of Rodney King said during their trial that they used such force because they believed King might have been "dusted"—under the influence of PCP.

The mechanism of PCP's action on the brain was a mystery for several years, because PCP alters many neurotransmitter systems but does not appear to act directly on any of them. In

1979, it was reported that a specific receptor for PCP was present in the brain, and in 1981 the identity between the receptor and another that had previously been considered a subtype of opiate receptor was reported.[62] The drug cyclazocine, which has some opiate activity and has also been reported to produce hallucinations, binds well to this PCP receptor, but morphine, naloxone, and other opiates do not. Thus, the receptor is probably better characterized as being selective for PCP, ketamine, and other similar drugs rather than as a type of opiate receptor. The presence of such a receptor has led to speculation about a possible endogenous substance, facetiously called "angel-dustin," that would normally act on the receptor. It is not far from there to the speculation that excessive amounts of this hypothetical "angel-dustin" in some individuals might be responsible for schizophrenia, but as of yet there is no good clinical evidence in support of such a notion.

The PCP receptor is found in close association with receptors for glutamate, an excitatory neurotransmitter, where PCP antagonizes the excitatory action of the normal transmitter. Thus, the mechanism by which PCP produces its effects is becoming clearer even if the proposed endogenous PCP-like substance has not yet been found.

ANTICHOLINERGIC HALLUCINOGENS

The potato family contains all the naturally occurring agents to be discussed in this section. Three of the genera—*Atropa, Hyoscyamus,* and *Mandragora*—have a single species of importance and were primarily restricted to Europe. The fourth genus, *Datura,* is worldwide and has many species containing the active agents.

The family of plants in which all these genera are found is *Solanaceae,* "herbs of consolation," and three pharmacologically active alkaloids are responsible for the effects of these plants. *Atropine,* which is *dl*-hyoscyamine, scopolamine or *l*-hyoscine, and *l*-hyoscyamine are all potent

central and peripheral cholinergic blocking agents. These drugs occupy the acetylcholine receptor site but do not activate it; thus, their effect is primarily to block muscarinic cholinergic neurons, including the parasympathetic system.

These agents have potent peripheral and central effects, and some of the psychological responses to these drugs are probably a reaction to peripheral changes. These alkaloids block the production of mucus in the nose and throat. They also prevent salivation, so the mouth becomes uncommonly dry, and perspiration stops. Temperature can increase to fever levels (109°F has been reported in infants with atropine poisoning), and heart rate can show a 50-beat-per-minute increase with atropine. Even at moderate doses these chemicals cause considerable dilation of the pupils of the eyes, with a resulting inability to focus on nearby objects. With large enough doses, there develops a behavioral pattern that resembles toxic psychosis; there is delirium, mental confusion, loss of attention, drowsiness, and loss of memory for recent events. These two characteristics—a clouding of consciousness and no memory for the period of intoxication—plus the absence of vivid sensory effects separate these drugs from the indole and catechol hallucinogens. Instead of phantastica, a better term for the anticholinergics might be *deliriants.*

Belladonna

Atropine, which was isolated in 1831, is the active ingredient in deadly nightshade, *Atropa belladonna.* The name of the plant reflects two of its major uses in the Middle Ages and before. The genus name reflects its use as a poison. Deadly nightshade was one of the plants used extensively by both professional and amateur poisoners; 14 of its berries contain enough of the alkaloid to cause death.

Belladonna, the species name, meaning "beautiful woman," comes from the use of the extract of this plant to dilate the pupils of the eyes. Interestingly, ancient Roman and Egyptian women knew something that science did not learn until more recently. In the 1950s, it was demonstrated, by using pairs of photographs identical except for the amount of pupil dilation, that most people judge the girl with the more dilated eyes to be prettier.

Of more interest here than pretty girls or poisoned men is the sensation of flying reported by witches. The first step toward completing this experiment is to make an ointment. Although there are many recipes, a good one seems to be infant's fat, juice of water parsnip, aconite, cinquefoile, deadly nightshade, and soot. When the ointment is made, it is rubbed on the body and especially liberally between the legs and on a stick that is to be straddled. This stick served as a phallic symbol during the ceremony of the Sabbat. The Sabbat, or Black Mass, worshipped Satan, and both men and women engaged in a nightlong orgy. Straddling the stick and hopping and shrieking around a circle, they felt able "to be carried in the aire, to feasting, singing, dansing, kissing, culling, and other acts of venerie, with such youths as they love and desire most!"[64] The feeling of levitation perhaps comes from the irregular heartbeat in conjunction with drowsiness. Some have reported that changes in heart rate coupled with falling asleep sometimes results in a sensation of falling (or flying),[65] but a more likely explanation is simply the power of suggestion.

Other actions were important in causing the effects of the Sabbat. The pounding of the heart would certainly convey excitement, and the excitement might cause sexual arousal. One of the reputations of belladonna was as an aphrodisiac, so it might all fit together. Perhaps the physiological effects of the agents coupled with a good placebo effect was enough for the witches who attended the Sabbat.

Mandrake

The *mandrake* plant *(Mandragora officinarum)* contains all three alkaloids. Although many drugs can be traced to the Bible, it is particularly important to do so with mandrake because its close association with love and lovemaking has persisted from Genesis to recent times:

> In the time of wheat-harvest Reuben went out and found some mandrakes in the open country and brought them to his mother Leah. Then Rachel asked Leah for some of her son's mandrakes, but Leah said, "Is it so small a thing to have taken away my husband, that you should take my son's mandrakes as well?" But Rachel said, "Very well, let him sleep with you tonight in exchange for your son's mandrakes." So when Jacob came in from the country in the evening, Leah went out to meet him and said, "You are to sleep with me tonight; I have hired you with my son's mandrakes." That night he slept with her.[66]

The mandrake root is forked and, if you have a vivid imagination, resembles a human body. The root contains the psychoactive agents and was endowed with all sorts of magical and medical properties. The association with the human form is alluded to in Shakespeare's Juliet's farewell speech: "And shrieks like mandrakes torn out of the earth, That living mortals hearing them run mad."

Henbane

Compared with deadly nightshade and mandrake, *Hyoscyamus niger* has had a most uninteresting life. This is strange, because it is pharmacologically quite active and contains both scopolamine and *l*-hyoscyamine. Other plants of this genus contain effective levels of the alkaloids, but it is *Hyoscyamus niger* that appears throughout history as *henbane,* a highly poisonous substance and truly the bane of hens, as well as other animals.

Pliny in A.D. 60 said, "For this is certainly known, that, if one takes it in drink more than four leaves, it will put him beside himself." Shakespeare's Hamlet's father must have had more than four leaves because it was henbane that was used to poison him.

Datura

The distribution of the many *Datura* species is worldwide, but they all contain the three alkaloids under discussion—atropine, scopolamine, and hyoscyamine—in varying amounts. Almost as extensive as the distribution are its uses and its history. Although it is not clear when the Chinese first used *Datura metel* as a medicine to treat colds and nervous disorders, the plant was important enough to become associated with Buddha:

> The Chinese valued this drug far back into ancient times. A comparatively recent Chinese medical text, published in 1590, reported that "when Buddha preaches a sermon, the heavens bedew the petals of this plant with rain drops."[67]

Halfway around the world 2,500 years before the Chinese text, virgins sat in the temple to Apollo in Delphi and, probably under the influence of *Datura*,[67] mumbled sounds that holy men interpreted as predictions that always came true. The procedure was straightforward, and

> preliminary to the divine possession, she appears to have chewed leaves of the sacred laurel . . . prior to speaking . . . she was supposed to be inspired by a mystic vapour that arose from a fissure in the ground.[68]

Probably either the plant material eaten was one of the *Datura* species or the burning seeds and leaves of the *Datura* plant formed the mystic vapor she inhaled. It should not go unnoticed, as we search for the beyond within, that engraved on the temple at Delphi were the words "Know thyself."

Datura is associated with the worship of Shiva in India, where it has long been recognized as an ingredient in love potions and has been known as "deceiver" and "foolmaker." In Asia the practice of mixing the crushed seeds of *Datura metel* in tobacco, cannabis, and food persists even today.

The ever-busy chronicler Hernandez mentioned the use of *Datura inoxia* (loco weed) by the Aztecs, and the use of various *Datura* species by Indians of the United States Southwest for magical and religious purposes is well substantiated.[36] One of the interesting uses of *Datura stramonium*, which is native and grows wild in the eastern United States, was devised by the Algonquin Indians. They used the plant to solve the problem of the adolescent search for identity:

> The youths are confined for long periods, given ". . . no other substance but the infusion or decoction of some poisonous, intoxicating roots . . ." and "they became stark, staring mad, in which raving condition they were kept eighteen or twenty days." These poor creatures drink so much of that water of Lethe that they perfectly lose the remembrance of all former things, even of their parents, their treasure, and their language. When the doctors find that they have drunk sufficiently of the wysoccan . . . they gradually restore them to their senses again. . . . Thus they unlive their former lives and commence men by forgetting that they ever have been boys.[67]

The same plant is now called Jamestown weed, or jimsonweed, as a result of an incident in the seventeenth century. This was recorded for history in the book *The History and Present State of Virginia*,[69] published first in 1705 by Robert Beverly.

> The *James-Town* Weed (which resembles the Thorny Apple of *Peru*, and I take to be the Plant so call'd) is supposed to be one of the greatest Coolers in the World. This being an early Plant, was gather'd very young for a boil'd Salad, by some of the Soldiers sent thither, to pacifie the Troubles of *Bacon;* and some of them eat plentifully of it, the Effect of which was a very pleasant Comedy; for they turn'd natural Fools upon it for several Days.

Although there has been some recent abuse of jimsonweed, the unpleasant and dangerous side effects of this plant limit its recreational use.

Synthetic Anticholinergics

Anticholinergic drugs were once used to treat Parkinson's disease (before the introduction of *L*-dopa) and are still widely used to treat the pseudoparkinsonism produced by antipsychotic drugs (see Chapter 10). Particularly in older people there is concern about inadvertently producing an "anticholinergic syndrome," characterized by excessive dry mouth, elevated temperature, delusions, and hallucinations. Anticholinergic drugs such as trihexyphenidyl (Artane) and benztropine (Cogentin) have only rarely been abused for their delirium-producing properties.

AMANITA MUSCARIA

The *Amanita muscaria* mushroom is also called "fly agaric," probably because of what it does to flies. It doesn't kill them, but when they suck its juice, it puts them into a stupor for 2 to 3 hours. It is one of the common poisonous mushrooms found in forests in many parts of the world. The older literature suggests that eating 5 to 10 *Amanita* mushrooms results in severe effects of intoxication, such as muscular twitching, leading to twitches of limbs and raving drunkenness, with agitation and vivid hallucinations. Later follow many hours of partial paralysis with sleep and dreams.

When the ancient Aryan invaders swept down from the north into India 3,500 years ago, they took Soma, itself considered a deity. The cult of Soma ruled India's religion and culture for many years—the poems of the Rig Veda celebrate the sacramental use of this substance. It has only been within the past 30 years that scholars have discovered and agreed on the identity of Soma as *Amanita*.[1]

The suggestion has been made that the ambrosia ("food of the gods") mentioned in the secret rites of the god Dionysius in Greece was a solution of the *Amanita* mushroom.[70] And based on paintings representing the "tree of life" found in ancient European cave paintings, it has been

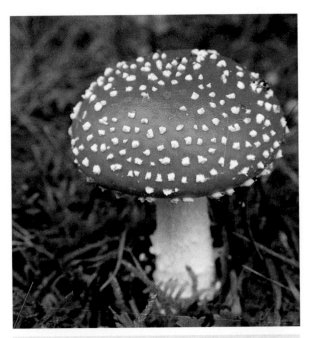

The red- and white-speckled mushroom *Amanita muscaria* played a major role in the early history of Indo-European and Central American religions.

suggested that *Amanita muscaria* use formed a basis for the cult that originated about 2,000 years ago and today calls itself Christianity.[71]

Until the Russians introduced them to alcohol, many of the isolated nomadic tribes of Siberia had no intoxicant but *Amanita:*

> Use of the Amanita mushroom by Siberian tribes continues today largely free from social control of any sort. Use of the drug has a Shamanist aspect, and forms the basis for orgiastic communal indulgences. Since the drug can induce murderous rages in addition to more moderate hallucinogenic experiences, serious injuries frequently result.[72]

In the frozen northland, these mushrooms are expensive; sometimes several reindeer are exchanged for an effective number of the mushrooms. However, they have the unique property of being reusable, and during the long winter

Drugs in Depth

Toadlicking: An Urban Legend

In the late 1980s, a story was going around about a substance called *bufotenin*, an indole that looks as if it might be hallucinogenic and was originally identified in the skins of toads (genus *Bufo*). In one version of the story, hippies living in the hills of Northern California were chasing toads through the woods and licking them to get high: California was said to have listed one species of toad as a controlled substance. In another version, it was the infamous cane toad of Australia, said to be licked or ingested both by aborigines and by Australian hippies.

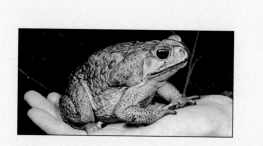

It's a great story, seemingly plausible enough, and certainly colorful enough to repeat. It found its way into drug-abuse lectures and at least one textbook, and the Australian version was passed along as fact by *USA Today* in 1988. The idea even became the plot for one episode of the television program *LA Law*. The only problem is that the story wasn't true.

Bufotenin was studied experimentally back in the 1950s, during the heyday of research on hallucinogens as models of schizophrenia. Probably it was studied because it was found in *Amanita* mushrooms, and they were known to have been used as hallucinogens. However, when bufotenin was given to "volunteer" prison inmates (by injection, not licking) it was found to be a not very potent hallucinogen. It may have been toxic in other ways because the experimental subjects became quite cyanotic (meaning they turned blue, although the researcher in charge says it was more of a deep purple). That basically ended human research with bufotenin. It can't be proved that nobody ever licked a toad in California, but there is no documented evidence for this as a regular practice of any group at any time, nor is there any documented evidence that hallucinatory effects can be gotten in this way.

This legend could have tragic consequences, in that toads do have a variety of toxins in their skins that protect them from being eaten by predators. If a person actually were to eat toad skins or somehow obtain and use pure bufotenin, he or she could become quite ill or even die. One Australian youth is reported to have died after eating cane toad eggs.

This story is such a graphically gross one that it doesn't want to go away, in spite of a small story debunking the myth published in *Scientific American* in 1990. Even after that came out, a Georgia legislator referred to "the extreme danger of cane-toad licking becoming the designer drug of choice." A warning was published in the *British Journal of Psychiatry* (November 1990) that "the Australian cane toad is popularly kept as a pet in the US, and licked by its owners for the resulting hallucinatory effects," with the note that two English toads also have the potential to be used in this way. The legend may be explained with a related truth (not uncommon). It was recently reported that the Sonoran desert toad, *Bufo alvarius*, secretes large amounts of 5-methoxy DMT, which is a potent hallucinogen, in its venom. Although the venom is toxic when eaten, the substance can be smoked to obtain the psychoactive effect. The authors speculated that anthropologists had long ago mistakenly concluded that the more common toad *Bufo marinus* was the one being referred to in their interviews with the native people of the region and depicted in pre-Columbian art of Central America.[74]

Two pieces of advice: don't lick strange toads, and be especially cautious about believing any weird story you hear that involves hallucinogenic drugs, unless there is documented evidence (who, what, when, where, why, how, and how much?). The "mystical" nature of these substances has, no doubt, inspired more untrue legends than any other type of drug.

months they might be worth the price. The mushrooms themselves are not reusable; once eaten, they're gone. But this is a hallucinogen that is excreted unchanged in the urine. When the effect begins to wear off, "midway in the orgy the cry of 'pass the pot' goes out."[73] The active ingredient can be reused four or five times in this way.

There is evidence that *Amanita* was also used as a holy plant by several tribal groups in the Americas, ranging from Alaska and the Great Lakes to Mexico and Central America. In several of the legends, its origin is associated with thunder and lightning.[1]

For many years the active agent in this mushroom was thought to be *muscarine* (for which the muscarinic cholinergic receptors were named). This substance activates the same type of acetylcholine receptor that is blocked by the anticholinergics. However, pharmacological studies with other cholinergic agonists did not produce similar psychoactive effects. Next, attention focused on *bufotenin*, an indole that is found in high concentrations in the skins of toads (see the Drugs in Depth box). However, the hallucinogenic properties of bufotenin have been in doubt, and *Amanita* species contain only small amounts of it. In the mid-1960s, meaningful amounts of two chemicals were found: ibotenic acid and muscimol.

The effects of *Amanita* ingestion are not similar to those of other hallucinogens, and that helped confuse the picture with regard to the mechanism. Muscimol can act as an agonist at GABA receptors, which are inhibitory and found throughout the CNS. Muscimol is more potent than ibotenic acid, and drying of the mushroom, which is usually done by those who use it, promotes the transformation of ibotenic acid to muscimol. Muscimol has been given to humans, resulting in confusion, disorientation in time and place, sensory disturbances, muscle twitching, weariness, fatigue, and sleep.[38]

It should be stressed that, although *Amanita muscaria* and other related poisonous mushrooms

are found in North America, they are a particularly dangerous type of plant with which to experiment.

SUMMARY

- Hallucinogenic plants have been used for many centuries, not only as medicines but for spiritual and recreational purposes as well.
- LSD, a synthetic hallucinogen, alters perceptual processes and enhances emotionality, so that the real world is seen differently and is responded to with great emotion.
- Other chemicals that contain the indole nucleus, such as psilocybin (from the Mexican mushroom), have effects similar to those of LSD.
- Mescaline, from the peyote cactus, and synthetic derivatives of the amphetamines represent the catechol hallucinogens. They have psychological effects quite similar to those of the indole types.
- MDMA is the only catechol hallucinogen that appears likely to be capable of producing permanent brain damage in its users.
- PCP, or angel dust, produces more changes in body perception and fewer visual effects than LSD.
- Anticholinergics are found in many plants throughout the world and have been used not only recreationally, medically, and spiritually but also as poisons.

REVIEW QUESTIONS

1. What are the distinctions among phantastica, psychedelics, psychotomimetics, entheogens, and hallucinogens?
2. What is the precise relationship between ergotism and LSD?

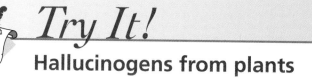

Try It!

Hallucinogens from plants

Match the plants on the left with the appropriate hallucinogenic chemical on the right:

ayahuasca

peyote

sacred mushrooms (from Mexico)

morning glories

belladonna

Amanita

mescaline

muscimol

∂-lysergic acid amide

atropine

DMT and harmaline

psilocybin

Web Watch

Check Out Publications on Hallucinogens

The National Clearing House for Drug and Alcohol Information offers a listing of publications about certain types of drugs. Go to www.health.org/catalog/catalog.asp?key=7&detail=false to find and, if you wish, order brochures or other publications about hallucinogens.

Read an LSD Overview

At www.cocaineaddiction.com/other_lsd.html, read the overview of LSD. You will find information on the history of LSD, its effects, study results, and related statistics.

How Dangerous Is Ecstasy?

Also known as MDMA, "Adam," and "XTC," Ecstasy is a mind-altering synthetic drug. At www.cocaineaddiction.com/other_ecstasy.html, find information on the history of Ecstasy, its effects, study results, and related statistics.

3. Why was LSD used in psychoanalysis in the 1950s and 1960s? How does this relate to its proposed use by the army and the CIA?

4. Describe the addictive potential of LSD in terms of tolerance, physical dependence, and psychological dependence.

5. What are three adverse psychological reactions that have been associated with LSD use?

6. What is the active agent in the "magic mushrooms" of Mexico, and is it an indole or a catechol?

7. Besides the psychological effects, what other effects are reliably produced by peyote?

8. Contrast MDMA and PCP in terms of how they appear to make people feel about being close to others.

9. Which of the hallucinogenic plants was most associated with witchcraft?

10. Describe what is actually known about bufotenin and the "toad-licking" phenomenon.

REFERENCES

1. Schultes RE, Hofmann A: *Plants of the gods*. New York: McGraw-Hill, 1979.
2. Hordern A: Psychopharmacology: Some historical considerations. In Joyce CRB, editor: *Psychopharmacology: Dimensions and perspectives*. Philadelphia: J. B. Lippincott, 1968.
3. Caporael LR: Ergotism: The Satan loosed in Salem, *Science* 192:21–26, 1976.
4. Gottlieb J, Spanos NP: Ergotism and the Salem village witch trials, *Science* 194:1390–1394, 1976.
5. Hofmann A: Psychotomimetic agents. In Burger A, editor: *Drugs affecting the central nervous system* (Vol. 2). New York: Marcel Dekker, 1968.
6. Horowitz M: Interview with Albert Hofmann, *High Times* pp 24–81, July 1976.
7. Clark W: Psychedelic research: Obstacles and values, *Journal of Humanistic Psychology* 15(3):5–17, 1975.
8. Segal J, editor: *Research in the service of mental health, research on drug abuse*, National Institute on Mental Health, Pub. No. (ADM) 75-236, U.S. Department of Health, Education, and Welfare, Washington, DC: U.S. Government Printing Office, 1975.
9. Johnston L: Ford signs grant of $750,000 in LSD death in CIA test, *New York Times* p C43, Oct 14, 1976.
10. Treaster JB: Mind-drug test a federal project for almost 25 years, *New York Times* p M42, Aug 11, 1975.
11. CIA considered big LSD purchase, *Washington Star* Aug 4, 1975. See also Knight M: LSD creator says army sought drug, *New York Times* Aug 1, 1975.
12. Taylor JR, Johnson WN: *Use of volunteers in chemical agent research*, Inspector General Report No. DAIGIN 21-75, Washington, DC: U.S. Department of Army, Mar 10, 1976.
13. Weil AT: The strange case of the Harvard drug scandal, *Look* pp 38–48, Nov 5, 1963.
14. Blumenthal R: Leary drug cult stirs Millbrook, *New York Times* p 49, June 14, 1967.
15. Celebration #1, *New Yorker* 42:43, 1966.
16. Masters REL: Sex, ecstasy, and the psychedelic drugs, *Playboy* pp 94–226, /1967.
17. Council on Mental Health and Committee on Alcoholism and Drug Dependence: Dependence on LSD and other hallucinogenic drugs, *JAMA* 202:141–144, 1967.
18. Leary, once an LSD advocate, paroled, *New York Times* p 25, Apr 21, 1976.
19. Leary and Liddy, debating specialists, *New York Times* p B26, Sept 3, 1981.
20. Hamon M: Common neurochemical correlates to the action of hallucinogens. In Jacobs BL, editor: *Hallucinogens: neurochemical, behavioral and clinical perspectives*. New York: Raven Press, 1984.

21. Aghajanian GK: LSD and serotonergic dorsal raphe neurons: Intracellular studies in vivo and in vitro. In Jacobs BL, editor: *Hallucinogens: Neurochemical, behavioral and clinical perspectives*. New York: Raven Press, 1984.

22. Appel JB, Rosecrans JA: Behavioral pharmacology of hallucinogens in animals: Conditioning studies. In Jacobs BL, editor: *Hallucinogens: neurochemical, behavioral and clinical perspectives*. New York: Raven Press, 1984.

23. Nichols DE, Glennon RA: Medicinal chemistry and structure-activity relationships of hallucinogens. In Jacobs BL, editor: *Hallucinogens: Neurochemical, behavioral and clinical perspectives*. New York: Raven Press, 1984.

24. Voellenweider FX and others: Psilocybin induces schizophrenia-like psychosis in humans via a serotonin-2 agonist action, *Neuroreport* 9:3897–3902,1998.

25. Siegel RK: The natural history of hallucinogens. In Jacobs BL, editor: *Hallucinogens: Neurochemical, behavioral and clinical perspectives*. New York: Raven Press, 1984.

26. Krippner S: Psychedelic experience and the language process, *Journal of Psychedelic Drugs* 3(1):41–51, 1970.

27. Levine J, Ludwig AM: The LSD controversy, *Comprehensive Psychiatry* 5(5):318–319, 1964.

28. Forsch WA, Robbins ES, Stern M: Untoward reactions to lysergic acid diethylamide (LSD) resulting in hospitalization, *New England Journal of Medicine* 273:1235–1239, 1965.

29. Abraham HD, Wolf E: Visual function in past users of LSD: Psychophysical findings, *Journal of Abnormal Psychology* 97:443–447, 1988.

30. Zegans LS, Pollard JC, Brown D: The effects of LSD-25 on creativity and tolerance to regression, *Archives of General Psychiatry* 16:740–749, 1967.

31. Spitzer M and others: Increased activation of indirect semantic associations under psilocybin, *Biological Psychiatry* 39:1055–1057, 1996.

32. Hollister LE, Shelton J, Krieger G: A controlled comparison of lysergic acid diethylamide (LSD) and dextroamphetamine in alcoholics, *American Journal of Psychiatry* 125:1352–1357, 1969.

33. NIMH research on LSD, Extramural programs fiscal year 1948 to present, prepared Sept 1, 1975.

34. Crahan ME: God's flesh and other preColumbian phantastica, *Bulletin of the Los Angeles County Medical Association* 99:17, 1969.

35. Wolbach AB Jr., Isbell H, Miner EJ: Cross tolerance between mescaline and LSD-25, with a comparison of the mescaline and LSD reactions, *Psychopharmacologia* 3:1–14, 1962.

36. Leary T: The religious experience: Its production and interpretation, *Journal of Psychedelic Drugs* 1(2):3–23, 1967–1968.

37. Delgado PL, Moreno FA: Hallucinogens, serotonin, and obsessive-compulsive disorder, *Journal of Psychoactive Drugs,* 30:359–366, 1998.

38. Schultes RE, Hofmann A: *The botany and chemistry of hallucinogens*. Springfield, IL: Charles C Thomas, 1980.

39. Al-Assmar SE: The Seeds of the Hawaiian baby woodrose are a powerful hallucinogen [letter], *Archives of Internal Medicine* 159:2090, 1999.

40. Strassman RJ and others: Differential tolerance to biological and subjective effects of four closely-spaced doses of N,N-dimethyltryptamine in humans, *Biological Psychiatry* 39:784–795, 1996.

41. Grob CS and others: Human psychopharmacology of hoasca, a plant hallucinogen used in ritual context in Brazil, *Journal of Nervous and Mental Disease* 184:86–94., 1996.

42. LaBarre W: *The peyote cult.* Hamden, CT: Shoe String Press, 1964.

43. Slotkin JS: Religious defenses (the Native American Church), *Journal of Psychedelic Drugs* 1(2):77–95, 1967–1968.

44. Bergman RL. Navajo peyote use: Its apparent safety, *American Journal of Psychiatry* 128:695–699, 1971.

45. Greenhouse L: Court is urged to rehear case on ritual drugs, *New York Times* pp May 11, 1990.

46. Dobkin de Rios M, Cardenas M: Plant hallucinogens, shamanism, and Nazca ceramics, *Journal of Ethnopharmacology* 2:233–246, 1980.

47. De Ropp RS: *Drugs and the mind.* New York: Grove Press, 1957.

48. Ellis H: Mescal: A study of a divine plant, *Popular Science Monthly* 61:59, 65, 1902.

49. Huxley A: *The doors of perception*. New York: Harper & Row, 1954.

50. Smith D, Meyers F: The psychotomimetic amphetamine with special reference to STP (DOM) toxicity. In Smith D, editor: *Drug abuse papers, 1969, Section 4.* Berkeley: University of California, 1969.

51. MDMA: Compound raises medical, legal issues, *Brain/Mind Bulletin* Apr 15, 1985.

52. Peroutka SJ and others: Subjective effects of 3,4-methylenedioxymethamphetamine in recreational users, *Neuropsychopharmacology* 1:273–277, 1988.

53. Curran HV: Is MDMA ("Ecstasy") neurotoxic in humans? An overview of evidence and of methodological problems in research, *Neuropsychobiology* 42:34–41, 2000.

54. McGann UD, Ricuarte GA: Reinforcing subjective effects of 3,4-methylenedioxymethamphetamine ("Ecstasy") may be separable from its neurotoxic actions: Clinical evidence, *Journal of Clinical Psychopharmacology* 13:214, 1993.

55. Greer GR, Tolbert R: A method of conducting therapeutic sessions with MDMA, *Journal of Psychoactive Drugs* 30:371–379, 1998.

56. Luby E and others: Study of a new schizophrenomimetic drug—Sernyl, *American Medical Association Archive of Neurological Psychiatry* 81: 113–119, 1959.

57. Jevtovic-Todorovic V and others: Ketamine potentiates cerebrocortical damage induced by the common

anaesthetic agent nitrous oxide in adult rats, *British Journal of Pharmacology* 130:1692–1698, 2000.

58. Siegel RK: Phencyclidine and ketamine intoxication: A study of four populations of recreational users. In Petersen RC, Stillman RC, editors: *Phencyclidine (PCP) abuse: An appraisal,* NIDA Research Monograph No. 21, Washington, DC: U.S. Department of Health and Human Services, 1978.

59. Balster RL, Chait LD: The behavioral effects of phencyclidine in animals. In Petersen RC, Stillman RC, editors: *Phencyclidine (PCP) abuse: An appraisal,* NIDA Research Monograph No. 21. Washington, DC: U.S. Department of Health and Human Services, 1978.

60. Siegel RK: PCP and violent crime: The people vs. peace, *Journal of Psychedelic Drugs* 12(3–4):317, 1980.

61. Overend W: PCP: Death in the "dust," *Los Angeles Times* Sept 26, 1977.

62. Quirion R and others: Phencyclidine (angel dust)/sigma "opiate" receptor: Visualization by tritium-sensitive film, *Proceedings of the National Academy of Sciences* 78:5881–5885, 1981.

63. Glick SD and others: 18-Methoxycoronaridine (18-MC) and ibogaine: Comparison of antiaddicitive efficacy, toxicity, and mechanisms of action, *Annals of the New York Academy of Sciences* 914:369–386, 2000.

64. Briggs KM: *Pale Hecate's team.* New York: Humanities Press, 1962.

65. Langdon-Brown W: *From witchcraft to chemotherapy.* Cambridge: Cambridge University Press, 1941.

66. Genesis 30:14–16, *The New English Bible,* Oxford University Press and Cambridge University Press, 1970.

67. Schultes RE: The plant kingdom and hallucinogens (Part III), *Bulletin on Narcotics* 22(1):43–46, 1970.

68. Encyclopedia Brittanica, vol 16, 1929

69. Beverly R: *The history and present state of Virginia, 1705.* Chapel Hill: University of North Carolina Press, 1947.

70. Graves R: *Steps.* London: Cassell, 1958.

71. Allegro JM: *The sacred mushroom and the cross.* New York: Doubleday, 1970.

72. Wasson RG: Fly agaric and man. In Efron DH, editor: *Ethnopharmacologic search for psychoactive drugs.* Washington, DC: National Institute of Mental Health, 1967. See also Wasson RG: *Soma, divine mushroom of immortality.* New York: Harcourt Brace Jovanovich, 1971.

73. Hallucinogens, *Columbia Law Review* 68(3):521–560, 1968.

74. Weil AT, Davis W: *Bufo alvarius:* A potent hallucinogen of animal origin, *Journal of Ethnopharmacology* 41:1–8, 1994.

Chapter 18

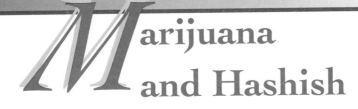

Marijuana and Hashish

KEY TERMS

- *Cannabis*
- hashish
- sinsemilla
- THC
- anandamide
- dronabinol
- Marinol

Online Learning Center Resources

www.mhhe.com/ray

Log on to our Online Learning Center (OLC) for access to these additional resources.

- Chapter definitions
- Learning objectives
- Student interactive question-and-answer sites
- Self-scoring chapter quiz

The OLC also offers web links for study and exploration of health topics. Here are some examples of what you'll find:

www.medmjscience.org

This site presents several articles on marijuana. It also displays polls about marijuana use.

wilkes1.wilkes.edu/~kklemow/Cannabis.html

Check out this site to learn the medical attributes of Cannabis. Slang terms are listed, as well as industrial, recreational, and medicinal uses.

www.mpp.org

This is the home page for the Marijuana Policy Project. It includes project explanations, recent news, and details about legislation. You can sign up for e-mail updates or information via mail.

Drugs in the Media

Medical Marijuana in the News

Probably no single psychoactive drug topic has received more publicity in the past few years than the issue of medical marijuana, which has been placed as a referendum on the ballot in at least eight states. Each time, there are stories about the plight of people with AIDS who say they need marijuana to stimulate their appetites.

Drugs in the Media Continued. . .

And each time there are stories reflecting the views of local police and federal drug-control officials who say that medical marijuana is just an excuse for people who want to grow and use an illegal substance. Here is a sampling of recent headlines that reveal the complexity of the issues raised when these laws are considered and then passed:

FEW SEEK APPLICATIONS FOR MEDICAL MARIJUANA, by Treena Shapiro, *Honolulu Star-Bulletin,* December 29, 2000. After some six months of waiting, medical marijuana applications weren't in high demand yesterday, with only about 10 physicians requesting them from the state Department of Public Safety.

EDITORIAL, *News Journal,* Mansfield, Ohio, December 26, 2000: The approval of the medicinal use of marijuana is a hot political topic. Voters across the United States have considered the legalization of "medicinal" marijuana.

BUSH BACKS STATES' RIGHTS ON MARIJUANA, by Susan Feeney, *The Dallas Morning News,* October 20, 1999. Bush opposes medical use but favors local control.

WASHINGTON (D.C.) BACKS MEDICAL USE OF MARIJUANA, by Irving Molotsky, *New York Times,* September 20, 1999. Congressional opponents of the measure had blocked a count of the initiative, but Judge Richard W. Roberts of Federal District Court here ruled on Friday that the restriction was illegal.

MARIJUANA MAY BE GOOD MEDICINE, BUT THIS IS A BAD LAW, by John W. Porter, *Press Herald,* Portland, Maine, October 13, 1999. Marijuana should be made available to patients, but Question 2 is the wrong way to do it.

Judging from the small but increasing number of states that permit seriously ill patients to grow and use marijuana under medical supervision (California took the lead in 1996), the issue isn't going away any time soon. And this is separate from the issue of general legalization. Currently, marijuana maintains a slot alongside heroin and methamphetamine as a "drug of concern" in its listing on the federal Drug Enforcement Administration's website.

The average American so far seems uninterested in a serious national debate on the use of marijuana. The mere mention of legalizing any illegal drug means political suicide for any politician willing to broach the subject. A notable exception is New Mexico Governor Gary Johnson, a Republican. An outspoken advocate for legalizing pot, Johnson is also a triathlete who maintains steady popularity ratings in his state. Although most U.S. citizens may not be ready to embrace his stance, we will certainly be seeing more arguments in the media for legalizing medical marijuana use.

Marijuana has meant so many things to so many people over the years that it is hard to describe it from a single perspective. We wind up behaving like that famous committee of blind men examining an elephant: the way you describe it depends on where you're standing. The matter of classifying marijuana among the other psychoactive drugs is so complex that we, like most authors, avoid the issue by setting it off by itself. Marijuana can produce some sedative-like effects, some pain relief, and, in large doses, hallucinogenic effects. Thus, many of its users treat it as a depressant; it has been called a narcotic (for both pharmacological, as well as political, reasons); and it is often included among descriptions of hallucinogenic plants. The effects it produces when used as most people use it are, however, sufficiently different from those of other psychoactive drugs to justify its consideration as a unique substance.

CANNABIS, THE PLANT

Marijuana (or *marihuana;* either spelling is correct) is a preparation of leafy material from the **Cannabis** plant that is used by smoking. The question is, which *Cannabis* plant, because there is still botanical debate over whether there is one, three, or more species of *Cannabis*. In previous years, there were legal arguments over this issue because the laws mentioned only *Cannabis sativa.* Does that include all marijuana or not? The evidence is strong that there are three separate species. *Cannabis sativa* originated in Asia but now grows worldwide and primarily has been used for its fibers, from which hemp rope is made. This is the species that grows as a weed in the United States and Canada. *Cannabis indica* is grown for its psychoactive resins and is cultivated in many areas

of the world, including selected planters and backyards of the United States. The third species, *Cannabis ruderalis,* grows primarily in Russia and not at all in America. The plant Linnaeus named *C. sativa* in 1753 is what is still known as *C. sativa.*[1]

It was *C. sativa* that George Washington grew at Mount Vernon, most likely not to get high but to make rope and possibly for medicinal uses. From his fields and many others like it, *C. sativa* spread across the nation, growing spontaneously.

C. sativa that is cultivated for use as hemp grows as a lanky plant up to 18 feet high. *C. indica* plants cultivated for their psychoactive effects are more compact and usually only 2 or 3 feet tall. The psychoactive potency results from an interaction between genetics and environmental conditions. Plants of different species grown under identical conditions produce different amounts of psychoactive material, and the same plants vary in potency from year to year, depending on the amount of sunshine, warm weather, and moisture.

PREPARATIONS FROM *CANNABIS*

The primary psychoactive agent, delta-9-tetrahydrocannabinol (THC), is concentrated in the resin of *cannabis;* most of the resin is in the flowering tops, less is in the leaves, and there is little in the fibrous stalks. The psychoactive potency of a *Cannabis* preparation depends on the amount of resin present and therefore varies, depending on the part of the plant used. There are three traditional *Cannabis* preparations from India, each of which corresponds roughly to preparations available in the United States. The most potent of these is called *charas* in India, and it consists of pure resin that has been carefully removed from the surface of leaves and stems. **Hashish,** or hasheesh, is a substance widely known around the world and in its purest form is pure resin, like charas. It may be less pure, depending on how carefully the resin has been separated from the plant material.

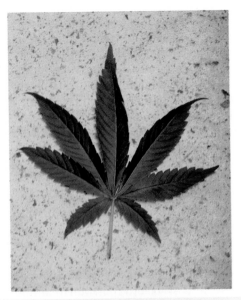
A leaf of the *Cannabis* (marijuana) plant.

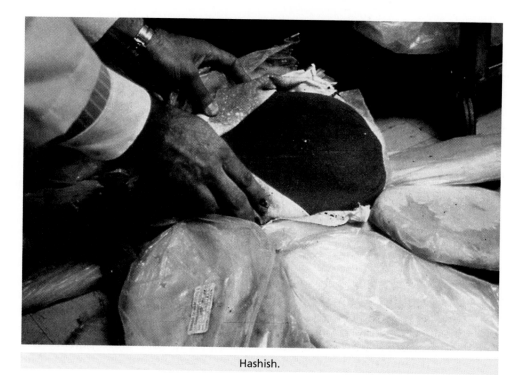

Hashish.

Samples of hashish available in the United States vary widely in their THC content, averaging about 7 or 8 percent and ranging up to about 14 percent THC.

The second most potent preparation is traditionally called *ganja* in India, and it consists of the dried flowering tops of plants with pistillate flowers (female plants). The male plants are removed from the fields before the female plants can become pollinated and put their energy into seed production; this increases the potency of the female plants. This method of production has become increasingly popular in recent years in the United States for producing high-grade marijuana known as **sinsemilla** (Spanish *sin semilla,* "without seeds"). The flowering top portion of the plant is referred to as the "bud" by American growers. Sinsemilla samples from the United States also vary widely in THC content, averaging around 4 or 5 percent, usually not over 7 or 8 percent maximum, although

occasionally samples have been reported as high as 10 or 11 percent.

The weakest form in India is *bhang,* which is made by using the entire remainder of the plant after the top has been picked, then drying it and grinding it into a powder. The powder can then be mixed into drinks or candies.[1] Americans don't usually see this type of preparation, but we might consider it somewhat analogous to low-grade marijuana, which consists of the leaves of

Cannabis: (*can* a biss) the genus of plant known as marijuana.

hashish: (hash *eesh* or *hash* eesh) concentrated resin from the *Cannabis* plant.

sinsemilla: (sin se *mee* ya) "without seeds"; a method of growing more potent marijuana.

a plant, perhaps even a *sativa* plant found growing as a weed. Some of this low-grade marijuana contains less than 1 percent THC.

Manually scraping exuded resin off the plant to make hashish is a tedious process, and a more efficient method of separating the resin from plants has been known for many years. The plants are boiled in alcohol, then the solids filtered out and the liquid evaporated down to a thick, dark substance once known medically as "red oil of cannabis" and now referred to as *hash oil*. Again, this product varies widely in its potency but can contain more than 50 percent THC. Until fairly recently, both the medical and the psychological effects of *Cannabis* preparations were variable. All the traditional methods could do was produce relatively pure plant resin, but that resin could vary considerably in its THC content.

If we consider only the marijuana available for smoking in the United States, we can see that it can vary widely in potency from a low-grade product containing less than 1 percent THC to a high-grade sinsemilla containing 8 percent or more THC. The usual range of potency for marijuana seems to be 2 to 5 percent, however. Since the mid-1980s there have been repeated statements to the effect that the marijuana available on the streets today is "10 times" more potent than the marijuana of the 1960s. The political message behind this is that the marijuana of the 1960s may have been relatively harmless, but the current marijuana is more dangerous. In fact, the entire range of these traditional preparations has been known, and scientific, literary, and medical descriptions of the wide range of effects have been based on this entire range of potencies, for 150 years. It is true that U.S. marijuana growers are becoming more sophisticated and producing more sinsemilla, but the overall range of potencies of marijuana available on the streets is still from under 1 percent to about 8 percent, just as in the early 1970s.[2]

A strange kind of success story surrounds modern-day American growers of marijuana. In the 1970s, domestic marijuana was typically inexpensive, low-grade *sativa* leaves, and higher-grade marijuana was usually imported from Mexico, Colombia, or other warm growing regions. As U.S. efforts to arrest drug smugglers intensified, smugglers turned to cocaine, which was easier to conceal and more profitable. U.S. growers attempting to produce sinsemilla figured out that *C. sativa* doesn't flower well in northern climates and focused on *C. indica*, planting crops in gardens and in small, isolated fields. The Drug Enforcement Administration (DEA) and local law enforcement agencies countered with large-scale efforts to eradicate these plants, driving many growers indoors to use hydroponics, "grow lights," and other technological advances. Experimentation and cross-breeding of *indica* and *sativa* plants has resulted in the most sophisticated growers being able to produce very small plants that take up little room but produce large buds within two months or so. These days, the most potent, and most expensive, marijuana comes from American growers. Marijuana is considered to be America's number one cash crop, earning about $30 billion per year.[3]

HISTORY

Early History

The earliest reference to *Cannabis* is in a pharmacy book written in 2737 B.C. by Chinese emperor Shen Nung. Referring to the euphoriant effects of *Cannabis,* he called it the "Liberator of Sin." There were some medical uses, however, and he recommended it for "female weakness, gout, rheumatism, malaria, beriberi, constipation and absent-mindedness."[4] Social use of the plant had spread to the Muslim world and North Africa by A.D. 1000. In this period in the eastern Mediterranean area, a legend developed around a religious cult that committed murder for political reasons. The cult was called "hashishiyya," from which our word *assassin* developed. In 1299, Marco Polo told the story he had heard of this group and its leader. It was a marvelous tale and had all the ingredients necessary for a tale to survive through the ages: intrigue, murder, sex, the use of drugs, and mysterious lands. The story of this group and its activities was told in many ways over the years, and Boccaccio's *Decameron* contained one story based on it. Stories of this cult, combined with the frequent reference to the power and wonderment of hashish in *The Arabian Nights,* were widely circulated in Europe over the years.

The Nineteenth Century: Romantic Literature and the New Science of Psychology

At the turn of the nineteenth century, world commerce was expanding. New and exciting reports from the world travelers of the seventeenth and eighteenth centuries introduced new cultures and new ideas to Europe. Asia and the Middle East had yielded exotic spices, as well as the stimulants coffee and tea. Europe was ready for another new sensation, and got it. The returning veteran, as usual, gets part of the blame for introducing what Europe was ready to receive:

> Napoleon's campaign to Egypt at the beginning of the nineteenth century increased the Romantic's acquaintance with hashish and caused them to associate it with the Near East. . . . Napoleon was forced to give an order forbidding all French soldiers to indulge in hashish. Some of the soldiers brought the habit to France, however, as did many other Frenchmen who worked for the government or traveled in the Near East.[5]

By the 1830s and 1840s, everyone who was anyone was using, thinking about using, or decrying the use of mind-tickling agents such as opium and hashish. One of the earliest (1844) popular accounts of the use of hashish is in *The Count of Monte Cristo* by Alexander Dumas. The story includes a reference to the Assassins story and contains statements about the characteristics of the drug that still sound contemporary. During the 1840s, a group of artists and writers gathered monthly at the Hotel Pimodan in Paris's Latin Quarter to use drugs. This group became famous because one of the participants, Gautier, wrote a book, *Le Club de Hachischins,* that described their activities. From this group have come some of the best literary descriptions of hashish intoxication. These French Romantics, like the Impressionist painters of a later period, were searching for new experiences, new sources of creativity from within, and new ways of seeing the world outside. A few of the regulars were well-known writers, including Baudelaire, Gautier, and Dumas.

Baudelaire used hashish and was an astute observer of its effects in himself and in others. In his book *Artificial Paradises,* he echoed what Dumas had written about the kind of effect to expect from hashish:

> The intoxication will be nothing but one immense dream, thanks to intensity of color and the rapidity of conceptions; but it will always preserve the particular tonality of the individual. . . . The dream will certainly reflect its dreamer. He is only the same man grown larger . . . sophisticate and ingenu . . . will find nothing miraculous, absolutely nothing but the natural to an extreme.[6]

The extent of Baudelaire's actual experience with hashish is debatable, but he did identify (and exaggerate) three stages of intoxication after oral intake. These are still being rediscovered:

> At first, a certain absurd, irresistible hilarity overcomes you. The most ordinary words, the simplest ideas assume a new and bizarre aspect. This mirth is intolerable to you; but it is useless to resist. The demon has invaded you. . . .
>
> It sometimes happens that people completely unsuited for word-play will improvise an endless string of puns and wholly improbable idea relationships fit to outdo the ablest masters of this preposterous craft. But after a few minutes, the relation between ideas becomes so vague, and the thread of your thoughts grows so tenuous, that only your cohorts . . . can understand you.
>
> Next your senses become extraordinarily keen and acute. Your sight is infinite. Your ear can discern the slightest perceptible sound, even through the shrillest of noises.

The strangest ambiguities, the most inexplicable transpositions of ideas take place. In sounds there is color; in colors there is a music. . . . You are sitting and smoking; you believe that you are sitting in your pipe, and that *your pipe* is smoking *you*; you are exhaling *yourself* in bluish clouds.

This fantasy goes on for an eternity. A lucid interval, and a great expenditure of effort, permit you to look at the clock. The eternity turns out to have been only a minute.

The third phase . . . is something beyond description. It is what the Orientals call *kef*; it is complete happiness. There is nothing whirling and tumultuous about it. It is a calm and placid beatitude. Every philosophical problem is resolved. Every difficult question that presents a point of contention for theologians, and brings despair to thoughtful men, becomes clear and transparent. Every contradiction is reconciled. Man has surpassed the gods.[6]

As the end of the nineteenth century approached, the use of the anxiety-relieving drugs increased, but the hashish experience held little interest for the dweller in middle America. Just beginning, however, was the new science of psychology, whose interest was in the workings of the mind. The writings of William James and others introduced the possibility of using psychoactive agents in studying psychological processes. In 1899, one of the psychologists who had been using *Cannabis* in experiments said, "To the psychologist it [*Cannabis*] was as useful as the microscope to the naturalist; it magnifies psychological states and in this way is an aid to its study."[7]

"Marijuana, Assassin of Youth"

At the beginning of the twentieth century, public interest in *Cannabis* and its use was not very widespread. In the early 1920s, there were a few references in the mass media to the use by Mexican Americans of something the newspapers called marijuana, but public concern was not aroused. In 1926, however, a series of articles associating marijuana and crime appeared in a New Orleans newspaper. As a result, the public began to take an interest in this "new" drug.

The U.S. commissioner of narcotics, Harry Anslinger, said that in 1931 the Bureau of Narcotics' file on marijuana was less than 2 inches thick. The same year, the Treasury Department stated:

> A great deal of public interest has been aroused by the newspaper articles appearing from time to time on the evils of the abuse of marijuana, or Indian hemp. This publicity tends to magnify the extent of the evil and lends color to an inference that there is an alarming spread of the improper use of the drug, whereas the actual increase in such use may not have been inordinately large.[4]

Even so, by 1935, there were 36 states with laws regulating the use, sale, and/or possession of marijuana. By the end of 1936, all 48 states had similar laws. The Federal Bureau of Narcotics also changed its tune. In 1937, at congressional hearings, Anslinger stated that "traffic in marihuana is increasing to such an extent that it has come to be the cause for the greatest national concern."[8] In the 1931 to 1937 period, the use of marijuana had spread throughout the country, but there is no evidence that there was extensive use in most communities. The primary motivation for the congressional hearings on marijuana came not because of the use of marijuana as an inebriant or a euphoriant but because of reports by police and in the popular literature stating, "Most crimes of violence are laid to users of marihuana."[9]

Scientific American reported in March 1936:

> Marijuana produces a wide variety of symptoms in the user, including hilarity, swooning, and sexual excitement. Combined with intoxicants, it often makes the smoker vicious, with a desire to fight and kill.[10]

And *Popular Science Monthly* in May 1936 contained a lengthy article with such statements as this:

The Chief of Philadelphia County detectives declared that whenever any particularly horrible crime was committed—and especially one pointing to perversion—his officers searched first in marijuana dens and questioned marijuana smokers for suspects.[11]

It hardly seemed necessary for readers to be told that marijuana had arrived as "the foremost menace to life, health, and morals in the list of drugs used in America."[11]

In this period the association was repeatedly made between crime, particularly violent and/or perverted crime, and marijuana use. A typical report, cautiously phrased, as were all of them, follows:

> In Los Angeles, Calif., a youth was walking along a downtown street after inhaling a marijuana cigarette. For many addicts, merely a portion of a "reefer" is enough to induce intoxication. Suddenly, for no reason, he decided that someone had threatened to kill him and that his life at that very moment was in danger. Wildly he looked about him. The only person in sight was an aged boot-black. Drug-crazed nerve centers conjured the innocent old shoe-shiner into a destroying monster. Mad with fright, the addict hurried to his room and got a gun. He killed the old man, and then, later, babbled his grief over what had been wanton, uncontrolled murder.
>
> "I thought someone was after me," he said. "That's the only reason I did it. I had never seen the old fellow before. Something just told me to kill him!"
>
> That's marijuana![12]

However, not all articles condemned marijuana as the precipitator of violent crimes. An article in *The Literary Digest* reported that the chief psychiatrist at Bellevue Hospital in New York City had reviewed the cases of more than 2,200 criminals convicted of felonies. Referring to marijuana, he said, "None of the assault cases could be said to have been committed under the drug's influence. Of the sexual crimes, there was none due to marihuana intoxication. It is quite probable that alcohol is more responsible as an agent for crime than is marihuana."[13]

There was very poor documentation of the relationship between marijuana and crime, which in the 1930s was stated as if it had been proved. A thorough review of Commissioner Anslinger's writings on marijuana concluded:

> In the works of Mr. Anslinger, there are either no references or references to volumes which my assistants and I have checked and which, in our checking, we find to be based upon much hearsay and little or no experimentation. We found a mythology in which later writers cite the authority of earlier writers, who also had little evidence. We have found, by and large, what can most charitably be described as a pyramid of prejudice, with each level of the structure built upon the shaky foundations of earlier distortions.[14]

Examples of this "pyramid of prejudice" abound, but here's one way it worked: one of Mr. Anslinger's Treasury agents would testify before Congress and relate one of the outrageous stories of marijuana-induced violence. Next, the testimony would be referred to in an editorial in a medical journal, such as the *Journal of the American Medical Association* (*JAMA*). Then Anslinger or one of his people would write a magazine article, citing the prestigious *JAMA* as the source of the information.

With such poor evidence supporting the relationship between marijuana use and crime, it seems strange that the true story was never told. There are probably several reasons. One was the Great Depression, which made everyone acutely sensitive to, and wary of, any new and particularly foreign influences. The fact that it was lower-class Mexican Americans and African Americans who had initiated use of the drug made the drug doubly dangerous to the white middle class.

Another contributing factor probably was the regular reference in associating marijuana and crime to the murdering cult of Assassins as suggestive of the characteristics of the drug. The 1936 *Popular Science Monthly* reference to the Assassins is the most concise:

> The origin of the word "assassin" has two explanations, but either demonstrates the menace of Indian hemp. According to one version, members of a band of Persian terrorists committed their worst atrocities while under the influence of hashish. In the other version, Saracens who opposed the Crusaders were said to employ the services of hashish addicts to secure secret murderers of the leaders of the Crusades. In both versions, the murderers were known as "haschischin," "hashshash" or "hashishi" and from those terms comes the modern and ominous "assassin."[11]

In none of the original stories and legends were the murders committed by individuals under the influence of hashish; rather, hashish may have been part of the reward for carrying out various crimes. No matter. As the 1930s rolled on, fear of marijuana users and of marijuana itself increased, as did state marijuana-control laws. In the mid-1930s, the Narcotics Bureau acted to support federal legislation, and in the spring of 1937 congressional hearings were held.

The Marijuana Tax Act of 1937

Passage of the Marijuana Tax Act was a foregone conclusion. There were few witnesses to testify other than law enforcement officers. People dealing in birdseed had the act modified so they could import sterilized *Cannabis* seed for use in their product. An official of the American Medical Association (AMA) testified on his own behalf, not representing the AMA, against the bill. His reasons for opposing the bill were multiple. Primarily, he thought the state antimarijuana laws were adequate and that the social-menace case against *Cannabis* had not been proved at all. It might be that most other medical doctors didn't associate the old remedies based on *Cannabis* with this new, foreign-sounding drug marijuana. The bill was passed in August and became effective on October 1, 1937.

The general characteristics of the law followed the regulation-by-taxation theme of the Harrison Act of 1914. The federal law did not outlaw *Cannabis* or its preparations; it just taxed the grower, distributor, seller, and buyer and made it, administratively, almost impossible for anyone to have anything to do with *Cannabis*. In addition, the Bureau of Narcotics prepared a uniform law that many states adopted. The uniform law on marijuana specifically named *C. sativa* as the species of plant whose leafy material is illegal. In later years, there were some court cases in which the defense argued that the material confiscated by the police had come from *C. indica* and thus was not illegal. In the usual specimens obtained by police or presented in court, all distinguishing characters between species are either not present or are obliterated by drying and crushing. Because the cannabinoids are present in all species, there is no way of telling what species one has at hand with most confiscated marijuana. The current federal and uniform laws refer only to *Cannabis*.

The state laws made possession and use of *Cannabis* illegal per se. In May 1969, 32 years later, the U.S. Supreme Court declared the Marijuana Tax Act unconstitutional and overturned the conviction of Timothy Leary because there was

> in the Federal anti-marijuana law—a section that requires the suspect to pay a tax on the drug, thus incriminating himself, in violation of the Fifth Amendment: and a section that assumes (rather than requiring proof) that a person with foreign-grown marijuana in his possession knows it is smuggled.[15]

After the Marijuana Tax Act

Passage of the Marijuana Tax Act had an amazing effect. Almost immediately there was a sharp reduction in the reports of heinous crimes committed under the influence of marijuana. The price of the merchandise increased rapidly (the war came along, too), so that five years after

Exploring Your Spirituality

Diversity and Dialog

We've recently seen a plethora of films—*Grass, Eyes Wide Shut, Wonder Boys, Saving Grace,* and *American Beauty*—in which marijuana plays an integral part in the story line. In almost every case, pot is portrayed in a positive manner, or at least as a deeply rooted reality that thrives in the shadow of unpopular laws. In *Grass,* a documentary history of marijuana in America, the drug is presented as a scapegoat in an ongoing American war of values, attitudes, and subcultures. It is a symbolic difference between fun-loving types (college students, hippies, musicians) and alarmists who fret if anyone is having a good time (1930s prohibitionists, 1950s witch hunters, the 1960s "silent majority").

Other types that might evoke as much of a reaction and spirited discussion among your classmates as the issue of drug use are abortion, religion, and the meaning of life. Are you comfortable discussing controversial issues such as these and recognizing the diversity of opinion? As we mature, we experience personal growth through forming a unique and independent adult identity, while being enriched through exposure to the ideas and experiences of others. A key to emotional and spiritual health is being able to take more control of the outcomes of our experiences and stand our ground when necessary. This way we learn about our own emotional responses and sometimes reframe our perceptions based on new information. With new insights, knowledge, and perspective, we continue to grow as human beings.

One way to increase your chances of positive interaction with others is to use good communication skills. Use the following tips to improve your skills:

- Schedule conversations so that you and the other person are prepared for them.
- Choose a neutral setting to lessen the possibility of hostility.
- Set aside any preoccupations before having the discussion.
- State your position clearly and nonaggressively.
- Be respectful in your tone, manner of speaking, and body language.
- Focus on the topic at hand.
- Be specific when you praise or criticize.
- Listen to what the other person is communicating—not only the words but also the feelings behind them.
- Avoid using trigger words that might turn a discussion into an argument.
- Suggest and ask for ideas about a course of action that will help resolve any problems.

By following these suggestions, you take into account the psychological well-being of the other person and yourself.

Every student is unique. Some students are willing to step outside their individual comfort zones and celebrate the diversity that surrounds them. For them, the college years can be a time of accelerated emotional and spiritual growth that prepares them to interact socially and work effectively with others throughout life.

---

passage of the act the cost of a marijuana cigarette—a reefer—had increased 6 to 12 times and cost about a dollar.

The year after the law was enacted, 1938, Mayor Fiorello LaGuardia of New York City remembered what no one else wanted to recall. What he recalled were two army studies on marijuana use by soldiers in the Panama Canal Zone around 1930. Both reports had found marijuana to be innocuous and had said that its reputation as a troublemaker "was due to its association with alcohol which was always found the prime agent."[16] Mayor LaGuardia asked the New York Academy of Medicine to study marijuana, its

use, its effects, and the necessity for control. The report, issued in 1944, was intensive and extensive and a very good study for its time. The complete report is available,[17] so the following is only a part of the summary:

It was found that marihuana in an effective dose impairs intellectual functioning in general. . . .

Marihuana does not change the basic personality structure of the individual. It induces a feeling of self-confidence, but this expressed in thought rather than in performance. There is, in fact, evidence of a diminution in physical activity. . . .

Those who have been smoking marihuana for a period of years showed no mental or physical deterioration which may be attributed to the drug.[17]

This 1944 report, which was completed by a very reputable committee of the New York Academy of Medicine, brought a violent reaction. The AMA stated in a 1945 editorial:

> For many years medical scientists have considered cannabis a dangerous drug. Nevertheless, a book called "Marihuana Problems" by New York City Mayor's Committee on Marihuana submits an analysis of seventeen doctors of tests on 77 prisoners and, on this narrow and thoroughly unscientific foundation, draws sweeping and inadequate conclusions which minimize the harmfulness of marijuana. Already the book has done harm. One investigator has described some tearful parents who brought their 16 year old son to a physician after he had been detected in the act of smoking marihuana. A noticeable mental deterioration had been evident for some time even to their lay minds. The boy said he had read an account of the LaGuardia Committee report and that this was his justification for using marihuana.[18]

As in all such reports and reactions to reports, there is little dispute over the facts, only over the interpretation. The LaGuardia Report is in substantial agreement with the Indian Hemp Commission Report of the 1890s, the Panama Canal Zone reports of the 1930s, and the comprehensive reports in the 1970s by the governments of New Zealand, Canada, Great Britain, and the United States, in addition to the 1981 report to the World Health Organization and the 1982 report by the National Academy of Science to the Congress of the United States, so it is likely that the conclusions of the LaGuardia Report were and are for the most part valid.

The 1950s and 1960s were a unique period in the history of marijuana. There was a hiatus in scientific research on *Cannabis,* but experimentation in the streets increased. With the arrival of the "psychedelic sixties," the popular press emphasized the more sensational hallucinogens. Marijuana, however, became the most common symbol of youthful rejection of authority and identification with a new era of personal freedom. According to the annual high school senior survey and the NIDA household survey (see Chapter 1), marijuana apparently peaked in popularity in the United States around 1980.

During the 1980s and early 1990s, marijuana use became much less popular than it had been in the 1970s, but the mid-1990s saw the beginning of a significant rise in the number of young people using marijuana or hashish.

PHARMACOLOGY

Cannabinoid Chemicals

The chemistry of *Cannabis* is quite complex, and the isolation and extraction of the active ingredient are difficult even today. The active agent in *Cannabis* is unique among psychoactive plant materials in that it contains no nitrogen and thus is not an alkaloid. Because *Cannabis* lacks nitrogen, the nineteenth-century chemists who had been so successful in isolating the active agents from other plants were unable to identify its active component.

There are over 400 chemicals in marijuana, but only 61 of them are unique to the *Cannabis* plant—these are called cannabinoids. One of them, delta-9-tetrahydrocannabinol (**THC**), was isolated and synthesized in 1964 and is clearly the most pharmacologically active. Structures of some of these chemicals are shown in Figure 18.1. The major active metabolite in the body of THC is 11-hydroxy-delta-9-THC.

Take special note that the relationship of THC to *Cannabis* is probably more similar to the relationship of mescaline to peyote than of alcohol to beer, wine, or distilled spirits. Alcohol is the only behaviorally active agent in alcoholic beverages, but there might be several active agents in *Cannabis.*

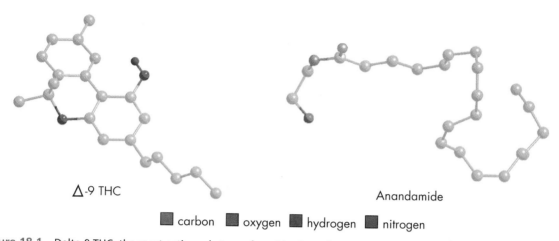

Δ-9 THC

Anandamide

■ carbon ■ oxygen ■ hydrogen ■ nitrogen

Figure 18.1   Delta-9 THC, the most active substance found in *Cannabis,* and anandamide, isolated from brain tissue.

Absorption, Distribution, and Elimination

When smoked, THC is rapidly absorbed into the blood and distributed first to the brain, then redistributed to the rest of the body, so that within 30 minutes much is gone from the brain. The psychological and cardiovascular effects occur together, usually within 5 to 10 minutes. The THC remaining in the blood has a half-life of about 19 hours, but metabolites (of which there are at least 45), primarily 11-hydroxy-delta-9-THC, are formed in the liver and have a half-life of 50 hours. After one week, 25 to 30 percent of the THC and its metabolites might still remain in the body. Complete elimination of a large dose of THC and its metabolites might take 2 or 3 weeks. THC taken orally is slowly absorbed, and the liver transforms it to 11-hydroxy-delta-9-THC; therefore, much less THC reaches the brain after oral ingestion, and it takes much longer for it to have psychological effects.

The high lipid solubility of THC means that it (like its metabolites) is selectively taken up and stored in fatty tissue to be released slowly. Excretion is primarily through the feces. All of this has two important implications: (1) there is no easy way to monitor (in urine or blood)

THC/metabolite levels and relate them to behavioral and/or physiological effects, as can be done with alcohol, and (2) the long-lasting, steady, low concentration of THC and its metabolites on the brain and other organs might have effects not yet determined.

With the advent of isolated THC, dose-response relationships could be determined and the differential response to oral and inhalation modes of intake evaluated:

> Threshold doses of 2 mg. smoked and 5 mg. orally produced mild euphoria; 7 mg. smoked and 17 mg. orally, some perceptual and time sense changes occurred; and at 15 mg. smoked and 25 mg. orally, subjects reported marked changes in body image, perceptual distortions, delusions and hallucinations.[19]

Oral intake is more frequently followed by nausea, physical discomfort, and hangover, and the dose level cannot be titrated as accurately as is possible when smoking. There might be other

THC: delta-9-tetrahydrocannabinol, the most active chemical in marijuana.

differences in effects between comparable oral and smoking intake, although this has not been studied extensively.

Cannabis is a drug that has primarily been used in two dosage forms of very different potency. Hashish and *Cannabis* extracts that give rise to the experiences reported by Baudelaire and others are potent hallucinogenic agents. The drug delivery system that spread through the United States in the 1920s and 1930s was a much less potent form, marijuana. The active ingredient is the same; the amount differs. Both marijuana and hashish are available and used in the United States today, although the great majority of users restrict themselves to marijuana.

Mechanism of Action

Scientists searched for years for a key to help them unlock the mystery of marijuana's action on the nervous system. Of course, the identification and purification of delta-9-THC was a necessary step. A significant breakthrough was made by researchers at the NIMH laboratories in 1988. They developed a technique to identify and measure highly specific and selective binding sites for THC and related compounds in rat brains. One result was the development and testing of more potent marijuana analogues.[20] Another result was the 1992 discovery of a natural substance produced in the body that has marijuana-like effects when administered to animals. This substance, (Figure 18.1) called **anandamide** (*ananda* is sanskrit for "bliss"), started the search for other related "endocannabinoids."[21] In 1996, it was reported that chocolate contains chemicals that are structurally and biochemically related to anandamide, but whether these chemicals have similar effects or are present in sufficient amounts remains unclear. Eventually these discoveries will lead to greater understanding of how we naturally cope with stress, pain, and nausea and might lead to the development of selective drugs that will be more practical than THC.

THC and other cannabinoids are known to bind to two receptors, designated CB1 and CB2.[22] There are substantial differences in the structures of these two receptors and their anatomical distribution in the body. CB1 receptors are found throughout the body, but primarily in the brain. CB2 receptors are found mainly in immune cells, suggesting a possible mechanism THC-mediated modulation of the immune response.

Physiological Effects

Thus far the study of the effects of THC on the physiology of the body has done little more than quantify earlier reports in which resin extracts were used. The established physiological effects of *Cannabis* are dose-related, are for the most part minor, are of indeterminate importance for the psychological effects, and are of unknown toxicological significance. For many years there has been substantial agreement on the short-term physiological effects of *Cannabis:*

> Physiological changes accompanying marijuana use at typical levels of American social usage are relatively few. One of the most consistent is an increase in pulse rate. Another is reddening of the eyes at the time of use. Dryness of the mouth and throat are uniformly reported. Although enlargement of the pupils was an earlier impression, more careful study had indicated that this does not occur. Blood pressure effects have been inconsistent.[23]

Except for bronchodilation, acute exposure to marijuana has little effect on breathing as measured by conventional pulmonary tests. Heavy marijuana smoking over a much longer period could lead to clinically significant and less readily reversible impairment of pulmonary function. The smoking of marijuana causes changes in the heart and circulation that are characteristic of stress. But there is no evidence to indicate that it exerts a permanently deleterious effect on the normal cardiovascular system. Marijuana increases the work of the heart, usually by increasing heart rate, and in some persons by increasing blood pressure. This increase in workload poses a threat to patients with hypertension, cerebrovascular disease, and coronary atherosclerosis.[23]

Behavioral Effects

Almost all writers emphasize that a new user has to learn how to smoke marijuana. The first step involves deeply inhaling the smoke and holding it in the lungs for 20 to 40 seconds. Then the user has to learn to identify and control the effects and, finally, to label the effects as pleasant. Because of this learning process, most first-time users do not achieve the euphoric "stoned" or "high" condition of the repeater.

The effects accompanying marijuana smoking by the experienced user are relatively well established:

A cannabis "high" typically involves several phases. The initial effects are often somewhat stimulating and, in some individuals, may elicit mild tension or anxiety which usually is replaced by a pleasant feeling of well-being. The later effects usually tend to make the user introspective and tranquil. Rapid mood changes often occur. A period of enormous hilarity may be followed by a contemplative silence.[18]

One investigator had experienced marijuana smokers indicate how frequently their marijuana intoxication included each of 206 effects listed on a sheet. Although there are great difficulties in looking for generalizations among idiosyncratic responses, the investigator was able to summarize 124 common subjective effects:

Sense perception is often improved, both in intensity and in scope. Imagery is usually stronger but well controlled, although people often care less about controlling their actions. Great changes in perception of space and time are common, as are changes in psychological processes

such as understanding, memory, emotion, and sense of identity. . . .

To the extent that the described effects are delusory or inaccurate, the delusions and inaccuracy are widely shared. It is interesting, too, that nearly all the common effects seem either emotionally pleasing or cognitively interesting, and it is easy to see why marijuana users find the effects desirable regardless of what happens to their external behavior.[24]

The subjective effects of smoking marijuana—the high—are quite difficult to study. First, because tolerance does develop, experienced smokers should show *less* effect than beginning smokers. But almost everyone suggests that you have to learn to use marijuana, and you have to learn to appreciate the psychological effects that occur. This means that experienced smokers should show *more* effect than beginning smokers. In addition to these factors, or maybe as part of them, there is much learning and association of the high with the smell, feel, taste, and rituals of using marijuana. This suggests that an experienced user would report *more* effect from a placebo cigarette than would a beginning user. The placebo cigarette would elicit the feelings associated with (conditioned to) the use of marijuana, and there should be more of these associations in the experienced user. It might also be expected that frequent marijuana users would be *less* sensitive than infrequent users to THC itself, because more of their expectations are involved in the factors related to smoking marijuana. Tables 18.1 and 18.2 speak to these issues. Placebo cigarettes were made for these studies by extracting the THC and other cannabinols from marijuana with alcohol. The marijuana contained 0.9 percent THC, and the

anandamide: (an *and* a mide) a chemical isolated from brain tissue that has marijuana-like properties.

cigarettes were made so that they contained 9 mg THC, of which about 5 mg would be delivered to the user. This was midrange potency, compared with what was being sold on the streets of San Francisco, where these double-blind studies were done.[25]

Table 18.1 shows that, although experienced users report more intoxication from using a THC-containing marijuana cigarette, there is a moderate level of intoxication reported after the use of a similarly smelling, tasting, and feeling cigarette without THC. It might be possible to fool the psyche, but not the soma. The physiological changes from use of the active cigarette are what you would expect: increase in heart rate, drying of mouth, reddening of eyes. These changes do not occur with the placebo.

The interaction of learning and of tolerance are clear in Table 18.2. When the THC-containing cigarettes were smoked, the infrequent users reported a bigger effect than the frequent users (tolerance). But when the placebo cigarettes were smoked, the frequent users got a much larger effect than the infrequent users (conditioned

TABLE 18.1

Reports of Intoxication and Measured Physiological Changes from Experienced Users Smoking Marijuana and Placebo Cigarettes ($n = 100$)

Intoxication level (0 sober, 100 maximum)	Number of Subjects Reporting	
	Marijuana	Placebo
0–19	15	35
20–39	11	28
40–59	20	21
60–79	32	12
80–100	22	4
Average	61	34

Average physiological change (pre- to post-smoking)	Marijuana*	Placebo†
Pulse rate (beats/min)	+24.00	−4.00
Salivary flow (ml/5 min)	−1.60	+0.80
Redness of eye (0–4 scale)	+1.92	+0.04

*All significant, $p < 0.05$

†None significant

TABLE 18.2

Reports of Intoxication and Measured Physiological Changes in Frequent and Infrequent Marijuana Users

	Infrequent users (less than two cigarettes a month)	Frequent users (more than seven cigarettes a month)
Reported level of intoxication after using (averages, range 0–100)		
A. Marijuana cigarette	67	52
Placebo cigarette	22	48
B. Marijuana cigarette	62	56
Oral extract (25 mg THC)	72	32
Placebo cigarette	26	51
Placebo oral extract	2	5
Physiological changes		
Pulse rate (beats/min)	+31.0*	+17.0
Salivary flow (ml/5 minutes)	−1.8*	−0.9
Redness of eye (0–4 scale)	+2.1	+1.5

*Significant differences, $p < 0.05$, between infrequent and frequent users

effect). The same type of response shows up in part B of Table 18.2, but it is also interesting that the frequent users responded much less to the oral THC than did the infrequent users. This is probably a combination of tolerance and absence of the usual associations with getting high ("If I don't see, smell, and feel these things, then I can't be intoxicated"). Even though the subjective effects varied with expectancy and other factors, the physiological effects followed the physiology, and the frequent users showed smaller physiological changes to the oral THC than the infrequent users did.

One of the most consistent effects is on short-term memory—that is, tasks such as learning and remembering new information or remembering and following a sequence of directions. In everyday use while intoxicated, the marijuana user is unable to easily recall information he or she learned just seconds or minutes before. This memory lapse affects the general thread of conversation among a group of users, as Baudelaire noted. On this issue one of the truly grand old men of the study of drug effects, A. Wikler, commented:

> The drunkard staggers—
> only when he walks,
> The pothead forgets—
> only when he talks.

This impairment of short-term memory is probably the basis for the changes in time sense frequently reported. The user feels that more time has passed than actually has. Such overestimation of the passage of time is the most commonly reported psychological effect of marijuana smoking and has been validated in many experiments.

One particularly important finding is that, although reaction time is not greatly affected, if affected at all, there is a great impairment in the ability to engage in *tracking* behavior, such as keeping a pointer on a spot on a rotating turntable. Tracking behavior requires sustained attention, and this ability is decreased considerably by marijuana. Loss of concentration is

perhaps also demonstrated by the finding that the quality of interpersonal communication (the richness of the language and attention to feedback from the other person) diminishes under the influence of marijuana.

MEDICAL USES OF *CANNIBIS*

Cannabis has never attained the medical status of opium, so its medical report is spotted, but the first report of medical use was by Shen Nung in 2737 B.C. About 2,900 years after the Shen Nung report, another Chinese physician, Hoa-tho (A.D. 200) recommended *Cannabis* resin mixed with wine as a surgical anesthetic. Although *Cannabis* preparations were used extensively in medicine in India and after about A.D. 900 in the Near East, there was almost nothing about it in European medicine until the 1800s.

Early reports in European medical journals, such as de Sacy's 1809 article titled "Intoxicating Preparations Made with Cannabis," awakened more interest in the writers and artists of the period than in medical men. In 1839, however, a lengthy article, "On the Preparations of the Indian Hemp, or Gunjah," was published by a British physician working in India.[26] He reviewed the use of *Cannabis* in Indian medicine and reported on his own work with animals, which suggested that *Cannabis* preparations were quite safe. Having shown *Cannabis* to be nontoxic, he used it clinically and found it to be an effective anticonvulsant and muscle relaxant, as well as a valuable drug for the relief of the pain of rheumatism.

In 1860, the Ohio State Medical Society's Committee on *C. indica* reported its successful use in the treatment of stomach pain, chronic cough, and gonorrhea. One physician felt he had to "assign to the Indian hemp a place among the so-called hypnotic medicines next to opium."[27] In the 1890s, a medical text included this statement: "Cannabis is very valuable for the relief of pain, particularly that depending on nerve disturbances."[4]

One of the difficulties that has always plagued the scientific, medical, and social use of *Cannabis* is the variability of the product. An 1898 brochure reviewed the assay and standardization techniques used with many of the common plant drugs and stated: "In Cannabis Indica we have a drug of great importance and one which all of materia medica is undoubtedly the most variable."[28] Four years later, Parke, Davis,[29] using new standardization procedures, claimed that "each lot sent out upon the market by us is of full potency and to be relied upon." The company listed a variety of *Cannabis* products available for medical use, including "a Chocolate Coated Tablet Extract Indian Cannabis 1/4 grain."

Passage of the Marijuana Tax Act of 1937 resulted in all 28 of the legal *Cannabis* preparations being withdrawn from the market, and in 1941 *Cannabis* was dropped from *The National Formulary* and *The U.S. Pharmacopeia*. Note that the decline in the medical use of *Cannabis* occurred long before 1937 and that the law did not eliminate an actively used therapeutic agent. Four factors, however, certainly contributed to the declining prescription rate of this plant. One was the development of new and better drugs for most illnesses. Second was the variability of the available medicinal preparations of *Cannabis*, which was repeatedly mentioned in the 1937 hearings.[8] Third, *Cannabis* is very insoluble in water and thus not amenable to injectable preparations. Last, taken orally it has an unusually long (one- to two-hour) latency to onset of action.

With the recent renewed interest in marijuana as a social drug has come some reevaluation of the implications of some of the older therapeutic reports. Scientists have looked again at some of the most interesting reported therapeutic effects of *Cannabis*. One is its anticonvulsant activity. A 1949 report[30] found it effective in some cases in which phenytoin (Dilantin), the anticonvulsant of choice both then and now, was ineffective. The fact that both Queen Victoria's physician and Sir William Osler, as well as others, found *Cannabis* to be very effective

against tension and migraine headaches has caused some interest.[31]

A 1972 report showed that marijuana smoking was effective in reducing the fluid pressure of the eye in a glaucoma patient.[32] That report became a cause célebre in 1975, when a glaucoma patient was arrested for growing marijuana plants on his back porch for medical purposes. Fifteen months later, this man (1) saw the charges against him dropped, (2) had his physician certify that the only way for him to avoid blindness was to smoke five joints a day, and (3) had these marijuana joints legally supplied to him by the United States government.[33] This began a very limited program in which the National Institute on Drug Abuse (NIDA) provided medical-grade marijuana cigarettes to patients with the FDA's approval of a "compassionate use" protocol.

A second possible important medical use was reported in 1975. Medication containing THC, the active ingredient in marijuana, was the only kind that was effective in reducing the severe nausea caused by certain drugs used to treat cancer. A 1982 report from the National Academy of Sciences stated:

> Cannabis and its derivatives have shown promise in the treatment of a variety of disorders. The evidence is most impressive in glaucoma . . . ; in asthma. . . ; and in the nausea and vomiting of cancer chemotherapy . . . and might also be useful in seizures, spasticity, and other nervous system disorders.[23]

On the other hand, Dr. Gabriel Nahas, a medical researcher and prominent foe of marijuana, felt that

> for each of these uses, there are other modern drugs with greater bioavailability, specificity, and effectiveness. . . . Reproducible absorption, consistent and predictable pharmacological effects may not be achieved. . . . It appears that it will not become a useful therapeutic agent.[34]

In 1985, the FDA licensed a small drug company, Unimed, Inc., to begin producing a capsule containing THC for sale to cancer chemotherapy patients who are experiencing nausea. The drug is referred to by the generic name **dronabinol** and the brand name **Marinol.** Dronabinol has helped cancer chemotherapy patients gain weight, and in 1993 the FDA also approved its use for stimulating appetite in AIDS patients.[35] The National Organization for the Reform of Marijuana Laws (NORML) wants marijuana cigarettes themselves approved, under the theory that the dose can be better controlled and smoking is therefore safer. Its position received some support from the DEA's chief administrative law judge in 1988, who recommended that the DEA move marijuana from Schedule I to Schedule II, so that physicians could use it to treat the nausea produced by cancer chemotherapy and to relieve suffering in cases of multiple sclerosis. He called natural marijuana "one of the safest therapeutically active substances known to man."[36] The DEA finally decided in 1992 that there was insufficient evidence to justify rescheduling marijuana to Schedule II, so it will remain officially "without medical usefulness"; part of the DEA's reasoning was that, because "pure" THC was now available by prescription, there was no justification for providing the raw plant material to be smoked.

Also in 1992, apparently in response to a number of "compassionate use" requests from AIDS patients seeking improved appetites, the FDA terminated the process of reviewing any new compassionate use protocols for marijuana cigarettes.[37] Although 36 states had approved legislation allowing for medical use of marijuana under a physician's prescription, only 13 patients had received FDA approval in the 17 years the program was in effect.

The question of medical usefulness for marijuana seemed to some to have been taken away from federal agencies and put in the hands of the public when, in November 1996, both Arizona and California voters passed ballot initiatives allowing physicians to recommend marijuana for serious illnesses and allowing patients to possess and use marijuana if their physicians recommend it.[38] There was still no legal way for patients to purchase marijuana, of course, and no legal growers or distributers. More than half the states had previously passed laws allowing medicinal use of marijuana, so in a sense this was not new. However, those previous laws had passed in the 1970s, when decriminalization and even legalization of marijuana were being debated openly. By the mid-1990s, when record numbers of arrests were being made for marijuana law violations, such action by voters came as a big surprise and elicited some strong reactions from the federal government (see the Taking Sides box).

The Institute of Medicine (IOM) of the prestigious National Academy of Sciences had issued a comprehensive report on marijuana in 1982.

In 1998, in response to public pressure to allow the medical use of marijuana, the White House Office of National Drug Control Policy funded another study by the IOM to perform a comprehensive review of the scientific evidence for potential benefits and risks of using marijuana as a medicine. The resulting 1999 report has been pointed to by proponents of medical marijuana as supporting the idea that marijuana is a relatively safe and effective medicine for patients suffering from chronic conditions, such as AIDS wasting syndrome or chronic pain. However, the report also recommends more research on cannabinoid biology, additional clinical studies on marijuana and synthetic cannabinoids and the development of an effective inhaler to solve the problem of poor oral absorption of THC. In the meantime, the panel recommended that the compassionate use of smoked marijuana cigarettes be allowed for no more than six

---

dronabinol: (dro *nab* i noll) the generic name for prescription THC in oil in a gelatin capsule.

Marinol: (*mare* i noll) the brand name for dronabinol.

Taking Sides

Should Medical Patients Have Access to Marijuana?

The 1996 Arizona and California ballot initiatives allowing patients to use marijuana on the advice of their physicians reawakened public interest in this topic. The best-demonstrated effects of marijuana (and of THC) are the reduction of the nausea caused by chemotherapy for cancer and the stimulation of appetite, which might benefit AIDS patients. With such serious illnesses involved, many feel that the compassionate thing is to allow marijuana to be used if it might help, since the risk of dependence seems to be a rather small issue in such cases. In fact, *"Cannabis* buyers clubs" sprang up in many large cities—most notably, San Francisco—and patients who had notes from the physicians could purchase from them. These clubs were illegal, but local law enforcement agencies for the most part left them alone, not wanting to arrest seriously ill patients. Of course, because the clubs were illegal and informally operated, there was no guarantee that everyone purchasing marijuana was, in fact, seriously ill.

Following the passage of the ballot initiatives, the U.S. government in December 1996 announced that it would move to revoke the DEA registration of any physician who advised a patient to use illegal drugs. This caused some to wonder about violations of the tradition of privileged communications between doctors and patients, and so far the legality of all of this is open to question. In early 1998, the U.S. Justice Department announced plans to shut down all *Cannabis* buyers clubs in California.

In September 2000, the U.S. District Court in San Francisco issued an injunction permanently barring the government from revoking a physician's license to prescribe medicine "merely because the doctor recommends medical marijuana to a patient based on a sincere medical judgement." The court also prevented the government from initiating an investigation of a doctor's other prescribing practices solely because he or she had recommended marijuana.

In November 2000, at the White House's request, the U.S. Supreme Court issued an emergency ban (by a vote of seven to one) on the distribution of marijuana for medical purposes. The Court struck down the U.S. Court of Appeals ruling in San Francisco, which would have made "medical necessity" a defense against violation of federal drug statutes. The Court is deciding whether to consider the case.

Do you think medical necessity is a compelling argument for the use of marijuana? Why or why not?

For more on this topic, log on to www.dushkin.com/online for current news and links to other popular and informative sites, as well as time-saving web search strategies and study tools.

---

months for patients with debilitating, intractable pain or vomiting, when the following conditions are met:

- The failure of approved medications to provide relief has been documented.
- The symptoms can reasonably be expected to be relieved by rapid-onset cannabinoid drugs.
- Such treatment is administered under medical supervision in a manner that allows for the assessment of treatment effectiveness.
- An oversight strategy is in place to approve or reject requests within 24 hours after a physician seeks permission to provide marijuana to a patient for a specified use.

The entire report can be found on the Internet at books.nap.edu/catalog/9586.html.

CAUSES FOR CONCERN

Dependence Potential

Tolerance

For years there was debate over whether tolerance developed to the effects of THC and/or marijuana. Whereas animal studies repeatedly demonstrated tolerance to the behavioral disruption produced by large doses of marijuana, the experiences of human marijuana smokers seemed to indicate that experienced users could get high more readily than inexperienced users, possibly implying reverse tolerance or sensitization to the drug. We now know that learning plays an important role in the psychological reaction, particularly to low doses of marijuana. That, combined with the fact that THC can build up in the tissues of chronic users, might account for any increased reaction. However, a number of human studies have now demonstrated clear evidence of tolerance to some of the physiological effects of THC (Review Table 18.2). If high levels of marijuana are used regularly over a sustained period of time, tolerance will be obvious.

Physical Dependence

Physical dependence has been demonstrated in laboratory experiments with humans given large doses of THC every 4 hours for 10 to 20 days. Beginning several hours after the last oral dose, subjects have shown irritability, restlessness, nausea, and vomiting. These symptoms peak at 8 hours and declined over the next 3 days. Sleep disturbances and loss of appetite have also been reported.[39] Such withdrawal symptoms are virtually never reported outside the research laboratory. One reason for this might be that the drug is so long-lasting. Withdrawal signs are always more dramatic when a drug leaves the body quickly. The development of a specific antagonist for the marijuana (or anandamide) receptor has made it possible to demonstrate clear withdrawal symptoms in laboratory animals, because administration of an antagonist has the effect of removing the drug from its receptors almost instantaneously.[40] In animal studies, the withdrawal symptoms resemble those of opiate withdrawal to some extent and might have some mechanisms in common.

Psychological Dependence

The strength of a drug's tendency to produce behavioral dependence can be estimated by looking at how many of its users develop patterns of daily, repeated use. With a highly addicting practice such as cigarette smoking, the majority of users are daily users of multiple doses. With alcohol and many other drugs, most users avoid such a pattern, but a few develop strong dependence. The marijuana pattern seems to be more similar to that of alcohol use than of cigarette smoking or heroin injection. As Dr. David E. Smith of the Haight-Ashbury Medical Center said in 1982, "Regular heavy users who smoke more than 10 joints a day may be rare, but they do exist."[41]

The picture that emerges is that addiction, in the sense of a constant craving, high-frequency use, the buildup of tolerance, and possible withdrawal symptoms, is not an issue for the majority of marijuana users who engage in occasional smoking of one or two marijuana cigarettes. However, a small fraction of marijuana users do become dependent on daily use of marijuana. This probably has a lot to do with psychosocial variables and is not seen by most researchers as an inevitable consequence of exposure to marijuana. Whatever the causes, drug treatment programs do have clients whose primary drug of abuse is marijuana, and some are voluntary clients seeking help for what can reasonably be called marijuana addiction. As Smith said, it doesn't happen to most users, but it does happen.

Toxicity Potential

Acute Physiological Effects

The acute physiological effects of marijuana, primarily an increase in heart rate, have not been thought to be a threat to health. However, as the marijuana-using population ages, there is concern that individuals with high blood pressure, heart disease, or hardening of the arteries might be harmed by smoking marijuana.[23] The lethal dose of THC has not been extensively studied in animals, and no human deaths have been reported from "overdoses" of *Cannabis*.

Impaired Driving Ability

Behaviorally, the intoxication produced by marijuana does present some danger, especially if the user is driving. Early experiments using

HealthQuest Activities

In Module 9, look under *Specifics On* and read "Unknown Drug Use/Abuse." This article provides an extensive list of herbal substitutes and details about each. Identify herbal substitutes for marijuana. Take a survey to find out how common this knowledge is among your fellow students. Make a list of herbal substitutes and ask students to tell you if they know of or do not know of each substance. Also, ask students if they have ever tried to use these substitutes and what kind of reactions they experienced.

Look under *Drug Interactions, Illicit Drugs* and read about marijuana. Get together with a group of classmates and discuss marijuana's interactions with other drugs. How many in the group have used marijuana? Have they ever used it in conjunction with other drugs? Now that they know the dangers of interaction, are they willing to restrict their use of this drug or to quit using it altogether?

weak marijuana and simple reaction-time driving tests found small effects, which experienced users seemed to be able to overcome (behavioral tolerance). However, there have now been a large number of studies using more complex and realistic driving tests, which show definite impairments with marijuana. In either computer-controlled driving simulators or actual driving tests on a closed course, these impairments have been found to be dose-related. In such studies, the ability to maintain concentration, correct for wind gusts, and maintain a steady speed were all impaired, as was judgment. A telephone survey of nearly 6,000 teenagers found that those who reported driving 6 or more times per month after smoking marijuana were 2.4 times more likely to be involved in traffic accidents than those who did not drive after smoking marijuana. Studies based on measurements of drugs in the blood of drivers involved in accidents also indicated a role for marijuana in causing accidents, but

most who tested positive for THC also tested positive for alcohol, so the results were inconclusive. Laboratory studies have found that smoking two marijuana cigarettes containing fairly high amounts of THC (3.6 percent) does impair performance on standard roadside sobriety tests of balance and coordination.[42]

Panic reactions

The other major behavioral problem associated with acute marijuana intoxication is the panic reaction. Much like many of the bad trips with hallucinogens, the reaction is usually fear of loss of control and fear that things will not return to normal. Even Baudelaire understood this and advised his readers to surround themselves with friends and a pleasant environment before using hashish. Although many people do seek emergency medical treatment for marijuana-induced panic and are sometimes given sedatives or tranquilizers, the best treatment is probably "talking down," or reminding the person of who and where they are, that the reaction is temporary, and that everything will be all right.

Chronic Lung Exposure

Since a large number of Americans began using marijuana chronically in the 1960s and 1970s, there has been a great deal of concern about the possible long-term effects of chronic marijuana use. A couple of physiological concerns merit attention. One is the effect on lung function and the concern about lung cancer. Experiments have shown that chronic, daily smoking of marijuana impairs air flow in and out of the lungs.[43] It is hard to tell yet whether years of such an effect results in permanent, major obstructive lung disease in the same way that smoking tobacco cigarettes does. Also, there is no direct evidence linking marijuana smoking to lung cancer in humans. Remember that it took many years of cigarette smoking by millions of Americans before the links between tobacco and lung cancer and other lung diseases were shown.

Marijuana smoke has been compared with tobacco smoke.[23] Some of the constituents differ (there is no nicotine in marijuana smoke and no THC in tobacco), but many of the dangerous components are found in both. Total tar levels, carbon monoxide, hydrogen cyanide, and nitrosamines are found in similar amounts (except for tobacco-specific nitrosamines, which are carcinogens). Another potent carcinogen, *benzopyrene,* is found in greater amounts in marijuana than in tobacco. Everyone suspects that marijuana smoking will eventually be shown to cause cancer, but how much of a problem this will be compared with tobacco is hard to say. On the one hand, few marijuana smokers smoke 20 marijuana cigarettes every day, whereas tobacco smokers regularly smoke this much. On the other hand, the marijuana cigarette is not filtered and the user generally gets as much concentrated smoke as possible as far down in the lungs as possible and holds it there. So, while some of us wait and see when the data will come out, others are participating in the experiment.

Reproductive Effects

Another area of concern is reproductive effects in both men and women. Heavy marijuana smoking can decrease testosterone levels in men, although the levels are still within the normal range and the significance of those decreases is not known. There have been reports of diminished sperm counts and abnormal sperm structure in heavy marijuana users, but

again the clinical significance of these reports is not clear.[44] A number of studies have reported either lower birth weight or shorter length at birth for infants whose mothers smoked marijuana during pregnancy.[45] Although these effects are small and inconsistent from one study to the next, it is, of course, wise to avoid the use of all drugs during pregnancy.

The Immune System Effects

There have also been reports that marijuana smoking impairs some measures of the functioning of the immune system.[46] Animal studies have found that THC injections can reduce immunity to infection, but at doses well above those obtainable by smoking marijuana. Some human studies of marijuana smokers have suggested reduced immunity, but most have not. If the effect were real, it could result in marijuana smokers' being more susceptible to infections, cancer, and other diseases, such as genital herpes. One might suspect that such problems would eventually be reflected in the overall death rate of marijuana users. However, a 1997 report examining 10 years of mortality data for more than 65,000 people found no relationship between marijuana use and overall death rates.[47]

Amotivational Syndrome

Since 1971, when some psychiatric case reports were published identifying an *amotivational* syndrome in marijuana smokers, there has been concern about the effect of regular marijuana use on behavior and motivation. A number of experiments and correlational studies have been aimed at answering this question. One thing to remember is the long half-life of marijuana in the body, so that daily smokers can be chronically intoxicated and exhibit behavioral or motivational impairments even before their daily dose. There does seem to be evidence for this diminished motivation, impaired ability to learn, and school and family problems in some adolescents who are chronic, heavy marijuana smokers. If they stop smoking and remain in counseling, the condition improves.[41] This probably implies a constant

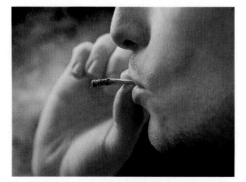
Inhaling marijuana smoke.

Drugs in Depth

Long-term Effects of Marijuana Smoke in Monkeys

Although there have been some well-controlled, convincing reports that chronic THC exposure may produce permanent changes in neurons in the hippocampus of rats, there have not yet been comparable studies in any primate species. Earlier reports of synaptic changes in the brains of rhesus monkeys have been widely criticized because proper control and sampling techniques were not used.

Some results have been reported from a long-term study[56] in which rhesus monkeys were exposed to marijuana smoke through a mask over their faces. The study was well controlled: some monkeys received the smoke from one cigarette each day for a year, others received smoke only on weekends, and others received daily exposure to the smoke from a marijuana cigarette from which the THC has been extracted.

One of the measures taken was how hard the monkeys would work for banana-flavored food pellets: each day each monkey could get one pellet by pressing a plate on the wall of the test cage. The second pellet required two presses, the third three presses, and so on (a progressive-ratio schedule of reinforcement). At some point each day the ratio would become so large that the monkey would stop pressing. At first the monkeys receiving active marijuana were unaffected; however, after several weeks of daily exposure they began to receive fewer pellets than the control monkeys. This effect persisted for a few weeks after the marijuana smoke was stopped. The authors interpreted these results to be a model of the amotivational syndrome reported in human marijuana smokers and indicated that the persistent effect might have been due to residual metabolites slowly clearing out of the brain tissue. When the monkeys' brains were examined, neither permanent neurochemical changes[57] nor structural changes in the neurons[58] could be found.

state of intoxication rather than a long-lasting change in brain function or personality (see also the Drugs in Depth box).

Insanity

The connection between marijuana use and insanity was one of the main arguments for outlawing the drug in the 1930s, and the notion still remains that marijuana can cause a type of psychosis. There have been reports of psychotic "breakdowns" occurring with rare frequency after marijuana has been smoked, but the causal relationship is in question. The psychotic episodes are generally self-limiting and seem to occur in individuals with a history of psychiatric problems.[41]

Brain Damage

For about 25 years, it has been speculated that amotivational or prolonged psychotic reactions could reflect an underlying damage to brain tissue produced by marijuana. For example, a 1972 report from England indicated that two individuals who demonstrated cerebral atrophy had a history of smoking marijuana. They also had a history of using many other illicit drugs, plus other medical problems, but it was suggested that the brain damage might have been caused by the marijuana. Several experiments have since been done, and all have failed to find a relationship between marijuana smoking and cerebral atrophy.

There have been other incomplete or poorly controlled reports of potential brain damage from animal research, and it has been possible to dismiss most of them as inconclusive. However, two experiments on rats, one appearing in 1987 and the other in 1988, gave stronger evidence that THC causes permanent changes in the structure of neurons in the hippocampus. One of the reports related these changes to a persistent deficit in the rats' performance on a radial arm maze. The doses used were in the range of what a very heavy marijuana smoker might obtain, and the treatment was given to the rats every day for 90 days. It's not clear what the implications might be for human beings smoking less heavily and only occasionally.

Ironically, some of the nonpsychoactive ingredients in marijuana, including cannabidiol, have been shown to have powerful antioxidant properties that protect brain cells from the toxic effects of other chemicals.[48] This effect was strong enough that the NIMH filed a patent in 1988 entitled "Cannabinoids as Antioxidants and Neuroprotectants."

There is probably no area of science in which emotion has played such an obvious and influential role. Scientists on both sides have become crusaders for their cause. Some individuals seem to think it is their professional duty to seek out and publicize every potential evil associated with marijuana, even if there is not strong scientific evidence in support of their views. Others seem to automatically question the negative reports and look for ways to discredit them. We can predict that the emotion, the premature announcements of new scary findings, the repeating of long discredited stories, and the conflicting reports will continue.

MARIJUANA AND AMERICAN SOCIETY

Remember that our patterns of drug use are but one facet of our evolving society. Our drug use affects and is affected by other social trends in our life. You should at least make note of a couple of important themes from the 1980s, and we'll see how they related to marijuana use.

One trend was the increased emphasis on physical health. Jogging, working out, dieting, drinking less alcohol and caffeine, and smoking less all were reflections of our national concern over shaping up. The health trend obviously worked against marijuana use: how many people who wouldn't smoke tobacco felt good about inhaling marijuana smoke? Second, the 1980s saw a move toward social and political conservatism, which worked against such counterculture behavior as marijuana smoking. And, of course, drug use tends to be faddish. If marijuana was the fashionable drug of the 1970s, then it couldn't be the fashionable drug of the

1980s. However, in the 1990s the drug came back into fashion, at least somewhat.

Data from the yearly survey of high school seniors shows the trends most clearly. After peaking in 1978–1979, the number of high school seniors who had ever smoked marijuana dropped from just over 60 percent to 32 percent in 1992, then rebounded to almost 50 percent by the class of 1997. Equally dramatic were the trends in daily use, which went from 11 percent in 1978 to 2 percent in 1992 and back to almost 6 percent by 1997.[49] The earlier decreases in marijuana use went along with a steady increase in the belief among these students that "people risk harming themselves if they smoke marijuana regularly." Whereas just over one-third of the high school seniors agreed with that statement in 1978, over three-fourths agreed in 1992. Fads being what they are, this downward trend in marijuana use had to end sometime, and the turnaround was seen in the high school senior class of 1992. Significant increases in marijuana use in the 1992–1997 period were accompanied by decreased estimates of risk (see Chapter 1).

Although marijuana is not used by most Americans, it is still remarkable how many people have used and continue to use a substance that shouldn't exist at all in our society, according to the Controlled Substances Act and the DEA. That a large fraction of the society continues to violate the laws regarding marijuana is a matter for concern. It is easy to look back and wish that the 1937 Marijuana Tax Act had never happened. Marijuana use was spreading slowly across the United States and, with any luck, it might have become acculturated. Society would have adapted to marijuana and adapted marijuana to society. Soon it would have become part of society: perhaps most people would never have used it regularly; of those who did use it, most would have known how to use it; some, of course, would have abused it. It has happened before with coffee, tea, tobacco, and alcohol.

The 1937 law prevented all that. It didn't affect most Americans a great deal until the 1960s, when a large number of young people began experimenting with drugs. Marijuana, more than anything else, convinced many young people that the government had been lying to them about drugs. They had been told that marijuana would make them insane, enslave them in drug addiction, and lead to violence and perverted sexual acts. Their experience told them that marijuana was pretty innocuous, compared with those stories, and it became an important symbol: smoking marijuana struck a blow for truth and freedom. The problem was that laws existed that allowed young people to be sent to jail for 20 years for striking this blow, and that didn't sit well with some people. Voice was given to the millions of marijuana users in 1970 when a young Washington lawyer established the National Organization for the Reform of Marijuana Laws (NORML) with a grant from the Playboy Foundation. As the founder of NORML put it, "The only people working for reform then were freaks who wanted to turn on the world, an approach that was obviously doomed to failure. I wanted an effective, middle-class approach, not pro-grass but antijail."

Also, in 1970 the Comprehensive Drug Abuse Prevention and Control Act of 1970 established the Commission on Marijuana and Drug Abuse. Its 1972 report recommended some legislative changes:

> The Commission recommended that federal and state laws be changed so that private possession of small amounts of marihuana for personal use, and casual distribution of small amounts without monetary profit, would no longer be offenses, though marihuana possessed in public would remain contraband. Cultivation, distribution for profit, and possession with intent to sell would remain felonies. Criminal penalties would be retained for disorderly conduct associated with marihuana intoxication and driving under the influence of marihuana, and a plea of marihuana intoxication would not be a defense to any criminal act committed under its influence.[50]

The year 1972 was a turning point in the fight to decriminalize marijuana. In June the American Medical Association came out in favor of dropping penalties for possession of "insignificant amounts" of marijuana and noted that "there is no evidence supporting the idea that marijuana leads to violence, aggressive behavior, or crime."[51] In August the American Bar Association called for the reduction of criminal penalties for possession, and a year later the organization recommended decriminalization. Both traditional liberals and conservatives could support the idea, not to declare marijuana legal but to make possession of marijuana a civil offense, punishable only by a fine. A week before Christmas in 1972, the best known and most literate of American conservatives, William F. Buckley, proclaimed in favor of the decriminalization of marijuana, saying,

> It isn't silly to say that the user should not be molested, even though the pusher should be put in jail. It was so, mostly, under prohibition, when the speakeasy operators were prosecuted, not so the patrons. Thus it is, by and large, in the case of prostitution; and even with gambling; and most explicitly with pornography, the Supreme Court having ruled that you can't molest the owner, even though you can go after the peddler.[52]

In October 1973, Oregon abolished criminal penalties for marijuana use, substituting civil fines of up to $100. Marijuana offenders were given citations that are processed as traffic tickets. Did marijuana use increase in Oregon as a result of the decriminalization? Yes. By leaps and bounds? No. From the fall of 1974, a year after decriminalization, to the fall of 1977, the percentage of adults over 18 who had ever used marijuana went from 19 percent to 25 percent. Current users went from 9 percent to 10 percent over the same period. However, marijuana use was increasing toward its 1978 to 1979 peak all over the country at the same time. Possession of a small amount of marijuana was made only a civil offense by 8 other states: Maine, Colorado, California, Ohio, Minnesota, Mississippi, New York, and North Carolina. In Alaska, private possession of up to 4 ounces of marijuana was not illegal at all. One consequence of changing marijuana possession from a felony to a misdemeanor was that it saved money on court costs, juries, and jails. It has been estimated that the state of California enjoyed an average annual savings of over $95 million between 1976 and 1985 as a result of its citation plan for marijuana possession.[53]

At the federal level, action picked up in 1977. In January, Rosalynn Carter joined her husband, the president, in calling for the decriminalization of marijuana and revealed that their oldest son had been discharged from the navy for smoking marijuana. Bills to decriminalize marijuana possession were introduced into both houses of Congress, and in August President Carter sent a message to Congress in which he asked them to abolish all federal criminal penalties for the possession of small amounts of marijuana.

If the truth were known, in the late 1970s de facto decriminalization had already occurred in many areas of the country. Law enforcement agencies in many of the larger cities of the United States had stopped arresting marijuana users and did not search out those with small amounts for personal use.

When the Reagan administration came into office in 1980, any hope of federal decriminalization was gone, replaced by a "get tough" attitude toward all illegal drugs. Marijuana was no exception. In addition to increased efforts to intercept marijuana shipments from abroad, a nationwide effort was launched in 1985 to combat the cultivation of marijuana plants. Over 100 million plants were tugged out of the ground in 1987 by state, local, and federal law enforcement teams.[54] Add to that the zero tolerance seizures of boats, cars, and planes containing even traces of marijuana and the 1988 legislation putting extra pressure on the user (e.g., $10,000 fines at the federal level; see Chapter 4), and we can see that the pendulum had definitely swung back. The states began to follow suit: in 1989, Oregon raised its civil penalty for possession from a $100 maximum to a $500 minimum. In 1990, Alaska voters approved the recriminalization of marijuana possession, making it a misdemeanor punishable by a jail term and up to a $1,000 fine. Increased penalties for the distribution of controlled substances has brought us back to a situation in which about one-sixth of all federal prisoners are incarcerated for marijuana offenses, and longer sentences are often given for selling marijuana than for murder.[55] In 1999, more than 700,000 arrests were made in the United States for violating marijuana laws.

SUMMARY

- *Cannabis* has a rich history relating both to its medicinal use and to its recreational uses.
- Marijuana became famous as the "Assassin of Youth" in the 1930s and was outlawed in 1937.
- *Cannabis* contains many active chemicals, but the most active is delta-9-THC.
- THC is absorbed rapidly by smoking but slowly and incompletely when taken by mouth.
- THC has a long half-life of elimination, and its metabolites can be found in the body for up to several weeks after THC enters the body.
- Selective THC receptors exist in brain tissue, leading to the discovery of a naturally occurring brain cannabinoid, anandamide.
- Marijuana causes an increase in the heart rate and reddening of the eyes as its main physiological effects.
- Psychologically, THC has some sedative properties, produces some analgesia, and at high doses can produce hallucinations.
- In recreational use, some of marijuana's most important behavioral effects probably relate to its impairment of memory.
- Marijuana is useful in the treatment of glaucoma, the reduction of nausea in patients undergoing cancer chemotherapy, and the increase of appetite in AIDS patients. A legal form of THC is available by prescription.

Web Watch

Are You Abusing Marijuana?
Complete the Marijuana Self-Assessment at www.mtholyoke.edu/offices/health/ADAP/marassess. htm. If you use marijuana, you can find out some of the ways the drug affects your health and lifestyle. Learn about dependence on marijuana as well.

Check Out Publications on Marijuana
The National Clearing House for Drug and Alcohol Information offers a listing of publications about certain types of drugs. Go to www.health.org/catalog/ catalog.asp?key=1&detail=false to find and, if you wish, order brochures or other publications about marijuana.

Read a Marijuana Overview
At www.cocaineaddiction.com/other_marijuana.html, read the overview of marijuana. You will find information on addiction, the history of marijuana, its effects, treatment, study results, and related statistics.

- Although strong behavioral dependence is not common, it does occur in some individuals.
- Marijuana can impair driving, and there is evidence that smoking marijuana leads to an increased frequency of accidents.
- Most experts agree that chronic smoking of marijuana impairs lung function somewhat and probably increases the risk of lung cancer.
- Long-standing concerns about marijuana-induced brain damage have received some limited support from animal studies.

REVIEW QUESTIONS

1. What are the major differences between *C. sativa* and *C. indica*?
2. How are hashish and sinsemilla produced?
3. What were the three stages of hashish intoxication described by Baudelaire?
4. Why were Harry Anslinger's writings on marijuana referred to as a "pyramid of prejudice"?
5. What were the general conclusions of the 1944 LaGuardia Commission?
6. What is meant by "cannabinoid," and about how many are there in *Cannabis*? What is the cannabinoid found in brain tissue?
7. How is the action of THC in the brain terminated after about 30 minutes, when the half-life of metabolism is much longer than that?
8. What are the two most consistent physiological effects of smoking marijuana?
9. What two medical uses have been approved by the FDA for dronabinol?
10. What seems to be the best explanation for amotivational syndrome?

REFERENCES

1. Schultes RE, Hofmann A: *The botany and chemistry of hallucinogens*. Springfield, IL: Charles C Thomas, 1980.
2. Mikuriya TH, Aldrich MR: Cannabis 1988: Old drug, new dangers—the potency question, *Journal of Psychoactive Drugs* 20:47–55, 1988.
3. Pollan M: How pot has grown. *New York Times Magazine* p 31, Feb 13, 1995.
4. Snyder SH: What we have forgotten about pot, *New York Times Magazine* p 27, Dec 13, 1970.
5. Mickel EJ: *The artificial paradises in French literature*, Chapel Hill: University of North Carolina Press, 1969.
6. Baudelaire CP: *Artificial paradises; on hashish and wine as means of expanding individuality,* translated by Ellen Fox. New York: Herder & Herder, 1971.
7. Unpublished material in the Archives of the American Psychological Association, Department of Psychology, University of Akron, Akron, Ohio.
8. *Taxation of marihuana, hearings before the Committee on Ways and Means, House of Representatives, Seventy-fifth Congress, First Session, on HR 6385, April 27–30 and May 4, 1937*. Washington, DC: U.S. Government Printing Office.
9. Parry A: The menace of marihuana, *American Mercury* 36:487–488, 1935.
10. Marihuana menaces youth, *Scientific American* 154:151, 1936.

11. Wolf W: Uncle Sam fights a new drug menace . . . marijuana, *Popular Science Monthly* 128:14, 1936.

12. Anslinger HJ, Cooper CR: Marijuana: Assassin of youth, *The American Magazine* 124:19, 153, 1937.

13. Facts and fancies about marihuana, *Literary Digest* 122:7–8, 1936.

14. Whitlock L: Review: Marijuana, *Crime and Delinquency Literature* 2(3):367, 1970.

15. Fort J: Pot: A rational approach, *Playboy,* pp 131, 154, Oct 1969.

16. The marihuana bugaboo, *Military Surgeon* 93:95, 1943.

17. Mayor LaGuardia's Committee on Marijuana. In Solomon D, editor: *The marihuana papers.* New York: New American Library, 1966.

18. Marijuana problems, *JAMA* 127:1129, 1945.

19. *Marihuana and health,* Department of Health, Education, and Welfare. Washington, DC: U.S. Government Printing Office, 1971.

20. Howlett AC and others: The cannabinoid receptor: Biochemical, anatomical and behavioral characterization, *Trends in Neuroscience* 13:420–423, 1990.

21. DiMarzo V and others: Formation and inactivation of endogenous cannabinoid anandamide in central neurons, *Nature* 372:686, 1994.

22. Pertwee RG: Cannabis and cannabinoids: Pharmacology and rationale for clinical use. *Forsch. Komplementarmed* 6: 12-5, 1999.

23. *Marijuana and health,* Institute of Medicine, National Academy of Sciences. Washington, DC: National Academy Press, 1982.

24. Tart CT: Marijuana intoxication: Common experiences, *Nature* 226:701–704, 1970.

25. Jones RT: Tetrahydrocannabinol and the marijuana-induced social "high," or the effects of the mind on marijuana. In Singer AJ, editor: *Marijuana: Chemistry, pharmacology, and patterns of social use, Annals of New York Academy of Science* 191:155–165, 1971.

26. O'Shaughnessy WB: On the preparations of the Indian hemp, or gunja, *Transactions of the Physical and Medical Society of Bengal,* pp 71–102, 1838–1840; pp 421–461, 1842.

27. Mikuriya TH: Marijuana in medicine: Past, present and future, *California Medicine* 110:34–40, 1969.

28. *Standardization of drug extracts,* promotional brochure, Detroit: Parke, Davis & Co, 1898.

29. Letter to EP Delabarre, 9 Arlington Ave, Providence, RI, from Parke, Davis & Co, Manufacturing Department, Main Laboratories, Detroit, Superintendent's Office, Control Department, Mar 10, 1902.

30. Davis JP, Ramsey HH: Antiepileptic action of marihuana-active substances, *Federation Proceedings* 8:284–285, 1949.

31. Lieberman DM, Lieberman BW: Marihuana—a medical review, *New England Journal of Medicine* 284:88–91, 1971.

32. Marijuana smoking said to have power to deter glaucoma, *New York Times* July 28, 1972.

33. Medical therapy, legalization issues debated at Marijuana Reform Conference, *National Drug Reporter* 7(1):3–5, 1977.

34. Nahas GG: The medical use of cannabis. In Nahas, GG, editor: *Marijuana in science and medicine.* New York: Raven Press, 1984.

35. Levine K: Drug approved for treating appetite loss in AIDS patients, *Drug Topics* Feb 8, 1993.

36. Conlan MF: Top drug cop weighs use of marijuana as an Rx drug, *Drug Topics* Dec 12, 1988.

37. Karel R: Hopes of many long-term sufferers dashed as FDA ends medical marijuana program, *Psychiatric News* May 1, 1992.

38. Trebach AS: Arizona and California voters seize initiatives, *The Drug Policy Letter,* Winter/Spring 1997.

39. Jones RT, Benowitz N: The 30-day trip-clinical studies of cannabis tolerance and dependence. In Braude MC, Szara S, editors: *Pharmacology of marijuana.* New York: Raven Press, 1976.

40. Swan N: Marijuana antagonist reveals evidence of THC dependence in rats, *NIDA Notes* Nov/Dec 1995.

41. Smith DE, Seymour RB: Clinical perspectives on the toxicology of marijuana: 1967–1981. In *Marijuana and youth: Clinical observations on motivation and learning.* Washington, DC: U.S. Department of Health and Human Services, U.S. Government Printing Office, 1982.

42. Mathias R: Marijuana impairs driving-related skills and workplace performance, *NIDA Notes* Jan/Feb, 1996.

43. Tashkin DP and others: Respiratory status of seventy-four habitual marijuana smokers, *Chest* 78:699–706, 1980.

44. Nahas GG: Toxicology and pharmacology. In Nahas GG, editor: *Marijuana in science and medicine.* New York: Raven Press, 1984.

45. Tennes K and others: Marijuana: Prenatal and postnatal exposure in the human. In Pinkert TM, editor: *Consequences of maternal drug abuse,* NIDA Research Monograph No. 59. Washington, DC: U.S. Government Printing Office, 1985.

46. Hollister LE: Health aspects of cannabis, *Pharmacological Review* 38:1–20, 1986.

47. Sidney S, Beck JE, Friedman GD: Marijuana use and mortality, *American Journal of Public Health* 87:585–590, 1997.

48. Hampson AJ and others. Neuroprotective antioxidants from marijuana. *Annals of the New York Academy of Sciences* 899:274–282, 2000.

49. Johnston LD and others: *University of Michigan press release on National High School Senior Survey,* Dec 18, 1997.

50. Farnsworth DL: Summary of the Report of the National Commission on Marijuana and Drug Abuse, *Tracks,* 9:1–2, 1972.

51. The AMA and pot, Stash Capsules 4(4), Aug 1972.

52. Buckley WF, Jr.: Pot, legalization of, conservative division, *New York Times* pp Dec 18, 1972.
53. Aldrich MR, Mikuriya T: Savings in California marijuana law enforcement costs attributable to the Moscone Act of 1976—a summary, *Journal of Psychoactive Drugs* 20:75–81, 1988.
54. *1987 Domestic cannabis eradication/suppression program final report,* Drug Enforcement Administration, US Department of Justice, 1987.
55. Schlosser E: Reefer madness, *Atlantic Monthly* Aug 1994.
56. Paule MG and others: Chronic marijuana smoke exposure in the rhesus monkey II: Effects on progressive ratio and conditioned position responding, *Journal of Pharmacology and Experimental Therapeutics* 260:210–222, 1992.
57. Ali SF and others: Chronic marijuana smoke exposure in the rhesus monkey IV: Neurochemical effects and comparison to acute and chronic exposure to D-9-tetrahydrocannabinol (THC) in rats, *Pharmacology Biochemistry and Behavior* 40:677–682, 1991.
58. Scallet AC: Neurotoxicology of cannabis and THC: A review of chronic exposure studies in animals, *Pharmacology Biochemistry and Behavior* 40:671–676, 1991.

Try It!

Short-term Memory

One of the most consistent findings about the effects of marijuana is that it impairs short-term memory. To learn more about short-term memory and get an idea of the types of tests that are used to measure it, go to the following website, which has an interactive test for short-term memory: faculty.washington.edu/ chudler/stm0.html. You can use this chart to record your responses.

Trial #	The letters I remember are
1	
2	
3	
4	
5	
6	

Chapter 19

Steroids and Other Drugs in Sport

KEY TERMS

- stimulants
- amphetamines
- steroids
- ergogenic
- anabolic
- androgenic
- human growth hormone
- creatine

Drugs in the Media

Banned Substances and How to Avoid Them

Television and other news from the 2000 Olympics Games in Syndey, Australia, reported many instances of athletes being disqualified for using banned substances. In some cases, the disqualification was not contested, but in

Drugs in the Media Continued. . .

others the athletes thought they had been disqualified unfairly because they had taken something prescribed for them or something that they were not aware had been banned. The following list, from an article in *Technique* magazine by Jack Swarbick, lawyer for USA Gymnastics, includes some tips for athletes on how to avoid the problem. Even if you aren't an Olympic competitor, these tips should give you an idea of how complex and difficult this problem can be.

1. Be familiar with the International Olympic Committee's banned substances list. This means knowing not only what drugs are on the list but also the types of medications or even foods in which those drugs are often found.
2. Make certain that others who ought to know, such as the athlete's parents, physician, and school nurse, are also familiar with the banned substances list.
3. Know what medications you are using. Athletes should consult with the United States Olympic Committee (USOC) regarding the potential for any medications to contain elements of banned substances and should be careful to list all medications when completing the screening form as part of the USOC's drug-testing program.
4. At competitions, drink only out of containers that were sealed when you got

them, and once you have begun drinking out of a container do not leave it unattended. Several sports have implemented fairly rigorous security measures for the handling of coolers and water bottles.
5. When you are required to produce a urine sample as part of the drug-testing procedures, never surrender possession of the sample or leave it unattended until after you have sealed it inside the shipping canister provided by the USOC.
6. If there are any irregularities in the process by which you give a urine sample and place that sample in the sealed container (e.g., a cracked beaker, a spilled sample, or unauthorized individuals on-site), immediately bring those irregularities to the attention of the USOC drug-control administrator on-site.
7. If you are informed that you have tested positive for a banned substance (and you dispute that result), you will be invited to witness the testing of the second half (i.e., the "B sample") of your urine sample. Attend the test of the B sample, take with you an individual qualified to evaluate the process, and consider videotaping the test.

Why is there so much concern over drug use by athletes? Why not focus on drug use by clarinet players or muffler repair people? There are several answers to this question, and together they demonstrate that there are special reasons to be concerned about drug use in sport. First, there are those well-known athletes who are seen as role models for young people, portraying youth, strength, and health. When a famous athlete is

reported to be using cocaine or some other illicit substance, there is concern that impressionable young people will see drug use in a more positive light. After all, haven't corporate sponsors paid these athletes to endorse their products, from shoes to breakfast cereal, based on this presumed influence over young consumers?

Second, some of the drugs used by athletes are intended to give the user an advantage over the competition, an advantage that is clearly viewed as being unfair. This is inconsistent with our tradition of fair play in sports, and widespread cheating of any kind tends to diminish a sport and to diminish public interest in it. Professional wrestling, which is widely viewed as being rigged or staged, is enjoyed more as a form of comic entertainment than as an athletic contest. Most professional and amateur sportspeople guard their honor carefully, and the use of performance-enhancing drugs is seen as a threat to that honor.

Third, there is a concern that both the famous and the not-so-famous athletes who use drugs are endangering their health and perhaps their lives for the sake of a temporary burst of power or speed. To the extent that there are risks associated with the use of these drugs, athletes should be aware of those risks. Because these drugs are often obtained illicitly, we can assume that the providers of the drugs do not present a balanced cost/benefit analysis to the potential user but, instead, probably maximize any possible benefit and minimize the dangers.

HISTORICAL USE OF DRUGS IN ATHLETICS

Ancient Times

Although we tend to think of drug use by athletes as a recent phenomenon, the use of chemicals to enhance performance might be as old as sport itself. As with many early drugs, some of these concoctions seemed to make sense at the time but probably had only placebo value. We no longer think that the powdered hooves of an ass will make our feet fly as fast as that animal's, but perhaps it was a belief in that powder that helped the ancient Egyptian competitor's self-confidence. Also, if all the others are using it, why take chances?

The early Greek Olympians did use various herbs and mushrooms that might have had some pharmacological actions as stimulants, and

Aztec athletes used a cactus-based stimulant resembling strychnine. Athletic competitions probably developed in tribal societies as a means of training and preparing for war or for hunting, and various psychoactive plants were used by tribal peoples during battles and hunts, so it is not surprising that the drugs were also used in "sport" from the beginning.

Early Use of Stimulants

During the 1800s and early 1900s, three types of stimulants were reported to be in use by athletes. *Strychnine*, which became famous as a rat poison, can at low doses act as a central nervous system stimulant. However, if the dose is too high, seizure activity will be produced in the brain. The resulting convulsions can paralyze respiration, leading to death. At least some boxers were reported to have used strychnine tablets. This might have made them more aggressive and kept them from tiring very quickly, but it was a dangerous way to do it. We'll never know how many of those rugged heroes were killed in this way, but there must have been a few. Thomas Hicks won the marathon in the 1904 St. Louis Olympics, then collapsed and had to be revived. His race was partly fueled by a mixture of brandy and strychnine.[1] Although the availability of amphetamines later made dangerous drugs such as strychnine less attractive, there is some evidence that the occasional use of strychnine continued at the level of world competition into the 1960s.

Cocaine was also available in the 1800s, at first in the form of Mariani's Coca Wine (used by the French cycling team), which was referred to in some advertisements as "wine for athletes."[2] When pure cocaine became available, athletes quickly adopted this more potent form. Many athletes used coffee as a mild stimulant, and some added pure *caffeine* to their coffee or took caffeine tablets. There were numerous reports of the suspected doping of swimmers, cyclists, boxers, runners, and other athletes during

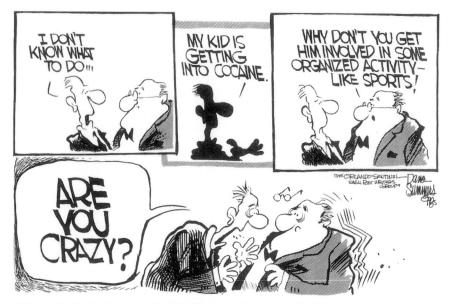

this period. Then, as now, some of the suspicions were raised by the losers, who might or might not have had any evidence of doping. Our use of the word *dope* for illicit drugs is derived from a Dutch word used in South Africa to refer to a cheap brandy, which was sometimes given to racing dogs or horses to slow them down. From this came the idea of doping horses and then people, more often in an effort to improve rather than impair performance. Dogs and horses received all the substances used by humans, including coca wine and cocaine, before the days of testing for drugs.

Amphetamines

It isn't clear when athletes first started using amphetamines for their stimulant effects, but it was probably not long after the drugs were introduced in the 1930s. Amphetamines were widely used throughout the world during World War II, and in the 1940s and 1950s there were reports of the use of these pep pills by professional soccer players in England and Italy. Boxers and cyclists also relied on this new synthetic energy source. More potent than caffeine, longer-lasting than cocaine, and safer than strychnine, it seemed to be the ideal **ergogenic** (energy-producing) drug for both training and competition.

In 1952, the presence of syringes and broken ampules in the speed-skating locker room at the Oslo Winter Olympics was an indication of amphetamines' presence in international competition. There were other reports from the 1952 summer games in Helsinki and the 1956 Melbourne Olympics. Unfortunately, several deaths during this period were attributed to overdoses of amphetamines or other drugs. By the time of the 1960 Rome games, amphetamine use had spread around the world and to most sports. On opening day a Danish cyclist died during time trials. An autopsy revealed that his death resulting from "sunstroke" was aided by the presence of amphetamines, which reduces blood flow to the skin, making it more difficult for the body to cool itself. Three other cyclists collapsed that day, and two were hospitalized.[1] This and other examples of amphetamine abuse led to investigations and to antidoping laws in France and Belgium. Other nations, including the United States, seemed less concerned.

International Drug Testing

Some sports, especially cycling, began to test competitors for drugs on a sporadic basis. Throughout the 1960s, there were instances of athletes refusing to submit to tests or failing tests and being disqualified. These early testing efforts were not enough to prevent the death of cyclist Tommy Simpson, an ex-world champion, who died during the 1967 *Tour de France*. His death was seen on television, and weeks later it was reported that his body contained two types of amphetamines and that drugs had been found in his luggage. This caused the International Olympic Committee in 1968 to establish rules requiring the disqualification of any competitor who refuses to take a drug test or who is found guilty of using banned drugs. Beginning with fewer than 700 urine tests at the 1968 Mexico City Olympics, each subsequent international competition has had more testing, more disqualifications, and more controversy.

American Football

Most Americans did not seem to be very concerned about drug use by athletes until reports surfaced in the late 1960s and early 1970s that professional football players were using amphetamines during games. Before that time, people might not have been very concerned about it even if they had known. You should remember from Chapter 8 that the amphetamines underwent a major status change in the United States during the 1960s. For years an increasing number of Americans had used amphetamines to keep them awake, to provide extra energy, or to lose weight. They were seen by most people as legal, harmless pep pills. It was in that context that the physicians for professional football teams ordered large quantities of the drugs as a routine part of their supplies, and trainers dispensed them liberally.

At the end of the 1960s, amphetamines were widely considered to be drugs of abuse, dangerous drugs that could lead to violent behavior. In this context, revelations that many professionals were playing high made for sensational headlines. Several National Football League (NFL) players sued their teams for injuries received while playing under the influence of drugs, and the NFL officially banned the distribution of amphetamines by team physicians and trainers in 1971. Although the drugs were no longer condoned by the league, the NFL did little at that time to enforce the ban, except to request copies of each team's orders for medical supplies. Athletes who wanted amphetamines still obtained and used them, often through a legal prescription from their own physicians. The attitude seemed to be that, if the players wanted to use pep pills and obtained them on their own, that was their business, but team physicians and trainers shouldn't be using medications to push the athletes beyond their normal endurance. The current NFL policy, of course, restricts all use of amphetamines, as well as many other drugs, no matter where they are obtained.

Steroids

During and after World War II, it was found that malnourished people could gain weight and build themselves up more rapidly if they were given the male hormone testosterone. It appears that the Soviets were the first to put this hormone to use on a wide scale to build up their athletes. An American team physician at the 1956 Olympics reported that the Soviet athletes were using straight testosterone, sometimes in

ergogenic: (er go *gen* ic) producing work or energy; a general term for performance enhancement.

Exploring Your Spirituality

Promoting Overall Fitness

A sharp rise in the use of illegal anabolic steroids by teenage girls, which some attribute to "reverse anorexia," has health authorities worried. This new interest in steroids among girls, experts say, reflects their desire to excel in high school sports, as well as a gradual change in fashion, attitude, and peer pressure away from a preoccupation with thinness. The desired style is to look more healthy and somewhat muscular, leading some girls to a compulsion for fitness and larger muscles. In pursuit of sports stardom or the perfect body, they expose themselves to the same severe health risks as boys taking steroids, but with the added complications of unwanted masculinizing effects.[5]

Young girls are not the only ones who may succumb to an addiction to the mirror. Researchers at Harvard Medical School's McLean Hospital recently completed a study of 32 women bodybuilders, 17 of whom showed signs of an emotional disorder called "body dysmorphism," or the excessive preoccupation with a trait or traits of the body viewed as defective or ugly, whether they are or not. The researchers found that several of the women studied were so addicted to working out that they cut off close personal relationships and job opportunities to do so.[5]

Although these cases take building a better body to an unhealthy extreme, most of us would agree that overall body fitness helps us feel better, mentally and physically. Even a modest increase in our daily activity level can be rewarding, reducing stress, decreasing

susceptibility to illness, and providing more energy to keep up the pace of school, family activities, and work. And an increase in physical well-being often goes hand in hand with the spiritual and emotional benefits of good health.

How can we increase self-esteem in young athletes and educate them about the long-term benefits of avoiding steroid use? Unless young people are taught to know that it's not right to try to win at all costs or to try to look good at all costs, they won't listen when they hear that steroids put their lives at risk. A program called Atlas, supported by the National Institute on Drug Abuse, is aimed at reducing steroid use among young male athletes by getting them to teach one another about the problems. After the program was instituted 31 high schools in Oregon and Washington—involving 3,200 male athletes—the number of male students who reported having used steroids within the past year was cut by 50 percent. A similar program for girls is under development.[5]

An additional deterrent is for role models to take a public stance against steroid use, as was done in the campaign kicked off by a group of former Olympians from a variety of sports. Gold medal winners Jim Ryan, Edwin Moses, Frank Shorter, Donna de Varona, John Nabor, and Bruce Baumgartner have made the point that it's possible to achieve athletic success through hard work, personal sacrifice, and determination. The power of the mind and spirit can sustain us through tough times and help us rise to our best.

---

excessive doses and with unfortunate side effects. Testosterone helps both men and women become more muscular, but its masculinizing effects on women and enlargement of the prostate gland in men are definite drawbacks. The American physician at the 1956 Olympics returned to the United States and helped develop and test **anabolic** steroids, which were quickly adopted by American weight lifters and bodybuilders.[3]

American and British athletes in events such as discus and shotput were the first to acknowledge publicly that they had used steroids, and there was evidence that steroid use was widespread during the 1960s in most track and field

events. These drugs were not officially banned, nor were they tested for in international competition until the early 1970s, mainly because a sensitive urine test was not available until then. Of the 2,000 urine samples taken during the 1976 Olympics, fewer than 300 were tested for the presence of steroids, and 8 of those were positive.[1] The first international athletes to be found guilty of taking steroids were a Bulgarian discus thrower, a Romanian shotputter, a Polish discus thrower, and weight lifters from several countries. By that time, individual Western athletes might have chosen to use steroids, but some of the Eastern European countries seemed to have adopted their use almost as a matter of official policy. When the East German swimming coach was asked during the 1976 Olympics why so many of their women swimmers had deep voices, the answer was, "We have come here to swim, not sing."[4]

Cocaine

During the 1980s, public revelations of drug use by athletes became commonplace and cocaine was often mentioned. Professional basketball, baseball, and football players in the United States were being sent into treatment centers for cocaine dependence, and several either dropped out or were kicked out of professional sports. Most amateur and professional sports organizations adopted longer and more complicated lists of banned substances and rules providing for more and more participants to be tested. For example, in 1986, the U.S. National Collegiate Athletic Association (NCAA) adopted a list of more than 3,000 brand-name drugs containing banned substances. All participants are to be tested during the championship contest and after all postseason football games. In many events around the world, all contestants must now be subjected to urine tests as a matter of routine.

At the end of the 1980s, some were beginning to question the wisdom of trying to test every athlete for everything. In spite of the enormous expense to which sports organizations have gone, the use of steroids, stimulants, and other performance-enhancing substances seems to be as great as ever. So far, however, both the extent of testing and the ingenuity of athletes trying to beat the tests continue to escalate.

STIMULANTS AS PERFORMANCE ENHANCERS

The first question to be answered about the use of a drug to increase energy or otherwise enhance athletic performance is, Does it work? We might not worry so much about unfair competition if we didn't feel that the use of a drug would

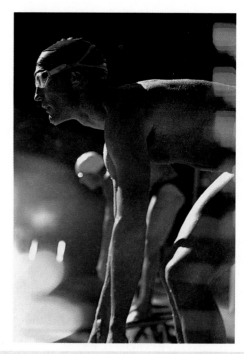

Stimulants have been shown to improve endurance.

really help the person using it. There is another reason it would be nice if these drugs were ineffective: if we could prove that, then we could presumably convince young people not to take the risk of using drugs because there would be no gain to be had. It is worthwhile pointing out that experiments can never prove that a drug has no effect—you might have done a hundred experiments and not used the right dose or the right test (peak output? endurance? accuracy?). The possibility always exists that someone will come along later with the right combination to demonstrate a beneficial effect. Therefore, be wary when someone tries to use scientific evidence to argue that a drug doesn't work, has no effect, is not toxic, or is otherwise inactive.

anabolic: (an a *ball* ick) promoting constructive metabolism; building tissue.

We've had a pretty good idea of the effectiveness of the amphetamines since 1959, when Smith and Beecher published the results of a double-blind study comparing amphetamines and placebo in runners, swimmers, and weight throwers.[6] Their conclusion was that most of the athletes performed better under amphetamines, but the improvement was small (a few percentage points' improvement). Several studies have reported no differences or very small differences in performance, and some medical experts in the 1960s wanted to argue that amphetamines were essentially ineffective and there was no reason for people to use them. An excellent 1981 review of the existing literature put it all into perspective. Pointing out that it had been taking athletes an average of about seven years for each 1 percent improvement in the world record speed for the mile run, if amphetamines produced even a 1 percent improvement they could make an important difference at that level of competition. Their conclusion was that there is an amphetamine margin. It is usually small, amounting to a few percent under most circumstances. But even when that tiny, it can surely spell the difference between a gold medal and sixth place."[7]

Whether amphetamines or other stimulants increase physical ability (provide pep or energy) or produce their actions only through effects on the brain is an interesting question, which might not be answerable. Surely a person who feels more confident will train harder, compete with a winning attitude, try harder, and keep trying longer. With amphetamines, improvements have been seen both in events requiring brief, explosive power (shotput) and in events requiring endurance, such as distance running. In laboratory studies, increases have been found in isometric strength and in work output during endurance testing on a stationary bicycle (the subjects rode longer under amphetamine conditions). This endurance improvement could be due to the masking of fatigue effects, allowing a person to compete to utter exhaustion.

HealthQuest Activities

In Module 9, find *Drug F/X Exploration* and determine your risk of dependence on and the effects of anabolic steroids. Have you ever taken anabolic steroids? Do you have any friends who have? What was their reaction? Take a poll of athletes on your campus. Ask them the following questions: Have you ever used steroids? Do you believe it's wrong to use steroids or other performance-enhancing drugs to improve your athletic performance? Do you believe it's dangerous to use them? Share your results in class.

In the same module, look under *Specifics On*. Read "Performance-Enhancing Drugs." Get together with a group of your classmates to discuss the issues surrounding performance-enhancing drugs. In a newspaper or sports magazine, you can find articles about the use of these substances among athletes. A suggestion might be the controversy surrounding Olympic athletes who tested positive for drugs and were not allowed to compete or had to return their medals. Discuss whether you think these regulations are fair or unfair.

Caffeine has also been shown to improve endurance performance under laboratory conditions. In one experiment, 330 mg of caffeine (approximately equivalent to 3 cups of brewed coffee) increased the length of a stationary bicycle ride by almost 20 percent. In another experiment, when subjects rode for 2 hours, their total energy output was 7 percent higher after 500 mg caffeine than in the control condition.[8] The effectiveness of caffeine might depend on other factors: for example, one study reported no benefit from caffeine when athletes ran long distances (12 miles) in hot, humid conditions.[9] Small amounts of caffeine are acceptable in most sports, but a urine level above 12 micrograms/mL will lead to disqualification in many competitions. The doses needed to produce large performance increases produce much higher levels than that, but there could still be a slight improvement even at legal levels.

Apparently there have not been any controlled laboratory or field experiments testing the performance-enhancing capabilities of cocaine, but especially during the 1980s there were many athletes who believed in its power. Cocaine's stimulant properties are generally similar to those of the amphetamines, so we can assume that cocaine would be effective under some circumstances. Given cocaine's shorter duration of action, it would not be expected to improve endurance over a several-hour period as well as either amphetamines or caffeine.

With all these and several other CNS stimulants banned by most sports associations, some athletes have continued to use them during training, to allow them to run, ride, or swim harder. They then do not use the drug for several days before the competition or during the competition, hoping that traces of the substance will not appear in the urine test. This might make sense, but no one knows whether training under one drug condition has an effect on com-petition under another condition. Also, overexertion under the influence of a fatigue-masking drug might be most dangerous during training, leading to muscle injury, a fall or another accident, or heat exhaustion.

Athletes and others who use amphetamines or cocaine regularly run the risk of developing a dependence on the drug, developing paranoid or violent behavior patterns, and suffering from the loss of energy and psychological depression that occur as the drugs wear off (see Chapter 8).

STEROIDS

The male sex hormone testosterone has two major types of effects on the developing man. **Androgenic** effects are masculinizing actions: initial growth of the penis and other male sex glands, deepening of the voice, and increased facial hair are examples. This steroid hormone also has anabolic effects. These include increased muscle mass, increases in the size of various internal organs, control of the distribution of body fat, increased protein synthesis, and increased calcium in the bones. In the 1950s, drug companies began to synthesize various steroids that have fewer of the androgenic effects and more of the anabolic effects than testosterone. These are referred to as *anabolic steroids,* although none of them is entirely free of some masculinizing effect.

Whether or not these drugs are effective in improving athletic performance has been controversial: for many years the medical position was that they were not, whereas the lore around the locker room was that they would make anyone bigger, stronger, and more masculine-looking. A lot of people must have had more faith in the locker-room lore than in the official word. The 1989 *Physician's Desk Reference* contained the

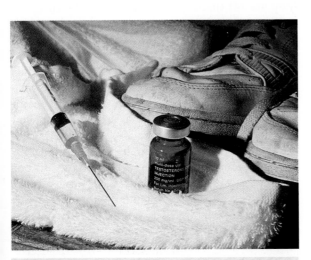

Testosterone, a male sex hormone, is sometimes abused by athletes for its protein-building (anabolic) effect.

androgenic: (an drow *gen* ick) masculinizing.

following statement in bold-face type: "**Anabolic Steroids Have Not Been Shown to Enhance Athletic Ability**." Try telling that to Ben Johnson, the disqualified winner of the 1988 Olympic gold medal in the 100-meter run or to the people who ran against him. That disclaimer is no longer required by the FDA.

There is no doubt that testosterone has a tremendous effect on muscle mass and strength during puberty, and experiments on castrated animals clearly show the muscle-developing ability of the synthetic anabolics.[10] What is not so clear is the effect of adding additional anabolic stimulation to adolescent or adult males who already have normal circulating levels of testosterone.

Laboratory research on healthy men who are engaged in weight training and are maintained on a proper diet has often found that anabolic steroids produce small increases in lean muscle mass and sometimes small increases in muscular strength. There is no evidence for an overall increase in aerobic capacity or endurance in those studies. However, it might never be possible to conduct experiments demonstrating the effectiveness of the high doses used by some athletes. Many athletes report that they take 10 or more times the dose of a steroid that has been tested and recommended for treatment of a deficiency disorder.[11] It is also common practice for athletes to take more than 1 steroid at a time (both an oral and an injectable form, for example). This practice is known as "stacking." To expose research subjects to such massive doses would clearly be unethical.

Another impediment to doing careful research on this topic is that these steroids produce detectable psychological effects. When double-blind experiments have been attempted, almost always the subjects have known when they were on steroids, thus destroying the blind control.[12] This is important because steroid users report that they feel they can lift more or work harder when they are on the steroids. This may be due to CNS effects of the steroids leading to a stimulant-like feeling of energy and loss of fatigue or to increased aggressiveness expressed as more aggressive training. There is a further possibility of what is known as an *active placebo effect*, with a belief in the power of steroids, enhanced by the clear sensation that the drug is doing something because one can "feel" it. Until recently, many of the scientists studying steroid hormones believed that their main effects were psychological, combined with a "bloating" effect on the muscle, in which the muscle retains more fluids, is larger, weighs more, but has no more physical strength.[1]

Psychological Effects of Steroids

The reported psychological effects of steroids, including a stimulant-like high and increased aggressiveness, might be beneficial for increasing the amount of work done during training and for increasing the intensity of effort during competition. However, there are also concerns that these psychological effects might produce great problems, especially at high doses. One concern is that a psychological dependence seems to develop in some users, who feel well when they are on the steroids but become depressed when they are off them. Many users take the drugs in cycles, and their mood swings can interfere with their social relationships and other life functions.

There has been a great deal of discussion about "roid rage," a kind of manic rage that has been reported by some steroid users.[13] We should be careful about attributing instances of violence to a drug on the basis of uncontrolled retrospective reports, especially when the perpetrator of a violent crime might be looking for an excuse.[14] However, there is a sufficient number of reports of violent feelings and actions among steroid users for us to be concerned and to await further research. Says Dr. William Taylor, a leading authority on anabolic steroids, "I've seen total personality changes. A passive, low-key guy goes on steroids for muscle enhancement, and the next thing you know, he's being arrested for assault or disorderly conduct."[15]

Drugs in Depth

Nutritional Ergogenic Aids

If athletes can't get or refuse to use pharmacological aids in athletic competition, most believe that certain foods or nutritional supplements are a "natural" way to enhance their performance. Following is a very abbreviated description of a more complete review of this topic by Melvin H. Williams, Ph.D. (*Nutrition Today*, pp 7–14, Jan/Feb 1989).

Amino acids are the natural building blocks of muscle, and one certainly requires a basic minimum intake of them in order to maintain normal protein synthesis and other functions (including the synthesis of some neurotransmitters). However, there is no scientific evidence to support the idea that supplementing with amino acids or extra protein above the recommended daily allowance will have any beneficial effect at all on muscle development, strength, speed, or endurance. Marketers of these "muscle-building" dietary supplements walk a fine line by avoiding making specific claims on the product labels, so they do not fall under the FDA's rules for demonstrating effectiveness. Usually nearby posters or pamphlets link amino acids to the idea of muscle growth. These supplements are probably of little or no value to an athlete who is receiving proper nutrition.

Carbohydrates are burned as fuels, especially during prolonged aerobic exercise. Carbohydrates taken immediately before or during an endurance performance lasting for more than an hour may enhance the performance by maintaining blood glucose levels and preventing the depletion of muscle stores of glycogen. Carbohydrate loading before marathon runs consists of resting for the last day or two while ingesting extra carbohydrates, increasing both muscle and liver stores of carbohydrates. In either case, there is not much evidence to support the value of carbohydrate supplements for athletic performances lasting less than an hour.

Fats, in experiments with fat supplements, have not been found to be a useful ergogenic aid.

Vitamins, especially the water-soluble B vitamins, are necessary for normal utilization of food energy.

Deficiencies in these vitamins, such as might result when a wrestler is dieting to meet a weight limit, can clearly impair physical performance. However, once the necessary minimum amount is available for metabolic purposes, further supplements are of no value. Many experiments have been done with supplements of C, E, and B-complex vitamins or with multivitamin supplements, the so-called vitamin B_{15}, and with bee pollen, and there is no evidence for enhanced performance or faster recovery after workouts. Again, these supplements are probably of no value to an athlete who is receiving proper nutrition.

Minerals, in the form of various mineral supplements, are widely used by athletes. Once again, most are probably not needed or useful, but there may be some exceptions. Electrolyte drinks are designed to replace both fluids and electrolytes, such as sodium and chloride that are lost in sweat. Actually, sweat contains a lower concentration of these electrolytes than does blood, so it is more important to replace the fluids than the electrolytes under most circumstances. Sodium supplementation may be useful for those engaged in ultraendurance events, such as 100-mile runs.

Iron supplements are helpful in athletes who are iron-deficient, as may occur especially in female distance runners. However, if iron status is normal, there is probably no value in iron supplements.

The jury is still out on whether sodium bicarbonate (baking soda) enhances performance in anaerobic events, such as 400- to 800-meter runs. Some studies indicate improvements, whereas others do not. The same may be said for phosphate loading, which is currently receiving some research attention.

Water is needed by endurance athletes to keep their body temperatures down, especially in a warm environment. Drinking water both before and during prolonged exercise can deter dehydration and improve performance.

Adverse Effects on the Body

There are many concerns about the effects of steroid use on the body. In young users who have not attained their full height, steroids can cause premature closing of the growth plates of the long bones, thus limiting their adult height. For all users the risk of peliosis hepatitis (bloody cysts in the liver) and the changes in blood lipids possibly leading to atherosclerosis, high blood pressure, and heart disease are potentially serious concerns. Acne and baldness are reported, as are atrophy of the testes and breast development in men using anabolic steroids.

There are also considerations for women who use anabolic steroids. Because women usually have only trace amounts of testosterone produced by the adrenals, the addition of even relatively small doses of anabolic steroids can have dramatic effects, in terms of both muscle growth and masculinization. Some of the side effects, such as mild acne, decreased breast size, and fluid retention, are reversible. The enlargement of the clitoris might be reversible if steroid use is stopped soon after it is noticed. Other effects, such as increased facial hair and deepening of the voice, might be irreversible.[12]

Regulation

As we found in Chapter 2, when a drug produces dependence, violent crime, and toxic side effects, society may feel justified in trying to place restrictions on the drug's availability. In 1988, congressional hearings were held on the notion of placing anabolic steroids on the list of controlled substances. Evidence was presented that a large black market had developed for these drugs, amounting to perhaps $100 million per year. In addition, there was concern that adolescent boys, many of whom were not athletic at all, had begun to use steroids in the belief that they would quickly become more muscular and "macho" looking.[16] As part of the Omnibus Crime Control Act of 1990, anabolic steroids became listed as a Schedule III controlled substance, requiring more record-keeping and limited prescription refills.[17]

OTHER HORMONAL MANIPULATIONS

Whereas the anabolic steroids have been in wide use, other treatments have been experimented with on a more limited basis. Female sex hormones have been used to feminize men, so that they could compete in women's events. The women's gold medal sprinter in the 1964 Olympics was shown by chromosome testing to have been a man, and he had to return the medal. Hormone receptor–blocking drugs have probably been used to delay puberty in female gymnasts. In women, puberty shifts the center of gravity lower in the body and changes body proportions in ways that adversely affect performance in some gymnastic events. Smaller women appear to be more graceful, spin faster on the uneven bars, and generally have the advantage, which is why top female gymnasts are usually in their teens. However, the Soviets were suspected of tampering with nature: their top three international gymnasts in 1978 were all 17 or 18 years old, but the following were their heights and weights: 53 inches, 63 pounds; 60 inches, 90 pounds; and 57 inches, 79 pounds.

We have certainly not seen the end of growth-promoting hormonal treatments. **Human growth hormone,** which is released from the pituitary gland, can potentially increase the height and weight of an individual to gigantic proportions, especially if administered during childhood and adolescence. In fact, in rare instances the excessive production of this hormone creates giants well over 7 feet tall. These giants usually die at an early age because their internal organs continue to grow. However, administration of a few doses of this hormone at the right time might produce a more controlled increase in body size. Likewise, the growth-hormone-releasing hormone, and some of the

Taking Sides

Has Creatine Killed Wrestlers?

In 1997, three wrestlers died while in training, and traces of creatine were found in one of the young men. Sensational news articles followed, in which the death was linked to creatine use. However, a look at what this athlete had done might indicate a different explanation.[20] Jeff Reese, the 21-year-old wrestler who was found to have elevated levels of creatine in his blood, had worked out for 2 hours in a 92°F gym wearing a rubber suit, in an attempt to lose 12 pounds in a single day. The other two wrestlers were undertaking similar extreme measures when they died, and there is no evidence they were using creatine. Clearly, we cannot say that creatine caused Reese's death. With thousands of creatine users, the risk of acute toxicity appears to be small. What we don't yet know is the effect of chronic use for months or years at a time. Although creatine is considered a dietary supplement, it is being used in a druglike manner: a pure chemical taken in doses well above normal physiological ranges. No matter how safe creatine appears to be now, we should be cautious about long-term use until more is known.

For more on this topic, log on to www.dushkin.com/online for current news and links to other popular and informative sites, as well as time-saving web search strategies and study tools.

cellular intermediary hormones by which growth hormone exerts its effects, might work to enhance growth. It is not currently possible to test for the presence of these substances. In spite of the possible dangers, the lure of an otherwise capable basketball player growing a couple of inches taller or of a football player being 30 pounds heavier has no doubt caused many young athletes to experiment with these substances. Experiments in which growth hormone was given to men found no increase in muscle protein synthesis or in strength.[18] The 1990 legislation that placed anabolic steroids on the list of controlled substances also made it a crime to distribute human growth hormone for nonmedical purposes.

BETA-2 AGONISTS

At the beginning of the 1992 Olympics, the leader of the British team was disqualified because of the detection of a new drug. Clenbuterol was developed as a treatment for asthma and is a relative of several other bronchodilators that are found in prescription inhalers. These drugs have sympathomimetic effects on the bronchi of the lungs but are designed to be more specific than older sympathomimetics, such as ephedrine or the amphetamines (see Chapter 8). Their specificity comes from a selective stimulation of the beta-2 subtype of adrenergic receptors. Research with cows had revealed an increase in muscle mass, and there was beginning to be speculation that this might represent a new type of nonsteroidal anabolic agent. Apparently someone in Great Britain was keeping an eye on the animal research literature and decided to try out the anabolic actions on at least one Olympic athlete. Presumably it was hoped that such a new drug would not be tested for, but the Olympic officials were also well informed and ready, at least for clenbuterol. More recent human studies have shown some increases in strength of selected muscle types with clenbuterol or a similar drug, but there is no evidence that beta-2 agonists improve athletic performance.[19]

human growth hormone: a pituitary hormone responsible for some types of giantism.

CREATINE

The big news for bodybuilders has been creatine, a natural substance found in meat and fish. This is a legal product sold as a food supplement. There is clear evidence that creatine helps regenerate ATP, which provides the energy for muscle contractions. Users of creatine tend to gain some weight, some of which is water weight. There is considerable evidence that the use of creatine can improve strength and short-term speed in sprinting. However, studies of longer-distance running, cycling, and swimming often find no effect, and in one case a significant slowing was reported, probably due to weight gain.[3]

SUMMARY

- Performance-enhancing drugs have been used by athletes throughout history.
- Athletic use of stimulants appears to have increased and spread to most sports with the use of amphetamines during the 1950s and 1960s.
- Amphetamines and caffeine have both been shown to increase work output and to mask the effects of fatigue.
- Some athletes continue to use stimulants for training, in spite of the dangers of injury and overexertion.
- Anabolic steroids are capable of increasing muscle mass and probably strength, although it has been difficult to separate the psychological stimulant-like effect of these drugs from the physical effects on the muscles themselves.
- Anabolic steroids can also produce a variety of dangerous and sometimes irreversible side effects.
- It is difficult to do ethical and well-controlled research on the effects of steroids.
- Misuse of human growth hormone and related substances might be the next problem to arise.

Web Watch

Do You Mix Drugs and Sports?
Go to www.antibully.org.uk/drsport.htm and read the information about drugs and sport. You'll learn about the physical and social effects of using steroids and other performance-enhancing drugs.

Who Uses Anabolic Steroids?
At www.nida.nih.gov/NIDA_Notes/NNVol15N3/Initiative.html, read the article "NIDA Initiative Targets Increasing Teen Use of Anabolic Steroids." Read about the ways the NIDA (National Institute on Drug Abuse) is attempting to educate young people about the risks of anabolic steroids. Do you think this initiative could be successful in helping young people avoid the negative effects of steroids?

Check Out Publications on Anabolic Steroids
The National Clearing House for Drug and Alcohol Information offers a listing of publications about certain types of drugs. Go to www.health.org/catalog/catalog.asp?key=13&detail=false to find and, if you wish, order brochures or other publications about anabolic steroids.

- Creatine is a legally available nutritional supplement that can increase strength but might slow distance runners because of resultant weight gain.

REVIEW QUESTIONS

1. What was the first type of stimulant drug reported to be used by boxers and other athletes in the 1800s? *Cocaine*
2. What was the first type of drug known to be widely used in international competition and that led to the first Olympic urine-testing programs? *Anabolic Steroids*
3. When and in what country were the selective anabolic steroids first developed?

Try It!

How Would You Run the Race?

Imagine that you have gone out for the track team. You compete in the 3,000-meter races and have been training hard for the past two years. It seems as though you have worked as hard as you could every day, yet it's clear that your times have gotten as fast as they're going to get. The conference championships are tomorrow. Your parents have traveled 300 miles to see you run, and lots of your friends will be there, cheering you on. You know your own times, and you know the competition, and, although you expect a close race for the top three spots, you figure to come in fourth. You yourself have never used any type of stimulant drug, but you have heard rumors that several of the fastest runners take amphetamines before the race, and you suspect that it is true. Your conference has not yet adopted a drug-screening program for track, however, so there's no way to know for sure.

Under these circumstances, what would you do if

1. Someone you don't know very well but who you heard is a drug dealer offers you some "speed" just for the race?

2. A friend of yours has some prescription diet pills that contain amphetamines, and the friend offers you one?

3. You are offered some cocaine to snort right before the race?

4. You are offered an OTC asthma pill that contains ephedrine?

5. You are offered coffee or tea?

Or would you rather not take artificial stimulants at all, come in fourth, and know you did your best and ran a clean race?

4. Do amphetamines and caffeine actually enhance athletic performance? If so, how much?

5. What muscle effect do we know for certain that anabolic steroids can produce in healthy men?

6. What is meant by roid rage, and what double-blind studies have been done on this phenomenon?

7. What specific effect of anabolic steroids might be of concern to young users? to females?

8. How might the Soviets have kept their female gymnasts under 5 feet tall?

9. Why do "pituitary giants" often die at an early age?

10. How does creatine increase strength?

REFERENCES

1. Donohue T, Johnson N: *Foul play: Drug abuse in sports.* Oxford, England: Basil Blackwell, 1986.
2. Asken MJ: *Dying to win: The athlete's guide to safe and unsafe drugs in sports.* Washington, DC: Acropolis, 1988.
3. Eichner ER: Ergogenic aids: What athletes are using—and why, *Physician and Sportsmedicine* 25:70–83, 1997.
4. Goldman B: *Death in the locker room.* South Bend, IN: Icarus Press, 1984.
5. Noble HB: Steroid use by teen-age girls is rising, *New York Times* pp June 1, 1999.
6. Smith GM, Beecher HK: Amphetamine sulfate and athletic performance, *JAMA* 170:542–557, 1959.
7. Laties VG, Weiss B: The amphetamine margin in sports, *Federation Proceedings* 40:2689–2692, 1981.
8. Noble BJ: *Physiology of exercise and sport.* St Louis: Mosby, 1986.
9. Cohen BS and others: Effects of caffeine ingestion on endurance racing in heat and humidity, *European Journal of Applied Physiology* 73:358–363, 1996.
10. Williams MH: *Ergogenic aids in sports.* Champaign, IL: Human Kinetics, 1983.
11. Marshall E: The drug of champions, *Science* 242:183–184, 1983.
12. Taylor WN Hormonal manipulation: a new era of monstrous athletes. Jefferson, NC, McFarland & Co., 1985
13. Pope HG, Katz DL: Affective and psychotic symptoms associated with anabolic steroid use, *American Journal of Psychiatry* 145:487–490, 1988.
14. Lubell A: Does steroid abuse cause—or excuse—violence? *Physician and Sportsmedicine* 17:176–185, 1989.
15. Fultz O: 'Roid rage, *American Health* 10:60, 1991.
16. Toufexis A: Shortcut to the Rambo look, *Time* p 78, Jan 30, 1989.
17. Nightingale SL: Anabolic steroids as controlled substances, *JAMA* 265:1229, 1991.
18. Yarasheski KE and others: Short-term growth hormone treatment does not increase muscle protein synthesis in experienced weight lifters, *Journal of Applied Physiology* 74:3073–3076, 1993.
19. Spann S: Effect of clenbuterol on athletic performance, *Annals of Pharmacotherapy* 29:75, 1995.
20. Tarlach GM: Creatine controversy, *Drug Topics* pp Feb 2, 1998.

Appendix A

Drug Names

acetaminophen: OTC analgesic. Similar to aspirin in its effects.

acetophenazine: Tindal. Antipsychotic.

acetylsalicylic acid: aspirin. OTC analgesic.

Adapin: doxepin. Tricyclic antidepressant.

alprazolam: Xanax. Benzodiazepine sedative.

Alurate: aprobarbital. Barbiturate sedative-hypnotic.

Amanita muscaria: hallucinogenic mushroom.

amitriptyline: Elavil, Endep. Tricyclic antidepressant.

amobarbital: Amytal. Barbiturate sedative-hypnotic.

amoxapine: Asendin. Tricyclic antidepressant.

amphetamine: Benzedrine. CNS stimulant and sympathomimetic.

Amytal: amobarbital. Barbiturate sedative-hypnotic.

Anavar: oxandrolone. Anabolic steroid.

angel dust: street name for PCP.

Antabuse: disulfiram. Alters metabolism of alcohol; used to treat alcoholism.

aprobarbital: Alurate. Barbiturate sedative-hypnotic.

Artane: trihexyphenidyl. Anticholinergic used to control extrapyramidal symptoms.

Asendin: amoxapine. Tricyclic antidepressant.

aspirin: acetylsalicylic acid. OTC analgesic.

Ativan: lorazepam. Benzodiazepine sedative.

atropine: anticholinergic.

Aventyl: nortriptyline. Tricyclic antidepressant.

belladonna: poisonous anticholinergic plant.

Benzedrine: amphetamine. CNS stimulant and sympathomimetic. Brand name no longer used.

benzodiazepines: class of sedative-hypnotics that includes diazepam (Valium).

benztropine: Cogentin. Anticholinergic used to control extrapyramidal symptoms.

bromide: group of salts with sedative properties.

bupropion: Wellbutrin. Atypical antidepressant. Also Zyban, to reduce craving during tobacco cessation.

butabarbital: Butisol. Barbiturate sedative-hypnotic.

Butisol: butabarbital. Barbiturate sedative-hypnotic.

caffeine: mild stimulant found in coffee and in OTC preparations.

Catapres: clonidine. Antihypertensive drug shown to reduce narcotic withdrawal symptoms.

chloral hydrate: Noctec. Nonbarbiturate sedative-hypnotic.

chlordiazepoxide: Librium. Benzodiazepine sedative.

chlorpheniramine maleate: OTC antihistamine.

chlorpromazine: Thorazine. Antipsychotic.

chlorprothixene: Taractan. Antipsychotic.

Cibalith: lithium citrate. Salt used in treating mania and bipolar affective disorders.

clenbuterol: an alpha-2 adrenergic agonist developed to treat asthma, but used by athletes to build muscle.

clonidine: Catapres. Antihyperintensive drug shown to reduce narcotic withdrawal symptoms.

clorazepate: Tranxene. Benzodiazepine sedative.

clozapine: Clozaril. Atypical antipsychotic.

Clozaril: clozapine. Atypical antipsychotic.

cocaine: CNS stimulant and local anesthetic.

codeine: narcotic analgesic found in opium.

Cogentin: benztropine. Anticholinergic used to control extrapyramidal symptoms.

Compazine: prochlorperazine. Antipsychotic.

creatine: natural substance found in meat and fish that might have anabolic properties and is used by athletes.

Cylert: pemoline. Stimulant used to treat ADD with hyperactivity.

Dalmane: flurazepam. Benzodiazepine hypnotic.

Darvon: propoxyphene. Narcotic analgesic.

Datura: genus of plants, many of which are anticholinergic.

Demerol: meperidine. Narcotic analgesic.

desipramine: Norpramin, Pertofrane. Tricyclic antidepressant.

Desoxyn: methamphetamine. CNS stimulant and sympathomimetic.

Desyrel: trazodone. Atypical antidepressant.

Dexedrine: dextroamphetamine. CNS stimulant and sympathomimetic.

dexfenfluramine: Redux. Appetite suppressant, removed from the market in 1997.

dextroamphetamine: Dexedrine. CNS stimulant and sympathomimetic.

dextromethorphan: OTC cough supressant.

diazepam: Valium. Benzodiazepine sedative.

diethylpropion: Tenuate, Tepanil. Amphetamine-like appetite supressant.

dihydrocodeine: narcotic analgesic.

Dilaudid: hydromorphone. Narcotic analgesic.

diphenhydramine: antihistamine.

disulfiram: Antabuse. Alters metabolism of alcohol; used to treat alcoholism.

DMT: dimethyltryptamine. Hallucinogen.

Dolophine: methadone. Narcotic analgesic.

DOM: hallucinogen.

doxepin: Adapin, Sinequan. Tricyclic antidepressant.

dronabinol: Marinol. Prescription form of delta-9-tetrahydrocannabinol.

Effexor: venlafaxine. Antidepressant (SSRI).

Elavil: amitriptyline. Tricyclic antidepressant.

Endep: amitriptyline. Tricyclic antidepressant.

endorphin: endogenous substance with effects similar to those of the narcotic analgesics.

enkephalin: endogenous substance with effects similar to those of the narcotic analgesics.

ephedrine: sympathomimetic used to treat asthma.

Equanil: meprobamate. Nonbarbiturate sedative-hypnotic.

Eskalith: lithium carbonate. Salt used in treating mania and bipolar affective disorders.

fenfluramine: Pondimin. Appetite suppressant, removed from the market in 1997.

fentanyl: Sublimaze. Potent synthetic analgesic.

flunitrazepam: Rohypnol. Benzodiazepine hypnotic, not sold in the U.S. Known as a "date-rape" drug.

fluoxetine: Prozac. Antidepressant (SSRI).

fluphenazine: Permitil, Prolixin. Antipsychotic.

flurazepam: Dalmane. Benzodiazepine hypnotic.

GHB: gamma hydroxybutyrate. CNS depressant, produced naturally in small amounts in the human brain. Has been used recreationally and, in combination with alcohol, has some reputation as a "date-rape" drug.

Halcion: triazolam. Benzodiazepine hypnotic.

Haldol: haloperidol. Antipsychotic.

haloperidol: Haldol. Antipsychotic.

henbane: poisonous anticholinergic plant.

heroin: Diacetylmorphine. Narcotic analgesic.

hydrocodone: narcotic analgesic.

hydromorphone: Dilaudid. Narcotic analgesic.

ibogaine: hallucinogen, also proposed to reduce craving in drug addicts.

ibuprofen: analgesic and anti-inflammatory.

imipramine: Janimine, Tofranil. Tricyclic antidepressant.

isocarboxazid: Marplan. MAO inhibitor used as antidepressant.

Janimine: imipramine. Tricyclic antidepressant.

Ketalar: ketamine. Dissociative anesthetic.

ketamine: Ketalar. Dissociative anesthetic.

LAAM: L-alpha-acetyl-methadol. Long-lasting synthetic narcotic used in maintenance treatment of narcotic addicts.

laudanum: tincture (alcohol solution) of opium.

Librium: chlordiazepoxide. Benzodiazepine sedative.

Lithane: lithium carbonate.

lithium carbonate, lithium citrate: salts used in treating mania and bipolar affective disorders.

Lithobid: lithium carbonate.

lorazepam: Ativan. Benzodiazepine sedative.

loxapine: Loxitane. Antipsychotic.

Loxitane: loxapine. Antipsychotic.

LSD: lysergic acid diethylamide. Hallucinogen.

Ludiomil: maprotiline. Tricyclic antidepressant.

Luminal: phenobarbital. Barbiturate sedative-hypnotic.

mandrake: anticholinergic plant.

maprotiline: Ludiomil. Tricyclic antidepressant.

Marinol: dronabinol. Prescription form of delta-9-tetrahydrocannabinol.

Marplan: isocarboxazid. MAO inhibitor used as antidepressant.

Mazanor: mazindol. Appetite suppressant.

mazinodol: Mazanor, Sanorex. Appetite suppressant.

MDA: hallucinogen.

MDMA: hallucinogen.

Mebaral: mephobarbital. Barbiturate sedative-hypnotic.

Mellaril: thioridazine. Antipsychotic.

meperidine: Demerol. Narcotic analgesic.

mephobarbital: Mebaral. Barbiturate sedative-hypnotic.

meprobamate: Equanil, Miltown. Nonbarbiturate sedative-hypnotic.

mescaline: hallucinogen found in peyote cactus.

mesoridazine: Serentil. Antipsychotic.

methadone: Dolophine. Narcotic analgesic.

methamphetamine: Desoxyn, Methedrine. CNS stimulant and sympathomimetic.

methaqualone: Quaalude, Sopor. Nonbarbiturate sedative-hypnotic.

methylphenidate: Ritalin. Stimulant used to treat ADD with hyperactivity.

Metrazol: pentylenetetrazol. Convulsant formerly used in convulsive therapy.

Miltown: meprobamate. Nonbarbiturate sedative-hypnotic.

mirtazapine: Remeron. Atypical antidepressant.

Moban: molindone. Antipsychotic.

molindone: Moban. Antipsychotic.

morphine: narcotic analgesic.

naloxone: Narcan. Narcotic antagonist.

naltrexone: Trexan, reVIA. Narcotic antagonist. Used in treating alcoholism.

Narcan: naloxone. Narcotic antagonist.

Nardil: phenelzine. MAO inhibitor used as antidepressant.

Navane: thiothixene. Antipsychotic.

Nembutal: pentobarbital. Barbiturate sedative-hypnotic.

Noctec: chloral hydrate. Nonbarbiturate sedative-hypnotic.

Norpramin: desipramine. Tricyclic antidepressant.

nortriptyline: Aventyl, Pamelor. Tricyclic antidepressant.

Numorphan: oxymorphone. Narcotic analgesic.

olanzepine: Zyprex. Atypical antipsychotic.

opium: narcotic analgesic.

oxandrolone: Anavar. Anabolic steroid.

oxazepam: Serax. Benzodiazepine sedative.

oxycodone: Percodan. Narcotic analgesic.

oxymorphone: Numorphan. Narcotic analgesic.

Pamelor: nortriptyline. Tricyclic antidepressant.

paraldehyde: nonbarbiturate sedative-hypnotic.

paregoric: tincture (alcohol solution) of opium.

Parnate: tranylcypromine. MAO inhibitor used as antidepressant.

paroxetine: Paxil. Antidepressant (SSRI).

Paxil: paroxetine. Antidepressant (SSRI).

PCP: phencyclidine, angel dust. Hallucinogen.

pemoline: Cylert. Stimulant used to treat ADD with hyperactivity.

pentazocine: Talwin. Narcotic analgesic.

pentobarbital: Nembutal. Barbiturate sedative-hypnotic.

pentylenetetrazol: Metrazol. Convulsant formerly used in convulsive therapy.

Percodan: oxycodone. Narcotic analgesic.

Permitil: fluphenazine. Antipsychotic.

perphenazine: Trilafon. Antipsychotic.

Pertofrane: desipramine. Tricyclic antidepressant.

peyote: cactus containing mescaline (hallucinogenic).

phencyclidine: PCP, angel dust. Hallucinogen.

phendimetrazine: amphetamine-like appetite suppressant.

phenelzine: Nardil. MAO inhibitor used as antidepressant.

phenmetrazine: Preludin. Amphetamine-like appetite suppressant.

phenobarbital: Luminal. Barbiturate sedative-hypnotic.

phentermine: Amphetamine-like appetite suppressant.

phenylpropanolamine (PPA): OTC appetite suppressant.

Pondimin: fenfluramine. Appetite suppressant, removed from the market in 1997.

Preludin: phenmetrazine. Amphetamine-like appetite suppressant.

prochlorperazine: Compazine. Antipsychotic.

Prolixin: fluphenazine. Antipsychotic.

propoxyphene: Darvon. Narcotic analgesic.

protriptyline: Vivactil. Tricyclic antidepressant.

Prozac: fluoxetine. Antidepressant (SSRI).

pseudoephedrine: OTC sympathomimetic.

psilocybin: hallucinogen from the Mexican psilocybe mushroom.

Quaalude: methaqualone. Nonbarbiturate sedative-hypnotic.

Redux: dexfenfluramine. Appetite suppressant, removed from the market in 1997.

Remeron: mirtazapine. Atypical antidepressant.

Restoril: temazepam. Benzodiazepine hypnotic.

reVIA: naltrexone. Narcotic antagonist used in treating alcoholism.

Risperdal: risperidone. Atypical antipsychotic.

risperidone: Risperdal. Atypical antipsychotic.

Ritalin: methylphenidate. Stimulant used to treat ADD with hyperactivity.

Rohypnol: flunitrazepam. Benzodiazepine hypnotic, not sold in the U.S., known as a "date-rape" drug.

Sanorex: mazindol. Appetite suppressant.

scopolamine: anticholinergic.

secobarbital: Seconal. Barbiturate sedative-hypnotic.

Seconal: secobarbital. Barbiturate sedative-hypnotic.

Serax: oxazepam. Benzodiazepine sedative.

Serentil: mesoridazine. Antipsychotic.

Sernyl: former brand name for PCP.

sertraline: Zoloft. Antidepressant (SSRI).

Sinequan: doxepin. Tricyclic antidepressant.

Sopor: methaqualone. Nonbarbiturate sedative-hypnotic.

stanozolol: Winstrol. Anabolic steroid.

Stelazine: trufluoperazine. Antipsychotic.

Sublimaze: fentanyl. Potent synthetic analgesic.

Talwin: pentazocine. Narcotic analgesic.

Taractan: chlorprothixene. Antipsychotic.

temazepam: Restoril. Benzodiazepine hypnotic.

Tenuate: diethylpropion. Amphetamine-like appetite suppressant.

Tepanil: diethylpropion. Amphetamine-like appetite suppressant.

Teslac: testolactone. Anabolic steroid.

testolactone: Teslac. Anabolic steroid.

theophylline: mild stimulant found in tea; used to treat asthma.

thioridazine: Mellaril. Antipsychotic.

thiothixene: Navane. Antipsychotic.

Thorazine: chlorpromazine. Antipsychotic.

Tindal: acetophenazine. Antipsychotic.

Tofranil: imipramine. Tricyclic antidepressant.

Tranxene: clorazepate. Benzodiazepine sedative.

tranylcypromine: Parnate. MAO inhibitor used as an antidepressant.

trazodone: Desyrel. Atypical antidepressant.

Trexan: naltrexone. Narcotic antagonist.

triazolam: Halcion. Benzodiazepine hypnotic.

trifluoperazine: Stelazine. Antipsychotic.

triflupromazine: Vesprin. Antipsychotic.

trihexyphenidyl: Artane. Anticholinergic used to control extrapyramidal symptoms.

Trilafon: perphenazine. Antipsychotic.

Valium: diazepam. Benzodiazepine sedative.

venlafaxine: Effexor. Antidepressant (SSRI).

Vesprin: triflupromazine. Antipsychotic.

Vivactil: protriptyline. Tricyclic antidepressant.

Wellbutrin: bupropion. Atypical antidepressant.

Winstrol: stanozolol. Anabolic steroid.

Xanax: alprazolam. Benzodiazepine sedative.

Zoloft: Sertraline. Antidepressant (SSRI).

Zyban: bupropion. To reduce craving during tobacco cessation.

Zyprex: olanzepine. Atypical antipsychotic.

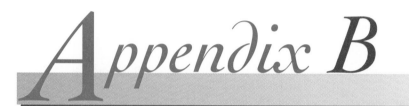

*A*ppendix *B*

Resources for Information and Assistance

FEDERAL GOVERNMENT AGENCIES

National Clearinghouse for Alcohol and Drug
   Information
Office of Substance Abuse Prevention (OSAP)
P.O. Box 2345
Rockville, MD 20852
(301) 468-2600
1-800-729-6686

Drugs & Crime Data Center
Bureau of Justice Statistics
1600 Research Blvd.
Rockville, MD 20850
1-800-666-3332

NIDA Cocaine Hot Line
1-800-662-HELP
Office on Smoking and Health
5600 Fishers Lane
Rockville, MD 20857
(301) 443-1575

ALCOHOL

Alcohol Research Information Service
1106 E. Oakland
Lansing, MI 48906
(517) 485-9900

Alcoholics Anonymous World Services
P. O. Box 459, Grand Central Station
New York, NY 10163
(212) 686-1100

American Council on Alcoholism
5024 Campbell Blvd., Suite H
Whitemarsh Business Center
Baltimore, MD 21236
(301) 529-9200

American Health and Temperance Society
6830 Eastern Ave., N.W.
Washington, DC 20012
(202) 722-6736

BACCHUS of the U.S.
(Boost Alcohol Counsciousness Concerning the
   Health of University Students)
P.O. Box 10430
Denver, CO 80210
(303) 871-3068

Licensed Beverage Information Council
1250 I St., Suite 900
Washington, DC 20005
(202) 628-3544

MADD (Mothers Against Drunk Driving)
669 Airport Fwy., Suite 310
Hurst, TX 76053
(817) 268-6233

National Alcohol Hot Line
1-800-ALCOHOL

National Council on Alcoholism
12 W. 21st St.
New York, NY 10010
(212) 206-6770

National Woman's Christian Temperance Union
1730 Chicago Ave.
Evanston, IL 60201
(312) 864-1396

RID (Remove Intoxicated Drivers)
P.O. Box 520
Schenectady, NY 12301
(518) 372-0034

SMOKING

ASH (Action on Smoking and Health)
2013 H St., N.W.
Washington, DC 20006
(202) 659-4310

Smoking Control Advocacy Resource Center
1730 Rhode Island Ave., N.W.
Washington, DC 20036
(202) 659-8475

Tobacco Institute
1875 I St., N.W.
Washington, DC 20006
(202) 457-4800

DRUGS

Alcohol and Drug Problems Association of North
America
444 N. Capitol St., N.W., Suite 706
Washington, DC 20001
(202) 737-4340

American Council for Drug Education
204 Monroe St., Suite 110
Rockville, MD 20850
(301) 294-0600

Do It Now Foundation
Box 27568
Tempe, AZ 85285
(602) 257-0797

Drug Policy Foundation
4801 Massachusetts Ave., N.W., Suite 400
Washington, DC 20016-2087

Fair Oaks Hospital
19 Prospect St. Box 100
Summit, NJ 07901
(201) 552-7000
1-800-COCAINE

Narcotic Educational Foundation of America
5055 Sunset Blvd.
Los Angeles, CA 90027
(213) 663-5171

National Drug Information Center of Families in
Action, Inc.
2296 Henderson Mill Rd., Suite 204
Atlanta, GA 30345
(404) 934-6364

National Federation of Parents for a Drug-Free Youth
1423 N. Jefferson
Springfield, MO 65802-1988
(407) 836-3709

NIDA (National Institute on Drug Abuse)
5600 Fishers Lane
Rockville, MD 20857

NORML (National Organization for the Reform of
Marijuana Laws)
2001 S. St., N.W., Suite 640
Washington, DC 20009
(202) 483-5500

PRIDE (Parent Resource Institute for Drug
Education)
100 Edgewood Ave., Suite 1002
Atlanta, GA 30303
1-800-241-7946

DRUG INFORMATION ON THE INTERNET

There is a great deal of information, opinion, misinformation, and discussion about drugs available on the Internet. It is possible to learn about the latest drug fads, to get involved in arguments about drug policy, and occasionally even to learn some solid facts by browsing on the Internet. But be warned that there is no quality control on many of these computer sites—they represent the ultimate in free expression! You're liable to find such things as a bogus recipe for making LSD from Foster's Beer, warnings about water addiction, and other foolishness mixed in with potentially useful information, so take care. Brief lists of some relevant Internet sites are found in the WebWatch in each chapter.

Glossary

A

abstinence   Refraining completely from the use of alcohol or another drug. Complete abstinence from alcohol means no drinking at all. Abstinence syndrome: see *withdrawal syndrome*.

abstinence violation effect   The tendency of a person who has been abstaining (as from alcohol), and "slips," to go on and indulge fully, because the rule of abstinence has been broken.

acetaldehyde   The chemical product of the first step in the liver's metabolism of alcohol. It is normally present only in small amounts because it is rapidly converted to acetic acid.

acetylcholine   Neurotransmitter found in the parasympathetic branch and in the cerebral cortex.

acute   In general, "sharp." In medicine, "rapid." Referring to drugs, the short-term effects or effects of a single administration, as opposed to *chronic*, or long-term, effects of administration.

additive effects   When the effects of two different drugs add up to produce a greater effect than either drug alone. As contrasted with *antagonistic* effects, in which one drug reduces the effect of another, or *synergistic* effects, in which one drug greatly amplifies the effect of another.

adenosine   A chemical believed to be a neurotransmitter in the CNS, primarily at inhibitory receptors. Caffeine might act by antagonizing the normal action of adenosine on its receptors.

ADHD   Attention deficit hyperactivity disorder, a learning disability. Terminology of the *DSM-IV*.

affective disorder   A disorder of mood or emotion, in contrast to disorders of thought. Depression, mania, and bipolar (formerly manic-depressive) disorders are examples.

affective education   In general, education that focuses on emotional content or emotional reactions, in contrast to *cognitive* content. In drug education, one example is learning how to achieve certain "feelings" (of excitement or belonging to a group) without using drugs.

aftercare   In drug or alcohol treatment programs, the long-term follow-up or maintenance support that follows a more intense period of treatment.

AIDS   Acquired immunodeficiency syndrome, a disease in which the body's immune system breaks down, leading eventually to death. Because the disease is spread through the mixing of body fluids, it is more prevalent in intravenous drug users who share needles. The infectious agent is the human immunodeficiency virus (HIV).

alcohol   Generally refers to grain alcohol, or ethanol, as opposed to other types of alcohol (for example, wood or isopropyl alcohol), which are too toxic to be drinkable.

alcohol abuse   In the *DSM-IV*, defined as a pattern of pathological alcohol use that causes impairment of social or occupational functioning. Compare with *alcohol dependence*.

alcohol dehydrogenase   The enzyme that metabolizes almost all of the alcohol consumed by an individual. It is found primarily in the liver.

alcohol dependence   In the *DSM-IV*, alcohol dependence is considered a more serious disorder than alcohol abuse, in that dependence includes either tolerance or withdrawal symptoms.

alcoholic personality   Personality traits, such as immaturity and dependency, that are frequently found in alcoholics in treatment. Many of these consistent traits might be a result of years of heavy drinking rather than a cause of alcoholism.

Alcoholics Anonymous   A worldwide, loosely organized group of alcoholics who try to help each other abstain from the use of alcohol.

alcoholism   The word has many definitions and therefore is not a precise term. Definitions might refer to pathological drinking behavior (e.g., remaining drunk for two days), to impaired functioning (e.g., frequently missing work), or to physical dependence. See also *alcohol abuse* and *alcohol dependence*.

alternatives (to drugs)   Assuming that there are motives for drug use, such as the need to be accepted by a group, many prevention and treatment programs teach alternative methods for satisfying these motives.

Alzheimer's disease   A progressive neurological disease that occurs primarily in the elderly. It causes loss of memory and then progressively impairs more aspects of intellectual and social functioning. Large acetylcholine-containing neurons of the brain are damaged in this disease.

Amanita muscaria   The fly agaric mushroom, widely used in ancient times for its hallucinogenic properties.

amotivational syndrome   A hypothesized loss of motivation that has been attributed to chronic marijuana use.

anabolic   Promoting constructive metabolism; building tissue.

anabolic steroids   Substances that increase anabolic (constructive) metabolism, one of the functions of male sex hormones. The result is increased muscle mass.

analgesic   Pain-relieving. An analgesic drug produces a selective reduction of pain, whereas an *anesthetic* reduces all sensation.

anandamide   A naturally occurring brain chemical with marijuana-like properties.

androgenic   Masculinizing.

anesthetic   Sense-deadening. An anesthetic drug reduces all sensation, whereas an *analgesic* drug reduces pain.

angel dust   A street name for phencyclidine (PCP).

animism   The belief that objects and plants contain spirits that move and direct them.

Antabuse   Brand name for dusulfiram, a drug that interferes with the normal metabolism of alcohol, so that a person who drinks alcohol after taking disulfiram will become quite ill. Antabuse interferes with the enzyme aldehyde dehydrogenase, so that there is a buildup of acetaldehyde, the first metabolic product of alcohol.

antecedents   In the context of Chapter 1, behaviors or individual characteristics that can be measured before drug use and might therefore be somewhat predictive of drug use. These are not necessarily causes of the subsequent drug use.

anticonvulsant   A drug that prevents or reduces epileptic seizures.

antidepressant   A group of drugs used in treating depressive disorders. The MAO inhibitors, the tricyclics, and the SSRIs are the major examples.

antihistamines   A group of drugs that act by antagonizing the actions of histamine at its receptors. Used in cold and sinus remedies and in OTC sedatives and sleep aids.

anti-inflammatory   Reducing the local heat, swelling, and redness caused by injury or infection. Aspirin has anti-inflammatory properties.

antipsychotics   A group of drugs used to treat psychotic disorders, such as schizophrenia. Also called neuroleptics or major tranquilizers.

antipyretic   Fever-reducing. Aspirin is a commomly used antipyretic.

antitussive   Cough-reducing. Narcotics have this effect. OTC antitussives generally contain dextromethorphan.

anxiety disorders   Mental disorders characterized by excessive worry, fears, avoidance, or a sense of impending danger. At pathological levels, these disorders can be debilitating.

anxiolytics   Drugs, such as Valium, used in the treatment of anxiety disorders. Literally, "anxiety-dissolving."

aphrodisiac   Any substance that is said to promote sexual desire.

aspirin   Originally Bayer's brand name for acetylsalicylic acid, now a generic name for that chemical.

assassin   The story is that this term for a hired killer is derived from a hashish-using cult, the hashshiyya.

ataxia   Loss of coordinated movement; for example, the staggering gait of someone who has consumed a large amount of alcohol.

attention deficit hyperactivity disorder   A learning disability accompanied by hyperactivity. More common in male children. This *DSM-IV* diagnostic category replaces *hyperkinetic syndrome* and *minimal brain dysfunction*.

autonomic nervous system   The branch of the peripheral nervous system that regulates the visceral, or automatic, functions of the body, such as heart rate and intestinal motility. In contrast to the *somatic*, or voluntary, nervous system.

aversion therapy   A form of treatment that attempts to suppress an undesirable behavior by punishing each instance of the behavior. For example, the drinking of alcohol might be punished by electric shocks or by a drug that causes nausea.

B

BAC   Blood alcohol concentration, also called blood alcohol level (BAL). The proportion of blood that consists of alcohol. For example, a person with a BAC of 0.10 percent has alcohol constituting one-tenth of 1 percent of the blood and is legally intoxicated in all states.

balanced placebo A research design in which alcohol is compared with a placebo beverage, and subjects either believe they are drinking alcohol or believe they are not.

barbiturate A major class of sedative-hypnotic drugs, including amobarbital and sodium pentothal.

basal ganglia A part of the brain containing large numbers of dopamine synapses. Responsible for maintaining proper muscle tone as a part of the *extrapyramidal motor system*. Damage to the basal ganglia, as in Parkinson's disease, produces muscular rigidity and tremors.

behavioral tolerance Repeated use of a drug can lead to a diminished effect of the drug (tolerance). When the diminished effect occurs because the individual has learned to compensate for the effect of the drug, it is called behavioral tolerance. For example, a novice drinker might be unable to walk with a BAC of 0.20 percent, whereas someone who has practiced walking while intoxicated would be able to walk fairly well at the same BAC.

behavioral toxicity Refers to the fact that a drug can be toxic because it impairs behavior and amplifies the danger level of many activities. The effect of alcohol on driving is an example.

benzodiazepine The group of drugs that includes Valium (diazepam) and Librium (chlordiazepoxide). They are used as *anxiolytics* or *sedatives*, and some types are used as sleeping pills.

benzoylecgonine A metabolite of cocaine that can be detected in urine samples.

bhang A preparation of cannabis (marijuana) that consists of the whole plant, dried and powdered. The weakest of the forms commonly used in India.

binding The interaction between a molecule and a receptor for that molecule. Although the molecules float onto and off the receptor, there are chemical and electrical attractions between a specific molecule and its receptor, so that there is a much higher probability that the receptor will be occupied by its proper molecule than by other molecules.

bioavailability The availability of molecules of a drug at the site of the drug's action in the body.

An important concept in comparing different brands of the same generic drug, because one preparation might dissolve better or be absorbed more readily than the other, thus producing greater bioavailability.

bipolar disorder One of the major affective, or emotional, disorders. Periods of mania and periods of depression have occurred in the same individual. Also called *manic-depressive illness*.

blackout A period of time during which a person was behaving, but of which the person has no memory. The most common cause of this phenomenon is excessive alcohol consumption, and blackouts are considered to indicate pathological drinking.

black tar A type of illicit heroin usually imported from Mexico.

blood alcohol concentration A measure of the concentration of alcohol in the blood, expressed in grams per 100 ml (percentage).

blood-brain barrier Refers to the fact that many substances, including drugs, that can circulate freely in the blood do not readily enter the brain tissue. The major structural feature of this barrier is the tightly jointed epithelial cells lining blood capillaries in the brain. Drug molecules cannot pass between the cells but must instead go through their membranes. Small molecules and molecules that are lipid- (fat-) soluble cross the barrier easily. Obviously, all psychoactive drugs must be capable of crossing the blood-brain barrier.

brain stem The medulla oblongata, pons, and midbrain. Located between the spinal cord and the forebrain, and generally considered to contain the "oldest" (in an evolutionary sense) and most primitive control centers for such basic functions as breathing, swallowing, and so on.

brand name The name given to a drug by a particular manufacturer and licensed only to that manufacturer. For example, *Valium* is a brand name for diazepam. Other companies may sell diazepam, but Hoffman-LaRoche, Inc., owns the name *Valium*.

bright Light-colored, flue-cured tobacco. Compare with *burley*.

British system Generally refers to the fact that heroin addicts in Great Britain may register as addicts and be prescribed legal narcotics, including heroin.

burley Dark-colored, air-cured tobacco. Compare with *bright*.

C

caffeinism Habitual use of large amounts of caffeine, usually in coffee.

Camellia sinesis The plant from which tea is made.

Cannabis Genus of plants known as marijuana, or hemp. Includes *C. indica* and *C. sativa*.

carbon monoxide A poisonous gas found in cigarette smoke.

catheter A piece of plastic or rubber tubing that is inserted into a vein or other structure.

central nervous system Brain and spinal cord.

charas A preparation of cannabis, or marijuana, that is similar to hashish. The most potent form of marijuana commonly used in India.

chemical name For a drug, the name that is descriptive of its chemical structure. For example, the chemical name *sodium chloride* is associated with the *generic* name *table salt*, of which there may be several *brand* names, such as *Morton's*.

China white A street name for one of the potent synthetic narcotics.

chipper An individual who uses heroin occasionally.

chronic Occurring over time. Chronic drug use is long-term use; chronic drug effects are persistent effects produced by long-term use.

chronic obstructive lung disease A group of disorders that includes emphysema and chronic bronchitis. Cigarette smoking is a major cause of these disorders.

cirrhosis A serious, largely irreversible, and frequently deadly disease of the liver. Usually caused by chronic heavy alcohol use.

coca The plant *Erythroxylon coca*, from which cocaine is derived. Also refers to the leaves of this plant.

cocaethylene A potent stimulant formed when cocaine and alcohol are used together.

cocaine hydrochloride The most common form of pure cocaine; it is stable and water soluble.

coca paste A paste derived from the coca leaf in the process of making cocaine. It is sometimes smoked in South and Central America and Mexico.

codeine A narcotic chemical present in opium.

coma A state of unconsciousness from which the individual cannot be aroused.

congeners In general, members of the same group. With respect to alcohol, the term refers to other chemicals that are produced in the process of making a particular alcoholic beverage.

controlled drinking The concept that individuals who have been drinking pathologically can be taught to drink in a controlled, nonpathological manner.

controlled substance A term coined for the 1970 federal law that revised previous laws regulating *narcotics and dangerous drugs*. Heroin and cocaine are examples of controlled substances.

correlate A variable that is statistically related to some other variable, such as drug use.

crack A smokable form of cocaine. Also called *rock*.

crank Street name for illicitly manufactured methamphetamine.

crash Originally referred to the rapid emotional descent after a binge of amphetamine use. One symptom is prolonged sleep, and eventually sleeping in general was referred to as crashing.

crystal meth Street term for a form of methamphetamine crystals, also called *ice*.

cumulative effects Drug effects that increase with repeated administrations, usually due to the buildup of the drug in the body.

D

DARE Drug Abuse Resistance Education, the most popular prevention program in schools.

date-rape drug A substance given to someone without her knowledge to cause unconsciousness in order to have nonconsensual sex. Rohypnol and GHB have become known for such use. A 1996 U.S. law provides serious penalties for using drugs in this manner.

Datura A plant genus that includes many species used for their hallucinogenic properties. These plants contain anticholinergic chemicals.

DAWN Drug Abuse Warning Network, a federal government system for reporting drug-related medical emergencies and deaths.

DEA United States Drug Enforcement Administration.

delirium tremens Alcohol withdrawal symptoms, including tremors and hallucinations.

demand reduction Efforts to control drug use by reducing the demand for drugs, as opposed to efforts aimed at reducing the supply of drugs.

Demand reduction efforts include education and prevention programs, as well as increased punishments for drug users.

depressant Any of a large group of drugs that generally depress the CNS and at high doses induce sleep. Includes alcohol, the barbiturates, and other sedative-hypnotic drugs.

depression A major type of mood disorder.

detoxification The process of allowing the body to rid itself of a large amount of alcohol or another drug. Often the first step in a treatment program.

deviance Behavior that is different from established social norms and that social groups take steps to change.

diagnosis The process of identifying the nature of an illness. A subject of great controversy for mental disorders.

distillation The process by which alcohol is separated from a weak alcohol solution to form more concentrated distilled spirits. The weak solution is heated, and the alcohol vapors are collected and condensed to a liquid form.

dopamine A neurotransmitter found in the basal ganglia and other regions of the brain.

dose-response curve A graph showing the relationship between the size of a drug dose and the size of the response (or the proportion of subjects showing the response).

drug Any substance, natural or artificial, other than food, that by its chemical nature alters structure or function in the living organism.

drug abuse The use of a drug in such a manner or in such amounts or in situations such that the drug use causes problems or greatly increases the chance of problems occurring.

drug disposition tolerance The reduced effect of a drug, which can result from more rapid metabolism or excretion of the drug.

drug misuse The use of prescribed drugs in greater amounts than, or for purposes other than, those prescribed by a physician or dentist.

drug therapy The use of a drug in an effort to treat an illness.

DSM-IV *Diagnostic and Statistical Manual of Mental Disorders*, fourth edition, published by the American Psychiatric Association. It has become a standard for naming and distinguishing among mental disorders.

dysentery A bowel infection that causes severe diarrhea, pain, and fever.

E

Ecstasy Street name for the hallucinogen MDMA. Also called "XTC."

ECT Electroconvulsive therapy, or electroconvulsive shock treatment. A procedure in which an electrical current is passed through the head, resulting in an epileptic-like seizure. Although this treatment is now used infrequently, it is still considered to be the most effective and rapid treatment for severe depression.

ED_{50} The effective dose for half the subjects in a drug test.

effective dose The dose of a drug that produces a certain effect in some percentage of the subjects. For example, an ED_{50} produces the effect in 50 percent of the subjects. Note that the dose will depend on the effect that is monitored.

EMIT Enzyme multiplied immunoassay test. The most commonly used urine-screening technique for detecting the presence of various drugs.

emphysema A lung disease in which tissue deterioration results in increased air retention and reduced exchange of gases. The result is difficulty breathing and shortness of breath. An example of a *chronic obstructive lung disease*, often caused by smoking.

employee assistance program A program within a company or an organization that provides counseling and/or treatment services to employees.

endorphins Opiate-like chemicals that occur naturally in the brains of humans and other animals. There are several proper endorphins, and the term is also used generically to refer to both the endorphins and the enkephalins.

enkephalins Opiate-like chemicals that occur naturally in the brains of humans and other animals. The enkephalins are smaller molecules than the endorphins.

enzyme A large, organic molecule that works to speed up a specific chemical reaction. Enzymes are found in brain cells, where they are needed for most steps in the synthesis of neurotransmitter molecules. They are also found in the liver, where they are needed for the metabolism of many drug molecules.

ephedrine A drug derived from the Chinese medicinal herb *ma huang* and used to relieve breathing difficulty in asthma. A sympathomimetic from which amphetamine was derived.

epilepsy A disorder of the nervous system in which recurring periods of abnormal electrical activity in the brain produce temporary malfunction. There might or might not be loss of consciousness or convulsive motor movements.

ergogenic Energy-producing. Refers to drugs or other methods (e.g., blood doping) designed to increase an athlete's energy output.

ergotism A disease caused by eating grain infected with the ergot fungus. There are both psychological and physical manifestations.

ethical In pharmacy, medicines dispensed only by prescription.

expectancies Learned beliefs about the effects of alcohol or another drug.

extrapyramidal system A motor control system in the central nervous system that is responsible for maintaining muscle tone and posture. Parkinson's disease causes damage to this system. Antipsychotic drugs also interfere with the extrapyramidal system, often producing symptoms similar to those of Parkinson's disease.

F

false transmitter One method by which a drug can affect the nervous system. The drug is taken into a neuron and acted on by enzymes to produce a substance resembling the natural neurotransmitter but differing from it functionally.

FAS Fetal alcohol syndrome.

FDA United States Food and Drug Administration.

fen-phen A combination of two prescription weight-control medications, fenfluramine and phentermine. No longer prescribed, due to concerns with toxicity to heart valves.

fermentation The process by which sugars are converted into grain alcohol through the action of yeasts.

fetal alcohol effect Individual developmental abnormalities associated with the mother's alcohol use during pregnancy.

fetal alcohol syndrome Facial and developmental abnormalities associated with the mother's alcohol use.

fibrocystic breast disease A benign (noncancerous) but painful disorder characterized by lumps (fibrocysts) in the breasts. There is controversy as to whether caffeine consumption is related to this problem.

flashback An experience reported by some users of LSD in which portions of the LSD experience recur at a later time without the use of the drug.

fly agaric mushroom *Amanita muscaria*, a hallucinogenic mushroom that is also considered poisonous.

freebase In general, when a chemical salt is separated into its basic and acidic components, the basic component is referred to as the free base. Most psychoactive drugs are bases that normally exist in a salt form. Specifically, the salt cocaine hydrochloride can be chemically extracted to form the cocaine free base, which is volatile and can therefore be smoked.

functional disorder A mental disorder for which there is no known organic cause. Schizophrenia is a form of psychosis that is considered to be a functional disorder.

G

GABA An inhibitory neurotransmitter; gamma-aminobutyric acid.

ganja A preparation of *cannabis* (marijuana) in which the most potent parts of the plant are used.

gateway substances Substances, such as alcohol, tobacco, and sometimes marijuana, that most users of illicit substances will have tried before their first use of cocaine, heroin, or other less widely used illicit drugs.

generic name For drugs, a name that specifies a particular chemical without being chemically descriptive. As an example, the *chemical name* sodium chloride is associated with the *generic name* table salt, of which there may be several *brand names,* such as Morton's.

genetic marker A chemical or physiological characteristic that is known to be caused by a particular gene and that is highly correlated with some disease state.

GRAE "Generally recognized as effective"; a term defined by the FDA with reference to the ingredients found in OTC drugs (see also *GRAS*).

GRAHL "Generally recognized as honestly labeled" (see also *GRAE* and *GRAS*).

grain neutral spirits Ethyl alcohol distilled to a purity of 190 proof (95 percent).

grand mal   An epileptic seizure that results in convulsive motor movements and loss of consciousness.

GRAS   "Generally recognized as safe"; a term defined by the FDA with reference to food additives and the ingredients found in OTC drugs.

H

hallucinogen   A drug, such as LSD or mescaline, that produces profound alterations in perception.

hashish   A potent preparation of *cannabis* (marijuana).

hash oil   A slang term for oil of cannabis, a liquid extract from the marijuana plant.

henbane   A poisonous plant containing anticholinergic chemicals and sometimes used for its hallucinogenic properties. *Hyoscyamus niger*.

heroin   Originally Bayer's name for diacetylmorphine, a potent narcotic analgesic synthesized from morphine.

HIV   Human immunodeficiency virus. The infectious agent responsible for AIDS.

homeostasis   A state of physiological balance maintained by various regulatory mechanisms.

hormone   A chemical substance formed in one part of the body that stimulates action in another part of the body.

human growth hormone   A pituitary hormone responsible for some types of giantism.

hyperactive   Refers to a disorder characterized by short attention span and a high level of motor activity. The *DSM-IV* term is *attention-deficit hyperactivity disorder*.

hypnotic   Sleep-inducing. For drugs, refers to sleeping preparations.

hypodermic syringe   A device to which a hollow needle can be attached, so that solutions can be injected through the skin.

hypothalamus   A group of nuclei found at the base of the brain, just above the pituitary gland.

I

ibogaine   A hallucinogen that has been shown to reduce self-administration of cocaine and morphine in rats and is proposed to reduce craving in drug addicts.

ibuprofen   An aspirin-like analgesic and anti-inflammatory.

ice   The street name for crystals of methamphetamine hydrochloride.

immunoassay   A method for measuring an organic chemical by inducing an animal to develop an antibody to it, then purifying the antibody and using it to measure the chemical in another tissue sample.

IND   Approval to conduct clinical investigations on a new drug, filed with the FDA after animal tests are complete.

indole   A type of chemical structure. The neurotransmitter serotonin and the hallucinogen LSD both contain an indole nucleus.

inhalants   Any of a variety of volatile solvents or other products that can be inhaled to produce intoxication.

insomnia   Inability to sleep. The most common complaint is difficulty falling asleep. Often treated with a hypnotic drug.

interferon   A chemical produced by the body in response to viral infections. Interferon treatments have been shown to reduce the risk of catching a cold.

intramuscular   A type of injection in which the drug is administered into a muscle.

intravenous   A type of injection in which the drug is administered into a vein.

K

kretek   A clove cigarette.

L

laissez-faire   A theory that government should not interfere with business or other activities.

LD_{50}   The lethal dose for half the animals in a test.

lethal dose   The dose of a drug that produces a lethal effect in some percentage of the animals on which it is tested. For example, LD_{50} is the dose that would kill 50 percent of the animals to which it was given.

leukoplakia   A whitening and thickening of the soft tissues of the mouth. The use of chewing tobacco is associated with an increase in leukoplakia, considered to be a "precancerous" tissue change.

limbic system   A system of various brain structures that are involved in emotional responses.

lipid solubility   The tendency of a chemical to dissove in oil, as opposed to in water.

lithium   A highly reactive metallic element, atomic number 3. Its salts are used in the treatment of mania and *bipolar disorder*.

liver microsomal enzyme   An enzyme associated with a particular subcellular component (the microsomal fraction) of liver cells. There are many such enzymes that are important for drug metabolism.

longitudinal   A study done over a period of time (months or years).

look-alikes   Drugs sold legally, usually through the mail, that are made to look like controlled, prescription-only drugs. The most common types contain caffeine and resemble amphetamine capsules or tablets.

M

ma huang   A Chinese herb containing ephedrine, which is a sympathomimetic drug from which amphetamine was derived.

major depression   A serious mental disorder characterized by a depressed mood. A specific diagnostic term in the *DSM-IV*.

malting   The process of wetting a grain and allowing it to sprout, to maximize its sugar content before fermentation to produce an alcoholic beverage.

mandrake   *Mandragora officinarum*, a plant having a branched root that contains anticholinergic chemicals. Now classed among the other anticholinergic hallucinogens, this plant was widely believed to have aphrodisiac properties.

marijuana   Also spelled marihuana; dried leaves of the cannabis plant.

MDMA   Methylenedioxy methamphetamine, a catechol hallucinogen related to MDA. Called "Ecstasy" or "XTC" on the street.

medial forebrain bundle   A group of neuron fibers that projects from the midbrain to the forebrain, passing near the hypothalamus. Now known to contain several chemically and anatomically distinct pathways, including dopamine and norepinephrine pathways.

medical model   With reference to mental disorders, a model that assumes that abnormal behaviors are *symptoms* resulting from a *disease*.

mental illness   A term that, to some theorists, implies acceptance of a medical model of mental disorders.

mesolimbic pathway   A group of dopamine-containing neurons that have their cell bodies in the midbrain and their terminals in the forebrain, on various structures associated with the limbic system. Believed by some theorists to be important in explaining the therapeutic effects of antipsychotic medications. Also believed by some theorists to be important for many types of behavioral reinforcers.

metabolism   (of drugs) The breakdown of drug molecules by enzymes, often in the liver.

metabolite   A product of enzyme action on a drug.

methadone maintenance   A program for treatment of narcotic addicts in which the synthetic drug methadone is provided to the addicts in an oral dosage form, so that they can maintain their addiction legally.

Mexican brown   A form of heroin that first appeared on American streets in the mid-1970s. Because the heroin is made from the hydrochloride salt of morphine, it is brown in its pure form.

moist snuff   A type of oral smokeless tobacco that is popular among young American men. A "pinch" of this chopped, moistened, flavored tobacco is held in the mouth, often between the lower lip and the gum.

monoamine oxidase (MAO) inhibitor   A drug that acts by inhibiting the enzyme monoamine oxidase (MAO). Used as an antidepressant.

morphinism   An older term used to describe dependence on the use of morphine.

motivational interviewing   A technique for encouraging alcoholics or addicts to seek treatment by first assessing their degree of dependence and then discussing the assessment results. Direct confrontation is avoided.

N

narcolepsy   A form of sleep disorder characterized by bouts of muscular weakness and falling asleep involuntarily. The most common treatment employs stimulant drugs such as amphetamine to maintain wakefulness during the day.

narcotic   See *opiate*.

narcotic antagonists   Drugs that can block the actions of narcotics.

Native American Church   A religious organization active among American Indians, in which the hallucinogenic peyote cactus is used in conjunction with Christian religious themes.

NDA In FDA procedures, a New Drug Application. This application, demonstrating both safety and effectiveness of a new drug in both animal and human experiments, must be submitted by a drug company to the FDA before a new drug can be marketed.

neuroleptic A general term for the antipsychotic drugs (also called *major tranquilizers*).

neurosis A type of mental disorder, mostly now referred to as *anxiety disorders*.

neurotransmitter A chemical that is released by one neuron and that alters the electrical activity in another neuron.

Nicotiana Any of several types of tobacco plant, including *N. tobacum* and *N. rustica*.

nicotine The chemical contained in tobacco that is responsible for its psychoactive effects and for tobacco dependence.

nigrostriatal pathway A group of dopamine-containing neurons that have their cell bodies in the *substantia nigra* of the midbrain and their terminals in the *corpus striatum* (basal ganglia), which is part of the extrapyramidal motor system. It is this pathway that deteriorates in Parkinson's disease and on which antipsychotic drugs act to produce side effects resembling Parkinson's disease.

nitrosamines A group of organic chemicals, many of which are highly carcinogenic. At least four are found only in tobacco, and these might account for much of the cancer-causing property of tobacco.

nonspecific effects Effects of a drug that are not changed by changing the chemical makeup of the drug. Also referred to as placebo effects.

norepinephrine A neurotransmitter that might be important for regulating waking and appetite.

NORML National Organization for the Reform of Marijuana Laws.

NSAIDs Nonsteroidal anti-inflammatory drugs, such as ibuprofen and naproxen.

nucleus basalis A group of large cell bodies found just below the basal ganglia and containing acetylcholine. These cells send terminations widely to the cerebral cortex. In Alzheimer's disease, there is a loss of these neurons and a reduction in the amount of acetylcholine in the cortex.

O

opiate One of a group of drugs similar to morphine, also referred to as narcotics, and used medically primarily for their analgesic effects. The Greek root for *narcotics* meant "numbness," and in early pharmacology writings the term was used for many psychoactive drugs that were thought to reduce pain or dull the senses. Also, by extrapolation from the Bureau of Narcotics, the term *narcotic* came into popular use to refer to any illegal drug (now replaced by the term *controlled substance* in legal writings).

opiate antagonist Any of several drugs that are capable of blocking the effects of drugs. Used in emergency medicine to treat overdose and in some addiction treatment programs to block the effect of any illicit opiate that might be taken. Nalorphine and naltrexone are examples.

opium A sticky substance obtained from the seed pods of the opium poppy and containing the narcotic chemicals morphine and codeine.

organic disorder For mental disorders, those with a known physical cause (e.g., psychosis caused by long-term alcohol use).

OTC Over-the-counter. OTC drugs are those drugs that can be purchased without a prescription.

P

Papaver somniferum The opium poppy.

paraphernalia In general, the equipment used in some activity. Drug paraphernalia include such items as syringes, pipes, scales, or mirrors.

parasympathetic The branch of the autonomic nervous system that has acetylcholine as its neurotransmitter and, for example, slows the heart rate and activates the intestine.

Parkinson's disease A disease of the extrapyramidal motor system, specifically involving damage to the nigrostriatal dopamine system. Early symptoms include muscular rigidity, tremors, a shuffling gait, and a masklike face. Occurs primarily in the elderly.

passive smoking The inhalation of tobacco smoke from the air by nonsmokers.

patent medicines Proprietary medicines. Originally referred to medicines that were, in fact, treated as inventions and patented in Great Britain. In America, the term came to refer to medicines sold directly to the public.

PCP Phenycyclidine; 1-(1-phenylcyclohexl) piperidine. The brand name Sernyl is no longer in use because it is not legally available for human use. This hallucinogen is often referred to as angel dust.

PDR *Physician's Desk Reference*, a book listing all prescription drugs and giving prescribing information about each. Updated yearly.

pekoe A grade of tea.

peptide A class of chemicals made up of sequences of amino acids. Enkephalins are small peptides containing only five amino acids, whereas large proteins may contain hundreds.

peyote A hallucinogenic cactus containing the chemical mescaline.

phantastica Hallucinogens that produce altered perceptions but do not generally impair communication with the real world.

pharmacodynamic tolerance Reduced effectiveness of a drug resulting from an altered tissue reaction to the drug.

phenothiazines A group of chemicals that includes several antipsychotic medications.

physical dependence Defined by the presence of a consistent set of symptoms when use of a drug is stopped. These withdrawal symptoms imply that homeostatic mechanisms of the body had made adjustments to counteract the drug's effects and without the drug the system is thrown out of balance.

placebo An inactive drug, often used in experiments to control for nonspecific effects of drug administration.

postsynaptic Refers to structures associated with the neural membrane on the receiving side of a synapse.

potency Relates to how little of a drug is required to produce a given effect.

precursor Something that precedes something else. In biochemistry, a precursor molecule may be acted upon by an enzyme and changed into a different molecule. For example, the dietary amino acid tryptophan is the precursor for the neurotransmitter serotonin.

prodrugs Drugs that are administered in an inactive form and become effective after they are chemically modified in the body by enzymes.

Prohibition The period 1920–1933, during which the sale of alcoholic beverages was prohibited in the United States.

proof A measure of a beverage's alcohol content; twice the alcohol percentage.

proprietary A medicine that is marketed directly to the public. Also called *OTC, patent*, or *nonprescription* medicines.

prostaglandins Local hormones, some of which are synthesized in response to cell injury and are important for initiating pain signals. Aspirin and similar drugs inhibit the formation of prostaglandins.

protein binding The combining of drug molecules with blood proteins.

psychedelic Another name for hallucinogenic drugs. Has a somewhat positive connotation of mind viewing or mind clearing.

psychoactive A term used to describe drugs that have their principal effect on the CNS.

psychological dependence A strong tendency to repeat the use of a drug.

psychopharmacology Science that studies the behavioral effects of drugs.

psychosis A type of mental disorder characterized by a loss of contact with reality and by deterioration in social and intellectual functioning.

psychotomimetic Another name for hallucinogenic drugs. Has a negative connotation of mimicking psychosis.

Q

quid A piece of something to be chewed, such as a wad of chewing tobacco.

R

receptors Locations at which neurotransmitters or drugs bind, perhaps triggering a physiological response.

reinforcement The process of strengthening a behavioral tendency by presenting a stimulus contingent on the behavior. For example, the tendency to obtain and take a drug might be strengthened by the stimulus properties of the drug that occur after it is taken, thus leading to psychological dependence.

reuptake One process by which neurotransmitter chemicals are removed from synapses. The chemical is taken back up into the cell from which it was released.

Reye's syndrome A rare brain infection that occurs almost exclusively in children and adolescents. There is some evidence that it is more likely to occur in children who have been given aspirin during a bout of flu or chicken pox.

risk factors   Behaviors, attitudes, or situations that correlate with, and might indicate the development of, a deviance-prone lifestyle that includes drug or alcohol abuse. Examples are early alcohol intoxification, absence from school, and perceived peer approval of drug use.

rock   Another name for *crack*, a smokable form of cocaine.

S

salicylate   A class of chemicals that includes aspirin.

schizophrenia   A chronic psychotic disorder for which the cause is unknown.

sedative   A drug used to calm a person, reducing stress and excitement.

serotonin   A neurotransmitter found in the raphe nuclei that might be important for impulsivity and depression.

sidestream smoke   Smoke that comes off a cigarette or cigar from the ash.

sinsemilla   A process for growing marijuana that is especially potent in its psychological effects because of a high THC content.

smokeless tobacco   Various forms of chewing tobacco and snuff.

social influence model   A prevention model adapted from successful smoking-prevention programs.

somatic system   The part of the nervous system that controls the voluntary, skeletal muscles, such as the large muscles of the arms and legs.

specific effects   Those effects of a drug that depend on the amount and type of chemical contained in the drug.

speed   A street term used at one time for cocaine, then for injectable amphetamine, and later for all types of amphetamine. Probably shortened from *speedball*.

SSRI Selective serotonin reuptake inhibitor; a class of antidepressants that includes Prozac.

stages of change   Theoretical description of the cognitive stages through which an addict would go in moving from active use to treatment and abstinence:

precontemplation, contemplation, preparation, action, and maintenance.

stimulant   Any of a group of drugs that has the effect of reversing mental and physical fatigue.

street value   The theoretical value of an amount of drugs if sold in small quantities on the street.

subcutaneous   Under the skin. A form of injection in which the needle penetrates through the skin (about $3/_8$ inch) but does not enter a muscle or vein.

sulfanilamide   A type of antibiotic.

sympathetic nervous system   The branch of the autonomic nervous system that contains norepinephrine as its neurotransmitter and, for example, increases heart rate and blood pressure.

sympathomimetic   Any drug that stimulates the sympathetic nervous system—for example, amphetamine.

symptom   In medical terms, an abnormality that indicates a disease. When applied to abnormal behavior, seems to imply a medical model in which an unseen disease causes the abnormal behavior.

synesthesia   A phenomenon in which the different senses become mixed—for example, a sound is "seen." Might be reported by a person taking hallucinogens.

synthesis   The formation of a chemical compound. For example, some neurotransmitter chemicals must be synthesized within the neuron.

T

tachyphylaxis   A rapid form of tolerance in which a second dose of a drug has a smaller effect than a first dose taken only a short time before.

tar   With regard to tobacco, a complex mixture of chemicals found in cigarette smoke. After water, gases, and nicotine are removed from the smoke, the remaining residue is considered to be tar.

tardive dyskinesia   Movement disorders that appear after several weeks or months of treatment with antipsychotic drugs and that usually become worse if use of the drug is discontinued.

temperance   With reference to alcohol, temperance originally meant moderation. Eventually the temperance movement adopted complete abstinence as its goal and prohibition as the means.

tetrahydrocannabinol   The most active of the many chemicals found in cannabis (marijuana).

THC   Tetrahydrocannabinol.

theobromine   A mild stimulant similar to caffeine and found in chocolate; a xanthine.

theophylline   A mild stimulant similar to caffeine and found in tea; a xanthine.

tolerance   The reduced effectiveness of a drug after repeated administration.

toxic   Harmful, destructive, or deadly.

tricyclics   A group of chemicals used in treating depression.

truth serum   Any drugs used to "loosen the tongue," in association with either psychotherapy or interrogation. Although people might speak more freely after receiving some drugs, there is no guarantee that anything they say is true.

U

uptake   The process by which a cell expends energy to concentrate certain chemicals within itself. For example, precursor substances to be synthesized into neurotransmitters must be taken up by the neuron.

V

values clarification   A type of affective education that avoids reference to drugs but focuses on helping students define and defend their own values.

W

Wernicke-Korsakoff syndrome   Chronic mental impairments produced by heavy alcohol use over a long period of time.

wine cooler   A beverage made from mixing wine with a fruit-based soft drink.

withdrawal syndrome   The set of symptoms that occur reliably when someone stops taking a drug; also called *abstinence syndrome*.

X

xanthine   The chemical class that includes caffeine, theobromine, and theophylline.

Credits

Art & Photo Credits

Chapter 1

p.4: © Michael Krasowitz/FPG.

Chapter 2

p.35: © Annie Griffiths Belt/Corbis Images.

Chapter 3

p.50: © Telegraph Colour Library/FPG.

Chapter 4

p.71: © PhotoEdit.

Chapter 5

p.94: © Superstock; **p.109:** © Amy C. Etra/ PhotoEdit; **p.111:** © Michael Okoniewski/ The Image Works.

Chapter 6

Figure 6.10: © H. Sochurek, Medichrome/ Stock Shop, Inc.; **Figure 6.11:** Tom & Dee Ann McCarthy/PhotoEdit.

Chapter 7

p.153: © Telegraph Colour Library/FPG; **p.155:** © Telegraph Colour Library/FPG.

Chapter 8

p.172(left): © Johnny Crawford/The Image Works; **p.172(right):** © Charles Steiner/ The Image Works.

Chapter 9

p.208: © Superstock; **p.209:** © Superstock.

Chapter 10

p.230: © Superstock; **p.238:** © Superstock.

Chapter 11

p.245: © McGraw-Hill Higher Education; **p.248:** © Superstock; **p.264, Figure 11-4a&b:** Fletcher, C.D.M. and McKee, P.H. An Atlas of Gross Pathology. © 1987 Mosby-Wolfe Europe Limited, London, UK; **p.266, Figure 11.5:** © David Young-Wolff/PhotoEdit.

Chapter 12

p.279: © Superstock; **p.281:** © Superstock; **p.283:** © Superstock.

Chapter 13

p.305: © McGraw-Hill Higher Education; **p.306:** © Superstock; **p.311** © Superstock; **p.316:** © Conor Caffrey/SPL/Photo Researchers, Inc.

Chapter 14

p.330: © Superstock; **p.332:** © FPG; **p.335:** © North Wind Picture Archives.

Chapter 15

p.354: © Bonnie Kamin/PhotoEdit; **p.360:** © Superstock; **p.367:** © Superstock.

Chapter 16

p.388: © Superstock; **p.398:** © Superstock.

Chapter 17

p.421: © Superstock; **p.428:** © McGraw-Hill Higher Education/Red Diamond Stock Photos; **p.442:** © K.G. Vock/Okapia/Photo Researchers, Inc.; **p.443:** © Superstock.

Chapter 18

p.452: © Superstock; **p.543:** Courtesy of DEA/U.S. Dept. of Justice; **p.471:** © Superstock.

Chapter 19

p.487: © Superstock; **p.489:** © SPL/Photo Researchers, Inc.

Index

Note: Page numbers in *italics* refer to figures; page numbers followed by *t* refer to tables.